# NUTRITION and CANCER PREVENTION

# NUTRITION AND DISEASE PREVENTION

## Published Titles

**Genomics and Proteomics in Nutrition**
*Carolyn D. Berdanier*, Ph.D., Professor Emerita, University of Georgia, Athens,
   Watkinsville, Georgia
*Naima Moustaid-Moussa*, Ph.D., University of Tennessee, Knoxville, Tennessee

**Perinatal Nutrition: Optimizing Infant Health and Development**
*Jatinder Bhatia*, M.B.B.S., Medical College of Georgia, Augusta, Georgia

**Soy in Health and Disease Prevention**
*Michihiro Sugano*, Ph.D., Professor Emeritus, Kyushu University, Japan

**Nutrition and Cancer Prevention**
*Atif B. Awad*, Ph.D., University at Buffalo, The State University of New York,
   Buffalo, New York
*Peter G. Bradford*, Ph.D., University at Buffalo, The State University of
   New York, Buffalo, New York

# NUTRITION and CANCER PREVENTION

Edited by
## Atif B. Awad
## Peter G. Bradford

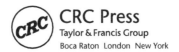

CRC Press
Taylor & Francis Group
Boca Raton  London  New York

CRC Press is an imprint of the
Taylor & Francis Group, an **informa** business

CRC Press
Taylor & Francis Group
6000 Broken Sound Parkway NW, Suite 300
Boca Raton, FL 33487-2742

First issued in paperback 2019

© 2006 by Taylor & Francis Group, LLC
CRC Press is an imprint of Taylor & Francis Group, an Informa business

No claim to original U.S. Government works

ISBN-13: 978-0-8493-3945-5 (hbk)
ISBN-13: 978-0-367-39212-3 (pbk)
Library of Congress Card Number 2005040594

### Library of Congress Cataloging-in-Publication Data

Nutrition and cancer prevention / edited by Atif B. Awad, Peter G. Bradford.
     p. cm. -- (Nutrition and disease prevention; 4)
  Includes bibliographical references and index.
  ISBN 0-8493-3945-6 (alk. paper)
    1. Cancer--Nutritional aspects. 2. Cancer--Chemoprevention. I. Awad, Atif B. II. Bradford, Peter G. III. Series.

RC268.45.N8742 2005
616.99'40654--dc22                                      2005040594

**Visit the Taylor & Francis Web site at
http://www.taylorandfrancis.com**

**and the CRC Press Web site at
http://www.crcpress.com**

# Preface

Nutrition plays an essential role in health and in the prevention of disease, including cancer. Epidemiological studies have estimated that approximately 35% of cancers are potentially avoidable by nutritional modification. These modifications include strategies such as caloric restriction and limitation of specific macronutrient groups. However, as this book reports, there is compelling evidence that essential foods contain micronutrient factors that confer protection from cancers, specifically the common cancers of the colon, breast, and prostate.

In *Nutrition and Cancer Prevention*, the top experts in the field present analyses of specific dietary components that may offer protection from common cancers. The book organizes these dietary components into the general classes of vitamins, minerals, phytosterols, polyphenols, isothiocyanates, saponins, and specialized lipids.

The introductory chapters update the descriptive epidemiology of the major cancers of the Western world as well as the general means by which diet may protect people from these cancers. Part II addresses the potential anticarcinogenic activities of vitamins A, D, E, C and folic acid, as well as some of their synthetic analogs. Part III focuses on studies of the minerals calcium and selenium: that calcium and calcium-sensing mechanisms in the gut affect colon cell differentiation and tumor formation and that diets of selenium-rich foods such as cereal grains, garlic, and broccoli are associated with reduced rates of cancers of the lung, colon, and prostate. Part IV discusses the phytosterols, plant compounds with chemical similarity to cholesterol. Diets rich in phytosterols are associated not only with reduced serum cholesterol and atherosclerosis, but also with decreased incidences of cancers of the breast and colon. Part V offers comprehensive analyses of the cancer chemoprotective activities of the class of nutrients broadly called polyphenols. Polyphenols include isoflavones from soy, flavonoids from soy and tea, catechins from green tea, resveratrol from grapes and red wine, lignans from flaxseed, and anthocyanins from berry fruits. Parts VI and VII detail the cancer chemoprotective effects of isothiocyanates and saponins. Isothiocyanates found in high amounts in broccoli, kale, and other cruciferous vegetables inhibit the metabolic activation of a variety of carcinogens. Saponins of ginseng and soy have antimutagenic and anticarcinogenic activities. Part VIII presents interesting evidence for the cancer chemoprotective potential of specialized dietary lipids, including omega-3 fatty acids, linoleic acid, and sphingolipids. Finally, Part IX addresses the roles of obesity and excess alcohol consumption in cancer development.

The book covers in detail those dietary components that have shown to have potential either in protection from cancer, in modulation of cancer development, or in the reduction of tumor metastasis. Supportive evidence includes epidemiological, experimental, and clinical studies. For each nutritional class, several leading experts present the scientific evidence addressing the potential mechanisms by which these dietary components may offer protection from cancer as well as future research directions.

**Atif B. Awad, Ph.D.**
**Peter G. Bradford, Ph.D.**

# About the Editors

**Atif B. Awad** is an associate professor of nutrition and biochemistry at the State University of New York at Buffalo. He obtained his Ph.D. degree in nutrition from Rutgers University, New Jersey, and completed postdoctoral training in biochemistry at the University of Iowa. He has supervised more than 75 M.S. and Ph.D. students. He has published 70 papers and has presented more than 70 abstracts at scientific meetings. His research focus is in the area of dietary lipids and disease prevention, including the effects of phytochemicals, such as phytosterols and phytoestrogens, on cardiovascular disease and cancer.

**Peter G. Bradford** is an associate professor of pharmacology and toxicology in the School of Medicine and Biomedical Sciences and an associate professor of oral biology in the School of Dental Medicine at the State University of New York at Buffalo. He is author or coauthor of more than 40 journal articles and book chapters. He served as visiting assistant professor at the Beijing Medical University in 1991. Dr. Bradford received a B.S. (1977) degree in biology from the University of Albany and his M.S. (1980) and Ph.D. (1982) degrees in biochemistry from the University of Rochester.

# Contributors

**Atif B. Awad**
Department of Exercise and Nutrition
  Sciences
School of Public Health and Health
  Professions
State University of New York at
  Buffalo
Buffalo, New York

**Maddalena Barba**
Department of Social and Preventive
  Medicine
School of Public Health and Health
  Professions
State University of New York at
  Buffalo
Buffalo, New York

**Peter G. Bradford**
Department of Pharmacology and
  Toxicology
School of Medicine and Biomedical
  Sciences
State University of New York at
  Buffalo
Buffalo, New York

**Subhas Chakrabarty**
Department of Molecular Pathology
Division of Pathology and Laboratory
  Medicine
M.D. Anderson Cancer Center
University of Texas
Houston, Texas

**Feng Chu**
Department of Cancer Biology
M.D. Anderson Cancer Center
University of Texas
Houston, Texas

**Guus S.M.J.E. Duchateau**
Unilever Health Institute
Unilever Research and Development
Vlaardingen, The Netherlands

**Barbara Fuhrman**
Department of Social and Preventive
  Medicine
School of Public Health and Health
  Professions
State University of New York at
  Buffalo
Buffalo, New York

**David A. Gewirtz**
Department of Medicine
Medical College of Virginia
Richmond, Virginia

**Vay Liang W. Go**
Department of Medicine
David Geffen School of Medicine at
  UCLA
Los Angeles, California

**Diane M. Harris**
UCLA Center for Human Nutrition
David Geffen School of Medicine at
  UCLA
Los Angeles, California

**Bruce J. Holub**
Department of Human Biology and
  Nutritional Sciences
University of Guelph
Guelph, Ontario, Canada

**Hiroko Inoue-Fruehauf**
Nutrition and Cancer Biology
  Laboratory
Jean Mayer USDA Human Nutrition
Research Center on Aging at Tufts
  University
Boston, Massachusetts

**David Jenkins**
Department of Nutritional Sciences
St. Michael's Hospital
University of Toronto
Toronto, Ontario, Canada

**Weiqin Jiang**
Cancer Prevention Laboratory
Colorado State University
Fort Collins, Colorado

**Kenji Jinno**
Internal Medicine
Shikoku Cancer Center
Matsuyama, Ehime, Japan

**Colin D. Kay**
Department of Human Biology and
  Nutritional Sciences
University of Guelph
Guelph, Ontario, Canada

**David D. Kitts**
Food, Nutrition and Health
University of British Columbia
Vancouver, British Columbia, Canada

**Roxanne LaBelle**
Department of Life Sciences
Faculty of Arts and Science
University of Toronto
Toronto, Ontario, Canada

**Chang Yong Lee**
Department of Food Science and
  Technology
Cornell University
Ithaca, New York

**Hyong Joo Lee**
Department of Food Science and
  Technology
School of Agricultural Biotechnology
Seoul National University
Seoul, South Korea

**Ki Won Lee**
Laboratory of Biochemistry and
  Molecular Toxicology
College of Pharmacy
Seoul National University
Seoul, South Korea

**Yiwei Li**
Department of Pathology
Karmanos Cancer Institute
Wayne State University School of
  Medicine
Detroit, Michigan

**Jen-Kun Lin**
Institute of Biochemistry & Molecular
  Biology
College of Medicine
National Taiwan University
Taipei, Taiwan

**Yang Mao**
Surveillance and Risk Assessment
  Division
Center of Chronic Diseases Prevention
  and Control
Public Health Agency of Canada
Ottawa, Ontario, Canada

**Mitsuharu Masuda**
Department of Biochemistry
Kyoto Prefectural University of
  Medicine
Kyoto, Japan

**John J. McGuire**
Department of Pharmacology and
  Therapeutics
Grace Cancer Drug Center
Roswell Park Cancer Institute
Buffalo, New York

**Marilyn E. Morris**
Department of Pharmaceutical
  Sciences
School of Pharmacy and
  Pharmaceutical Sciences
State University of New York at
  Buffalo
Buffalo, New York

**Xiao Yang Mou**
Department of Biochemistry
Kyoto Prefectural University of
  Medicine
Kyoto, Japan

**Michiaki Murakoshi**
Department of Biochemistry
Kyoto Prefectural University of
  Medicine
Kyoto, Japan

**Paola Muti**
Department of Social and Preventive
  Medicine
School of Public Health and Health
  Professions
State University of New York at
  Buffalo
Buffalo, New York

**Joseph L. Napoli**
University of California
Berkeley, California

**Jiri Neuzil**
Apoptosis Research Group
School of Medical Sciences
Griffith University
Southport, Queensland, Australia

**Hoyoku Nishino**
Department of Biochemistry
Kyoto Prefectural University of
  Medicine
Kyoto, Japan

**Catherine A. O'Brian**
Department of Cancer Biology
M.D. Anderson Cancer Center
University of Texas
Houston, Texas

**Yasuhito Ohsaka**
Department of Biochemistry
Kyoto Prefectural University of
  Medicine
Kyoto, Japan

**Sai Yi Pan**
Surveillance and Risk Assessment
  Division
Center of Chronic Diseases Prevention
  and Control
Public Health Agency of Canada
Ottawa, Ontario, Canada

**Yongsoon Park**
Nutrition Program
School of Culinary Arts and Food
  Management
Youngsan University
Pusan, Korea

**David G. Popovich**
Food, Nutrition and Health
University of British Columbia
Vancouver, British Columbia, Canada

**Krista A. Power**
Department of Nutritional Sciences
Faculty of Medicine
University of Toronto
Toronto, Ontario, Canada

**Bandaru S. Reddy**
Department of Chemical Biology
School of Pharmacy
Susan Lehman Cullman Cancer
  Research Laboratory
Rutgers, The State University of New
  Jersey
Piscataway, New Jersey

**Fazlul H. Sarkar**
Department of Pathology
Karmanos Cancer Institute
Wayne State University School of
  Medicine
Detroit, Michigan

**Yoshiko Satomi**
Department of Biochemistry
Kyoto Prefectural University of
  Medicine
Kyoto, Japan

**Eva M. Schmelz**
Karmanos Cancer Institute
Wayne State University School of
  Medicine
Detroit, Michigan

**Jeremy P.E. Spencer**
Molecular Nutrition Group
School of Food Biosciences
University of Reading
Reading, United Kingdom

**Jubilee R. Stewart**
Department of Cancer Biology
M.D. Anderson Cancer Center
University of Texas
Houston, Texas

**Sujatha Sundaram**
Department of Surgery
Dartmouth Medical School
Lebanon, New Hampshire

**Urvi Telang**
Department of Pharmaceutical
  Sciences
School of Pharmacy and
  Pharmaceutical Sciences
State University of New York at
  Buffalo
Buffalo, New York

**Barbara Teter**
Department of Social and Preventive
  Medicine
School of Public Health and Health
  Professions
State University of New York at
  Buffalo
Buffalo, New York

**Henry J. Thompson**
Cancer Prevention Laboratory
Colorado State University
Fort Collins, Colorado

**Lilian U. Thompson**
Department of Nutritional Sciences
Faculty of Medicine
University of Toronto
Toronto, Ontario, Canada

**Elke A. Trautwein**
Unilever Health Institute
Unilever Research & Development
Vlaardingen, The Netherlands

**Anne-Marie Ugnat**
Surveillance and Risk Assessment
  Division
Center of Chronic Diseases Prevention
  and Control
Public Health Agency of Canada
Ottawa, Ontario, Canada

**Saeri Wada**
Department of Biochemistry
Kyoto Prefectural University of
  Medicine
Kyoto, Japan

**Xiang-Dong Wang**
Nutrition and Cancer Biology
  Laboratory
Jean Mayer USDA Human Nutrition
  Research Center on Aging at Tufts
  University
Boston, Massachusetts

**Xiu-Fang Wang**
Apoptosis Research Group
School of Medical Sciences
Griffith University
Southport, Queensland, Australia

**P.D. Whanger**
Department of Environmental and
  Molecular Toxicology
Oregon State University
Corvallis, Oregon

**Kun Wu**
Department of Nutrition and Food
  Hygiene
School of Public Health
Harbin Medical University
Harbin, Heilongjiang Province, China

**Yan Zhao**
Department of Nutrition and Food
  Hygiene
School of Public Health
Harbin Medical University
Harbin, Heilongjiang Province, China

**Jin-Rong Zhou**
Nutrition/Metabolism Laboratory
Beth Israel Deaconess Medical Center
Harvard Medical School
Boston, Massachusetts

**Zongjian Zhu**
Cancer Prevention Laboratory
Colorado State University
Fort Collins, Colorado

# Contents

**PART I    Introduction**

**Chapter 1**  Epidemiology of Breast, Prostate, and Colon Cancers .................3
*Maddalena Barba, Barbara Fuhrman, Barbara Teter, and Paola Muti*

**Chapter 2**  How Dietary Components Protect from Cancer..........................27
*Diane M. Harris and Vay Liang W. Go*


**PART II    Dietary Components That Protect from Cancer: Vitamins**

**Chapter 3**  Vitamin A, β-Carotene, and Cancer..............................................61
*Joseph L. Napoli*

**Chapter 4**  Anticarcinogenic Activity of Natural and Synthetic
 Carotenoids ................................................................................75
*Hoyoku Nishino, Michiaki Murakoshi, Xiao Yang Mou, Saeri Wada,
Mitsuharu Masuda, Yasuhito Ohsaka, Yoshiko Satomi, and Kenji Jinno*

**Chapter 5**  Vitamin D and the Risk of Cancer ..............................................89
*Sujatha Sundaram and David A. Gewirtz*

**Chapter 6**  Vitamin E Analogs as Anticancer Agents....................................111
*Jiri Neuzil, Xiu-Fang Wang, Yan Zhao, and Kun Wu*

**Chapter 7**  Vitamin C Blocks Carcinogenic Tumor Formation....................139
*Ki Won Lee, Hyong Joo Lee, and Chang Yong Lee*

**Chapter 8**   Folic Acid, Folates, and Cancer ................................................... 153

*John J. McGuire*


## PART III   *Dietary Components That Protect from Cancer: Minerals*

**Chapter 9**   Calcium and Chemoprevention of Colon Cancer ...................... 177

*Subhas Chakrabarty*


**Chapter 10**   Relationship of Selenium Intake to Cancer ............................... 189

*P.D. Whanger*


## PART IV   *Dietary Components That Protect from Cancer: Phytosterols*

**Chapter 11**   Phytosterols: Sources and Metabolism ..................................... 223

*Elke A. Trautwein and Guus S.M.J.E. Duchateau*


**Chapter 12**   Phytosterols: Bioactivity on Cancer .......................................... 251

*Peter G. Bradford and Atif B. Awad*


## PART V   *Dietary Components That Protect from Cancer: Polyphenols*

**Chapter 13**   Classification, Dietary Sources, Absorption, Bioavailability, and Metabolism of Flavonoids ................................................... 273

*Jeremy P.E. Spencer*


**Chapter 14**   Isoflavones, Soybean Phytoestrogens, and Cancer .................... 295

*Fazlul H. Sarkar and Yiwei Li*

**Chapter 15** Implications of Flavonoids as a Sex Hormone Source ............313

*David Jenkins and Roxanne LaBelle*

**Chapter 16** Flavonoids as Inhibitors of Tumor Metastasis...........................325

*Jin-Rong Zhou*

**Chapter 17** Catechins and Inhibitory Activity against Carcinogenesis.........351

*Jen-Kun Lin*

**Chapter 18** Cancer Chemoprotective Activity of Stilbenes: Resveratrol......369

*Catherine A. O'Brian, Jubilee R. Stewart, and Feng Chu*

**Chapter 19** Flaxseed and Lignans: Effects on Breast Cancer......................385

*Krista A. Power and Lilian U. Thompson*

**Chapter 20** Anthocyanins and Cancer Prevention .......................................411

*Colin D. Kay and Bruce J. Holub*

## *PART VI    Dietary Components That Protect from Cancer: Isothiocyanates*

**Chapter 21** Isothiocyanates and Cancer Prevention ....................................435

*Marilyn E. Morris and Urvi Telang*

## *PART VII   Dietary Components That Protect from Cancer: Saponins*

**Chapter 22** Anticancer Activity of Ginseng and Soy Saponins....................457

*David G. Popovich and David D. Kitts*

# PART VIII   Dietary Components That Protect Cancer: Specialized Lipids

**Chapter 23** Omega-3 Fatty Acids and Cancer Prevention............................487
*Bandaru S. Reddy*

**Chapter 24** Conjugated Linoleic Acid and Cancer.......................................503
*Yongsoon Park*

**Chapter 25** Sphingolipids as Chemopreventive Agents.................................519
*Eva M. Schmelz*

# PART IX   Dietary Cancer Risk Factors

**Chapter 26** Obesity as a Cancer Risk Factor: Epidemiology........................541
*Yang Mao, Sai Yi Pan, and Anne-Marie Ugnat*

**Chapter 27** Obesity as a Cancer Risk Factor: Potential Mechanisms
     of Action ................................................................................565
*Henry J. Thompson, Weiqin Jiang, and Zongjian Zhu*

**Chapter 28** Alcohol and Cancer: Cellular Mechanisms of Action................579
*Xiang-Dong Wang and Hiroko Inoue-Fruehauf*

**Index** ........................................................................................597

# Part I

## Introduction

# 1 Epidemiology of Breast, Prostate, and Colon Cancers

*Maddalena Barba, Barbara Fuhrman,*
*Barbara Teter, and Paola Muti*

## CONTENTS

1.1 Introduction: Cancer Epidemiology ................................................................3
1.2 Female Breast Cancer in Western Countries .............................................6
    1.2.1 Descriptive Epidemiology ...............................................................6
    1.2.2 Reproductive Factors ......................................................................6
    1.2.3 Lifestyle Factors .............................................................................7
    1.2.4 Early Life Exposures .......................................................................8
    1.2.5 Endogenous Hormones ...................................................................8
    1.2.6 Exogenous Hormones ...................................................................10
    1.2.7 Markers of Risk .............................................................................11
    1.2.8 Mammographic Density and Breast Cancer ...............................12
1.3 Prostate Cancer in Western Countries .....................................................12
    1.3.1 Demographic Factors ....................................................................12
    1.3.2 Endocrine Factors .........................................................................13
    1.3.3 Genetic Factors .............................................................................14
    1.3.4 Dietary Components ......................................................................14
1.4 Colorectal Cancer .......................................................................................14
    1.4.1 Adenomatous Polyps ....................................................................16
    1.4.2 Familial and Hereditary Factors ..................................................16
    1.4.3 Dietary Factors .............................................................................16
    1.4.4 Role of Inflammation ...................................................................16
Acknowledgments ................................................................................................17
References ..............................................................................................................17

## 1.1 INTRODUCTION: CANCER EPIDEMIOLOGY

Cancers represent a heterogeneous group of diseases characterized by uncontrolled growth and spread of abnormal cells in the body. The disruptive behaviors of cancer cells reflect dynamic changes in their genomes and in gene expression that result in disruption of normal regulatory signaling circuits. Cancers vary on the basis of both the biologic features of the disease and the characteristics of the affected organism. The process by which normal cells are transformed into cancer cells is known as carcinogenesis.

Cancers are multifactorial diseases, with environmental and endogenous factors contributing at a different level in determining cancer risk. Epidemiology is the study of the distribution and determinants of diseases in populations. Cancer frequency is expressed by mean of measures of disease occurrence. Many sciences are aimed at the study of tumors, but in epidemiology the focus is on occurrence rather than natural history or any other aspect of the disease under investigation.

Incidence rate and prevalence represent the basic epidemiologic tools that allow us to quantify the disease occurrence. Incidence rate is the number of newly diagnosed cases of disease that occurs in a population during a specified period of time over person-year of observation. To define the incidence rate of a given disease, we indicate the population at risk for the disease of interest, the risk or event we are studying (e.g., disease occurrence), and the period over which we want to measure incidence. Every member of the population experiences a specific amount of time in the population over the risk period. Person-time represents the observational experience in which disease onset can be observed. The number of new cases of disease (incident number) divided by the person-time is the disease incidence rate in the considered population over the defined period:

$$\text{Incidence rate} = \text{No. disease onset/} \sum_{persons} \text{time spent in population}$$

The only events suitable to be counted in the numerator of an incidence rate are those that occur to persons who are contributing time to the denominator of the incidence rate at the time the disease onset occurs. The time contributed by each person to the denominator is known as the "time at risk," that is, time at risk of an event's occurring. People who contribute time to the denominator of an incidence rate are referred to as "the population at risk."

Prevalence may be defined as the ratio of number of cases of disease at a given time to the size of the population at that time. The population subset affected by the disease is known as the "prevalence pool." While incidence measures focus on events in a population at risk for the disease under investigation over a defined period of time, prevalence focuses on disease status in a prevalence pool at a specific point in time.

Given these definitions, disease prevalence and incidence rate appear to be related to each other. For a disease under investigation, a certain proportion of the population at risk of developing a specific cancer feeds the prevalence pool of persons affected by the cancer of interest at a specific point in time. The event occurrence (e.g., newly diagnosed breast cancer) influences the disease status at a population level.

An important role in the linkage between the measures of disease frequency is played by the mean duration of the disease under consideration. Diseases with large incidence rates may have low prevalence if they are rapidly fatal (e.g., SCLC or small cell lung cancer). On the other hand, cancer may be characterized at the same time by a high incidence rate and a quite long natural history, having a large prevalence in the population under consideration (e.g., prostate cancer). In defining the relationship between incidence rate and prevalence of a disease of interest, many factors, not only the disease mean duration, should be taken into account, since, in the same population, subgroups of individuals might deeply differ in terms of measures of disease occurrence on the basis of parameters such as gender, age, ethnicity, education, income, social class, disability, geographic location.[1]

Cancer determinants, as well as cancer frequency, represent a major topic in cancer epidemiology. Cancer is a multifactorial disease. The final risk of developing a pathologic condition depends on interactions of different risk factors. A risk factor is anything that increases the chances of getting a disease such as cancer. Different cancers have different risk factors. The role of genetic and environmental interaction in the occurrence of several common malignancies has been clearly demonstrated in many recent epidemiologic studies, as reviewed by Caporaso and Goldstein[2] and Strong and Amos.[3]

A small percentage of cancers (5 to 10%) can be attributed to the inheritance of one or more mutated genes that are carried in germ cells of parent and passed on to an offspring. As a result, all cells of the offspring show the same genetic defect, predisposing the individual to one or more specific cancer. Familial breast, ovarian, and prostatic cancers, linked to breast cancer susceptibility gene 1 (BRCA-1) and breast cancer susceptibility gene 2 (BRCA-2) gene mutations, and familial adenomatous polyposis predisposing to colon cancer, based on APC gene mutations, represent good examples of diseases caused by genetic factors.

A large proportion of cancers previously thought to be attributable to environmental factors alone are now considered the result of interaction between inherited susceptibility factors and environmental exposures. The study of gene–environment interaction has become one of the major topics in genetic epidemiology, a discipline integrating the principles and methodology of genetics and epidemiology.[4]

An understanding of disease etiology, supported by measures of disease occurrence at a population level, represents the basis of cancer therapy and prevention. Cancer epidemiology combines its interest in disease frequency and determinants in the elaboration and validation of hypotheses that can explain patterns of disease occurrence.

Even though scientific hypotheses are often posed as qualitative propositions, the testing of hypotheses is predicated on measurement. The importance of measurements has been reflected in the evolution of epidemiologic understanding. It was only when scientists began to measure the occurrence of diseases rather than merely reflect on what may have caused diseases that scientific knowledge about causation made impressive strides.[1]

Epidemiologic studies represent useful tools to collect data to elucidate the etiology of and risk factors for human diseases. Scientists design and conduct studies, which are critically important both in clinical medicine and in public health practice.

## 1.2  FEMALE BREAST CANCER IN WESTERN COUNTRIES

### 1.2.1  DESCRIPTIVE EPIDEMIOLOGY

Women in the U.S., New Zealand, the European Union, Israel, Canada, Australia, and Uruguay have breast cancer incidence rates that rank as the highest in the world.[5] Among women living in the U.S., breast cancer is the most commonly diagnosed cancer and the second leading cause of cancer-related mortality. Projections for 2004 show an expected 215,990 new cases of invasive breast cancer, representing 32% of all new cancer diagnoses, and 40,110 breast cancer-related deaths, accounting for 15% of cancer-related mortality.[6]

Breast cancer incidence has increased over the past 30 years in the U.S.[6] This trend is thought to reflect increased diagnosis due to mammographic screening,[7] and perhaps also to secular trends in the prevalence of obesity and hormone replacement therapy (HRT) use by postmenopausal women.[8] Over the same period, breast cancer mortality rates have declined, reflecting earlier breast cancer detection and treatment, and improvements in breast cancer therapies.[9]

The risk of breast cancer increases with age. There is a rapid rise in breast cancer incidence with age up to about age 50; then the rate of increase slows dramatically.[10]

In the U.S., breast cancer incidence and mortality rates vary by race and ethnicity. White women have the highest incidence rates of breast cancer, while Asian Americans and American Indians/Alaskan natives have the lowest incidence rates.[6] African American women have the highest breast cancer death rates, with mortality rates 30% higher than those of white women, in spite of significantly lower disease incidence.[11] These differences have been attributed to disparate use of screening services and diagnoses at later stages, higher rates of early and more aggressive cancers, and undertreatment of disease.[12]

Breast cancer rates vary widely among different countries. The countries cited above have incidence rates six times higher than countries in Asia and Africa. Migrant studies suggest the importance of early life experience in affecting breast cancer risk. Japanese women who were born in Japan and migrated to the U.S. have higher breast cancer rates in comparison to their counterparts in Japan. While Japanese women who migrated to the U.S. as young adults experience a modest increase in their breast cancer rates; those born in the U.S. have rates approaching their white counterparts.[13] International differences and migrant studies have pointed to the importance of environmental and lifestyle factors in determining breast cancer risk. Among the potential risk factors, we discuss those of particular interest.

### 1.2.2  REPRODUCTIVE FACTORS

Epidemiologic studies have been consistent in showing early age at menarche as a risk factor for breast cancer. A 5% decrease in breast cancer risk results from each year that menarche is delayed.[14] A number of studies have provided evidence that the timing of menarche is associated with levels of endogenous estrogens in later adulthood.[15] Early menarche results in early onset of regular ovulatory menstrual cycles,[16] and consequently into an extended exposure to reproductive hormones.[17] Over the past 100 years, age at menarche has progressively decreased in the U.S. and in most other areas of the world. It is possible that improved nutrition and control of infectious diseases of childhood may have led to lower ages at menarche, and increasing breast cancer incidence over the past century.

At the time of menopause, age-specific incidence rates of breast cancer slow markedly, and the rate of increase in the postmenopausal period is only about one sixth the rate of increase in the premenopausal period. In their study, Trichopolous and colleagues[18] found that women who experienced natural menopause (defined as cessation of periods) before age 45 had only one half the breast cancer risk of those whose menopause occurred after age 55.

Parity, and in particular early age at first full-term pregnancy, are associated with decreased breast cancer risk. Pregnancy causes a transient increase in breast cancer risk, followed by a lasting protective effect.[19] In one international case-control study, women with a first birth before the age of 20 had about one half the risk of nulliparous women.[20] The first full-term birth has the strongest effect on breast cancer risk; however, there is an additional protective effect of subsequent births.[21] The association of parity with a lasting decrease in breast cancer risk may be due to a favorable change in the susceptibility of breast tissue to carcinogenesis resulting from maturation and differentiation of breast tissue in response to hormonal events occurring during pregnancy.[22] It is also true that there are some lasting changes in hormonal milieu following pregnancy. Free estradiol and prolactin levels are lower and sex hormone-binding globulin (SHBG) levels are higher in parous compared to nulliparous women.[23,24]

Lactation is associated with a reduction in breast cancer risk. Nursing results in a delay in the reestablishment of ovulation after a full-term pregnancy. The Collaborative Group on Hormonal Factors in Breast Cancer conducted a pooled analysis of 47 epidemiologic studies done in 30 countries and found a decrease of 4.3% in breast cancer risk associated with each 12 months of breastfeeding, in addition to an independent decrease in risk associated with bearing each child.[25]

### 1.2.3 LIFESTYLE FACTORS

International differences in breast cancer occurrence might be partly explained on the basis of lifestyle factors, such as diet and alcohol consumption. Among the dietary factors, the most of the studies have focused on diet content of fat and fiber. As for micronutrients, phytoestrogens have been largely and still inconclusively investigated. Alcohol consumption has shown a moderate effect on breast cancer risk. The existing evidence about dietary components and alcohol intake in affecting breast cancer risk is discussed in detail further in the following chapters of this manuscript.

Numerous epidemiologic studies on the putative association between cigarette smoking and breast cancer have been conducted with mixed results.[26] An elegant paper by Band et al.[27] isolates the competing effects of cigarette smoking by stratifying smoking study subjects by menopausal status, and, among those who are parous, comparing the time of smoking initiation relative to first pregnancy. In contrast to postmenopausal women, circulating estrogen levels in premenopausal women do not appear to be strongly affected by smoking.[28] Among premenopausal women, the beginning of smoking before the first pregnancy occurrence was associated with an increased breast cancer risk (adjusted odds ratio [OR]: 1.47, 95% confidence interval [CI]: 1.02 to 2.10). According to the authors, this finding might reflect a different degree of susceptibility of the mammary gland to carcinogens, resulting from maturation and differentiation of breast tissue in response to hormonal events occurring during pregnancy. Among postmenopausal women, those who began smoking after their first pregnancy were relatively protected against breast cancer (adjusted OR: 0.63, 0.41 to 0.96). This suggests that an antiestrogenic effect of smoking can protect women whose breast tissue is relatively refractory to tobacco mutagens.

### 1.2.4 EARLY LIFE EXPOSURES

Among perinatal factors of interest, recent studies have linked high birth weight[29] and a negative history of breastfeeding in infancy[30] to an increased breast cancer risk, while most of the studies regarding birth rank and maternal age reported little or no association.[31] Fetal growth has been positively associated with concentrations of estrogens at the extremes of the corresponding distributions, although evidence for an association throughout the usual range of fetal growth is not clear.[32] Recent studies suggest that the role of early life factors in determining breast cancer risk may be more apparent in younger women, but this may be due to better recall in this group.[33] Differences in caloric intake, availability of specific nutrients, or possible hormonal and immunologic consequences of having been breastfed have been proposed as possible causes of a decreased breast cancer risk.[33–35]

### 1.2.5 ENDOGENOUS HORMONES

The hormone-responsive nature of many breast tumors has led many to hypothesize that endogenous hormones play a causal role in the pathogenesis of this disease. Indeed, this hypothesis has been supported both by animal models and *in vitro* research, but challenges in epidemiologic study design and implementation have postponed arrival at a consensus regarding even the most strongly implicated hormones, such as estrogens. The Collaborative Group on Hormonal Factors in Breast Cancer conducted a pooled analysis of nine prospective cohort studies that employed careful specimen collection, storage, and analytic procedures to investigate the relationship between sex-steroid hormone levels and risk of postmenopausal breast cancer.[36] They examined risk of postmenopausal breast cancer by quintiles of serum hormone levels and found that estrogens and androgens were significantly and independently associated with increases in breast cancer risk, with evidence of dose–response relationships. The relative risk for breast cancer for women in the highest quintile of estradiol compared with women in the lowest quintile was 2.00 (95% CI: 1.47 to 2.71). Relative risks in the highest quintile compared with the lowest quintile for the other estrogens (estrone and estrone sulfate) and the androgens (androstenedione, dehydroepiandrosterone, DHEAS, testosterone) were all approximately equal to 2, and the highest relative risks were in the highest quintiles of free estradiol [relative risk 2.58 (1.76 to 3.78)]. For SHBG, which modulates availability of estrogens to tissues, there was a significant inverse association with breast cancer risk [relative risk in top fifth 0.66 (0.43 to 1.00)].[37]

The evidence is mixed with respect to the effects of bioavailable estrogens on breast cancer risk in premenopausal women. Two prospective studies have found no effect;[38–40] another found a significant trend in breast cancer risk by quintiles of circulating estrogens associated with breast cancer risk;[41] and a fourth research study produced findings suggesting decreased estrogen excretion in the urine[42] and increased estrogens circulating in the blood of women who would go on to have premenopausal breast cancer compared to those who would not.[43]

Mixed findings in studies of premenopausal breast cancer may be attributable to either the small sample size or the biological variability in hormones determinations. Notably, in contrast to the earliest prospective studies reviewed, more recent studies adjusted for the interval between date of specimen collection and the start of the subsequent menstrual period. Thus, it is currently difficult to conclude whether endogenous estrogens play a role in the etiology of premenopausal breast cancer. Also, prospective studies have failed in demonstrating any significant association between premenopausal breast cancer and androgen levels.[38,41]

The mechanism by which estrogens may cause pre- and/or postmenopausal breast cancer is still an open question. The most commonly held hypothesis, based on the interaction between estrogen and estrogen receptor-$\alpha$ or estrogen receptor-$\beta$,[44,45] has been revisited at the light of a complementary hypothesis, according to which estrogens can be metabolized to genotoxic compounds and directly damage DNA.[46] The effects of androgens on risk of breast cancer are thought to be, at least in part, mediated through conversion by the enzyme aromatase to estrogens in peripheral tissues. This mechanism may be particularly important in obesity and in postmenopausal women.

New epidemiologic evidence has indicated that glucose metabolism, hyper-insulinemic insulin resistance, and insulin-like growth factor bioavailability may also play roles in breast cancer etiology. Insulin is a powerful mitogenic agent.[47] Moreover, insulin may also play a role in tumor promotion by upregulation of ovarian steroid secretion.[48] To date, three prospective studies have been conducted on serum insulin or C-peptide and breast cancer risk with inconsistent results.[49–51] Nonfasting condition at blood collection for these studies may, at least in part, explain the weakness of the observed association. There is consistent prospective epidemiological evidence of a close association between insulin-like growth factor-1 (IGF-1) and breast cancer risk, however, more often in premenopausal women.[50–53]

Melatonin (*N*-acetyl-5-methoxy-tryptamine) is proposed to be a factor in the etiology of breast cancer.[54] This hormone is secreted by the pineal gland and synthesized during darkness.[55] There are a number of proposed mechanisms by which melatonin could effect breast cancer development: induction of apoptosis,[56] inhibition of cell proliferation,[57,58] scavenging of reactive oxygen species, and immunomodulation.[55,59] Consistent with this theory, observational studies have shown evidence that women who work at night have an elevated risk of breast cancer, while residence in the Arctic, blindness, and visual impairment are all associated with decreased breast cancer risk.[60–65] However, a recent large prospective study found no evidence that the level of melatonin was associated with risk of breast cancer.[66]

The endogenous hormone prolactin is secreted by the anterior pituitary and its expression is regulated by the hypothalamus. Evidence about the role of prolactin in the etiology of breast cancer has been collected from both laboratory studies and epidemiologic studies.[67–69] Prolactin regulates the growth of breast epithelium,[70] promotes cell proliferation,[71] and protects human breast cancer cells against apoptosis.[67] Epidemiologic evidence about the relationship between prolactin and risk of postmenopausal breast cancer is inconsistent.[69,72,73] There is no evidence of such an association in premenopausal women affected by breast cancer.[69,73,74]

## 1.2.6 EXOGENOUS HORMONES

The association between oral contraceptive (OC) use and risk of breast cancer has been controversial. The Collaborative Group on Hormonal Factors in Breast Cancer[75] reviewed 54 studies (performed in 26 countries) on the relationship between OC use and risk of breast cancer. The combined studies included a total of 53,297 cases and 100,239 controls. The group concluded that oral contraceptive use conferred a small increase in risk of breast cancer for current OC users (RR 1.24; 95% CI: 1.15 to 1.33), and a trend for decreasing risk following cessation of use. In women who discontinued OC use within the previous 10 years, the reported pooled result was RR 1.07 (95% CI: 1.02 to 1.13) and no evidence of increased risk was reported for women who had discontinued use more than 10 years before.[75,76] However, cases were diagnosed in the 1980s, formulations of oral contraceptives (current estrogen dose between 20 to 30 µg vs. 100 µg in 1960), age at first use, and duration of use have changed greatly since that time.[77]

More recently, Marchbanks et al.[78] report null findings from the large Women's CARE study (Women's Contraceptive and Reproductive Experiences) that included more than 9000 subjects recruited in five U.S. sites. Although they found case subjects had significantly lower parity, older ages at first birth, higher reports of family history of breast cancer, later age at menopause, and less use of hormone replacement therapies, they found no significant association between current OC use (RR 1.0; 95% CI: 0.8 to 1.3) or former use (RR 0.9; 95% CI: 0.8

to 1.0) and risk of breast cancer.[78] Victory et al. (2004) reported findings from the large multicenter prospective WHI (Women's Health Initiative) study, which included 161,809 women with 40% having a history of OC use. After controlling for other risk factors, it was shown that OC use had no effect on risk of breast cancer regardless of HRT exposure and, further, that OC use significantly reduced the risk of endometrial or ovarian cancers.[79]

Postmenopausal hormone replacement regimens include a large number of different estrogen and progestin combinations, unopposed estrogen formulations, doses, and routes of therapy such as oral or transdermal. Since the 1990s numerous observational studies on the impact of HRT on breast cancer risk have been conducted. In the Women's CARE study, a large case-control study of 1847 postmenopausal women with incident breast cancer and 1932 control subjects, Norman et al.[79] reported a linear trend of an estimated 5% increased risk of breast cancer with each year of use of combined HRT, whereas no increase was found with use of estrogen-only regimens. Further evidence comes from two important prospective studies, which also found significant breast cancer risk associated with combined estrogen–progestin regimens and lower risk for estrogen-only therapies.[80–82] The WHI trial involving combined HRT was stopped by the safety monitoring board in 2002 when elevated breast cancer risk associated with combined HRT use became evident. Among 40 clinical centers, postmenopausal women aged 50 to 79 ($N = 16,608$) were randomly assigned to receive combined conjugated equine estrogens plus medroxyprogesterone acetate or placebo. Incident breast cancer cases in the treatment group compared to the placebo group resulted in a hazard ratio of 1.24 (95% CI: 1.02 to 1.50) compared to the placebo group. The WHI study investigating conjugated equine estrogens alone compared with placebo showed no increased risk of breast cancer.[83] It has also been shown that HRT increases breast density and therefore reduces the sensitivity and specificity of mammographic breast cancer screening.[84,85]

### 1.2.7 MARKERS OF RISK

In the U.S., 10 to 20% of patients with breast cancer and patients with ovarian cancer have a positive familial history, namely, a first- or second-degree relative with one of these diseases.[86] Two major genes associated with susceptibility to breast and ovarian cancer — BRCA-1 and BRCA-2 — have been identified to date.[87,88] Mutations in either of these genes confer a lifetime risk of breast cancer of between 60 and 85% and a lifetime risk of ovarian cancer of between 15 and 40%.[89] However, mutations in these genes account for only 2 to 3% of all breast cancers.[90]

Benign breast diseases include a heterogeneous group of diagnoses, which are categorized by their association with breast cancer risk. In particular, proliferative lesions without atypia are associated with a 1.5- to 2-fold increase in risk, whereas atypical hyperplasias are associated with a 4-fold to 5-fold increase in breast cancer risk.[91] Lesions not expressing either proliferative or hyperplastic features have not been explored extensively yet as for their relation with breast cancer risk, even though there is evidence of an increased risk of breast cancer associated with nonproliferative diagnoses, especially evident in women 50 years of age and older.[92]

### 1.2.8 MAMMOGRAPHIC DENSITY AND BREAST CANCER

Epithelium and stromal tissues that are strongly related to risk of breast cancer appear radiologically dense, whereas fat appears radiologically lucent.[93] The proportion of the mammographic image occupied by radiologically dense tissue is a composite measure of breast tissue composition. At present, the role of mammographic density in breast cancer etiology is not clear.[94] However, it has been established that mammographic density is an independent predictor of breast cancer risk, with associated relative risks between 4 and 6 for the highest vs. the lowest quartile of mammographic density. Evidence suggests that the magnitude of the increase in breast cancer risk is greater than that associated with nearly all other breast cancer risk factors after adjustment for age, body mass index (BMI), age at menarche, breast cancer family history, parity, menopausal status, and HRT use.[93,95]

## 1.3 PROSTATE CANCER IN WESTERN COUNTRIES

The incidence of prostate cancer in the U.S. and certain Western countries has risen sharply during the past decade. In U.S. men, between 1987 and 1992, prostate cancer incidence rate increased 85%, followed by a decline of 29% between 1992 and 1995, and then increasing again by 2.3% per year beginning in 1995. Recent prostate cancer incidence increased by 3.0% per year among white men and by 2.3% per year among black men.[96] Prostate cancer mortality in the U.S. stopped increasing in 1991, and decreased an average of 4.4% annually from 1994 through 1997.[97] Declines in prostate cancer mortality might reflect improvements in treatment and longer survival due to prostate specific antigen (PSA)-related early detection.[98]

### 1.3.1 DEMOGRAPHIC FACTORS

Prostate cancer is a disease that typically strikes older men. It is usually diagnosed in very few people aged younger than 50 years (<0.1% of all patients). The mean age of patients with this disorder is 72 to 74 years, and about 85% of patients are diagnosed after age 65.[99] There are striking international differences, as much as 90-fold, in prostate cancer incidence and mortality rates between highly developed countries and less-developed countries. The lowest rates are found in Asia, especially among Chinese men in Tianjin, China (1.9 per 100,000 per year), and the highest are in North America and Scandinavia, especially in African American men in the U.S. (137 per 100,000 per year).[100] Results of migrant studies appear to show some real shift in incidence toward the new host country, providing evidence that these international and racial differences in prostate cancer incidence are not based entirely on genetic predisposition or differences in health care and cancer registration. As an example, Japanese men who move from Japan (a country with low incidence) to the U.S. (high incidence) show an increased incidence of prostate cancer, that is to about 50% of the rate for white men and to 25% of that for African American men in the U.S.[101]

A disproportionate number of cancer deaths occur among racial/ethnic minorities, particularly African Americans, who, compared with whites, have a 33% higher risk of dying of cancer of the prostate, lung and bronchus, colon and rectum, oral cavity and pharynx, cervix, and stomach. Overall, age-adjusted cancer incidence is higher among African Americans compared to all other racial/ethnic groups.[102] Disparities in cancer mortality trends have also been noted. Mortality rates have been decreasing among both African Americans and whites overall, but decreases generally have been smaller and less consistent among African Americans than among whites,[102] and racial disparities in mortality have persisted.[103] This may be due to less use of prostate cancer screening among African American men, and consequently, later stage at diagnosis.[104]

Prostate cancer is notable among cancer sites in that there is considerable evidence, albeit from the minority of published studies on the topic, that race may be an independent factor in prognosis after equivalent treatment. However, it is not clear whether this observation is caused by underlying behavioral, biologic, or genetic factors associated with race or because of incomplete or inaccurate measurement of clinical risk or quality-of-care factors.[105]

The theory that socioeconomic status (SES) inequalities and other characteristics of the sociocultural environment are key determinants of health and could account for health differences among countries has become stronger in the past decades. It is still unclear to what extent and by which mechanisms social and environmental factors can account for racial and ethnic differences in rates of disease and death. There is evidence that SES could influence the pattern of survival in patients diagnosed with prostate cancer. Between 1988 and 1999, the proportion of localized and regional prostate cancer diagnoses increased, whereas the proportion of distant-stage prostate cancer decreased. In a monograph examining socioeconomic variations in cancer rates, researchers found that, although this trend holds across all socioeconomic groups, more distant-stage prostate cancers are diagnosed within census tracts with higher poverty rates.[106]

### 1.3.2 ENDOCRINE FACTORS

Human prostate carcinomas are often androgen sensitive and react to hormonal therapy by temporary remission, followed by relapse to an androgen-insensitive state. These well-established features of prostate cancer strongly suggest that steroid hormones, particularly androgens, play a major role in human prostatic carcinogenesis, but the precise mechanisms by which androgens affect this process are unknown. In addition, the possible involvement of estrogenic hormones is not entirely clear.[107] Estrogens induce mitosis of both normal and malignant prostatic epithelial cells in many species, including humans.[108,109] An important metabolic pathway of the estrogens is the formation of hydroxylated estrogens.

Muti et al.,[110] in a case-control study on urinary estrogen metabolites and prostate cancer risk, showed a protective effect of the metabolic pathway favoring 2-hydroxylation over 16-hydroxylation on risk of prostate cancer.

Two distinct lines of epidemiologic and basic science research have converged in the hypothesis that the somatotropic axis plays an important role in the development of prostate cancer. Insulin-like growth factor-1 (IGF-1) is an important hormone in the axis, conveying centrally regulated signals to the tissue level. IGF-1 is a mitogen that stimulates cell proliferation and inhibits apoptosis. Recent epidemiologic studies suggest an association between elevated blood levels of IGFs and risk of prostate cancer, although data are inconsistent across the studies.[111,112]

Although it is well known that growth hormone (GH) is a major factor regulating IGF levels, there is no evidence about how the physiological mechanisms regulating GH secretion on the basis of IGF-1 serum concentration may change in the presence of prostate cancer. From experimental studies, it appears that GH might be involved in regulating prostate function. The coexpression of GH and its receptor demonstrated by Chopin and colleagues[113] would enable an autocrine-paracrine pathway to exist in the prostate that would be able to stimulate prostate growth, either directly or indirectly via IGF production.

Briefly, scientific evidence suggests a multifactorial general hypothesis of prostate carcinogenesis, with androgens acting via androgen receptor-mediated mechanisms to enhance the carcinogenic activity of strong endogenous genotoxic carcinogens, such as reactive estrogen metabolites. In addition, the body of evidence is growing for a role of the IGF family members. In this hypothesis, all of these processes are modulated by a variety of environmental factors and genetic determinants.[107]

### 1.3.3 Genetic Factors

Familial aggregation (at least two cases in the family) is observed in about 20% of cases and a hereditary form of prostate cancer in 5%. This proportion increases with younger age at diagnosis. Familial types of prostate cancer account for about 40% of patients who present younger than 55 years and for up to 9% of those presenting at 85 years or older.[114]

### 1.3.4 Dietary Components

Given that dietary components are extensively discussed in subsequent chapters, the reader will easily find a clear referral to the role of vitamin D, dietary fat intake, selenium, vitamin E, and lycopene in affecting prostate cancer risk in the subsequent chapter of this book.

## 1.4 COLORECTAL CANCER

Because of their biological and epidemiologic similarities, colon and rectal cancers are often considered as a single disease entity. The progression of colorectal cancers from an early precancerous lesion (adenomatous polyps) to an invasive cancer has been well described at histologic and even molecular levels. Screening strategies for early detection have been successfully developed[115] and implemented on a large scale with subsequent declines seen in both incidence and mortality rates. Around the world, incidence rates for colorectal cancer can vary by as much as 20-fold. Currently, the highest incidence rates for colorectal cancer are reported in Australia and New Zealand, parts of Eastern and Northern Europe, and the U.S., whereas the lowest rates are reported in Africa and Asia.[5] In some low-incidence countries in Asia, colorectal cancer incidence appears to be increasing as lifestyles become increasingly Westernized. The incidence of colonic cancers varies internationally to a greater extent than that of rectal cancers. Rectal cancer is usually more common in males at all ages, with an age-standardized male:female incidence ratio of 1.5 to 2.0. In areas with low colon cancer incidence rates, such as India and Senegal, the rates for rectal cancer may exceed those for colon cancer.[116] Countries in which colon cancer incidence is high have a higher proportion of sigmoid cancers, while in countries with low incidence rates, cancers of cecum and ascendant colon predominate.[117]

In the U.S., colorectal cancer is the third leading cancer diagnosis and the third leading cause of cancer-related deaths among both men and women. Estimates for 2004 predict 106,370 new cases of colon cancer and 40,570 new cases of rectal cancer. Incidence rates have declined continuously from 1985 to 2000 and this may be attributable to increased screening and removal of precancerous polyps. Mortality attributed to colorectal cancer has declined in both men and women over this period, reflecting a concurrent fall in disease incidence and improvements in treatment and survival.[118]

The risk of colorectal cancer increases with age, with most cases diagnosed after age 50. In high-incidence countries like the U.S., age-specific incidence rates are higher among women, until about age 60, when they are outstripped by those for men.[119] Migrant studies have consistently demonstrated that risk of colorectal cancer changes quickly among those who move from low-risk to high-risk countries, within the first generation, or after 20 or more years of residence in the adopted country.[120–122] Significantly, the transition was shown to be slower for those groups of Puerto Rican migrants who traveled back and forth between the U.S. and their native land, suggesting that acculturation and associated environmental and lifestyle exposures are involved in the transition.[121] These findings suggest the importance of environmental factors in the development of colorectal cancer.[117]

In the U.S., colorectal cancer incidence and mortality rates vary among racial/ethnic groups. African Americans have the highest incidence of colorectal cancer of any racial/ethnic group. Compared with whites, African Americans are diagnosed with this disease at a younger age and have higher rates of proximal cancers. In contrast, Hispanics, Asian Americans, and native Americans have the lowest risk for colorectal cancers.[6] These differences may be due to differences in diet, physical activity, and smoking rates among different racial/ethnic groups. African Americans are also more likely than whites to present with late-stage disease perhaps due to lower screening rates and fewer diagnostic tests performed in this group.[123]

### 1.4.1 ADENOMATOUS POLYPS

The frequency of adenomas in various populations parallels the level of colorectal cancer incidence. The positive correlation coefficient worldwide for men and women combined is about 0.7. The malignant potential of an adenoma may be predicted by its size, the presence of high-grade dysplasia, and the predominance of villous features over tubular features.[124]

### 1.4.2 FAMILIAL AND HEREDITARY FACTORS

Inherited conditions account for approximately 10 to 15% of colorectal carcinomas in the general population; these include the rare autosomal syndrome of familial adenomatous polyposis (FAP) and the hereditary nonpolyposis colorectal cancer (HNPCC) syndromes. HNPCC is among the most common of all cancer predisposition syndromes and results from germ line mutations in mismatch DNA repair genes. It is characterized by early onset-colorectal cancer, but also confers increased risk of endometrial, gastric, and urogenital cancers.[125,126]

### 1.4.3 DIETARY FACTORS

Caloric intake and fiber deficiency have been the topics of greatest interest during the latest years. The collected evidence about their relationship with colorectal cancer risk is extensively illustrated in subsequent chapters of this book.

### 1.4.4 ROLE OF INFLAMMATION

Both case-control studies[127] and prospective cohort studies[128] have shown with good consistency that aspirin users experience lower risks of colorectal cancer compared to nonusers. These findings have emphasized the role of inflammation in carcinogenesis, and also suggested that nonsteroidal anti-inflammatory drugs (NSAIDs) are potential chemopreventive agents. Some randomized clinical trials have shown that aspirin can reduce the incidence of adenomas in participants with a history of adenomatous polyps[129] and may induce regression of adenomas in participants with FAP.[130] Caution must be advised in applying this preventive strategy since NSAIDs, and even very specific cyclooxygenase-2 (COX-2) inhibitors, when used regularly and at effective doses, could have adverse health effects that tip the balance of the risk–benefit equation.[131]

In molecular and animal studies, hyperinsulinemia and hyperglycemia[132,133] have been shown to be independent risk factors of colorectal carcinogenesis. Insulin and IGF-1 receptors are expressed by both normal colorectal epithelial cells and colon cancer tissue.[134,135] Therefore, both premalignant and cancerous stages can be affected by IGF-1. In a recent review, Chang and colleagues[136] summarize the epidemiologic literature with respect to hyperinsulinemia and hyperglycemia as risk factors for colorectal cancer. According to the authors, epidemiologic findings to date indicate a slightly increased risk of colorectal cancer for patients with diabetes; however, there are some inconsistencies across the study results. Possible explanations for these inconsistencies might include inadequate information about patients' diabetic disease and treatment status. A greater attention toward medical history, staging and treatment for hyperinsulinemia and hyperglycemia might be helpful to further our understanding of the role of hyperinsulinemia and hyperglycemia in colorectal carcinogenesis.[136]

## ACKNOWLEDGMENTS

Partly supported by the American Italian Cancer Foundation (AICF).

## REFERENCES

1. Rothman KJ, Greenland S. Measures of disease frequency. In: Rothman KJ, Greenland S, eds. *Modern Epidemiology*. Philadelphia: Lippincott/Williams & Wilkins; 1998:29–46.
2. Caporaso N, Goldstein A. Issues involving biomarkers in the study of genetics of human cancer. In: Toniolo PBP, Shuler DEG, Rothman N, Hulka B, Pearce N, eds. IARC Scientific Publications. Vol. 142. Lyon, France: International Agency for Research on Cancer; 1997:237–250.
3. Strong L, Amos C. Inherited susceptibility. In: Fraumeni, JF, Schottenfeld, D, eds. *Cancer Epidemiology and Prevention*. 2nd ed. New York: Oxford University Press; 1996: 559–583.
4. Zheng W. Epidemiologic studies of genetic factors for cancer. In: Nasca PC, Pastides H, eds. *Fundamentals of Cancer Epidemiology*. Gaithersburg, MD: Aspen; 2001:103–121.
5. Ferlay J, Bray F, Pisani P, Parkin DM. GLOBOCAN 2002: Cancer Incidence, Mortality and Prevalence Worldwide, Version 2.0. In: *IARC CancerBase*. No 5. Lyon, France: IARC Press; 2004.
6. Jemal A, Clegg LX, Ward E, Ries LA, Wu X, Jamison PM, Wingo PA, Howe HL, Anderson RN, Edwards BK. Annual report to the nation on the status of cancer, 1975–2001, with a special feature regarding survival. *Cancer* 2004; 101(1):3–27.
7. Nasseri K. Secular trends in the incidence of female breast cancer in the United States, 1973–1998. *Breast J* 2004; 10(4):380–380.
8. Ghafoor A, Jemal A, Ward E, Cokkinides V, Smith R, Thun M. Trends in breast cancer by race and ethnicity. *CA Cancer J Clin* 2003; 53(6):342–355.
9. Mariotto A, Feuer EJ, Harlan LC, Wun LM, Johnson KA, Abrams J. Trends in use of adjuvant multi-agent chemotherapy and tamoxifen for breast cancer in the United States: 1975–1999. *J Natl Cancer Inst* 2002; 94(21):1626–1634.
10. Pike MC. Age-related factors in cancers of the breast, ovary, and endometrium. *J Chronic Dis* 1987; 40 Suppl 2:59S–69S.
11. Stewart SL, King JB, Thompson TD, Friedman C, Wingo PA. Cancer mortality surveillance — United States, 1990–2000. *MMWR Surveill Summ* 2004; 53(3):1–108.

12. Chu KC, Lamar CA, Freeman HP. Racial disparities in breast carcinoma survival rates: separating factors that affect diagnosis from factors that affect treatment. *Cancer* 2003; 97(11):2853–2860.

13. Shimizu H, Ross RK, Bernstein L, Yatani R, Henderson BE, Mack TM. Cancers of the prostate and breast among Japanese and white immigrants in Los Angeles County. *Br J Cancer* 1991; 63(6):963–966.

14. Hunter DJ, Spiegelman D, Adami HO, van den Brandt PA, Folsom AR, Goldbohm RA, Graham S, Howe GR, Kushi LH, Marshall JR et al. Non-dietary factors as risk factors for breast cancer, and as effect modifiers of the association of fat intake and risk of breast cancer. *Cancer Causes Control* 1997; 8(1):49–56.

15. Apter D, Reinila M, Vihko R. Some endocrine characteristics of early menarche, a risk factor for breast cancer, are preserved into adulthood. *Int J Cancer* 1989; 44(5):783–787.

16. Apter D, Vihko R. Early menarche, a risk factor for breast cancer, indicates early onset of ovulatory cycles. *J Clin Endocrinol Metab* 1983; 57(1):82–86.

17. Henderson BE, Ross RK, Judd HL, Krailo MD, Pike MC. Do regular ovulatory cycles increase breast cancer risk? *Cancer* 1985; 56(5):1206–1208.

18. Trichopolous D, MacMahon B. The menopause and breast cancer risk. *J Natl Cancer Inst* 1972; 48:605.

19. Rosner B, Colditz GA, Willett WC. Reproductive risk factors in a prospective study of breast cancer: the Nurses' Health Study. *Am J Epidemiol* 1994; 139(8):819–835.

20. MacMahon B, Cole P, Lin TM, Lowe CR, Mirra AP, Ravnihar B, Salber EJ, Valaoras VG, Yuasa S. Age at first birth and breast cancer risk. *Bull World Health Organ* 1970; 43(2):209–221.

21. Lambe M, Hsieh C, Tsaih S, Ekbom A, Adami HO, Trichopoulos D. Maternal risk of breast cancer following multiple births: a nationwide study in Sweden. *Cancer Causes Control* 1996; 7(5):533–538.

22. Medina D, Sivaraman L, Hilsenbeck SG, Conneely O, Ginger M, Rosen J, Omalle BW. Mechanisms of hormonal prevention of breast cancer. *Ann NY Acad Sci* 2001; 952:23–35.

23. Yu MC, Gerkins VR, Henderson BE, Brown JB, Pike MC. Elevated levels of prolactin in nulliparous women. *Br J Cancer* 1981; 43(6):826–831.

24. Bernstein L, Pike MC, Ross RK, Judd HL, Brown JB, Henderson BE. Estrogen and sex hormone-binding globulin levels in nulliparous and parous women. *J Natl Cancer Inst* 1985; 74(4):741–745.

25. Collaborative Group on Hormonal Factors in Breast Cancer: Breast cancer and breastfeeding: collaborative reanalysis of individual data from 47 epidemiological studies in 30 countries, including 50302 women with breast cancer and 96973 women without the disease. *Lancet* 2002; 360(9328):187–195.

26. Terry PD, Rohan TE. Cigarette smoking and the risk of breast cancer in women: a review of the literature. *Cancer Epidemiol Biomarkers Prev* 2002; 11(10 Pt 1):953–971.

27. Band PR, Le ND, Fang R, Deschamps M. Carcinogenic and endocrine disrupting effects of cigarette smoke and risk of breast cancer. *Lancet* 2002; 360(9339):1044–1049.

28. Barrett-Connor E. Smoking and endogenous sex hormones in men and women. In: Wald N, Baron JA, eds. *Smoking and Hormonal-Related Disorders* Oxford: Oxford University Press; 1990:183–196.

29. Sanderson M, Williams MA, Malone KE, Stanford JL, Emanuel I, White E, Daling JR. Perinatal factors and risk of breast cancer. *Epidemiology* 1996; 7(1):34–37.

30. Janerich DT, Hayden CL, Thompson WD, Selenskas SL, Mettlin C. Epidemiologic evidence of perinatal influence in the etiology of adult cancers. *J Clin Epidemiol* 1989; 42(2):151–157.

31. Rothman KJ, MacMahon B, Lin TM, Lowe CR, Mirra AP, Ravnihar B, Salber EJ, Trichopoulos D, Yuasa S. Maternal age and birth rank of women with breast cancer. *J Natl Cancer Inst* 1980; 65(4):719–722.

32. Gerhard I, Fitzer C, Klinga K, Rahman N, Runnebaum B. Estrogen screening in evaluation of fetal outcome and infant's development. *J Perinat Med* 1986; 14(5):279–291.

33. Weiss HA, Potischman NA, Brinton LA, Brogan D, Coates RJ, Gammon MD, Malone KE, Schoenberg JB. Prenatal and perinatal risk factors for breast cancer in young women. *Epidemiology* 1997; 8(2):181–187.

34. Brinton LA, Hoover R, Fraumeni JF Jr. Reproductive factors in the aetiology of breast cancer. *Br J Cancer* 1983; 47(6):757–762.

35. Freudenheim JL, Marshall JR, Graham S, Laughlin R, Vena JE, Bandera E, Muti P, Swanson M, Nemoto T. Exposure to breastmilk in infancy and the risk of breast cancer. *Epidemiology* 1994; 5(3):324–331.

36. Collaborative Group on Hormonal Factors in Breast Cancer. Breast cancer and endogenous sex hormones in postmenopausal women: a collaborative re-analysis of data on 650 cases and 1700 controls from nine prospective studies. *J Natl Cancer Inst*, manuscript accepted.

37. Endogenous Hormones and Breast Cancer Collaborative Group. Breast Cancer and Endogenous Sex Hormones in Postmenopausal Women: a collaborative re-analysis of data on 650 cases and 1700 controls from nine prospective studies. *J Natl Cancer Inst*, in press.

38. Helzlsouer KJ, Alberg AJ, Bush TL, Longcope C, Gordon GB, Comstock GW. A prospective study of endogenous hormones and breast cancer. *Cancer Detect Prev* 1994; 18(2):79–85.

39. Wysowski DK, Comstock GW, Helsing KJ, Lau HL. Sex hormone levels in serum in relation to the development of breast cancer. *Am J Epidemiol* 1987; 125(5):791–799.

40. Rosenberg CR, Pasternack BS, Shore RE, Koenig KL, Toniolo PG. Premenopausal estradiol levels and the risk of breast cancer: a new method of controlling for day of the menstrual cycle. *Am J Epidemiol* 1994; 140(6):518–525.

41. Kabuto M, Akiba S, Stevens RG, Neriishi K, Land CE. A prospective study of estradiol and breast cancer in Japanese women. *Cancer Epidemiol Biomarkers Prev* 2000; 9(6):575–579.

42. Key TJ, Wang DY, Brown JB, Hermon C, Allen DS, Moore JW, Bulbrook RD, Fentiman IS, Pike MC. A prospective study of urinary oestrogen excretion and breast cancer risk. *Br J Cancer* 1996; 73(12):1615–1619.

43. Thomas HV, Key TJ, Allen DS, Moore JW, Dowsett M, Fentiman IS, Wang DY. A prospective study of endogenous serum hormone concentrations and breast cancer risk in premenopausal women on the island of Guernsey. *Br J Cancer* 1997; 75(7):1075–1079.

44. Preston-Martin S, Pike MC, Ross RK, Jones PA, Henderson BE. Increased cell division as a cause of human cancer. *Cancer Res* 1990; 50(23):7415–7421.

45. Yue W, Wang JP, Conaway M, Masamura S, Li Y, Santen RJ. Activation of the MAPK pathway enhances sensitivity of MCF-7 breast cancer cells to the mitogenic effect of estradiol. *Endocrinology* 2002; 143(9):3221–3229.

46. Cavalieri E, Frenkel K, Liehr JG, Rogan E, Roy D. Estrogens as endogenous genotoxic agents — DNA adducts and mutations. *J Natl Cancer Inst Monogr* 2000; 27:75–93.

47. Milazzo G, Giorgino F, Damante G, Sung C, Stampfer MR, Vigneri R, Goldfine ID, Belfiore A. Insulin receptor expression and function in human breast cancer cell lines. *Cancer Res* 1992; 52(14):3924–3930.

48. Osborne CK, Clemmons DR, Arteaga CL. Regulation of breast cancer growth by insulin-like growth factors. *J Steroid Biochem Mol Biol* 1990; 37(6):805–809.

49. Jernstrom H, Deal C, Wilkin F, Chu W, Tao Y, Majeed N, Hudson T, Narod SA, Pollak M. Genetic and nongenetic factors associated with variation of plasma levels of insulin-like growth factor-I and insulin-like growth factor-binding protein-3 in healthy premenopausal women. *Cancer Epidemiol Biomarkers Prev* 2001; 10(4):377–384.

50. Muti P, Quattrin T, Grant BJ, Krogh V, Micheli A, Schunemann HJ, Ram M, Freudenheim JL, Sieri S, Trevisan M et al. Fasting glucose is a risk factor for breast cancer: a prospective study. *Cancer Epidemiol Biomarkers Prev* 2002; 11(11):1361–1368.

51. Toniolo P, Bruning PF, Akhmedkhanov A, Bonfrer JM, Koenig KL, Lukanova A, Shore RE, Zeleniuch-Jacquotte A. Serum insulin-like growth factor-I and breast cancer. *Int J Cancer* 2000; 88(5):828–832.

52. Krajcik RA, Borofsky ND, Massardo S, Orentreich N. Insulin-like growth factor I (IGF-I), IGF-binding proteins, and breast cancer. *Cancer Epidemiol Biomarkers Prev* 2002; 11(12):1566–1573.

53. Hankinson SE, Willett WC, Colditz GA, Hunter DJ, Michaud DS, Deroo B, Rosner B, Speizer FE, Pollak M. Circulating concentrations of insulin-like growth factor-I and risk of breast cancer. *Lancet* 1998; 351(9113):1393–1396.

54. Anisimov VN. The role of the pineal gland in breast cancer development. *Crit Rev Oncol Hematol* 2003; 46(3):221–234.

55. Brzezinski A. Mechanisms of disease: melatonin in humans. *N Engl J Med* 1997; 336(3):186–195.

56. Blask D, Hill S. Effects of melatonin on cancer studies; studies of MCF-7 human breast cancer cells in culture. *J Neural Transm Suppl* 1986; 21:433–449.

57. Hill S, Blask D. Effects of the pineal hormone melatonin on the proliferation and morphological characteristics of human breast cancer cells (MCF-7) in culture. *Cancer Res* 1988; 48:6121–6126.

58. Tamarkin L, Danforth D, Lichter A, et al. Decreased nocturnal plasma melatonin peak in patients with estrogen receptor positive breast cancer. *Science* 1982; 216:1003–1005.

59. Reiter RJ, Calvo JR, Karbownik M, Qi W, Tan DX. Melatonin and its relation to the immune system and inflammation. *Ann N Y Acad Sci* 2000; 917:376–386.

60. Hansen J. Increased breast cancer risk among women who work predominantly at night. *Epidemiology* 2001; 12:74–77.

61. Reiter R. Electromagnetic fields and melatonin production. *Biomed Pharmacother* 1993; 47:439–444.

62. Glickman G, Levin R, Brainard G. Ocular input for human melatonin regulation: relevance to breast cancer. *Neuroendocrinol Lett* 2002; 23(Suppl 2):17–22.

63. Erren TC, Piekarski C. Does winter darkness in the Artic protect against cancer? The melatonin hypothesis revisited. *Med Hypotheses* 1999; 53(1):1–5.

64. Feychting M, Osterlund B, Ahlbom A. Reduced cancer incidence among the blind. *Epidemiology* 1998; 9(5):490–494.

65. Verkasalo PK, Pukkala E, Kaprio J, Heikkila KV, Koskenvuo M. Magnetic fields of high voltage power lines and risk of cancer in Finnish adults: nationwide cohort study. *Br Med J* 1996; 313(7064):1047–1051.

66. Travis RC, Allen DS, Fentiman IS, Key TJ. Melatonin and breast cancer: a prospective study. *J Natl Cancer Inst* 2004; 96(6):475–482.

67. Perks CM, Keith AJ, Goodhew KL, Savage PB, Winters ZE, Holly JMP. Prolactin acts as a potent survival factor for human breast cancer cell lines. *Br J Cancer* 2004; 91:305–311.

68. Wennbo H, Tornell J. The role of prolactin and growth hormone in breast cancer. *Oncology* 2000; 19(8):966–967.

69. Hankinson SE, Willett WC, Michaud DS, Manson JE, G.A. C, Longcope C, Rosner B, Speizer FE. Plasma prolactin levels and subsequent risk of breast cancer in postmenopausal women. *J Natl Cancer Inst* 1999; 91:629–634.

70. Maskarinec G, Williams AE, Kaaks R. A cross-sectional investigation of breast density and insulin-like growth factor 1. *Int J Cancer* 2003; 107:991–996.

71. Gutzman JH, Miller KK, Schuler LA. Endogenous human prolactin and not exogenous human prolactin induces estrogen receptor alpha and prolactin receptor expression and increases estrogen responsiveness in breast cancer cells. *J Steroid Biochem Mol Biol* 2004; 88:69–77.

72. Tworoger SS, Eliassen H, Rosner B, Sluss P, Hankinson SE. Plasma prolactin concentrations and risk of postmenopausal breast cancer. *Cancer Res* 2004; 64:6814–6819.

73. Manjer J, Johansson R, Berglund G, Janzon L, Kaaks R, Agren A, Lenner P. Postmenopausal breast cancer risk in relation to sex steroid hormones, prolactin, and SHBG. *Cancer Causes Control* 2003; 14(7):599–607.

74. Bernstein L, Ross RK. Endogenous hormones and breast cancer risk. *Epidemiol Rev* 1993; 15:48–65.

75. Collaborative Group on Hormonal Factors in Breast Cancer. Breast cancer and hormonal contraceptives: collaborative reanalysis of individual data on 53,297 women with breast cancer and 100,239 women without breast cancer from 54 epidemiological studies. *Lancet* 1996; 347:1713–1727.

76. Collaborative Group on Hormonal Factors in Breast Cancer. Breast cancer and hormonal contraceptives: further results [Review]. *Contraception* 1996; 54(3 Suppl):1S–106S.

77. Hankinson SE, Hunter D. Breast Cancer. In: Adami HO, Hunter D, Trichopoulos D, eds. *Textbook of Cancer Epidemiology.* New York: Oxford University Press; 2002.

78. Marchbanks PA, McDonald JA, Wilson JG, Folger SG, Mandel MC, Daling JR et al. Oral contraceptives and the risk of breast cancer. *N Engl J Med* 2002; 346(26):2052–2032.

78a. Victory R, D'Souza C, Diamond MP, McNeely SG, Vista-Deck D, Hendrix S. Reduced cancer risks in oral contraceptive users: results from the Women's Health Initiative. *Fertil Steril* 2004; 82(2 Suppl): S104–105.

79. Norman SA, Berlin JA, Weber AL, Strom BL, Daling JR, Weiss LK, Marchbanks PA, Bernstein L, Voight LF, McDonald JA et al. Combined effect of oral contraceptive use and hormone replacement therapy on breast cancer risk in postmenopausal women. *Cancer Causes Control* 2003; 14:933–943.

80. Schairer C, Lubin J, Troisi R, Sturgeon S, Brinton L, Hoover R. Menopausal estrogen and estrogen-progestin replacement therapy and breast cancer risk. *J Am Med Assoc* 2000; 283:485–491.

81. Colditz GA, Rosner B. Cumulative risk of breast cancer to age 70 years according to risk factor status: data from Nurses Health Study. *Am J Epidemiol* 2000; 152:950–964.

82. Nelson HD, Humphrey LL, Nygren P, Teutsch SM, Allan JD. Postmenopausal hormone replacement therapy. Scientific Review. *J Am Med Assoc* 2002; 288(7):872–881.

83. Chlebowski RT, Hendrix SL, Langer RD, Stefanick ML, Gass M, Lane D, Rodabough RJ, Gilligan MA, Cyr MG, Thomson CA et al. Influence of estrogen plus progestin on breast cancer and mammography in healthy postmenopausal women. The Women's Health Initiative Randomized Trial. *J Am Med Assoc* 2003; 289(24):3243–3253.

84. Sendag F, Terek MC, Ozsener S, Oztekin K, Bilgin O, Bilgen I, Memis A. Mammographic density changes during different postmenopausal hormone replacement therapies. *Fertil Steril* 2001; 76(3):445–450.

85. Greendale GA, Reboussin BA, Slone S, Wasilauskas C, Pike MC, Ursin G. Postmenopausal hormone therapy and change in mammographic density. *J Natl Cancer Inst* 2003; 95(1):30–37.

86. Madigan MP, Ziegler RG, Benichou J, Byrne C, Hoover RN. Proportion of breast cancer cases in the United States explained by well-established risk factors. *J Natl Cancer Inst* 1995; 87(22):1681–1685.

87. Miki Y, Swensen J, Shattuck-Eidens D, Futreal PA, Harshman K, Tavtigian S, Liu Q, Cochran C, Bennett LM, Ding W. A strong candidate for the breast and ovarian cancer susceptibility gene BRCA1. *Science* 1994; 266(5182):66–71.

88. Wooster R, Bignell G, Lancaster J, Swift S, Seal S, Mangion J, Collins N, Gregory S, Gumbs C, Micklem G. Identification of the breast cancer susceptibility gene BRCA2. *Nature* 1995; 378(6559):789–792.

89. Thompson D, Easton DF. Cancer Incidence in BRCA1 mutation carriers. *J Natl Cancer Inst* 2002; 94(18):1358–1365.

90. Ford D, Easton DF, Peto J. Estimates of the gene frequency of BRCA1 and its contribution to breast and ovarian cancer incidence. *Am J Hum Genet* 1995; 57(6):1457–1462.

91. Schnitt SJ. Benign breast disease and breast cancer risk: morphology and beyond. *Am J Surg Pathol* 2003; 27(6):836–841.

92. Wang J, Costantino JP, Tan-Chiu E, Wickerham DL, Paik S, Wolmark N. Lower-category benign breast disease and the risk of invasive breast cancer. *J Natl Cancer Inst* 2004; 96(8):616–620.

93. Boyd N, Lockwood G, Byng J, Tritchler D, Yaffe M. Mammographic densities and breast cancer risk. *Cancer Epidemiol Biomarkers Prev* 1998; 7:1133–1144.

94. Thurfjell E. Breast density and the risk of breast cancer. *N Engl J Med* 2002; 347(12):866.

95. Harvey JA, Bovbjerg VE. Quantitative assessment of mammographic breast density: relationship with breast cancer risk. *Radiology* 2004; 230(1):29–41.

96. Weir HK, Thun MJ, Hankey BF, Ries LA, Howe HL, Wingo PA, Jemal A, Ward E, Anderson RN, Edwards BK. Annual report to the nation on the status of cancer, 1975–2000, featuring the uses of surveillance data for cancer prevention and control. *J Natl Cancer Inst* 2003; 95(17):1276–1299.

97. Ries LA, Wingo PA, Miller DS, Howe HL, Weir HK, Rosenberg HM, Vernon SW, Cronin K, Edwards BK. The annual report to the nation on the status of cancer, 1973–1997, with a special section on colorectal cancer. *Cancer* 2000; 88(10):2398–2424.

98. Hsing AW, Devesa SS. Trends and patterns of prostate cancer: what do they suggest? *Epidemiol Rev* 2001; 23(1):3–13.

99. Gronberg H. Prostate cancer epidemiology. *Lancet* 2003; 361(9360):859–864.

100. *Cancer Incidence in Five Continents*, vol. VII. Lyon, France: IARC Scientific Publications; 1997.

101. Ries LAG, Eisner M, Kosary CL et al. *SEER Cancer Statistics Review*. Bethesda, MD: National Cancer Institute; 2002:973–999.

102. *SEER Cancer Statistics Review*, 1973–1998. Bethesda, MD: National Cancer Institute; 2001.

103. Chu KC, Tarone RE, Freeman HP. Trends in prostate cancer mortality among black men and white men in the United States. *Cancer* 2003; 97(6):1507–1516.

104. Gilligan T, Wang PS, Levin R, Kantoff PW, Avorn J. Racial differences in screening for prostate cancer in the elderly. *Arch Intern Med* 2004; 164(17):1858–1864.

105. Shavers VL, Brown ML. Racial and ethnic disparities in the receipt of cancer treatment. *J Natl Cancer Inst* 2002; 94(5):334–357.

106. Stat bite. Distant-stage prostate cancer diagnoses by ethnicity and socioeconomic status. *J Natl Cancer Inst* 2003; 95(19):1432.

107. Bosland MC. The role of steroid hormones in prostate carcinogenesis. *J Natl Cancer Inst Monogr* 2000; (27):39–66.

108. Castagnetta LA, Miceli MD, Sorci CM, Pfeffer U, Farruggio R, Oliveri G, Calabro M, Carruba G. Growth of LNCaP human prostate cancer cells is stimulated by estradiol via its own receptor. *Endocrinology* 1995; 136(5):2309–2319.

109. Carruba G, Miceli MD, Comito L, Farruggio R, Sorci CM, Oliveri G, Amodio R, di Falco M, d'Amico D, Castagnetta LA. Multiple estrogen function in human prostate cancer cells. *Ann NY Acad Sci* 1996; 784:70–84.

110. Muti P, Westerlind K, Wu T, Grimaldi T, De Berry J 3rd, Schunemann H, Freudenheim JL, Hill H, Carruba G, Bradlow L. Urinary estrogen metabolites and prostate cancer: a case-control study in the United States. *Cancer Causes Control* 2002; 13(10):947–955.

111. Stattin P, Rinaldi S, Biessy C, Stenman UH, Hallmans G, Kaaks R. High levels of circulating insulin-like growth factor-I increase prostate cancer risk: a prospective study in a population-based nonscreened cohort. *J Clin Oncol* 2004; 22(15):3104–3112.

112. Lacey JV Jr, Hsing AW, Fillmore CM, Hoffman S, Helzlsouer KJ, Comstock GW. Null association between insulin-like growth factors, insulin-like growth factor-binding proteins, and prostate cancer in a prospective study. *Cancer Epidemiol Biomarkers Prev* 2001; 10(10):1101–1102.

113. Chopin LK, Veveris-Lowe TL, Philipps AF, Herington AC. Co-expression of GH and GHR isoforms in prostate cancer cell lines. *Growth Horm IGF Res* 2002; 12(2):126–136.

114. Carter BS, Bova GS, Beaty TH, Steinberg GD, Childs B, Isaacs WB, Walsh PC. Hereditary prostate cancer: epidemiologic and clinical features. *J Urol* 1993; 150(3):797–802.

115. Smith RA, Cokkinides V, Eyre HJ. American Cancer Society guidelines for the early detection of cancer, 2004. *CA Cancer J Clin* 2004; 54(1):41–52.

116. Parkin DM. Cancer incidence in five continents. In: Whelan SL, Parkin DM, Masuyer E, Smans M, eds. IARC Scientific Publications, No. 120. New York: Oxford University Press; 1992:xviii.

117. Schottenfeld D, Winawer SJ. Cancers of the large intestine. In: Schottenfeld D, Joseph F. Fraumeni J, eds. *Cancer Epidemiology and Prevention*. 2nd ed. New York: Oxford University Press; 1996:813–840.

118. *Cancer Facts and Figures*, 2004. Atlanta, GA: American Cancer Society; 2004:1–56.

119. Kune S, Kune GA, Watson L. The Melbourne colorectal cancer study: incidence findings by age, sex, site, migrants and religion. *Int J Epidemiol* 1986; 15(4):483–493.

120. Whittemore AS, Zheng S, Wu A, Wu ML, Fingar T, Jiao DA, Ling CD, Bao JL, Henderson BE, Paffenbarger RS Jr. Colorectal cancer in Chinese and Chinese-Americans. *Natl Cancer Inst Monogr* 1985; 69:43–46.

121. Warshauer ME, Silverman DT, Schottenfeld D, Pollack ES. Stomach and colorectal cancers in Puerto Rican-born residents of New York City. *J Natl Cancer Inst* 1986; 76(4):591–595.

122. Moradi T, Delfino RJ, Bergstrom SR, Yu ES, Adami HO, Yuen J. Cancer risk among Scandinavian immigrants in the US and Scandinavian residents compared with US whites, 1973–89. *Eur J Cancer Prev* 1998; 7(2):117–125.

123. Gornick ME, Eggers PW, Riley GF. Associations of race, education, and patterns of preventive service use with stage of cancer at time of diagnosis. *Health Serv Res* 2004; 39(5):1403–1427.

124. Simons BD, Morrison AS, Lev R, Verhoek-Oftedahl W. Relationship of polyps to cancer of the large intestine. *J Natl Cancer Inst* 1992; 84(12):962–966.

125. Lynch HT, Schuelke GS, Kimberling WJ, Albano WA, Lynch JF, Biscone KA, Lipkin ML, Deschner EE, Mikol YB, Sandberg AA et al. Hereditary nonpolyposis colorectal cancer (Lynch syndromes I and II). II. Biomarker studies. *Cancer* 1985; 56(4):939–951.

126. Peltomaki P, Aaltonen LA, Sistonen P, Pylkkanen L, Mecklin JP, Jarvinen H, Green JS, Jass JR, Weber JL, Leach FS et al. Genetic mapping of a locus predisposing to human colorectal cancer. *Science* 1993; 260(5109):810–812.

127. Rosenberg L, Louik C, Shapiro S. Nonsteroidal antiinflammatory drug use and reduced risk of large bowel carcinoma. *Cancer* 1998; 82(12):2326–2333.

128. Garcia Rodriguez LA, Huerta-Alvarez C. Reduced incidence of colorectal adenoma among long-term users of nonsteroidal antiinflammatory drugs: a pooled analysis of published studies and a new population-based study. *Epidemiology* 2000; 11(4):376–381.

129. Tangrea JA, Albert PS, Lanza E, Woodson K, Corle D, Hasson M, Burt R, Caan B, Paskett E, Iber F et al. Non-steroidal anti-inflammatory drug use is associated with reduction in recurrence of advanced and non-advanced colorectal adenomas (United States). *Cancer Causes Control* 2003; 14(5):403–411.

130. Asano TK, McLeod RS. Non steroidal anti-inflammatory drugs (NSAID) and aspirin for preventing colorectal adenomas and carcinomas. *Cochrane Database Syst Rev* 2004; 2:CD004079.
131. Singh D. Merck withdraws arthritis drug worldwide. *Br Med J* 2004; 329(7470):816.
132. McKeown-Eyssen G. Epidemiology of colorectal cancer revisited: are serum triglycerides and/or plasma glucose associated with risk? *Cancer Epidemiol Biomarkers Prev* 1994; 3(8):687–695.
133. Giovannucci E. Insulin and colon cancer. *Cancer Causes Control* 1995; 6(2):164–179.
134. MacDonald RS, Thornton WH Jr., Bean TL. Insulin and IGE-1 receptors in a human intestinal adenocarcinoma cell line (CACO-2): regulation of $Na^+$ glucose transport across the brush border. *J Recept Res* 1993; 13(7):1093–1113.
135. Guo YS, Narayan S, Yallampalli C, Singh P. Characterization of insulinlike growth factor I receptors in human colon cancer. *Gastroenterology* 1992; 102(4 Pt 1):1101–1108.
136. Chang CK, Ulrich CM. Hyperinsulinaemia and hyperglycaemia: possible risk factors of colorectal cancer among diabetic patients. *Diabetologia* 2003; 46(5):595–607.

# 2 How Dietary Components Protect from Cancer

*Diane M. Harris and Vay Liang W. Go*

## CONTENTS

2.1 Introduction..................................................................................................28
2.2 Evidence Linking Diet to Cancer .............................................................28
2.3 Bioactive Dietary Components ..................................................................29
2.4 Pathogenesis of Cancer — Acquired Capabilities....................................32
2.5 Molecular Targets for Chemopreventive Action of Dietary
Components ..................................................................................................35
    2.5.1 Inhibition of Cellular Replication .................................................35
    2.5.2 Increased Response to Antigrowth Signals and Induction of
Differentiation................................................................................40
    2.5.3 Enhancement of Apoptosis.............................................................41
    2.5.4 Induction of Senescence.................................................................42
    2.5.5 Inhibition of Angiogenesis ............................................................43
    2.5.6 Inhibition of Tissue Invasion and Metastasis................................43
    2.5.7 Increased Antioxidant Capacity and Genomic Stability..............44
    2.5.8 Other Mechanisms..........................................................................45
        2.5.8.1 Inflammation .................................................................45
        2.5.8.2 Carcinogen Activation/Detoxification by Xenobiotic
Metabolizing Enzymes...................................................46
        2.5.8.3 Epigenetic Events..........................................................47
2.6 Example of Pleiotropic Actions of Nutrients — Vitamin D in Colon
Cancer..........................................................................................................48
2.7 Implications ................................................................................................50
Acknowledgments................................................................................................52
References ............................................................................................................52

## 2.1 INTRODUCTION

Cancer is a chronic disease of the genome that may be influenced at many stages in its natural history by nutritional factors that affect not only the prevention but also the progression and treatment of this devastating disease. The cancer phenotype is the result of the interaction of both genetic and environmental influences; the evidence for this is drawn on studies of human populations as well as from animal experiments that model the process of carcinogenesis.[1] Perhaps the strongest environmental influence is that of diet. It is estimated that up to 80% of colon, breast, and prostate cancer cases and one third of all cancer cases may be influenced by diet and associated lifestyle factors.[2] As our understanding of the pathogenesis of cancer progresses, we can better define the specific sites at which individual nutrients may influence the development of cancer.

## 2.2 EVIDENCE LINKING DIET TO CANCER

Chapter 1 describes the worldwide epidemiology of cancer. The estimated incidence rates for various cancers worldwide in 2002 found lung, colon/rectum, and stomach to be the most common cancers in both men and women, as well as prostate and liver cancer in men, and breast and cervical cancer in women.[3] The pattern of cancer distribution based on incidence and mortality rates varies geographically. In general, the predominant cancers in economically developing countries contrast to those in the industrially developed world. For Asia, Africa, and Latin America, there is a relatively high rate of cancer of the upper aerodigestive tract, stomach, liver, and cervix, whereas in Europe and North America there is a relatively high rate of cancer of the colon/rectum, breast, and prostate. These "Western" cancers have a strong environmental component, with diet and lifestyle factors particularly important, while in developing countries, infections with such agents as viral hepatitis and *Helicobacter pylori* play a key role. The geographic pattern differences in tumor incidence, prevalence, and natural history as related to food, diet, nutrition, and related lifestyle factors have been extensively reviewed by the World Cancer Research Fund and the American Institute for Cancer Research (AICR) and published in an expert report in 1997.[2] An updated second report is due in 2007.

Epidemiological studies in the U.S. have defined certain specific dietary factors as having highest impact on reduction of cancer risk. The most consistent relationship is an inverse relationship between cancer risk and intake of vegetables and fruits. Additional dietary factors with evidence for decreased cancer risk include whole grains, dietary fiber, certain micronutrients (e.g., selenium, vitamin E, vitamin D, and calcium), and certain types of fat (e.g., $n$-3 fatty acids, particularly $n$-3/$n$-6 ratios), as well as physical activity. Other diet-related factors that increase risk include high intakes of total fat and other types of fat (e.g., saturated fat), alcohol, certain food preparation methods such as smoking, salting, and pickling foods, and high-temperature cooking of meats, as well as obesity (high body mass index).[4] Results from these studies have led to organizations such as the AICR to compile specific dietary recommendations for individuals to reduce cancer risk. These general guidelines advise a reduction in fat intake (especially from animal sources), an increase in fiber intake and inclusion of a variety of vegetables and fruits in the daily diet, increased physical activity and maintenance of healthy body weight, moderation in alcoholic beverage intake, and minimization of salt-cured, salt-pickled, or smoked food.[2,4] Indeed, recent data from the Iowa Women's Health Study Cohort of 29,564 women studied for 13 years suggest that adherence to at least a subset (6 to 9) of cancer prevention recommendations as outlined by the AICR results in a reduction in cancer incidence, and, to a lesser extent, cancer mortality.[5] Based on the wealth of epidemiological and experimental data supporting a role of diet in cancer prevention, the 2005 USDA Dietary Guidelines for Americans are the first to include cancer prevention as an outcome in evaluating the evidence base for setting dietary guidelines.[6]

## 2.3  BIOACTIVE DIETARY COMPONENTS

All classical nutrient categories consist of bioactive dietary components, including carbohydrates, amino acids, fatty acids and structural lipids, minerals, and vitamins. In addition is an extensive list of non-nutrient components, particularly phytochemicals, which can have anticancer activity. Phytochemicals are components of a plant-based diet that possess substantial anticarcinogenic and antimutagenic properties.[7] An estimated 25,000 different chemical compounds occur in fruits, vegetables, and other plants eaten by humans.[8] They can encompass such diverse chemical classes as carotenoids, flavonoids, organosulfur compounds, isothiocyanates, indoles, monoterpenes, phenolic acids, and chlorophyll.[9] Table 2.1 lists a sampling of bioactive compounds, most of which are discussed more comprehensively in subsequent chapters of this book.

Cancer-preventive properties of the macronutrient (carbohydrate, protein, fat, and fiber) and micronutrient (vitamin and mineral) components of diets have been the object of study for a number of years, and the National Cancer Institute (NCI) has sponsored a number of human intervention trials with individual vitamins and minerals.[10] More recently, however, research efforts have extended to the non-nutritive phytochemicals. The NCI has determined that more than 35 plant-based foods and 1000 individual phytochemicals possess cancer-preventive activity in cell culture and animal models.[7] Well-studied food sources and representative phytochemicals include garlic (diallyl sulfide), soybeans (genistein), turmeric (curcumin), tomatoes (lycopene), grapes (resveratrol), green tea (epigallocatechin-3-gallate [EGCG]), and cruciferous vegetables (such as broccoli, cabbage, and Brussels sprouts; indole-3-carbinol, sulforaphane).[7] However, the repertoire of chemopreventive phytochemicals is vast, and foods, dietary supplements, and traditional herbal medicines with previously undocumented anticancer activities are continually being identified.

When discussing the activity of chemopreventive compounds derived from whole foods and dietary supplements, a couple of important principles should be recognized. First, whole foods contain a plethora of different constituents, each

**TABLE 2.1**
**Partial List of Bioactive Food Components with Cancer-Preventive Properties That Are Detailed in This Volume and Their Primary Food Sources**

| Class | Example Bioactive Compounds | Dietary Source |
|---|---|---|
| Vitamins | Vitamin A | Eggs, meat, dairy products, organ meats, fish oil |
| | Vitamin D | Dairy products, fish |
| | Vitamin E ($\alpha$- and $\gamma$-tocopherol) | Wheat germ, corn, nuts and seeds, olives, vegetable oils, leafy greens |
| | Vitamin C | Green peppers, citrus fruits and juices, strawberries, tomatoes, broccoli, turnip greens and other greens, sweet and white potatoes, and cantaloupe |
| | Folic acid | Beans and legumes, citrus fruits and juices, wheat bran and other whole grains, dark green leafy vegetables, poultry, pork, shellfish, liver |
| Minerals | Calcium | Dairy products, soybeans, spinach, kale |
| | Selenium | Fish, shellfish, red meat, grains, eggs, chicken, liver, garlic |
| Carotenoids | Lycopene | Tomatoes, guava, watermelon, pink grapefruit |
| | Lutein | Corn, egg yolks, green vegetables and fruits, such as broccoli, green beans, green peas, Brussels sprouts, cabbage, kale, collard greens, spinach, lettuce, kiwi and honeydew |
| | $\beta$-Carotene | Sweet potatoes, carrots, kale, spinach, collard greens |
| Phytosterols | $\beta$-Sitosterol | Rice bran, wheat germ, corn oils, soybeans |
| Polyphenols: | | |
| Isoflavones | Genistein, daidzein | Soybeans, legumes |
| Flavonones | Naringenin, hesperedin | Citrus fruits, prunes |
| Flavonols | Quercetin, kaempferol | Onions, kale, broccoli, apples, cherries, fennel, sorrel, berries, tea |
| Flavanols | Catechin, epicatechin, gallocatechin | Cocoa, chocolate, green tea, grapes, wine |
| Flavones | Luteolin, apigenin | Parsley, thyme, celery, sweet red pepper |
| Stilbenes | Resveratrol | Grapes, red wine |
| Lignans | Enterodiol, enterolactone | Flaxseeds, legumes, whole grains, fruits, and vegetables |
| Anthocyanidins | Pelargonidin, malvidin, cyanidin | Cherries, grapes |

*(continued)*

**TABLE 2.1 (CONTINUED)**
**Partial List of Bioactive Food Components with Cancer-Preventive Properties That Are Detailed in This Volume and Their Primary Food Sources**

| Class | Example Bioactive Compounds | Dietary Source |
|---|---|---|
| Isothiocyanates | Phenethyl isothiocyanate | Watercress |
| | Sulforaphane | Broccoli and other cruciferous vegetables |
| Saponins | Sapogenin, ginsenoside | Legumes, soybean, ginseng |
| Curcuminoids | Curcumin | Turmeric |
| Fatty Acids | | |
| Omega-3 fatty acids | Eicosapentaenoic acid, docosahexaenoic acid | Fish oils |
| Conjugated linoleic acids | *cis*-9, *trans*-11 and *trans*-10, *cis*-12 conjugated linoleic acid | Grass-fed beef, dairy products, eggs |
| Sphingolipids | Ceramide, sphingomyelin | Dairy foods, eggs, soybeans |

having one or several effects on the cellular mechanisms outlined below. For example, it has been estimated that more than 100 different phytochemicals can be provided in a single serving of vegetables.[7] These phytochemicals tend to run in families, so that a single serving of a fruit and vegetable provides not only the major bioactive component, but also a group of chemically related molecules plus other unrelated active compounds. For example, tomato paste provides not only lycopene and its isomers, but other carotenoids as well, including $\gamma$-, $\zeta$-, $\alpha$-, and $\beta$-carotene, neurosporine, lutein, phytofluene, and phytoene, as well as other vital nutrients including folate, vitamin C, and potassium.[11] Increasingly, experimental data indicate that increased intake of the whole food may be more efficacious and certainly exhibit less toxicity than the single compound administered in supraphysiological doses. A recently published study showed that when rats treated with *N*-methyl-*N*-nitrosourea and testosterone to induce prostate cancer were fed diets containing whole tomato powder or lycopene beadlets, the animals that were fed whole tomato powder had increased prostate cancer-free survival, while the lycopene-fed rats survived no longer than controls.[12] Furthermore, Liu[13] showed synergy among whole fruits and vegetables with different phytochemical profiles. In an *in vitro* assay of antioxidant capacity of fruit extracts, the combination of orange, apple, grape, and blueberry extracts showed a synergistic effect relative to the action of each alone. It should be noted that the interaction between individual nutrients might not necessarily be positive. For example, vitamin C has been reported to reduce selenium's effectiveness against carcinogen-induced mammary cancer in animals.[14] Dietary components differ in molecular size, polarity, and solubility, and these differences can affect the bioavailability and distribution of each constituent in the various cellular and tissue compartments.[15] Thus, bioactive dietary components work in a dynamic, constantly changing milieu *in vivo,* and defining the interactions between these factors over time is a challenge.[9]

Thus, because of the difficulty of studying the effects of groups of compounds, researchers tend to take a reductionist approach using one phytochemical to test in an assay system against one biological outcome. Those who advocate dietary supplements often extrapolate these results to produce products that provide high levels of a single compound in concentrated form. However, in reviewing the *in vitro* data on a given constituent, caution must be used when applying results to the *in vivo* condition. One consideration is that doses of compounds can be applied to cells in culture that are not physiologically achievable through use of whole foods or even concentrated dietary supplements, given issues of intake, bioavailability, and toxicity. Further testing in animal models is required to provide information on safety, efficacy, absorption, and metabolism of given compounds before moving to clinical trials. With the current increase in interest in dietary supplement use, information from animal and human trials is necessary to prevent long-term unanticipated adverse effects of high-dose dietary supplement use. An alternative is to provide the bioactive compounds in a whole food approach, which has a greater margin of safety, as there is little possibility of toxicity when a given nutrient is supplied as part of a food providing the full complement of beneficial nutrients rather than a supplement.[15,16] Therefore, a number of U.S. organizations involved with nutrition, health, and cancer prevention, including the National Cancer Institute and the 5-a-Day Program,[17] the AICR,[18] and the American Cancer Society[19] advocate daily consumption of a variety of whole vegetables and fruits to reduce cancer risk.

## 2.4  PATHOGENESIS OF CANCER — ACQUIRED CAPABILITIES

Research over the past 25 years has produced a deeper understanding of the molecular, biochemical, and cellular changes that occur as cells are transformed from normal cells to malignant cancers. The multiple genetic defects leading to cancer cell production can result from exposure to environmental, dietary, and lifestyle factors, as well as infectious agents. The multistep, multistage process of gradual carcinogenetic changes in the biological behavior of a clonogenic population of cells is illustrated schematically in Figure 2.1.[20] As indicated, this progression of cellular changes may span years or decades.[21] Among the epithelial cancers, such as colorectal, breast, prostate, lung, pancreas, and others, a diffuse genomic instability after exposure to damaging agents (inflammation, toxins, etc.), and increased epithelial hyperplasia is the initiating act. A single basal cell may develop one or more mutations of a number of critical oncogenic or tumor suppressor genes, allowing escape from regulatory controls on position, differentiation, and growth.[22] Oncogenes are genes that as proto-oncogenes are involved in signal transduction and execution of mitogenic signals. However, when their expression or protein function is altered, they demonstrate uncontrolled activity leading to unrestrained cellular growth. The normal function of tumor suppressor genes is in negative control of cell cycling; however, this control is released when the genes are mutated.[23] Specific genetic alterations involved with the transformation process have been defined for many cell types. For example, in colorectal cancer, particular events that are associated with initiation and progression include mutation or loss of the *Apc* gene (adenomatous polyposis coli, a tumor suppressor gene), mutation of K-*ras* (a proto-oncogene), and generalized disorganization of DNA methylation. Later events associated with malignant transformation include loss of tumor suppressor genes p53, SMAD4, and SMAD2 functions.[24] These four sequential genetic changes are necessary to ensure colorectal cancer evolution, and it appears that the temporal sequence, rather than accumulation of alterations, is most important in determining the neoplastic phenotype. However, the fact that K-*ras* mutations are found in only about 50% of colorectal cancers indicates that other unknown oncogenes, as well as epigenetic events such as alteration in DNA methylation patterns, may be involved (described further below).[24] Overall, loss-of-function mutations in tumor suppressor and DNA repair genes, as well as gain-of-function mutations in proto-oncogenes, result in transformed cells, which acquire selective advantage over normal cells.[25]

Neoplastic clonal expansion of transformed cells starts at one or more sites in an epithelium and progresses independently at different sites. This leads to the development of preinvasive intraepithelial neoplasia, or a multicellular mass that tends to distort surrounding normal cells. The onset of intraepithelial neoplasia is initiated by a monoclonal expansion, which progresses via clonal evolution; that is, the different mutated cell types with the fastest growth rate will overtake all others as they expand. This neoplastic promotion leads to increases in both total mass and extent of dissemination (known clinically as increase in stage and grade of the neoplasm with time).[22] The host tissue environment, particularly through the action of hormones and cytokines emanating from the stroma around the developing epithelial tumor, influences the tumor's development. Eventually the mass progresses to an invasive neoplasia defined by the presence of stromal invasion, and subsequent metastasis to distant sites is possible.[20] Again using colorectal cancer as an example, the histopathology of this process is seen as a progression from normal intestinal epithelial crypts to aberrant crypt foci, to adenomas or polyps (hyperplastic [nondysplastic] or adenomatous [dysplastic]), and to carcinoma.[24] Prevention models target the development of intraepithelial neoplasia due to the high likelihood of progression from dysplasia to invasive cancer, and because evidence indicates that reduction in the precancerous burden reduces cancer risk and/or the need for invasive interventions.[21]

Thus, tumorigenesis is a multistep process, and these steps reflect a succession of genetic changes, each of which confer a growth advantage that drives the progressive transformation of normal human cells into highly malignant cells. Hanahan and Weinberg[26] have postulated that the vast array of cancer cell genotypes can be defined as a manifestation of six essential alterations in cell physiology that cumulatively lead to malignant growth. These six changes are (1) self-sufficiency in growth signals; (2) insensitivity to growth-inhibitory

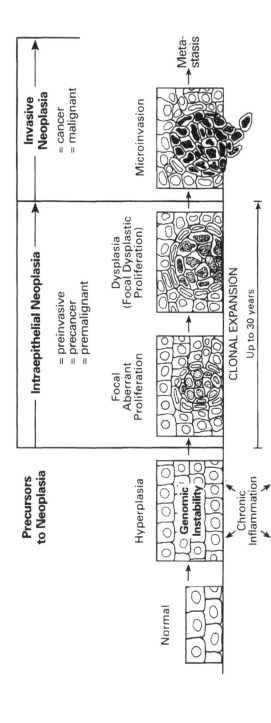

**FIGURE 2.1** Diagram illustrating the onset and progression of neoplasia through an intraepithelial phase to an invasive phase. The onset of intraepithelial neoplasia is heralded by a monoclonal expansion, which progresses via clonal evolution to the invasive phase. (From Go VL, Wong DA, Butrum R. Diet, nutrition and cancer prevention: where are we going from here? *J Nutr* 2001; 131:3123S. With permission).

signals; (3) evasion of programmed cell death (apoptosis); (4) limitless replicative potential; (5) sustained angiogenesis; and (6) tissue invasion and metastasis. The authors propose that these six capabilities are shared in common by most and perhaps all types of human tumors, and represent successful breaching of protective mechanisms normally in place to prevent uncontrolled growth.

## 2.5 MOLECULAR TARGETS FOR CHEMOPREVENTIVE ACTION OF DIETARY COMPONENTS

This outline of genetic changes can be used as a structure for illustrating the chemopreventive actions of dietary components in cancer prevention. Ample evidence exists to demonstrate that bioactive compounds can act in each of these areas. Table 2.2 cites several examples of molecular targets and representative nutritional factors that can act at these sites.[27,28] The overview presented in this chapter is by no means a comprehensive catalog of all bioactive compounds, nor of all of their defined mechanisms of actions. Note that most compounds have a pleiotropic action; that is, they can act at a number of sites in the carcinogenesis pathway. In addition, many different compounds can act on a single molecular target. We outline one example of a nutrient, the active form of vitamin D, $1\alpha,25$-dihydroxyvitamin $D_3$, with many different mechanisms of cancer preventive action. The activities of many other compounds are further detailed in later chapters. Note that all of the biochemical and genetic pathways described here do not operate in a linear fashion within a cell, but are intimately interwoven and represent a balance of opposing forces. An illustration of this integrated circuit of signaling pathways within the cell can be seen in the review by Hanahan and Weinberg.[26] In addition, this framework does not include some of the other important ways that nutrients and other compounds can be chemopreventive in a context broader than the individual cell. Figure 2.2 shows not only the cellular changes in the multistep carcinogenesis pathway during promotion and progression, but also the formation of carcinogens that can lead to DNA damage during the initiation phase.[20] Some additional factors to consider include effects on inflammation, carcinogen detoxification by xenobiotic metabolizing enzymes, and epigenetic events. These are reviewed briefly as well, and we recognize that other potential mechanisms exist, such as antibacterial and antiviral effects (e.g., suppression of *H. pylori* by various phytochemicals).

### 2.5.1 INHIBITION OF CELLULAR REPLICATION

Dividing cells undergo a series of steps of well-defined cellular changes referred to as the cell cycle. Mitogenic growth signals are required for cells to move from the resting or quiescent state ($G_0$) to the proliferative state, defined by a successive series of phases: initial gap ($G_1$), DNA synthesis (S), second gap ($G_2$), and mitosis (M). Each step is characterized by distinct cellular processes that are required for proper cell division. The formation of cyclin (a structural protein) with a cyclin-dependent kinase (CDK) into a complex regulates phase

**TABLE 2.2**
**Mechanisms for Chemoprevention by Diet-Derived Agents with Possible Molecular Targets**

| Mechanism | Possible Molecular Targets | Representative Agents |
|---|---|---|
| **Antimutagenesis** | | |
| Inhibit carcinogen uptake | Bile acids | Calcium |
| Inhibit formation/activation of carcinogen | Cytochrome P450s | PEITC, tea, indole-3-carbinol, soy isoflavones |
| | PG synthase hydroperoxidase, 5-lipoxygenase | Curcumin |
| | Bile acids | Urosdiol |
| Deactivate/detoxify carcinogen | GSH/GST | NAC, garlic/onion disulfides |
| Prevent carcinogen-DNA binding | Cytochrome P450s | Tea |
| Increase level or fidelity of DNA repair | Poly(ADP-ribosyl)transferase | NAC, protease inhibitors (Bowman–Birk) |
| **Antiproliferation/Antiprogression** | | |
| Modulate hormone/growth factor activity | Estrogen receptor | Soy isoflavones |
| | Steroid 5α-reductase | Tea |
| | IGF-1 | Soy isoflavones, retinoids, lycopene |
| | AP-1 | Retinoids |
| | PPARs | Retinoids |
| Inhibit oncogene activity | Farnesyl protein transferase | Perillyl alcohol, limonene, DHEA |
| Inhibit polyamine metabolism | ODC induction | Retinoids, curcumin, tea |
| Induce terminal differentiation | TGF-β | Retinoids, vitamin D, soy isoflavones |
| Restore immune response | T, NK lymphocytes | Selenium, tea |
| | Langerhans cells | Vitamin E |
| Reduce inflammation | NF-κB | Wogonin, EGCG, resveratrol, curcumin |
| Inhibit eicosanoid production | Cyclooxygenases and lipoxygenases | Tea, curcumin, resveratrol, EPA/DHA |
| Increase intercellular communication | Connexin 43 | Carotenoids (lycopene), retinoids |
| Induce apoptosis | TGF-β | Retinoids, soy isoflavones, vitamin D |
| | Ras farnesylation | Perillyl alcohol, limonene, DHEA |
| | Arachidonic acid | Retinoic acid |
| | Caspase | Retinoids |

*(continued)*

## TABLE 2.2 (CONTINUED)
## Mechanisms for Chemoprevention by Diet-Derived Agents with Possible Molecular Targets

| Mechanism | Possible Molecular Targets | Representative Agents |
|---|---|---|
| Induce senescence | Telomerase | Vitamin D, retinoids, EGCG, curcumin |
| Inhibit angiogenesis | FGF receptor tyrosine kinase | Soy isoflavones |
| | Thrombomodulin | Retinoids |
| Correct DNA methylation imbalances | CpG island methylation | Folic acid |
| Inhibit basement membrane degradation | Type IV collagenase | Protease inhibitors (Bowman–Birk), vitamin D |
| Inhibit DNA synthesis | Glucose 6-phosphate dehydrogenase | DHEA |

*Abbreviations:* PEITC, phenethyl isothiocyanage; PG, prostaglandin; GSH, glutathione; GST, glutathione-*S*-transferase; NAC, *N*-acetyl-L-cystein; IGF-1, insulin-like growth factor-1; AP-1, (transcription) activator protein-1; PPAR, peroxisome proliferator activated receptor; DHEA, dehydroepiandrosterone; EPA/DHA, eicosapentaenoic acid/ docosahexaenoic acid; ODC, ornithine decarboxylase; TGF-β, transforming growth factor-β; NK, natural killer; NF-κB, nuclear factor kappa B; RAS, *ras* oncogene product; FGF, fibroblast growth factor; CpG, cytosine-guanosine.

*Source:* Adapted from Kelloff GJ, Crowell JA, Steele VE et al. Progress in cancer chemoprevention: development of diet-derived chemopreventive agents. *J Nutr* 2000; 130:468S. With permission.

transitions. External stimuli (e.g., nutrients) and internal signals (e.g., DNA damage) regulate the formation of cyclin–CDK complexes via cyclin-dependent kinase inhibitors, which include the *cip/waf* family (p21, p27, p58). These regulated transitions are referred to as "checkpoints" and represent important targets for control.[29]

The most significant checkpoint occurs in late $G_1$, and when activated in response to DNA damage, entry into S-phase is delayed to allow time for DNA repair.[23] If irreparable DNA damage is present, the pathway for programmed cell death, or apoptosis, is activated. Critical to the function of this restriction point is the interaction between the retinoblastoma (Rb) protein and the E2F family of transcription factors. When hypophosphorylated, Rb binds E2F to form a silencing complex inhibiting transcription of genes necessary for cell cycle entry. With mitogen stimulation, e.g., by growth factors, D-type cyclases are synthesized with their associated kinases. Rb is thus phosphorylated, releasing the E2F factors and allowing transcription of genes essential to DNA synthesis as well as other cyclins and CDKs that maintain the phosphorylated state of Rb, allowing mitogen-independent passage through the remainder of the S-phase. Additional checkpoints are present at the $G_2/M$ transition prior to mitosis and during metaphase of mitosis.[23]

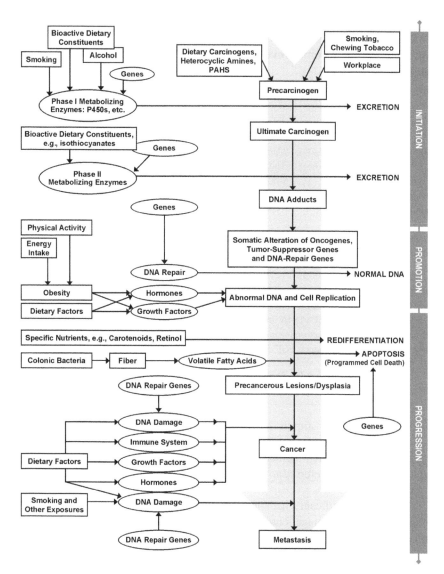

**FIGURE 2.2** Dietary factors, smoking, physical activity, and obesity in relation to the carcinogenesis process, from the initiation and promotion stages to metastasis or apoptosis. (From Go VL, Wong DA, Butrum R. Diet, nutrition and cancer prevention: where are we going from here? *J Nutr* 2001; 131:3123S. With permission).

Growth signals are transmitted by transmembrane receptors that bind different classes of signaling molecules, including growth factors, extracellular matrix components, and cell adhesion molecules. In addition, nuclear receptors (e.g., estrogen and androgen receptors, peroxisome proliferating receptors, retinoic acid receptors, vitamin D receptor) activated by steroid hormones and other lipophilic substances (e.g., prostaglandins, retinoids, vitamin D) act as transcription factors to regulate genes, including those involved with cellular proliferation. Normal cells proliferate in response to an array of growth factor signals produced from cells in the immediate environment or circulating hormones. Local factors can include epidermal growth factor (EGF), fibroblast growth factor (FGF), tumor growth factor-α (TGF-α), and platelet derived growth factor (PDGF).[23] Tumor cells characteristically show a decreased dependence on exogenous growth signals coming from the normal tissue environment by generating their own growth signals. In fact, many cancer cells acquire the ability to synthesize growth factors to which they are responsive, creating an autocrine-positive feedback loop. In addition, the components of the signal transduction pathways are perturbed. Changes include overexpression of growth factor receptors, which creates cells with an exaggerated response to growth signals, alteration in types of extracellular matrix receptors (integrins) expressed, and notably, modulation of the downstream cytoplasmic signaling pathways that define growth factor action resulting from ligand activation of growth factor receptors and integrins. Many growth factor receptors, when overexpressed, carry with them enhanced tyrosine kinase activities in their cytoplasmic domains. This overexpression may make cancer cells hyper-responsive to growth factor signals that under normal circumstances may not stimulate proliferation.[26]

Many of the proteins involved in growth regulation are proto-oncogenes; that is, they are oncogenic when mutated. For example, one central signaling pathway in proliferation is the mitogen-activated protein (MAP) kinase pathway. This pathway is overactive when the oncogenic form of *ras* proteins is mutated so that they are constitutively activated and disregulated from upstream regulators. *Ras* mutations are found in some 25% of human cancers.[26]

A comprehensive catalog of bioactive food components has been shown to inhibit cell proliferation *in vitro* at physiologically relevant doses, although there is specificity in the effects depending on dose, length of treatment, and cell type tested. A prominent example is genistein, an isoflavone and the major phytoestrogen in soybeans and other legumes. Genistein and other phytoestrogens have a chemical structure reminiscent of 17β-estradiol, can bind the estrogen receptors (ERα and ERβ), although with stronger affinity to ERβ, and exhibit estrogen-like biological activity.[9] Human breast and prostate cancer cell lines stimulated by EGF are inhibited by genistein independently of whether the cells express estrogen or androgen receptors. When all cell culture media are depleted of estrogens, genistein at concentrations <1 μmol/L acts as a growth stimulant to estrogen-dependent breast cancer cells; in the presence of 17β-estradiol (0.3 nmol/L, a physiological concentration) the effect of genistein is not additive. However, at concentrations >5 μmol/L, genistein causes a dose-dependent decrease in 17β-estradiol-induced cell proliferation.[30]

Genistein has been shown to inhibit cellular growth of a number of different cell types other than breast and prostate, including leukemia, lymphoma, neuroblastoma, gastric, lung, head, and neck squamous cancer cells; these lines vary in the presence of estrogen and androgen receptors and p53 status indicating effectiveness in cancer cells with varied molecular signatures. In a number of these cell types genistein induces a $G_2/M$ cell cycle arrest.[31] This effect is borne out in a decrease in cyclin B, which is important for the formation of the cyclin B/CDK complex to allow progression through $G_2/M$.[31] The CDK inhibitor p21[WAF1] was also upregulated in genistein-treated cells, which illustrates genistein's coordinated action in regulation of cell growth and the cell cycle.[32,33]

Genistein has also been postulated to have ER-independent action as well. Genistein was identified as a protein tyrosine kinase (PTK) inhibitor as it inhibited the EGF receptor PTK *in vitro*, and this function has been presumed to be a mechanism of genistein's antimitogenic action.[30] However, proliferation in several cell lines stimulated by EGF is inhibited by genistein without inhibition of EGF-R tyrosine autophosphorylation or tyrosine phosphorylation of other substrates involved with signaling pathways, suggesting alterations tyrosine phosphorylation may be an indirect effect of genistein's actions.[30] Alternatively, genistein may enhance production of TGF-$\beta$1, which is normally a growth-inhibitory factor, as described below.[34]

### 2.5.2 Increased Response to Antigrowth Signals and Induction of Differentiation

Normal cells within tissues are also responsive to antiproliferative signals that serve to maintain cellular quiescence and tissue homeostasis. These antigrowth signals are soluble factors or inhibitors embedded in the extracellular matrix. Signals are transmitted to the nucleus via intracellular signaling circuits that are in a balance with the positive growth signals. One of the most prominent negative growth signals in many cell types is TGF-$\beta$).[26]

Most antigrowth signals act on the tumor suppressor proteins, such as Rb. TGF-$\beta$ acts to prevent the phosphorylation that inactivates Rb, thus blocks advance through $G_1$.[26] When hypophosphorylated, Rb sequesters and inhibits E2F transcription factors that control the expression of genes required for progression from $G_1$ to S. Other tumor suppressor proteins include p53 (or TP53), which in the wild-type state suppresses tumor growth by initiating DNA repair and inducing death of irreparable cells. Generally, p53 is maintained at a low concentration, although it can be induced by physical or chemical DNA damage.[9] When p53 is mutated or suppressed by Mdm2, an oncogenic protein, proliferation of cells with DNA damage results.[23] Studies have shown that function of the p53 pathway is lost in most if not all of human cancers.[26] However, many other tumor suppressor genes have been defined and may be definitive for certain types of cancers, such as APC (adenomatous polyposis coli) in colorectal cancer[24] or BRCA in breast cancer.[35] For example, during human colon carcinogenesis, inactivation of APC/$\beta$-catenin pathway blocks the differentiation of the enterocytes in the colonic crypts, resulting in aberrant crypt foci.[26]

Antigrowth signals block proliferation by either forcing cells into quiescence or $G_0$, which is a reversible state upon activation by pro-growth signals, or by inducing differentiation, which, depending on cell type, is a permanent acquisition of specific phenotypic traits characteristic of the mature cell type. As cells move toward the differentiated state, the rate of proliferation slows, so that fully differentiated cells do not proliferate, or at least do so at a very slow rate. Cancer cells are poorly differentiated yet retain the potential to differentiate into more mature cells. Thus, induction of differentiation (or redifferentiation) is a cancer prevention and treatment strategy, although its effectiveness is lower for relatively slow-growing cancers like breast or prostate than for faster ones such as leukemia. Several nuclear acting nutrients, including vitamins D and A, have been the most comprehensively studied as differentiation-promoting agents, although a number of other compounds have been shown to induce cellular markers of differentiation *in vitro*, including a variety of flavonoids, the *n*-3 polyunsaturated fatty acids eicosapentaenoic acid (EPA) and docosahexaenoic acid (DHA), and resveratrol.[36]

## 2.5.3 ENHANCEMENT OF APOPTOSIS

The steady state of a normal tissue, or a tumor cell, is a balance between new cells acquired from mitotic division of precursor cells with the attrition of cells through apoptosis or programmed cell death. Apoptosis occurs when physiologic signals trigger a defined series of cellular changes resulting in disruption of the cellular membrane, disintegration of the cytoskeleton, extrusion of cytosol, degradation of chromosomes, and fragmentation of the nucleus.[26] This process induces cell destruction without the inflammatory responses characteristic of cell necrosis.[23] Although almost all cell types in the body have the capability to undergo apoptosis under appropriate developmental circumstances, apparently most, if not all, types of cancer cells acquire the capability to evade apoptosis, making activation of apoptosis a chemopreventive and therapeutic target.

Two families of membrane-associated death receptors are known. One is the FAS-receptor and another related set includes the tumor necrosis factor (TNF) and TNF-related apoptosis inducing ligand (TRAIL) receptors.[23] Several proteins have been identified to be intrinsic to the apoptotic pathway. *Bcl-2* (and related proteins Bcl-XL and Bcl-W) is an oncogenic protein that protects cancer cells by inhibiting apoptosis. Opposing *Bcl-2* is *Bax* (and related proteins *Bak*, *Bid*, and *Bim*), which competes with *Bcl-2* and acts as an inducer of apoptosis.[26] Upon sensing DNA damage, the p53 tumor suppressor protein elicits apoptosis by upregulating the expression of proapoptotic *Bax*, which then stimulates mitochondria to release cytochrome C and initiate programmed cell death. The ultimate effectors of apoptosis include the family of intracellular proteases, the caspases. Caspase-8 is activated by death receptors including FAS, and caspase-9 by cytochrome C released from mitochondria.[26] A number of other proapoptotic and antiapoptotic components are also involved; the complexity of this apoptotic signaling network is depicted by Gosslau and Chen.[37]

A plethora of natural compounds have been identified that can induce apoptosis by a number of different mechanisms. These include increasing signals to promote cell death (i.e., *Bax*) and by decreasing signals inhibiting cell death (i.e., *Bcl-2*). Death signals can be increased by cellular damage (at least *in vitro*), increased function of p53, and increased activity of antigrowth factors such as TGF-β. The opposing strategy involves inhibition of survival factors, including growth factors and their signaling pathways.[36] The proapoptotic effects of resveratrol have been extensively reviewed.[38] These effects include effects on induction of death receptors, activation of the mitochondrial pathway, effects on Rb phosphorylation, activation of p53 pathway, generation of the proapoptotic mediator ceramide, and more. Other phytochemicals that can induce apoptosis include lycopene and β-carotene, a number of flavonoids, the allyl-sulfur compounds of garlic, caffeic acid phenethyl ester from honeybee propolis, and curcumin.[37]

### 2.5.4 INDUCTION OF SENESCENCE

Normal cells in culture have a finite replicative potential. When these cell populations proceed through a set number of doublings, they undergo senescence, or a cessation of growth and eventually death via apoptosis. This process operates independently of the cell-to-cell signaling involved with proliferation and apoptosis. Cultured tumor cells are immortalized and exhibit limitless replicative potential. This suggests that, with the genetic changes occurring during the process of carcinogenesis, cells acquire traits resulting in a breach of the mortality barrier. The counting device for tallying replications has been found to be the ends of the chromosomes, called telomeres. With every replication, 50 to 100 base pairs are lost from the telomeres, until the unprotected chromosomal ends become involved in chromosomal aberrations and karyotypic disarray, stimulating cell death processes.[23] However, in nearly all malignant cells, telomeres are maintained through the action of telomerase, which adds nucleotides onto the ends of telomeric DNA. Human telomerase is composed of template RNA components and two proteins, telomerase-associated protein-1, and telomerase reverse transcriptase (hTERT), which are thought to be the enzyme's catalytic subunit.[39] Most human somatic cells do not have detectable telomerase activity and lack activity of hTERT. However, immortalized cells express hTERT and have detectable telomerase.[23]

Tumor growth is thought to require activation of telomerase, making it a target for chemoprevention.[39] Retinoids induce senescence in malignant and premalignant human and rat breast carcinoma cells, *in vitro* and *in vivo*.[40] Retinoids also synergize with vitamin D in inhibiting telomerase. The combination of vitamin $D_3$ and 9-*cis*-retinoic acid inhibited telomerase activity through direct interaction of the heterodimer of the vitamin $D_3$ receptor and retinoid X receptor (RXR) in prostate cancer cells.[41] Other nutritional factors, including EGCG and curcumin, also regulate telomerase activity. In nude mice models bearing both telomerase-dependent and -independent xenograft tumors cloned from a single human cancer progeny, only the telomerase-dependent tumors responded to prolonged oral administration of EGCG.[42] Furthermore, curcumin inhibits telomerase activity in MCF-7 breast cancer cells via downregulation of hTERT expression.[43]

## 2.5.5 INHIBITION OF ANGIOGENESIS

The growth of new blood vessels, angiogenesis, is a requirement of new organ growth. Capillary blood vessels must deliver oxygen and nutrients to cells, and withdraw cellular wastes, within a maximum diffusion distance of about 100 μm. This process is also necessary for tumorigenesis, as tumor size is dependent on the ability to develop new vasculature.[26] The process of angiogenesis involves the proliferation, migration, and capillary formation from existing vessels in response to multiple extracellular signals. A number of protein factors have been identified to both stimulate and inhibit angiogenesis. More than two dozen inducers and the same number of inhibitors have been identified, and *in vivo* it is thought that tumors activate angiogenesis by shifting the balance of inducers and inhibitors. The most prominent angiogenesis activating signals are vascular endothelial growth factor (VEGF) and acidic and basic fibroblast growth factors (FGF 1/2), while thrombospondin-1 is among the angiogenesis inhibitors.[26]

We have studied green tea and its catechin components, including EGCG, for their antiangiogenic properties. Green tea extract (GTE) as well as its individual catechin components inhibited MDA-MB231 breast cancer cell and human umbilical vein endothelial cell (HUVEC) proliferation. Furthermore, GTE suppressed breast cancer xenograft size and decreased the tumor vessel density *in vivo*.[44] GTE or EGCG also decreased levels of VEGF peptide secreted into conditioned media in HUVEC and MDA-MB231 human breast cancer cells and decreased RNA levels of VEGF in the cancer cells. This inhibition occurred at the transcriptional level and was accompanied by a significant decrease in VEGF promoter activity.[45]

In addition, lipoxygenase and cyclooxygenase products of *n*-6 fatty acid metabolism in the eicosanoid pathway are angiogenic in *in vitro* assays. As outlined below, the activity of both of these enzymes can be suppressed by resveratrol or *n*-3 polyunsaturated fatty acids EPA and DHA.[46]

## 2.5.6 INHIBITION OF TISSUE INVASION AND METASTASIS

The defining event of a malignancy is the ability of rogue cells to advance from the primary tumor, invade adjacent tissue, and travel to distant sites to found new colonies. Most cancer mortality is due to these distant metastases, which arise as amalgams of cancer cells and normal cells recruited from the host tissue. The mechanisms whereby tumor cells can undergo invasion and metastasis are complex and are still being defined. However, to elicit these migrations of cancer cells, it is clear that molecules involved in interactions between cells and between cells and their matrix must be involved. These proteins include the cell adhesion molecules (CAMs), which are members of the immunoglobulin and calcium-dependent cadherin families, and integrins, which link cells to their extracellular matrix. The most commonly observed altered protein is E-cadherin, which is normally expressed ubiquitously in epithelial cells, mediating cell-to-cell interactions; loss of cadherin is associated with metastasis in a majority of epithelial cancers. In addition, extracellular proteases, including the matrix metalloprotein-ases (MMPs) are upregulated, while protease inhibitors are downregulated in the metastatic process.[26]

As outlined above, green tea and EGCG are effective antiangiogenic agents. They also are found to inhibit genes related to adhesion, invasion, and metastasis, including urokinase, MMP-2, and MMP-9.[47,48] Interestingly, when black tea and a soy phytochemical concentrate were combined in a mouse model of orthotopic androgen-sensitive human prostate cancer, the combination resulted in a syner-gistic interaction to inhibit prostate tumorigenicity, final tumor weight, and metastases to lymph nodes *in vivo*.[49]

### 2.5.7 INCREASED ANTIOXIDANT CAPACITY AND GENOMIC STABILITY

The traits described thus far are acquired in the course of tumor progression via alterations in the genomes of cancer cells, resulting from DNA damage. Cells are exposed to a variety of oxidizing agents, termed reactive oxygen species (ROS), coming from exogenous and endogenous sources that can damage DNA. Oxidative damage of DNA, if left unrepaired, can lead to base mutations, single and double strand breaks, DNA cross-linking, chromosomal breaks and rearrange-ments.[50] An estimate of the daily rate of oxidative damage to DNA is $10^4$ hits per cell in humans.[51] Normally there is a balance between oxidizing and antiox-idizing molecules in the body and mutations in specific genes are kept in check by a number of DNA monitoring and repair systems that work to prevent and reverse alterations in specific genes.[50] However, an imbalance in the system due to overproduction of free radical oxidants or an inadequacy of antioxidants, can lead to oxidative damage of large biomolecules, including DNA, proteins, and lipids.[52] As described above, DNA damage activates p53 tumor suppressor protein to arrest the cell cycle to allow DNA repair or induce apoptosis when damage is too excessive.

Antioxidants common in fruits and vegetables can either prevent formation of, scavenge, or promote decomposition of ROS.[51] Classical antioxidant nutrients include vitamins E and C, β-carotene, and selenium. However, a large number of phytochemicals can accumulate within cells and act as either antioxidants or even pro-oxidants. Vegetables and fruits are rich in polyphenols such as epigal-locatechin gallate, quercetin, genistein, and taxifolin, which are excellent anti-oxidants *in vitro*.[52] The relationship between high consumption of antioxidants from fruits and vegetables and risk of a variety of cancer sites, including lung, colon, breast, cervix, esophagus, oral cavity, stomach, bladder, pancreas, and ovary, has been reviewed.[53] However, although vegetable and fruit intake can be approximated using current databases, total antioxidant activity is more difficult to determine due to large differences in antioxidant capabilities between plants and their edible parts, and even within a plant food due to agronomy and post-harvest conditions.[52] Wu et al. surveyed more than 100 different kinds of foods (also assessing variation due to geographic region, season, and processing), including fruits, vegetables, nuts, dried fruits, spices, cereals, infant food, and other foods for hydrophilic and lipophilic antioxidant capacities to arrive at a total antioxidant capacity.[54] These types of data are important for databases, which can be used to evaluate total antioxidant intake from nutrient as well as "nonnutrient" antioxidants and relate it to cancer risk. These data can be used to show an inverse correlation between total antioxidant capacity intake and risk of cancer, as was done recently for gastric cancer.[55]

## 2.5.8 OTHER MECHANISMS

The above analysis, focusing on the six essential alterations in cell physiology as defined by Hanahan and Weinberg[26] and their modification by nutrients, focuses mainly on the changes within the cancer cells themselves. However, the effects of nutrients on other aspects affecting cancer incidence and progression at the tissue and whole-body levels cannot be ignored. Some of these other factors include effects on inflammation, carcinogen detoxification by xenobiotic metabolizing enzymes, and epigenetic events.

### 2.5.8.1 Inflammation

Prostaglandins and other members of the eicosanoid pathway are thought to induce carcinogenesis through action on nuclear transcription sites and downstream gene products important in the control of cell proliferation. Eicosanoids are locally acting hormone-like compounds derived predominantly from arachidonic acid in tissue cells and tumor-infiltrating leukocytes.[56] The most well-known eicosanoids, prostaglandins, are produced by the action of the cyclooxygenases (COX), but the lipoxygenase group of enzymes produce the leukotrienes and hydroperoxyeicosatetraenoic acids, which also have important proinflammatory effects.[57] Substantial evidence from animal studies and human epidemiological and clinical trials show that nonsteroidal anti-inflammatory drugs (NSAIDs), which are inhibitors of COX, are associated with reduced risk of a number of cancers, including those of the colon-rectum, esophagus, stomach, pancreas, breast, lung, prostate, bladder, brain, and cervix.[57]

However, chronic NSAID use leads to toxicities, including gastric ulceration, perforation, or obstruction, which limit their therapeutic use.[57] Newer selective COX-2 inhibitors have been postulated to be safer, but the recent voluntary worldwide recall of Merck's product Vioxx® (rofecoxib) — and subsequently other NSAIDs — illustrates that the long-term safety of these drugs has yet to be established.[58] Therefore, research has focused on identifying and understanding the bioactivity of a number of natural, nontoxic agents to control inflammatory eicosanoids. Those agents that have been studied include $n$-3 polyunsaturated fatty acids EPA and DHA such as from fish oils, vitamin A, vitamin E, and a number of botanical anti-inflammatory agents, such as boswellia, bromelain, curcumin, resveratrol, quercetin, EGCG, and others.[57] One mechanism of action of these compounds is via inhibition of the inducible transcription factor nuclear factor kappa B (NF-κB), which is activated by pro-inflammatory signals and upregulates COX-2 expression.[59]

## 2.5.8.2 Carcinogen Activation/Detoxification by Xenobiotic Metabolizing Enzymes

Although this discussion has focused on the beneficial roles of certain dietary constituents, we must recognize the role of dietary carcinogens as well. A number of known or suspected dietary carcinogens are present in foods, including mycotoxins (moldy foods), polycyclic aromatic hydrocarbons and heterocyclic amines (grilled, fried, broiled, or charred meats and fish), N-nitrosoamines (foods preserved with nitrates and nitrites), alcohol (alcoholic beverages), as well as certain metals and pesticides.[60] The enzymes responsible for the oxidation, reduction, and conjugation of harmful and other dietary constituents, as well as endogenous hormones and other foreign compounds, are called drug metabolizing enzymes (DMEs). The Phase I enzymes, which include the cytochrome P450 mixed-function oxidases, act by oxidizing, reducing, or hydrolyzing toxins, creating biotransformed intermediates. This process exists in the cell to detoxify compounds by rendering them more water soluble for excretion in the urine. However, as a consequence certain foreign compounds, termed xenobiotics, can be activated to increase their mutagenicity in the process. Phase II enzymes perform conjugation reactions that help to convert the biotransformed intermediates from Phase I into less-toxic, water-soluble substances for excretion from the body. These enzymes may also work independently of Phase I activity by acting directly on a drug or toxin. Phase II enzymes include glutathione-S-transferases (GSTs), UDP-glucuronosyl transferases, and quinone reductase. Phase I enzyme activity must be in balance with that of Phase II for effective elimination of biotransformed intermediates to prevent accumulation of toxins in the body. Another potentially damaging effect of the Phase I enzymes is the production of oxygen free radicals that occur as a result of cytochrome P450 activity.[61] Oxidative stress in the liver is prevented by adequate intake of antioxidants, such as vitamins C and E, and many naturally occurring phytochemicals can also act as antioxidants, as reviewed above.

Vegetables of the *Brassica oleracea* species (e.g., cabbage, broccoli, cauliflower, Brussels sprouts, kohlrabi, and kale; also called cruciferous vegetables) as well as many other genera that include a variety of food plants (e.g., arugula, radish, daikon, watercress, horseradish, and wasabi) are known to be rich in glucosinolates (β-thioglycoside-N-hydroxysulfates). These compounds are hydrolyzed by myrosinase, a plant enzyme released when plants are cut, ground, or chewed, releasing the biologically active isothiocyanates (ITC). Some naturally occurring forms of this phytochemical include 2-phenethyl isothiocyanate, benzyl isothiocyanate, and sulforaphanes.[62] ITCs are known to induce expression of Phase I and Phase II enzymes and, to a lesser extent, also directly inhibit the P450s; the effect is dependent on the individual ITC. However, in animal models and cell culture systems, combinations of ITC confer protection against genotoxic agents at levels that the individual compounds do not achieve alone.[63] A number of human epidemiological studies have shown an inverse relationship between cruciferous vegetable intake and risk of cancer. Importantly, this effect is dependent on individual polymorphisms in the biotransformation enzyme genes. The relationship with GST has been most studied. For example, in a case-control study, Lin et al. showed that individuals with the highest quartile of broccoli intake had the lowest risk for colorectal adenomas compared with individuals who never ate broccoli, but the effect was seen only in the GSTM1-null (an inactivating mutation in a GST class μ isozyme) genotype individuals.[64] This genetic polymorphism is theorized to result in longer circulating half-lives of ITC and potentially greater chemoprotective effects by activation of other GST enzymes.

### 2.5.8.3  Epigenetic Events

Much of the previous discussion has focused on genomic alterations by dietary constituents. However, a key role of nutrient action is epigenetic, referring to changes in the phenotype that are not due to changes in the genotype, or in other words, changes in gene expression that are transmissible through mitosis, but do not involve mutations of the primary DNA sequence itself.[65]

A critical mechanism for epigenetic gene regulation involves alterations in patterns of DNA methylation. DNA methylation, or the covalent addition of a methyl group to the 5-position of cytosine within CpG dinucleotides, is particularly important in epigenetic control by nutrients. Tumors commonly exhibit widespread global DNA hypomethylation, region-specific hypermethylation, and increased activity of *Dnmt* enzymes, which catalyze the transfer of methyl groups from *S*-adenosylmethionine (SAM) to cytosine residues in DNA. Global genomic hypomethylation is linked to induction of chromosomal instability while hypermethylation is associated with inactivation of most pathways of carcinogenesis, including DNA repair, cell cycle regulation, and apoptosis.[66]

Dietary factors may influence DNA methylation patterns in several ways. First, nutrient inadequacies will influence the supply of methyl groups for the formation of SAM. Dietary factors that are involved in one-carbon metabolism that influence the availability of SAM include folate, vitamin $B_{12}$ (cobalamin), vitamin $B_6$ (pyroxidine), vitamin $B_2$ (riboflavin), methionine, choline, and alcohol. Other nutrients including zinc, selenium, and retinoic acid will affect global DNA hypomethylation.[66] A second way is by altering the use of methyl groups, including altering DNA methyltransferase activity via *Dnmt* enzymes. Higher *Dnmt* activity has been observed in tumor cells compared to normal cells, and activity of these enzymes is upregulated with chronic methyl deficiency, in an apparent attempt to compensate for diminished SAM supply. In addition the DNA demethylation process, previously assumed to be passive, may be a regulated activity.[66] These changes in methylation patterns can influence activity of specific genes; this likely occurs through modifying transcription factor-gene interactions through methyl-DNA binding proteins.[66] For example, consumption of a chronic methyl-deficient diet in rats leads to hepatomas.[67] In this model, hypomethylation of specific CpG sites in several oncogenes, including c-*myc,* c-*fos,* and H-*ras,* results in elevated mRNA levels for these genes.[68,69] Also, in the same model, levels of p53 tumor suppressor mRNA is decreased in tumor tissue due to relative hypermethylation, although the level of p53 mRNA in preneoplastic nodules was increased and associated with hypomethylation in the coding region.[70]

## 2.6  EXAMPLE OF PLEIOTROPIC ACTIONS OF NUTRIENTS — VITAMIN D IN COLON CANCER

Vitamin D is an example of a nutrient that exhibits many of the mechanisms described above in inhibiting cancer development, particularly in inhibition of proliferation, induction of differentiation, activation of apoptosis, and blocking initiation. Vitamin D and its analogs have been investigated for some time for their anticancer properties in a number of cancers, including colorectal, prostate, breast, and leukemia.[9] The classical role of the most bioactive form of vitamin D, $1\alpha,25$-dihydroxyvitamin $D_3$ ($1\alpha,25(OH)_2D_3$), is to regulate calcium absorption in the intestine, maintain mineral homeostasis in the kidney, and regulate bone remodeling. This function can lead to toxic hypercalcemia when exogenous $1\alpha,25(OH)_2D_3$ is administered in therapeutic doses; therefore, a number of pharmaceutical analogs have been developed that retain their anticancer properties with minimal effects on circulating calcium.[71] Many tissues other than those involved with mineral metabolism have specific vitamin D nuclear receptors, suggesting alternative roles for vitamin D. Normal and cancer cells that express vitamin D receptors respond to $1\alpha,25(OH)_2D_3$ by decreasing proliferation and enhancing maturation or differentiation.[72] In addition, many cell types, including notably colon cancer cells,[73,74] can make $1\alpha,25(OH)_2D_3$, suggesting autocrine/paracrine actions in manipulating cell growth.

$1\alpha,25(OH)_2D_3$ has direct antiproliferative properties against many cancer cells *in vitro,* including colon,[75–78] breast,[79,80] prostate,[81,82] and hematopoietic cells.[83] Also, $1\alpha,25(OH)_2D_3$ and its metabolic precursor, $25(OH)_2D_3$, reduce crypt cell production in colonic tissue removed from individuals with familial adenomatous polyposis (an inherited cancer syndrome caused by a mutation in the *Apc* gene).[84] Whether the antiproliferative effects of vitamin D are totally independent of calcium level is not clear. For example, the effect of vitamin D in colon cancer cells *in vitro* varies by extracellular calcium concentration[85] and is reduced by addition of calcium channel blockers.[75]

The anticarcinogenic activity of $1\alpha,25(OH)_2D_3$ appears to be correlated with cellular vitamin D receptor (VDR) levels. VDRs belong to the superfamily of steroid-hormone zinc-finger receptors and share the common characteristic with other members of this family in that they are ligand-activated regulators of gene transcription. VDRs selectively bind $1\alpha,25(OH)_2D_3$ and RXR to form a heterodimeric complex that interacts with specific DNA sequences known as vitamin D-responsive elements (VDRE) to regulate gene expression. For example, the binding of $1\alpha,25(OH)_2D_3$ to the VDR in intestinal cells activates the transcription of the calcium-binding protein that enhances the absorption of calcium.

The VDR is expressed in colon tumor cells,[75,86] and the density of the vitamin D receptor is increased in hyperplastic polyps and in early stages of tumorigenesis, but declines in late-stage neoplasia.[74,87,88] With carcinogen treatment, rats show a decreased number of $1\alpha,25(OH)_2D_3$ binding sites in the colon.[89] The level of vitamin D receptor in wild-type, heterozygote, and vitamin D receptor null mice is inversely correlated with proliferating nuclear cell antigen and cyclin D1, markers of cellular proliferation, and positively correlated with 8-hydroxy-2′-deoxyguanosine levels, a marker of oxidative stress in the colon descendens.[90] These results implicate genomic $1\alpha,25(OH)_2D_3$ action in prevention of hyperproliferation and oxidative DNA damage.

The activated receptor recognizes specific vitamin D response elements in a number of vitamin D–regulated genes, including p21[WAF1] and the calcium-sensing receptor. However, vitamin D regulates a number of different proto-oncogenes and tumor suppressor genes related to proliferation and differentiation, including p27[KIP1], c-*myc*, laminin, tenascin, fibronectin, cyclin C, c-*fos*, c-*jun*, phospholipase C$\gamma$, ornithine decarboxylase, and members of the TGF-$\beta$ family.[91] As not all of these genes have vitamin D response element consensus sequences identified in their promoter regions, their regulation is thought to be indirect through regulation of upstream events or even activation of a putative membrane-bound receptor.

The anticancer effects restricting cellular growth are thought to involve various mechanisms, including effects on growth factor and cytokine synthesis and signaling, cell cycle progression, apoptosis, and differentiation. An example of the regulation by $1\alpha,25(OH)_2D_3$ of a growth-factor signaling pathway is that of TGF-$\beta$, which inhibits epithelial cell proliferation. SMAD3, a downstream protein in the TGF-$\beta$ signaling pathway, is a coactivator of the vitamin D receptor and positively regulates the vitamin D signaling pathway.[92–94] Cross talk between vitamin D and TGF-$\beta$1 has been demonstrated in the growth inhibition of human colon cancer–derived cells.[95] The antimitotic actions of vitamin D and its analogs seem to be mediated by the induction of $G_1$ cell cycle arrest, resulting from the upregulation of expression of p21[WAF1] and p27[KIP1].[96–98]

In addition to inhibiting tumor growth and progression, $1\alpha,25(OH)_2D_3$ has anticancer action by inducing apoptosis in various transformed cells, including colon cancer cells.[96,99] The mechanisms of the proapoptotic action in colon cells is not entirely clear, but in human colon adenoma and carcinoma cell lines the apoptotic action of vitamin D was associated with upregulation of the expression of the proapoptotic protein *Bak*.[100] The differentiation-promoting effect of $1\alpha,25(OH)_2D_3$ was demonstrated in a human colon carcinoma cell line, SW480, which expresses vitamin D receptors, but not in other similar lines that do not express the receptor. $1\alpha,25(OH)_2D_3$ induced the expression of proteins associated with the mature phenotype, such as E-cadherin and cell adhesion proteins, and repressed $\beta$-catenin signaling, which has an antitumor effect *in vivo*.[101]

The VDR also has been postulated to have a role in suppressing initiation of colon carcinogenesis. The VDR has been shown to have high affinity for the secondary bile acid lithocholic acid LCA and its metabolites, which are carcinogenic. By binding to the vitamin D receptor, both LCA and vitamin D may activate a feed-forward catabolic pathway that increases the expression of CYP3A, a cytochrome P450 enzyme that detoxifies LCA in the liver and intestines to clear LCA from the body.[102] This may provide one mechanism to explain how the protective pathway of vitamin D receptor activation may become overwhelmed by high-fat diets (which increase LCA levels) or compromised when vitamin D is deficient with inadequate sun exposure or intake.

Studies using carcinogen-induced intestinal cancer models show the effect *in vivo* of vitamin D alone or in combination with calcium on the development of intestinal cancer. Rats on a high-fat (20% corn oil) diet had increased tumor incidence after 1,2-dimethylhydrazine (DMH) treatment, and this increase was ameliorated by either supplemental calcium or vitamin D.[103,104] Conversely, vitamin D deficiency abolished the protective effects of calcium on colon cancer in DMH-treated rats.[105,106] $1\alpha,25(OH)_2D_3$ before treatment with DMH obliterated the peak in ornithine decarboxylase activity (a sign of increased mucosal cell proliferation) seen with DMH administration, and reduced by 50% the number of colon adenocarcinomas.[89] However, in this and a similar study,[107] $1\alpha,25(OH)_2D_3$ did not prevent tumor formation when administered *after* DMH. One mechanism of the chemopreventive action of $1\alpha,25(OH)_2D_3$ treatment elucidated in AOM-treated rats was an inhibition in angiogenesis, defined as a decrease in immunohistochemical staining for vascular endothelial growth factor and microvessel counts.[108] In our own studies using mutant mice, we found that administration of $1\alpha,25(OH)_2D_3$ and an analog of vitamin D to *Apc^min* mice, which have a germ line mutation in the Apc tumor suppressor gene, resulted in a significant decrease in total tumor area over the entire gastrointestinal tract in both the analog- and the $1\alpha,25(OH)_2D_3$-treated groups.[109]

## 2.7 IMPLICATIONS

Cancer is a genetic disease resulting from multiple genetic defects caused by exposure to environmental, dietary, and infectious agents as well as other lifestyle factors. Figure 2.2 presents a conceptual framework for these relationships, showing the molecular mechanisms of dietary constituents in the carcinogenesis pathway, from activation of procarcinogens to the initiation and promotion stages of carcinogenesis, and to tissue invasion and metastasis.[20]

The implications of our broadening knowledge of the biology of cancer and the impact of nutrient intake is that we can hope to utilize nutritional interventions to slow the progression of tumor development in the intraepithelial hyperplasia phase before tumor size becomes large enough for diagnosis and probability of metastasis increases (Figure 2.3).[110] Opportunity exists to stretch this prevention phase so that symptom-free life of the future patient with cancer is prolonged. Because the median age of cancer diagnosis in the U.S. is 70 years, and the average life expectancies are 74 years for men and 79 years for women, cancer delay may result in total prevention for many people.[111]

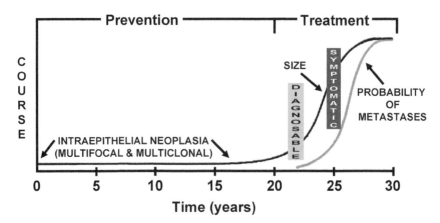

**FIGURE 2.3** Clinical course of epithelial tumors over time, from the intraepithelial neoplasia stage to metastases. (From Go VL, Butrum RR, Wong DA. Diet, nutrition, and cancer prevention: the postgenomic era. *J Nutr* 2003; 133:3834S. With permission.)

In the postgenomic era, new opportunities are arising from advances in nutrition sciences to understand the integrative biology of living organisms. The complexities of the interactions among genotype, diet, and environment are unraveling, and personalized nutrition recommendations for individuals will become feasible. Nutritional genomics, proteomics, and metabolic profiling use high throughput technologies that enable researchers to analyze thousands of genes and their interactions simultaneously. Nutritional genomics refers to the interface of plant biochemistry, genomics, and human nutrition for the purpose of understanding and manipulating nutrient reactions and interactions at the molecular or genomic level.[8] One mechanism involves gene-nutrient interactions in relation to specific gene polymorphisms among individuals have already been identified. The example of broccoli intake in relation to colon cancer risk in GSTM1-null genotype individuals was reviewed earlier. Another example involves certain polymorphisms in the methylenetetrahydrofolate reductase gene, a key enzyme in one-carbon metabolism, that have been associated with a lower risk of developing colorectal cancer, but only in persons with adequate folate status.[112]

The resulting data facilitate molecular analysis of bioactive food components and identification of appropriate biomarkers that target individuals who are at risk and predisposed to cancer. Ever-increasing evidence, including that presented in this volume, substantiate the beneficial effects of certain nutrients and interactions between nutrients in the carcinogenesis pathway, paving the way for modification of nutritional requirements as a cancer prevention strategy. In the future, diet, nutrition, and cancer prevention will be included in public health programs that target cancer risk management in the population at large, and on individual programs that focus on particular cancer risk profiles. Concomitantly, agricultural sciences will continue to develop improved plants through both traditional breeding techniques and genetic modification and food industries will provide functional foods enriched with beneficial nutrients.[9,20] Targeting cancer prevention with specific foods and/or bioactive components is a relatively non-toxic and cost-effective strategy for reducing cancer burden. However, the complexity of the human diet coupled with individual variation in the carcinogenesis process will make continued research in the area of diet and cancer prevention mandatory.[46]

## ACKNOWLEDGMENTS

Funding provided by the National Cancer Institute (NCI)/UCLA Clinical Nutrition Research Unit (CA42710) and NCI Grant CA109612. The authors would like to recognize the editorial assistance of Yu Wang, Tom Gossard, and Emily Besselink.

## REFERENCES

1. Heber D, Blackburn G, Go V. The principles of nutritional oncology. In: Heber D, Blackburn G, Go V, eds. *Nutritional Oncology.* San Diego, CA: Academic Press; 1999: 1–10.
2. World Cancer Research Fund and American Institute for Cancer Research. *Food, Nutrition and the Prevention of Cancer: A Global Perspective.* Washington, DC: American Institute for Cancer Research; 1997.
3. Ferlay J, Bray F, Pisani P, Parkin D. *GLOBOCAN 2002: Cancer Incidence, Mortality and Prevalence Worldwide.* 2004. IARC Press. IARC CancerBase No. 5, version 2.0. http://www-dep.iarc.fr/.
4. Greenwald P, Clifford CK, Milner JA. Diet and cancer prevention. *Eur J Cancer* 2001; 37(8):948–965.
5. Cerhan JR, Potter JD, Gilmore JM et al. Adherence to the AICR cancer prevention recommendations and subsequent morbidity and mortality in the Iowa Women's Health Study cohort. *Cancer Epidemiol Biomarkers Prev* 2004; 13(7):1114–1120.
6. U.S. Department of Health and Human Services, U.S. Department of Agriculture. *2005 Dietary Guidelines Advisory Committee Report.* Departments of Health and Human Services and Agriculture. 2005. http://www.healthierus.gov/dietaryguidelines/.
7. Surh YJ. Cancer chemoprevention with dietary phytochemicals. *Nat Rev Cancer* 2003; 3(10):768–780.
8. Milner JA. Functional foods and health: a US perspective. *Br J Nutr* 2002; 88(Suppl 2):S151–S158.
9. Milner JA, McDonald SS, Anderson DE, Greenwald P. Molecular targets for nutrients involved with cancer prevention. *Nutr Cancer* 2001; 41(1–2):1–16.
10. Greenwald P, Milner JA, Anderson DE, McDonald SS. Micronutrients in cancer chemoprevention. *Cancer Metastasis Rev* 2002; 21(3–4):217–230.
11. Khachik F, Carvalho L, Bernstein PS, Muir GJ, Zhao DY, Katz NB. Chemistry, distribution, and metabolism of tomato carotenoids and their impact on human health. *Exp Biol Med (Maywood)* 2002; 227(10):845–851.

12. Boileau TW, Liao Z, Kim S, Lemeshow S, Erdman JW Jr, Clinton SK. Prostate carcinogenesis in *N*-methyl-*N*-nitrosourea (NMU)-testosterone-treated rats fed tomato powder, lycopene, or energy-restricted diets. *J Natl Cancer Inst* 2003; 95(21):1578–1586.

13. Liu RH. Potential synergy of phytochemicals in cancer prevention: mechanisms of action. *J Nutr* 2004; 134(12Suppl):3479S–3485S.

14. Ip C. Interaction of vitamin C and selenium supplementation in the modification of mammary carcinogenesis in rats. *J Natl Cancer Inst* 1986; 77(1):299–303.

15. Liu RH. Health benefits of fruit and vegetables are from additive and synergistic combinations of phytochemicals. *Am J Clin Nutr* 2003; 78(3 Suppl):517S–520S.

16. Hasler CM, Bloch AS, Thomson CA, Enrione E, Manning C. Position of the American Dietetic Association: functional foods. *J Am Diet Assoc* 2004; 104(5):814–826.

17. National Cancer Institute. 5-a-Day. *National Cancer Institute*. 2005. http://5aday.gov/.

18. American Institute for Cancer Research. *Diet and Health Guidelines for Cancer Prevention*. American Institute for Cancer Research. 2005. http://www.aicr.org/.

19. American Cancer Society. *American Cancer Society Recommendations for Nutrition and Physical Activity for Cancer Prevention*. American Cancer Society. 2005. http://www.cancer.org/.

20. Go VL, Wong DA, Butrum R. Diet, nutrition and cancer prevention: where are we going from here? *J Nutr* 2001; 131(11 Suppl):3121S–3126S.

21. O'Shaughnessy JA, Kelloff GJ, Gordon GB et al. Treatment and prevention of intraepithelial neoplasia: an important target for accelerated new agent development. *Clin Cancer Res* 2002; 8(2):314–346.

22. Boone CW, Kelloff GJ. Cancer chemoprevention: subject cohorts with early neoplasia, agents, and intermediate marker endpoints in clinical trials evaluated by computer-assisted image analysis. In: Heber D, Blackburn G, Go V, eds. *Nutritional Oncology*. San Diego: Academic Press; 2004:343–378.

23. Bertram JS. The molecular biology of cancer. *Mol Aspects Med* 2000; 21(6):167–223.

24. Fodde R, Smits R, Clevers H. APC, signal transduction and genetic instability in colorectal cancer. *Nat Rev Cancer* 2001; 1(1):55–67.

25. Mathers JC. Nutrition and cancer prevention: diet–gene interactions. *Proc Nutr Soc* 2003; 62(3):605–610.

26. Hanahan D, Weinberg RA. The hallmarks of cancer. *Cell* 2000; 100(1):57–70.

27. Kelloff GJ, Crowell JA, Steele VE et al. Progress in cancer chemoprevention: development of diet-derived chemopreventive agents. *J Nutr* 2000; 130(2S Suppl):467S–471S.

28. Kelloff GJ, Sigman CC, Greenwald P. Cancer chemoprevention: progress and promise. *Eur J Cancer* 1999; 35(13):1755–1762.

29. Bohnsack BL, Hirschi KK. Nutrient regulation of cell cycle progression. *Annu Rev Nutr* 2004; 24:433–453.

30. Kim H, Peterson TG, Barnes S. Mechanisms of action of the soy isoflavone genistein: emerging role for its effects via transforming growth factor beta signaling pathways. *Am J Clin Nutr* 1998; 68(6 Suppl):1418S–1425S.

31. Sarkar FH, Li Y. Mechanisms of cancer chemoprevention by soy isoflavone genistein. *Cancer Metastasis Rev* 2002; 21(3–4):265–280.

32. Sarkar FH, Li Y. Soy isoflavones and cancer prevention. *Cancer Invest* 2003; 21(5):744–757.

33. Magee PJ, Rowland IR. Phyto-oestrogens, their mechanism of action: current evidence for a role in breast and prostate cancer. *Br J Nutr* 2004; 91(4):513–531.

34. Kim H, Xu J, Su Y et al. Actions of the soy phytoestrogen genistein in models of human chronic disease: potential involvement of transforming growth factor beta. *Biochem Soc Trans* 2001; 29(Pt 2):216–222.

35. Tutt A, Ashworth A. The relationship between the roles of BRCA genes in DNA repair and cancer predisposition. *Trends Mol Med* 2002; 8(12):571–576.

36. Boik J. *Natural Compounds in Cancer Therapy*. Princeton, MN: Oregon Medical Press, 2001.

37. Gosslau A, Chen KY. Nutraceuticals, apoptosis, and disease prevention. *Nutrition* 2004; 20(1):95–102.

38. Aggarwal BB, Bhardwaj A, Aggarwal RS, Seeram NP, Shishodia S, Takada Y. Role of resveratrol in prevention and therapy of cancer: preclinical and clinical studies. *Anticancer Res* 2004; 24(5A):2783–2840.

39. Pendino F, Flexor M, Delhommeau F, Buet D, Lanotte M, Segal-Bendirdjian E. Retinoids down-regulate telomerase and telomere length in a pathway distinct from leukemia cell differentiation. *Proc Natl Acad Sci USA* 2001; 98(12):6662–6667.

40. Shay JW, Roninson IB. Hallmarks of senescence in carcinogenesis and cancer therapy. *Oncogene* 2004; 23(16):2919–2933.

41. Ikeda N, Uemura H, Ishiguro H et al. Combination treatment with $1\alpha$,25-dihydroxyvitamin $D_3$ and 9-*cis*-retinoic acid directly inhibits human telomerase reverse transcriptase transcription in prostate cancer cells. *Mol Cancer Ther* 2003; 2(8):739–746.

42. Naasani I, Oh-Hashi F, Oh-Hara T et al. Blocking telomerase by dietary polyphenols is a major mechanism for limiting the growth of human cancer cells *in vitro* and *in vivo*. *Cancer Res* 2003; 63(4):824–830.

43. Aggarwal BB, Kumar A, Bharti AC. Anticancer potential of curcumin: preclinical and clinical studies. *Anticancer Res* 2003; 23(1A):363–398.

44. Sartippour MR, Heber D, Ma J, Lu Q, Go VL, Nguyen M. Green tea and its catechins inhibit breast cancer xenografts. *Nutr Cancer* 2001; 40(2):149–156.

45. Sartippour MR, Shao ZM, Heber D et al. Green tea inhibits vascular endothelial growth factor (VEGF) induction in human breast cancer cells. *J Nutr* 2002; 132(8):2307–2311.

46. Milner JA. Strategies for cancer prevention: the role of diet. *Br J Nutr* 2002; 87 Suppl 2:S265–S272.

47. Jung YD, Ellis LM. Inhibition of tumour invasion and angiogenesis by epigallocatechin gallate (EGCG), a major component of green tea. *Int J Exp Pathol* 2001; 82(6):309–316.

48. Adhami VM, Ahmad N, Mukhtar H. Molecular targets for green tea in prostate cancer prevention. *J Nutr* 2003; 133(7 Suppl):2417S–2424S.

49. Zhou JR, Yu L, Zhong Y, Blackburn GL. Soy phytochemicals and tea bioactive components synergistically inhibit androgen-sensitive human prostate tumors in mice. *J Nutr* 2003; 133(2):516–521.

50. Ogino T, Packer L, Traber MG. Oxidant stress and host oxidant defense mechanisms. In: Heber D, Blackburn G, Go V, eds. *Nutritional Oncology*. San Diego, CA: Academic Press; 2004: 253–275.

51. Stanner SA, Hughes J, Kelly CN, Buttriss J. A review of the epidemiological evidence for the "antioxidant hypothesis." *Public Health Nutr* 2004; 7(3):407–422.

52. Seifried HE, McDonald SS, Anderson DE, Greenwald P, Milner JA. The antioxidant conundrum in cancer. *Cancer Res* 2003; 63(15):4295–4298.

53. Block G, Patterson B, Subar A. Fruit, vegetables, and cancer prevention: a review of the epidemiological evidence. *Nutr Cancer* 1992; 18(1):1–29.

54. Wu X, Beecher GR, Holden JM, Haytowitz DB, Gebhardt SE, Prior RL. Lipophilic and hydrophilic antioxidant capacities of common foods in the United States. *J Agric Food Chem* 2004; 52(12):4026–4037.

55. Serafini M, Bellocco R, Wolk A, Ekstrom AM. Total antioxidant potential of fruit and vegetables and risk of gastric cancer. *Gastroenterology* 2002; 123(4):985–991.

56. Wargovich MJ, Woods C, Hollis DM, Zander ME. Herbals, cancer prevention and health. *J Nutr* 2001; 131(11 Suppl):3034S–3036S.

57. Wallace JM. Nutritional and botanical modulation of the inflammatory cascade — eicosanoids, cyclooxygenases, and lipoxygenases — as an adjunct in cancer therapy. *Integr Cancer Ther* 2002; 1(1):7–37.

58. U.S. Food and Drug Administration. Vioxx (rofecoxib) Drug Information Page. U.S. Food and Drug Administration. 2005. http://www.fda.gov/cder/drug/infopage/vioxx/default.htm.

59. Bremner P, Heinrich M. Natural products as targeted modulators of the nuclear factor-κB pathway. *J Pharm Pharmacol* 2002; 54(4):453–472.

60. Ferguson LR. Natural and man-made mutagens and carcinogens in the human diet. *Mutat Res* 1999; 443(1–2):1–10.

61. Heber D, Go V. Future directions in cancer and nutrition research: gene–nutrient interaction and the xenobiotic hypothesis. In: Heber D, Blackburn G, Go V, eds. *Nutritional Oncology*. San Diego, CA: Academic Press; 1999:613–619.

62. Kris-Etherton PM, Hecker KD, Bonanome A et al. Bioactive compounds in foods: their role in the prevention of cardiovascular disease and cancer. *Am J Med* 2002; 113(Suppl 9B):71S–88S.

63. Lampe JW, Peterson S. *Brassica*, biotransformation and cancer risk: genetic polymorphisms alter the preventive effects of cruciferous vegetables. *J Nutr* 2002; 132(10):2991–2994.

64. Lin HJ, Probst-Hensch NM, Louie AD et al. Glutathione transferase null genotype, broccoli, and lower prevalence of colorectal adenomas. *Cancer Epidemiol Biomarkers Prev* 1998; 7(8):647–652.

65. Jaenisch R, Bird A. Epigenetic regulation of gene expression: how the genome integrates intrinsic and environmental signals. *Nat Genet* 2003; 33(Suppl):245–254.

66. Ross SA. Diet and DNA methylation interactions in cancer prevention. *Ann N Y Acad Sci* 2003; 983:197–207.

67. Henning S, Swendseid ME. The role of folate, choline, and methionine in carcinogenesis induced by methyl-deficient diets. In: Heber D, Kritchevsky D, eds. *Dietary Fats, Lipids, Hormones, and Tumorigenesis*. New York: Plenum Press; 1996:143–155.

68. Bhave MR, Wilson MJ, Poirier LA. *c*-H-*ras* and *c*-K-*ras* gene hypomethylation in the livers and hepatomas of rats fed methyl-deficient, amino acid-defined diets. *Carcinogenesis* 1988; 9(3):343–348.

69. Zapisek WF, Cronin GM, Lyn-Cook BD, Poirier LA. The onset of oncogene hypomethylation in the livers of rats fed methyl-deficient, amino acid-defined diets. *Carcinogenesis* 1992; 13(10):1869–1872.

70. Pogribny IP, Miller BJ, James SJ. Alterations in hepatic p53 gene methylation patterns during tumor progression with folate/methyl deficiency in the rat. *Cancer Lett* 1997; 115(1):31–38.

71. Banerjee P, Chatterjee M. Antiproliferative role of vitamin D and its analogs — a brief overview. *Mol Cell Biochem* 2003; 253(1–2):247–254.

72. Holick MF. Vitamin D: importance in the prevention of cancers, type 1 diabetes, heart disease, and osteoporosis. *Am J Clin Nutr* 2004; 79(3):362–371.

73. Tangpricha V, Flanagan JN, Whitlatch LW et al. 25-Hydroxyvitamin D-1α-hydroxylase in normal and malignant colon tissue. *Lancet* 2001; 357(9269):1673–1674.

74. Cross HS, Bareis P, Hofer H et al. 25-Hydroxyvitamin $D_3$-1α-hydroxylase and vitamin D receptor gene expression in human colonic mucosa is elevated during early cancerogenesis. *Steroids* 2001; 66(3–5):287–292.

75. Lointier P, Wargovich MJ, Saez S, Levin B, Wildrick DM, Boman BM. The role of vitamin $D_3$ in the proliferation of a human colon cancer cell line *in vitro*. *Anticancer Res* 1987; 7(4B):817–821.

76. Glinghammar B, Rafter J. Carcinogenesis in the colon: interaction between luminal factors and genetic factors. *Eur J Cancer Prev* 1999; 9(Suppl 1):S87–S94.

77. Shabahang M, Buras RR, Davoodi F et al. Growth inhibition of HT-29 human colon cancer cells by analogues of 1α,25-dihydroxyvitamin $D_3$. *Cancer Res* 1994; 54(15):4057–4064.

78. Thomas MG, Tebbutt S, Williamson RC. Vitamin D and its metabolites inhibit cell proliferation in human rectal mucosa and a colon cancer cell line. *Gut* 1992; 33(12):1660–1663.

79. Brenner RV, Shabahang M, Schumaker LM et al. The antiproliferative effect of vitamin D analogs on MCF-7 human breast cancer cells. *Cancer Lett* 1995; 92(1):77–82.

80. Buras RR, Schumaker LM, Davoodi F et al. Vitamin D receptors in breast cancer cells. *Breast Cancer Res Treat* 1994; 31(2–3):191–202.

81. Campbell MJ, Reddy GS, Koeffler HP. Vitamin $D_3$ analogs and their 24-oxo metabolites equally inhibit clonal proliferation of a variety of cancer cells but have differing molecular effects. *J Cell Biochem* 1997; 66(3):413–425.

82. de Vos S, Holden S, Heber D et al. Effects of potent vitamin $D_3$ analogs on clonal proliferation of human prostate cancer cell lines. *Prostate* 1997; 31(2):77–83.

83. Koeffler HP, Amatruda T, Ikekawa N, Kobayashi Y, DeLuca HF. Induction of macrophage differentiation of human normal and leukemic myeloid stem cells by 1α,25-dihydroxyvitamin $D_3$ and its fluorinated analogues. *Cancer Res* 1984; 44(12 Pt 1):5624–5628.

84. Thomas MG. Luminal and humoral influences on human rectal epithelial cytokinetics. *Ann R Coll Surg Engl* 1995; 77(2):85–89.

85. Cross HS, Huber C, Peterlik M. Antiproliferative effect of 1α,25-dihydroxyvitamin $D_3$ and its analogs on human colon adenocarcinoma cells (CaCo-2): influence of extracellular calcium. *Biochem Biophys Res Commun* 1991; 179(1):57–62.

86. Frampton RJ, Suva LJ, Eisman JA et al. Presence of 1α,25-dihydroxyvitamin $D_3$ receptors in established human cancer cell lines in culture. *Cancer Res* 1982; 42:1116–1119.

87. Shabahang M, Buras RR, Davoodi F, Schumaker LM, Nauta RJ, Evans SR. 1α,25-dihydroxyvitamin D₃ receptor as a marker of human colon carcinoma cell line differentiation and growth inhibition. *Cancer Res* 1993; 53(16):3712–3718.

88. Sheinin Y, Kaserer K, Wrba F et al. *In situ* mRNA hybridization analysis and immunolocalization of the vitamin D receptor in normal and carcinomatous human colonic mucosa: relation to epidermal growth factor receptor expression. *Virchows Arch* 2000; 437(5):501–507.

89. Belleli A, Shany S, Levy J, Guberman R, Lamprecht SA. A protective role of 1α,25-dihydroxyvitamin D₃ in chemically induced rat colon carcinogenesis. *Carcinogenesis* 1992; 13(12):2293–2298.

90. Kallay E, Pietschmann P, Toyokuni S et al. Characterization of a vitamin D receptor knockout mouse as a model of colorectal hyperproliferation and DNA damage. *Carcinogenesis* 2001; 22(9):1429–1435.

91. Lamprecht SA, Lipkin M. Chemoprevention of colon cancer by calcium, vitamin D and folate: molecular mechanisms. *Nat Rev Cancer* 2003; 3(8):601–614.

92. Yanagisawa J, Yanagi Y, Masuhiro Y et al. Convergence of transforming growth factor-beta and vitamin D signaling pathways on SMAD transcriptional coactivators. *Science* 1999; 283(5406):1317–1321.

93. Gurlek A, Pittelkow MR, Kumar R. Modulation of growth factor/cytokine synthesis and signaling by 1α,25-dihydroxyvitamin D₃: implications in cell growth and differentiation. *Endocr Rev* 2002; 23(6):763–786.

94. Yanagi Y, Suzawa M, Kawabata M, Miyazono K, Yanagisawa J, Kato S. Positive and negative modulation of vitamin D receptor function by transforming growth factor-beta signaling through smad proteins. *J Biol Chem* 1999; 274(19):12971–12974.

95. Chen A, Davis BH, Sitrin MD, Brasitus TA, Bissonnette M. Transforming growth factor-beta 1 signaling contributes to Caco-2 cell growth inhibition induced by 1α,25(OH)₂D₃. *Am J Physiol Gastr Liver Physiol* 2002; 283(4):G864–G874.

96. Ylikomi T, Laaksi I, Lou YR et al. Antiproliferative action of vitamin D. *Vitam Horm* 2002; 64:357–406.

97. Scaglione-Sewell BA, Bissonnette M, Skarosi S, Abraham C, Brasitus TA. A vitamin D₃ analog induces a G₁-phase arrest in CaCo-2 cells by inhibiting cdk2 and cdk6: roles of cyclin E, p21[Waf1], and p27[Kip1]. *Endocrinology* 2000; 141(11):3931–3939.

98. Jensen SS, Madsen MW, Lukas J, Binderup L, Bartek J. Inhibitory effects of 1,25-dihydroxyvitamin D₃ on the G₁-S phase-controlling machinery. *Mol Endocrinol* 2001; 15(8):1370–1380.

99. Vandewalle B, Wattez N, Lefebvre J. Effects of vitamin D₃ derivatives on growth, differentiation and apoptosis in tumoral colonic HT29 cells: possible implication of intracellular calcium. *Cancer Lett* 1995; 97(1):99–106.

100. Diaz GD, Paraskeva C, Thomas MG, Binderup L, Hague A. Apoptosis is induced by the active metabolite of vitamin D₃ and its analogue EB1089 in colorectal adenoma and carcinoma cells: possible implications for prevention and therapy. *Cancer Res* 2000; 60(8):2304–2312.

101. Palmer HG, Gonzalez-Sancho JM, Espada J et al. Vitamin D₃ promotes the differentiation of colon carcinoma cells by the induction of E-cadherin and the inhibition of beta-catenin signaling. *J Cell Biol* 2001; 154(2):369–387.

102. Makishima M, Lu TT, Xie W et al. Vitamin D receptor as an intestinal bile acid sensor. *Science* 2002; 296(5571):1313–1316.

103. Pence BC, Buddingh F. Inhibition of dietary fat-promoted colon carcinogenesis in rats by supplemental calcium or vitamin $D_3$. *Carcinogenesis* 1988; 9(1):187–190.

104. Beaty MM, Lee EY, Glauert HP. Influence of dietary calcium and vitamin D on colon epithelial cell proliferation and 1,2-dimethylhydrazine-induced colon carcinogenesis in rats fed high fat diets. *J Nutr* 1993; 123(1):144–152.

105. Sitrin MD, Halline AG, Abrahams C, Brasitus TA. Dietary calcium and vitamin D modulate 1,2-dimethylhydrazine-induced colonic carcinogenesis in the rat. *Cancer Res* 1991; 51(20):5608–5613.

106. Llor X, Jacoby RF, Teng B-B, Davidson NO, Sitrin MD, Brasitus TA. K-*ras* mutations in 1,2-dimethylhydrazine-induced colonic tumors: effects of supplemental dietary calcium and vitamin D deficiency. *Cancer Res* 1991; 51:4305–4309.

107. Comer PF, Clark TD, Glauert HP. Effect of dietary vitamin $D_3$ (cholecalciferol) on colon carcinogenesis induced by 1,2-dimethylhydrazine in male Fischer 344 rats. *Nutr Cancer* 1993; 19(2):113–124.

108. Iseki K, Tatsuta M, Uehara H et al. Inhibition of angiogenesis as a mechanism for inhibition by 1α-hydroxyvitamin $D_3$ and 1α,25-dihydroxyvitamin $D_3$ of colon carcinogenesis induced by azoxymethane in Wistar rats. *Int J Cancer* 1999; 81(5):730–733.

109. Huerta S, Irwin RW, Heber D et al. 1α,25-$(OH)_2$-$D_3$ and its synthetic analogue decrease tumor load in the Apc*min* mouse. *Cancer Res* 2002; 62(3):741–746.

110. Go VL, Butrum RR, Wong DA. Diet, nutrition, and cancer prevention: the postgenomic era. *J Nutr* 2003; 133(11 Suppl 1):3830S–3836S.

111. Lippman SM, Hong WK. Cancer prevention by delay. Commentary re: J. A. O'Shaughnessy et al., Treatment and prevention of intraepithelial neoplasia: an important target for accelerated new agent development. *Clin Cancer Res* 2002 8:314–346; *Clin Cancer Res* 2002; 8(2):305–313.

112. Friso S, Choi SW. Gene–nutrient interactions and DNA methylation. *J Nutr* 2002; 132(8 Suppl):2382S–2387S.

# Part II

---

*Dietary Components That
Protect from Cancer: Vitamins*

# 3 Vitamin A, β-Carotene, and Cancer

*Joseph L. Napoli*

## CONTENTS

3.1 Vitamin A (all-*trans*-retinol) Homeostasis.................................................61
3.2 Systemic Functions of Vitamin A ...........................................................62
3.3 Mechanism of Vitamin A Action .............................................................63
3.4 Mechanisms of Complexity in Vitamin A Signaling..............................64
3.5 Vitamin A and Cancer in Experimental Animals ....................................65
3.6 Epidemiological Insight into Vitamin A, Carotenoids, and Cancer.........68
3.7 Clinical Trials with Retinoids .................................................................69
3.8 Conclusions...............................................................................................71
References ..........................................................................................................71

## 3.1 VITAMIN A (ALL-*TRANS*-RETINOL) HOMEOSTASIS

Insight into the sources, metabolism, and homeostasis of vitamin A will facilitate our ability to decipher whether vitamin A status in humans correlates inversely with cancer risk and supports its potential as a cancer chemopreventive agent. Vitamin A is the compound all-*trans*-retinol. All-*trans*-retinol, however, does not have biological activity in its own right. Rather, it serves as the substrate for producing metabolites that fulfill the functions of vitamin A. These metabolites include, but may not be limited to, the cofactor in rhodopsin, 11-*cis*-retinal, and the humoral transducer of systemic vitamin A action, all-*trans*-retinoic acid (RA).[1–5] The term *vitamin A*, therefore, pertains to a specific compound, all-*trans*-retinol. The term also denotes the spectrum of biological activity, as in "vitamin A activity," produced indirectly by retinol.[6] The term *retinoids* refers to all compounds, both naturally occurring and synthetic, which have vitamin A activity.[7]

Although vitamin A intake seems adequate in most of the population of North America and Europe, this appears to be an evolutionarily aberrant situation. Indeed, the usual situation, as evidenced by recurrent problems in countries outside of North America and Europe, seems to be limited vitamin A intake, resulting from generally poor, often nutritionally monotonous diets.[8] In North America and Europe preformed vitamin A accounts for 60 to 80% of vitamin A

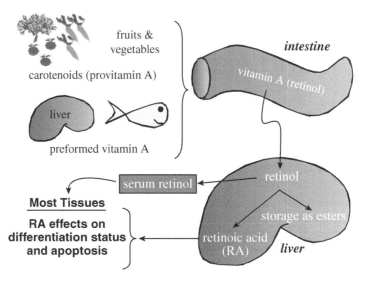

**FIGURE 3.1** A schematic depicting the sources of vitamin A and its uptake and storage in the liver as retinyl esters. Vitamin A is converted into RA in liver and delivered to extrahepatic tissues, and vitamin A itself is delivered to extrahepatic tissues and converted *in situ* into RA.

requirements, whereas in south Asia and Africa, carotenoids serve as the major vitamin A precursors. This confounds the issue whether dietary intake of vitamin A or carotenoids, or both, correlate with risk of various diseases. Common dietary sources of vitamin A include liver, dairy products, and fish, such as herring, sardines, and tuna. Common dietary sources of provitamin A carotenoids include carrots, yellow squash, corn, dark-green leafy vegetables, and red palm oil. Only ~50 of the 600 carotenoids found in nature have provitamin A activity, however. As a result, color is not a reliable indicator of the vitamin A value of vegetables. Regardless of the source, all-*trans*-retinol accounts for the quantitatively major circulating retinoid in serum. But unless it is very low or in excess, serum retinol does not reflect vitamin A status, because with adequate vitamin A stores in liver, the liver homeostatically controls plasma retinol levels. In addition, other factors can affect plasma vitamin A within the genetically and liver-stores determined range, such as infection and inadequate intake of other nutrients (e.g., zinc and protein) (Figure 3.1).

## 3.2  SYSTEMIC FUNCTIONS OF VITAMIN A

Normal reproduction occurs only in animals with adequate vitamin A status. The estrus cycle, normal epithelia in female reproductive organs (and therefore conception), spermatogenesis, placentation, and embryogenesis, all require retinoids for normal growth and function.[1,9] Retinoid deficiency in early pregnancy results in failure of placentation. Deficiency later in pregnancy, but in the first trimester, results in birth defects, especially heart and craniofacial defects. Deficiency postnatally impairs growth and fertility, depresses the immune response and neurofunction, and causes a host of problems related to abnormal stem cell differentiation and proliferation (e.g., squamous metaplasia of the epithelium). Maintenance of the appropriate differentiation state of many tissues/systems (epithelial, nerve, immune system) depends on retinoid status. Retinoids also regulate apoptosis in the immune system and during embryogenesis.

Contrasting skin with other epithelial cell-containing tissues provides an example of retinoid action. Retinoids prevent basal skin cells from terminally differentiating. Thus, the skin keratinizes during normal vitamin A status. In contrast, retinoids induce epithelial cells in the airways (and reproductive and digestive tracks) to terminally differentiate. Thus, intestine, trachea, etc., are soft, mucus-secreting tissues that do not keratinize. In the absence of retinoids, the trachea will fail to differentiate, resulting in squamous metaplasia — a proliferation of abnormal cells that cornify (keratinize), resulting in loss of integrity and function.

The first symptoms of vitamin A depletion are the readily reversible loss of peripheral vision and nyctalopia (night blindness). Long-term deficiency causes degeneration of the epithelial tissues including the cornea, resulting in xerophthalmia, i.e., ulceration of the cornea and inflammation of the eye that can lead to permanent corneal damage, progressing to irreversible blindness. Chronic toxicity can result after weeks to years of excessive vitamin A intake ($\geq$ tenfold the recommended daily allowance [RDA]), producing headaches, alopecia, dry and itching skin, cracked lips, hepatomegaly, bone and joint pain, and many other symptoms. Ultimately, permanent damage to liver, bone, and vision can occur, which can cause death. The most serious teratogenic effects of vitamin A include fetal resorbtion, abortion, birth defects, and permanent learning disabilities in offspring. Especially toxic are RA and the synthetic retinoids that have long biological elimination $t_{1/2}$.

## 3.3 MECHANISM OF VITAMIN A ACTION

RA and its isomer, 9-*cis*-retinoic acid (9cRA), serve as ligands that activate ligand-activated transcription factors that belong to a superfamily of nuclear receptors.[10] This superfamily of related genes expresses nuclear receptors for steroids (the female sex hormones estrogen and progesterone, the mineralocorticoid aldosterone, the glucocorticoid cortisol, the male sex hormones testosterone and dihydrotestosterone), prostanoids, the thyroid hormone, the hormonal form of vitamin D, calcitriol, and peroxisome proliferators. Additionally, more than 50 orphan receptors belong to this family. Two classes of retinoid receptors occur: retinoic acid receptors (RAR) and retinoid X receptors (RXR). Each has three different versions (α, β, and γ) encoded by distinct genes. Each version also has multiple isoforms resulting from differential promoter use and alternative RNA splicing. Thus, multiple forms of each occur (e.g., RARα1, RARα2, etc.). Moreover, RAR functions as a heterodimer with RXR. The multiple forms of both RAR and RXR predict 48 different combinations. Several other receptors (e.g., vitamin D receptor; peroxisome proliferator activated receptors; thyroid hormone receptor) function as heterodimers with RXR. RXRs therefore seem to serve as "master" permissive factors for several hormones. Vertebrates conserve each receptor, e.g., greater sequence similarity occurs between mouse and human RARα than between human RARα and RARβ.[10]

Despite the expectation of exquisite specificity fostered by the various discrete combinations of RAR and RXR isoforms, these receptors exhibit a great deal of apparent functional redundancy and/or ability to compensate for loss of another. In gene knockout experiments, more than one receptor can perform the same function *in vivo*, although this may represent an artifact of the knockouts and demonstrate what can happen, not necessarily what does occur.[11] Nevertheless, receptor ablation has provided enormous insight into receptor function. Deletion of the RARα gene results in postnatal lethality within 24 h: RARα-null mice represent only 3% of the population by 1 to 2 months of age. Of these, 60% have webbed digits on both fore and hind limbs. A few mice survive 4 to 5 months, but no males are fertile, and all have severe degeneration of the testis germinal epithelium. RARβ-null mice have locomotor defects, reminiscent of Parkinson's disease, but are fertile with normal longevity. RARβ-null mice have impaired hippocampal synaptic plasticity and compromised short-term learning (as do RXRγ-null mice). Also, the β2 isoform of RAR may serve as a tumor suppressor (see below). RARγ mutants show growth deficiency (40 to 80% of the weight of the wild-type mice), early lethality (50% dead by 1 to 3 weeks old and <40% surviving by 3 months) and male sterility due to squamous metaplasia of the seminal vesicles and prostate gland. No genitourinary defects occurred in null females, which are fertile. Mice with null mutations in either RXRα or RXRβ die between gestational ages 9.5 and 10.5 and display a wide range of abnormalities. Although the direct cause of death appears to be malformation of the placenta, RXR appear necessary for embryonic development before placentation. Mice null in RXRβ or RXRγ also have locomotor defects and blunted neuro responses, especially related to dopamine signaling.

## 3.4  MECHANISMS OF COMPLEXITY IN VITAMIN A SIGNALING

To fully appreciate the obstacles in using higher doses of exogenous retinoids in long-term chemotherapy, one must appreciate the complexity of retinoid signaling. First, precise concentrations of RA must be generated from retinol in a temporally and spatially specific manner.[12] This process involves not only several steps (retinyl ester hydrolysis, retinol dehydrogenation, retinal dehydrogenation), but multiple enzymes that catalyze each step.[13] After generation of RA, autoregulation also contributes to homeostasis through RA induction of degradative enzymes. In addition, multiple retinoid-specific binding proteins control substrate access to enzymes, RA concentrations, and RA access to receptors.[14,15] As mentioned earlier,

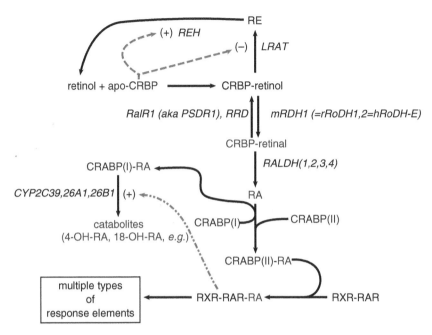

**FIGURE 3.2** An outline of vitamin A activation into RA and the degradation of RA illustrating the roles of retinoid-specific binding proteins. The abbreviations used are CRABP, cellular retinoic acid-binding protein; CRBP, cellular retinol-binding protein; CYP, cytochrome P450; LRAT, lecithin:retinol acyltransferase; RALDH, retinal dehydrogenase; RalR1 and RRD, retinal reductases; RDH and RoDH, retinol dehydrogenases; RE, retinyl esters; REH, retinyl ester hydrolase.

there are numerous potential combinations of RAR and RXR isoforms. In addition, the numerous genes regulated by RA manifest a variety of receptor heterodimer response elements. This entire system, illustrated in Figure 3.2, is subject to feedback and other types of control that are only beginning to be understood. Any imposition of exogenous retinoids, especially in high concentrations and for the long term, invites a plethora of compensatory and potentially adverse responses, which almost certainly will have unpredictable effects.

## 3.5 VITAMIN A AND CANCER IN EXPERIMENTAL ANIMALS

Vitamin A has long been associated with decreased cancer incidence in animals, especially of epithelial cancers. This concept was promoted by early insights into the effects of vitamin A depletion on animals. Wolbach[16] published studies in 1925 demonstrating that vitamin A deficiency resulted in squamous metaplasia and correlated with increased respiratory and upper alimentary canal cancer. Studies with laboratory animals, prompted by these early observations, revealed the conversion of mucous secreting and/or ciliated epithelium into squamous keratinizing epithelial as the most conspicuous effects of vitamin A deficiency. These observations focused attention of vitamin A function on epithelia, and gave birth to the conclusion that the primary systemic function of vitamin A was to control epithelial differentiation.[1] These observations also prompted multiple intervention studies with laboratory animals, which concluded that dosing with various retinoids (retinyl palmitate, retinyl acetate, RA) reduced the incidence of chemically induced (7,12-dimethyl-1,2-benzanthracene, benzo[a]pyrine, 3-methylcholanthrene, N-methyl-N-nitrosourea) lesions in several epithelial targets, including the respiratory tract, the stomach, the vagina, and skin.[17] Most likely because of poorly controlled protocols and/or different protocols that really were not comparable, the earliest animal studies reported mixed results of dietary vitamin A supplementation on the incidence of chemically caused carcinogenesis. Many studies, however, showed amazing reductions in cancer incidence using larger amounts of vitamin A in rodents exposed to chemical carcinogens. This stimulated great interest to pursue vitamin A and retinoid supplementation in cancer chemoprevention.

For example, as reviewed by De Luca,[17] a study with golden hamsters painted a 5% solution of DMBA twice weekly for 13 weeks on check pouches and either fed a vitamin A-depleted diet (but not necessarily deficient) or gave a pair-fed group (400 nmol) retinyl palmitate per week. Oddly, the death rate of the vitamin A-supplemented animals was twice as high as the depleted animals, but the cancer rate in the surviving vitamin A-dosed animals was fivefold lower.[18] A more clearly promising outcome was noted in a study in which hamsters were dosed with DMBA (10 mg/week) or BP (10 mg/week) with or without co-dosing with retinyl palmitate (100 mg/week = 190,000 nmol). The incidence of stomach cancer was 22 and 62% in the DMBA- and BP-dosed hamsters, respectively, and 0% in both carcinogen plus retinyl palmitate-dosed groups.[19] Note, however, that the recommended amount of vitamin A in the AIN93 rodent diet is 4 nmol retinol/g diet (1 nmol = 1 IU). Sequential dosing studies, perhaps, provided a more realistic model, at least of chemoprevention "after the fact." Retinyl palmitate (19,000 nmol/week for life) decreased respiratory tumors 66% and squamous tumors 90% in hamsters dosed with BP intratracheally. Higher concentrations of vitamin A (7700 nmol) started 1 week after BP exposure increased the incidence of respiratory tumors 40%, but the tumor incidence decreased 20% when the hamsters were placed in laminar flow hoods.[20]

These studies were characterized by high doses of carcinogens applied topically or dosed intragastrically to rodents, higher doses of vitamin A or its esters (not synthetic retinoids), and were done using stock diets, with few exceptions. They examined a variety of tissues. These variables made it difficult to draw clear conclusions, but the studies did demonstrate that under certain circumstances pharmacological doses of vitamin A can prevent chemically induced epithelial cancer in some rodent tissues. This is an intriguing conclusion, but left unresolved whether a lifetime of enhanced vitamin A nutrition would help prevent cancer and whether diet has a confounding influence on vitamin A effects.

As more animal studies were published and studies were broadened to include RA and synthetic retinoids, clearer patterns emerged in laboratory animals.[21] Perhaps the earliest, most consistent effects of vitamin A and other retinoids were obtained with the initiation/promotion model of skin carcinoma. Painting mice skin with a single dose of a carcinogen, such as DMBA, followed by one or more paintings with a promoter, such as croton oil or TPA, invariably produces many papillomas. Within 5 to 8 months, a few percent of the papillomas develop into carcinomas. Bollag[22] showed that intraperitoneally dosing with high amounts of RA (100 mg/kg = >300,000 nmol) reduced papilloma volume >80% relative to controls. In a subsequent study, Bollag[23] showed that oral dosing with RA (200 mg/kg every 2 weeks) during promotion also reduced the incidence of carcinomas by ~67%. These results presaged data, which consistently showed that retinol, retinyl palmitate, RA, and certain synthetic retinoids delayed appearance of skin papillomas, decreased their number and volume, and decreased their rate of progression into carcinomas in rabbits, mice, and rats. Mechanistic work on this phenomenon demonstrated that in this model retinoids function as antipromoters, specifically inhibiting induction of ornithine decarboxylase, an enzyme necessary for replication.[24] These insights were extended by the demonstration that skin basal cell carcinomas in humans regressed upon topical RA treatment.[23,25]

Retinyl acetate, fed in rather high amounts (250 to 750 nmol/g food) to rats also has a chemopreventive effect with respect to mammary tumors induced by chemical carcinogens including BP, DMBA, and MNU.[22] However, retinyl acetate causes hepatoxicity at effective doses. Fortunately, the synthetic retinoid N-(4-hydroxyphenyl)retinamide (fenretinide) also is effective, and tends to concentrate in the breast.[26] Curiously, dietary 13-*cis*-RA is not an effective chemopreventive of MNU-induced breast cancer. These results illustrate two issues concerning retinoids as chemopreventives: (1) doses/compounds effective against cancer in one tissue may have toxic effects in other tissues; (2) chemopreventive activity in test systems *in vitro* often does not predict actions in the intact mammal. Obviously, the pharmacology of a retinoid (tissue distribution, metabolism rate, etc.) has great impact on its chemopreventive action and toxicity *in vivo*.

The conclusion that specific retinoids act on cancer of specific tissues in experimental animals is extended by the observation of the impact of retinoids on bladder cancer.[27] For example, 13-*cis*-RA reduces the incidence of transitional cell carcinoma in rats initiated by N-butyl-N-(4-hydroxybutyl)nitrosamine, a bladder-specific carcinogen. Recall that dietary 13-*cis*-RA does not prevent MNU-induced breast cancer in rats. It is also important to note that transitional cell carcinoma accounts for the major type of human bladder cancer, rather than squamous cell carcinoma.

Lasnitski[28] developed organ culture of mouse prostate and demonstrated with it that RA and synthetic retinoids could inhibit or reverse MC-induced neoplastic changes. This, of course, generated a great deal of interest in the potential use of retinoids to prevent and/or treat prostate cancer. A subsequent study demonstrated that fenretinide, a retinoid active against carcinogen-induced breast cancer, caused a 76% decrease in prostate cancer in rats treated with the carcinogen MNU and testosterone.[29] In addition, RA and other retinoids at higher doses inhibited the growth of established prostate cancer cell lines and induced apoptosis.[30] Perhaps not surprisingly, given previous experience with retinoids and with established cell lines, retinoid effects on cultured prostate cancer cells are retinoid- and cell line-dependent. RA, for example, is effective with LNCaP cells, WPEI-NB11, and WEI-NB14 cells, but not with DU-145 or PC-3 cells. Fenretinide, however, was more effective than RA in the WPEI cell lines. Alas, these are established cancer cell lines. Regardless of these reports of success, and others like them,[27] a very recent review of the literature concluded that "no evidence" exists that vitamin A or synthetic retinoids can be used as prostate cancer chemopreventive agents, because of either toxicity or lack of efficacy.[31] Consistent with this conclusion, a review of clinical studies with RA concluded that only modest effects were obtained in inducing apoptosis of prostate cancer.[30]

To summarize: (1) there tends to be a degree of species, retinoid, carcinogen, and tissue specificity associated with the effects of retinoids on cancer chemoprevention in experimental animals; (2) *in vitro* models, especially cancer cells in culture, are not necessarily good predictors of retinoid chemopreventive effects in intact animals; (3) doses of retinoids that act chemopreventively at one site in intact animals may be toxic to other tissues. Nevertheless, retinoids still hold tremendous potential as cancer chemopreventive or therapeutic agents. Use of synthetic retinoids, as exemplified by fenretinide, may circumvent toxicity associated with naturally occurring retinoids.

## 3.6 EPIDEMIOLOGICAL INSIGHT INTO VITAMIN A, CAROTENOIDS, AND CANCER

Early epidemiological studies and limited measurements of blood retinol seemed to support an inverse relationship between vitamin A intake and cancer, and/or blood retinol and cancer, and/or β-carotene intake and cancer in humans (reviewed in References 32 and 33). The current body of knowledge, however, does not support such conclusions. First, as pointed out above, serum retinol is a poor indicator of vitamin A status and of vitamin A and carotenoid intake. Second, retinol in serum samples can be adversely affected easily by storage and handling, producing misleading results. Third, many of the epidemiological studies concluding that an inverse relationship existed between vitamin A and cancer, based their conclusions on an inverse relationship between colored vegetable intake and cancer. As mentioned above, color is not a reliable indicator of the vitamin A value of vegetables; in addition, each type of vegetable can contain up to 10,000 different phytochemicals. Certain of these phytochemicals seem to have potent anticancer activity. Lately, a focused study on bladder cancer (the Netherlands Cohort Study of >120,000 persons >6 years) has further uncoupled supplementation with dietary vitamin A and carotenoids with reducing cancer risk.[34]

## 3.7 CLINICAL TRIALS WITH RETINOIDS

Acute promyelocytic leukemia (APL) shows the most spectacular response to retinoid treatment, consistent with results in the cultured human APL cell line HL60.[35] Combined therapy with RA and conventional chemotherapy produces 70% long-term remission.[36] A few cases of APL develop resistance to RA therapy. In contrast, although RA alone has spectacular initial effects on patients with the form of APL that involves the t(15,17)-translocation, which produces the fusion protein PML-RARα, many of these patients relapse and become resistant to further RA therapy, for reasons still debated.

Oral retinol (25,000 nmol/day) reduces by 32% the development of squamous cell carcinomas of the skin in high-risk patients, with no apparent toxicity, as shown in a study that involved 5 years of treatment and nearly 4 years of follow-up.[37] In contrast, oral retinol had no effect on basal cell carcinoma, and neither retinol nor isotretinoin (13-*cis*-RA) affected the incidence of nonmelanoma skin cancers. An extension of this work demonstrated the safety and enhanced efficacy of using 50,000 and 75,000 nmol/day of vitamin A for 1 year in patients with sun-damaged skin.[38]

Organ transplant patients suffer from an increased incidence of premalignant skin lesions and from nonmelanoma skin cancers. The synthetic aromatic retinoid acitretin — Soriatane or all-*trans*-9-(4-methoxy-2,3,6-trimethylphenyl)-3,7-dimethyl-2,4,6,8-nonatetraenoic acid) — is effective systemically as a chemopreventive agent for skin premalignant lesions and cancer, but only during treatment. Like fenretinide, discontinuation of acitretin treatment results in complete loss of chemopreventive effects, indicating need for lifetime therapy.[39,40]

The RAR ligands RA, isotretinoin, etretinate, and acitretin have been used to treat disorders in which malignant T cells accumulate in skin, known as cutaneous T-cell lymphomas.[41] Depending on the retinoid used, the response rate with RAR agonists was as high as 85% and the complete response rate was as high as 33%. The RXR ligand bexarotene has been approved recently for clinical use for the same indication. Higher oral doses (650 mg/m$^2$) provide response rates as high as 67% and complete responses as high as 54%.[41-43] Lower toxicity compared to RAR ligands has been suggested as an anticipated benefit of bexoretine, because bexoretine produces only "laboratory abnormalities," such as hypertriglyceridemia, hypercholesterolemia, hypothyroidism, and leukopenia, which may be addressed with other drugs without discontinuing retinoid therapy.[41] In contrast, RAR ligands commonly produce side effects of dry skin, conjunctivitis, alopecia, headache, and bone changes. Not unexpectedly, the RAR ligands demonstrate vitamin A excess symptoms, whereas RXR ligands demonstrate consequences of activating nuclear receptors that heterodimerize with RXR, such as PPAR and LXR. Long-term studies should eventually determine the relative therapeutic indices of these two approaches.

Fenretinide represents one of the most promising cancer chemopreventive agents because of its activity in model systems, its lower toxicity compared to many other retinoids, and its tendency to show some tissue-specific uptake.

Disappointingly, in several Phase III clinical trials, fenretinide has not shown broad-based chemoprevention activity against cancer of the sites predicted as responders from studies in models, including breast, bladder, cervix, and head and neck. Two groups have concluded, however, that fenretinide may show an effect in reducing ovarian cancer, as long as treatment is continued, but not after, and possibly a reduction in second malignancies of the breast in premenopausal women, but not for second breast cancers in postmenopausal women.[44–46] Currently, there is hope for fenretinide, but final evaluation must await the outcome of further clinical investigation.

Isotretinoin has been evaluated fairly extensively for its ability to suppress second primary tumors in patients with head and neck squamous cell carcinoma.[47–49] High doses (50 to 100 mg/m$^2$/day) reduced by nearly fivefold the rate of second primary tumor occurrence over a 55 month period. The impact of isotretinoin continued for 2 years beyond cessation of dosing. Unfortunately, the majority of patients suffered from conjunctivitis, skin toxicities, and cheilitis and required dose reduction.[48] A trial to evaluate lower-dose use of isotretinoin (30 mg/day) for 3 years followed by another 4 years of appraisal in the absence of dosing reported no obvious anticancer effects.[49] Consistent with other studies, which often reveal retinoid-specific results, etretinate did not reduce the incidence of second primary tumors.[50] Treatment with retinyl palmitate for 2 years did not affect survival and second primary tumors formation in patients with head and neck cancer.[51]

Retinoids have been among the most widely tested agents for prevention of nonsmall cell lung cancer, reversal of premalignant lesions, and prevention of additional cancer in former lung cancer patients.[52–54] No large-scale, reproducible, randomized clinical trial has shown positive results, i.e., no impact of retinoids, including isotretinoin, fenretinide, etretinate, retinol, or retinyl palmitate, has been observed with respect to any of these three outcomes. In the Physician's Health, CARET, and ATBC studies, β-carotene alone had no impact or, in conjunction with α-tocopherol or retinol, was harmful. These data seem to indicate total gloom, but recent work relating RAR to lung tissue changes suggests continued studies might be warranted.[55] RAR, especially RARβ2, has been proposed as a tumor suppressor gene, because it is lost in squamous cell carcinomas and adenocarcinomas, is epigenetically silenced by hypermethylation in the early stages of lung cancer, and is not expressed in tumor samples of the esophagus, prostate, breast, and lung.[56] The effect of upregulating and activating RAR on the development of second primary lung cancers, however, seems related to whether the patients are current or former smokers. Only in former smokers was RAR upregulation and activation (unmethylated form) protective, through inhibiting carcinogenesis and inducing apoptosis. In current smokers, activation of RAR may enhance carcinogenesis.

Bladder cancer clinical trials with isotretinoin had too much toxicity to continue, whereas a double-blind trial with etretinate showed a modest overall impact, and has supported a call for large-scale trials with retinoids in superficial bladder cancer.[57]

## 3.8 CONCLUSIONS

Despite the indications by its functions and mechanisms of action that vitamin A should prevent cancer, and despite animal and *in vitro* work indicating that various retinoids are effective at chemoprevention, at this point it is easier to list the clinical trials that have been effective, than to relate the numerous failed attempts to apply the experimental science to humans without toxicity.[36] Nevertheless, besides the successes mentioned above, isotretinoin holds promise in neuroblastoma and in premalignant lesions, including oral leukoplakia and xeroderma pigmentosum.[58] The acylic retinoid analog polyprenoic acid reduces second primary hepatocarcinoma and 9-*cis*-RA (alitretinoin) shows promise for Kaposi's sarcoma. In hindsight, it is not surprising that progress has been slow, arising from the complexity of retinoid homeostasis and signaling, the pleiotropic functions of retinoids, retinoid toxicity, the complicated nature of cancer, and the intrusion of pharmacology on our desire to deliver retinoids selectively to cancer sites. Although the task appears formidable, compelling justification continues for pursuing use of retinoids in chemoprevention and therapy. Especially promising are the advent of additional synthetic retinoids that may be receptor specific, or show site-specific accumulation, or have more attractive therapeutic indices.

## REFERENCES

1. Wolf G. Multiple functions of vitamin A. *Physiol Rev* 1984; 64:873–937.
2. Olson JA. The irresistible fascination of carotenoids and vitamin A. *Am J Clin Nutr* 1993; 57:833–839.
3. Blomhoff R, Green MH, Green JB, Berg T, Norum KR. Vitamin A metabolism: new perspectives on absorption, transport, and storage. *Physiol Rev* 1991; 71:951–990.
4. Saari JC. Biochemistry of visual pigment regeneration: the Friedenwald lecture. *Invest Ophthalmol Vis Sci* 2000; 41:337–348.
5. Stephensen CB. Vitamin A, infection, and immune function. *Annu Rev Nutr* 2001; 21:167–192.
6. Olson JA. Needs and sources of carotenoids and vitamin A. *Nutr Rev* 1994; 52:S67–S73.
7. Olson, JA. Requirements and safety of vitamin A in humans. In: Livrea MA, ed. *Vitamin A and Retinoids: An Update of Biological Aspects and Clinical Applications, Molecular and Cell Biology Updates.* Boston: Birkhäuser Verlag; 2000:29–44.
8. Olson JA. Serum levels of vitamin A and carotenoids as reflectors of nutritional status. *J Natl Cancer Inst* 1984; 73:1439–1444.
9. Napoli JL. Vitamin A (retinoids). In: Lennarz WJ, Lane MD, eds. *Encyclopedia of Biological Chemistry.* New York: Elsevier; 2004: vol 4, 354–359.
10. Aranda A, Pascual A. Nuclear hormone receptors and gene expression. *Physiol Rev* 2001; 81:1269–1304.

11. Mark M, Ghyselinck NB, Wendling O, Dupe V, Mascrez B, Kastner P, Chambon P. A genetic dissection of the retinoid signaling pathway in the mouse. *Proc Nutr Soc* 1999; 58:609–613.

12. Maden M. Role of retinoic acid in embryonic and post-embryonic development. *Proc Nutr Soc* 2001; 59:65–73.

13. Napoli JL. Enzymology and biogenesis of retinoic acid, In: Livrea MA, ed. *Vitamin A and Retinoids: An Update of Biological Aspects and Clinical Applications, Molecular and Cell Biology Updates.* Boston: Birkhäuser Verlag; 2000:17–27.

14. Ong DE, Newcomer ME, Chytil F. Cellular retinoid-binding proteins. In: Sporn MB, Roberts AB, Goodman DS, eds. *The Retinoids: Biology, Chemistry and Medicine*, 2nd ed. New York: Raven Press; 1994: chapter 7, 283–318.

15. Napoli JL. Retinoic acid: its biosynthesis and metabolism. *Prog Nucl Acids Res* 2000; 63:139–188.

16. Wolbach SB. Tissues changes following deprivation of fat soluble A vitamin. *J Exp Med* 1925; 42:753–757.

17. De Luca L. Vitamin A. In: DeLuca HF, ed. *Handbook of Lipid Research 2*. New York: Plenum Press; 1978:47–53.

18. Rowe NH, Gorlin RJ. The effect of vitamin A deficiency upon experimental oral carcinogenesis. *J Dent Res* 1959; 38:72–83.

19. Chu EW, Malmgren RA. An inhibitory effect of vitamin A on the induction of tumors of forestomach and cervix in the Syrian golden hamster by carcinogenic polycyclic hydrocarbons. *Can Res* 1965; 25:884–895.

20. Smith DM, Rogers AE, Newberne PM. Vitamin A and benzo[a]pyrene carcinogenesis in the respiratory tract of hamsters fed a semi-synthetic diet. *Can Res* 1975; 35:1485–1488.

21. Hill DL, Grubbs CJ. Retinoids as chemopreventive and anticancer agents in intact animals (review). *Anticancer Res* 1982; 2:111–124.

22. Bollag W. Therapy of chemically induced skin tumors of mice with vitamin A palmitate and vitamin A acid. *Experientia* 1971; 27:90–92.

23. Bollag W. Prophylaxis of chemically induced benign and malignant epithelial tumors by vitamin A acid (retinoic acid). *Eur J Can* 1972; 8:689–693.

24. Verma AK. Retinoids in chemoprevention of cancer. *J Biol Regul Homeost Agents* 2003; 17:92–97.

25. Bollag W, Ott F. Vitamin A acid in benign and malignant epithelial tumours of the skin. *Acta Derm Venerol* 1975; Suppl 74:163–166.

26. Moon RC, Constantinou AI. Dietary retinoids and carotenoids in rodent models of mammary tumorigenesis. *Breast Cancer Res Treat* 1997; 46:181–189.

27. Moon RC, Mehta RG, Rao KVN. Retinoids and cancer in experimental animals. In: *The Retinoids*. New York: Raven Press; 1994: 573–595.

28. Lasnitski I. Reversal of methylcholanthrene-induced changes in mouse prostates in vitro by retinoic acid and its analogues. *Br J Cancer* 1976; 34:239–248.

29. Pollard M, Luckert PH, Sporn MB. Prevention of primary prostate cancer in Lobund-Wistar rats by N-(4-hydroxyphenyl)retinamide. *Can Res* 1991; 51:3610–3611.

30. Hammond LA, Brown G, Keedwell RG, Durham J, Chandraratna RAS. The prospects of retinoids in the treatment of prostate cancer. *Anti-Cancer Drugs* 2002; 13:781–790.

31. Kristal AR. Vitamin A, retinoids and carotenoids as chemopreventive agents for prostate cancer. *J Urol* 2004; 171:S54–S58.

32. Peto R, Doll R, Buckley JD, Sporn MB. Can dietary beta-carotene materially reduce human cancer rates? *Nature* 1981; 290:201–208.

33. Hong WK, Itri L. Retinoids and human cancer. In: *The Retinoids*. New York: Raven Press; 1994:597–658.

34. Zeegers MP, Goldbohn RA, van den Brandt PA. Are retinol, vitamin C, vitamin E, folate and carotenoids intake associated with bladder cancer risk? Results from the Netherlands cohort study. *Br J Cancer* 2001; 85:977–983.

35. Imaizumi M, Breitman TR. Retinoic acid-induced differentiation of the human promyelocytic leukemia cell line, HL-60, and fresh human leukemia cells in primary culture: a model for differentiation inducing therapy of leukemia. *Eur J Haematol* 1987; 38:289–302.

36. Freemantle SJ, Spinella MJ, Dmitrovsky E. Retinoids in cancer therapy and chemoprevention: promise meets resistance. *Oncogene* 2003; 22:7305–7315.

37. Stratton SP, Dorr RT, Alberts DS. The state-of-the-art in chemoprevention of skin cancer. *Eur J Cancer* 2000; 36:1292–1297.

38. Alberts D, Ranger-Moore J, Einspahr J, Saboda K, Bozzo P, Liu Y, Xu XC, Lotan R, Warneke J, Salasche S, Stratton S, Levine N, Goldman R, Islas M, Duckett L, Thompson D, Bartels P. Safety and efficacy of dose-intensive oral vitamin A in subjects with sun-damaged skin. *Clin Can* 2004; 10:1875–1880.

39. De Graaf YG, Euvrard S, Bouwes Bavinck JN. Systemic and topical retinoids in the management of skin cancer in organ transplant recipients. *Dermatol Surg* 2004; 30:656–661.

40. Smit JV, de Sevaux RG, Blokx WA, van de Kerkhof PC, Hoitsma AJ, de Jong EM. Acitretin treatment in (pre)malignant skin disorders of renal transplant recipients: histologic and immunohistochemical effects. *J Am Acad Dermatol* 2004; 50:189–196.

41. Zhang C, Duvic M. Retinoids: therapeutic applications and mechanisms of action in cutaneous T-cell lymphoma. *Dermatol Ther* 2003; 16:322–330.

42. Farol LT, Hymes KB. Bexarotene: a clinical review. *Expert Rev Anticancer Ther* 2004; 4:180–188.

43. Kempf W, Kettelhack N, Duvic M, Burg G. Topical and systemic retinoid therapy for cutaneous T-cell lymphoma. *Hematol Oncol Clin North Am.* 2000; 17:1405–1409.

44. Decensi A, Serrano D, Bonanni B, Cazzaniga M, Guerrieri-Gonzaga A. Breast cancer prevention trials using retinoids. *J Mammary Gland Biol Neoplasia* 2003; 8:19–30.

45. Malone W, Perloff M, Crowell J, Sigman C, Higley H. Fenretinide, a prototype cancer prevention drug. *Expert Opin Invest Drugs* 2003; 12:1829–1842.

46. Veronesi U, De Palo G, Marubini E, Costa A, Formelli F, Mariani L, Decensi A, Camerini T, Del Turco MR, Di Mauro MG, Muraca MG, Del Vecchio M, Pinto C, D'Aiuto G, Boni C, Campa T, Magni A, Miceli R, Perloff M, Malone WF, Sporn MB. Randomized trial of fenretinide to prevent second breast malignancy in women with early breast cancer. *J Natl Cancer Inst* 1999; 91:1847–1856.

47. Hong WK, Lippman SM, Itri LM, Karp DD, Lee JS, Byers RM, Schantz SP, Kramer AM, Lotan R, Peters LJ. Prevention of second primary tumors with isotretinoin in squamous-cell carcinoma of the head and neck. *N Engl J Med* 1990; 323:795–801.

48. Benner SE, Pajak TF, Lippman SM, Lippman SM, Hong WK, Schantz SP, Gallagher MJ, Shenouda G. Prevention of second primary tumors with isotretinoin in patients with squamous-cell carcinoma of the head and neck: follow-up. *J Natl Cancer Inst* (Bethesda) 1994; 86:140–141.

49. Khuri FR, Kim ES, Lee JJ, Winn RJ, Benner SE, Lippman SM, Fu KK, Cooper JS, Vokes EE, Chamberlain RM, Williams B, Pajak TF, Goepfert H, Hong WK. The impact of smoking status, disease stage, and index tumor site on second primary tumor incidence and tumor recurrence in the head and neck retinoid chemoprevention trial. *Cancer Epidemiol* 2001; 10:823–829.

50. Bolla M, Lefur R, Ton Van J, Domenge C, Badet JM, Koskas Y, Laplanche A. Prevention of second primary tumours with etretinate in squamous cell carcinoma of the oral cavity and oropharynx. Results of a multicentric double-blind randomised study. *Eur J Cancer* 1994; 30:767–772.

51. van Zandwijk N, Dalesio O, Pastorino U, de Vries N, van Tinteren H. Euroscan: a randomized trial of vitamin A and N-acetylcysteine in patients with head and neck or lung cancer. *J Natl Cancer Inst* 2000; 92:977–986.

52. Khuri FR, Cohen V. Molecularly targeted approaches to the chemoprevention of lung cancer. *Clin Cancer Res* 2004; 10:4249s–4253s.

53. van Zandwijk N, Hirsch FR. Chemoprevention of lung cancer: current status and future prospects. *Lung Cancer* 2003; 42 Suppl 1:S71–S9.

54. Kelley MJ, McCrory DC. Prevention of lung cancer: summary of published evidence. *Chest* 2003; 123(1 Suppl):50S–59S.

55. Khuri FR, Lotan R. Retinoids in lung cancer: friend foe, or fellow traveler? *J Clin Oncol* 2004; 22:3435–3477.

56. Soprano DR, Qin P, Soprano KJ. Retinoic acid receptors and cancer. *Annu Rev Nutr* 2004; 24:201–221.

57. Nutting C, Huddart RA. Rethinking the secondary prevention of superficial bladder cancer: is there a role for retinoids? *BJU Int* 2000; 85:1023–1026.

58. Niles RM. Recent advances in the use of vitamin A (retinoids) in the prevention and treatment of cancer. *Nutrition* 2000; 16:1084–1089.

# 4 Anticarcinogenic Activity of Natural and Synthetic Carotenoids

*Hoyoku Nishino, Michiaki Murakoshi,
Xiao Yang Mou, Saeri Wada,
Mitsuharu Masuda, Yasuhito Ohsaka,
Yoshiko Satomi, and Kenji Jinno*

## CONTENTS

Abstract .................................................................................................................76
Key Words ............................................................................................................76
4.1 Introduction ..................................................................................................76
4.2 Anticarcinogenic Activity of Vitamin A, Retinoids, and Rexinoids ........77
4.3 Anticarcinogenic Activity of Natural and Synthetic Carotenoids ............77
    4.3.1 β-Carotene (Synthetic) .................................................................78
    4.3.2 α-Carotene .....................................................................................78
    4.3.3 Lutein ............................................................................................79
    4.3.4 Zeaxanthin ....................................................................................80
    4.3.5 Lycopene .......................................................................................80
    4.3.6 β-Cryptoxanthin............................................................................82
    4.3.7 Other Carotenoids.........................................................................82
    4.3.8 Multicarotenoids ..........................................................................82
4.4 Production of Phytoene in Mammalian Cells.............................................84
    4.4.1 Establishment of Phytoene-Producing Mammalian Cells and
           Analysis of Their Properties .......................................................84
    4.4.2 Bio-Chemoprevention...................................................................85
4.5 Conclusion ...................................................................................................86
Acknowledgments ................................................................................................86
References ..............................................................................................................86

## ABSTRACT

Vitamin A deficiency has been known as a risk factor for various cancers, such as stomach cancer. Because long-term administration of vitamin A is practically difficult due to its hepatic toxicity, vitamin A analogs have been developed and applied for cancer prevention in clinical trials. Provitamin A carotenoids, which are widely distributed in vegetables and fruits, are also important nutritional factors as the source of vitamin A. These help to maintain our healthy condition, including risk reduction of cancer development. We should also pay attention to natural carotenoids other than provitamin A carotenoids, some of which were proved to have very potent anticarcinogenic activity. For example, lycopene is a very potent suppressor for liver cancer development. In the case of phytoene, the concept of "bio-chemoprevention," which means biotechnology-assisted method for cancer chemoprevention, may be applicable. In fact, establishment of mammalian cells producing phytoene was succeeded by the introduction of *crtB* gene, which encodes phytoene synthase, and these cells were proved to acquire the resistance against carcinogenesis. Antioxidative phytoene-containing animal foods may be classified as a novel type of functional food, which has the preventive activity against carcinogenesis, as well as the ability to reduce the accumulation of oxidative damage, which is hazardous for human health.

## KEY WORDS

vitamin A, natural carotenoids, multicarotenoids, cancer chemoprevention, bio-chemoprevention, functional foods

## 4.1  INTRODUCTION

Vitamin A as well as its precursor, provitamin A, are not synthesized by humans but must be supplied via diets. Because vitamin A is required for growth and various biological functions, its deficiency causes serious health problems. It has also been reported that vitamin A deficiency causes an increased rate of cancer development.

Information has accumulated indicating that diets rich in vegetables and fruits can reduce the risk of a number of chronic diseases, including cancer, cardiovascular disease, diabetes, and age-related macular degeneration. Various factors in plant foods, such as carotenoids, antioxidative vitamins, phenolic compounds, terpenoids, steroids, indoles, and fibers, have been considered responsible for the risk reduction. Among them, carotenoids have been studied widely and have proved to show diverse beneficial effects on human health. Initially, carotenoids in vegetables and fruits were suggested to serve as precursors of vitamin A. In this context, β-carotene has been studied most extensively, because β-carotene has the highest provitamin A activity among carotenoids.

Peto et al.[1] suggested that β-carotene could have a protective effect against cancer without converting to vitamin A. Then, carotenoids other than β-carotene may also contribute for the protection of cancer and various diseases. Of more than 600 carotenoids identified to date, about 40 carotenoids are found in our daily foods. However, as a result of selective uptake in the digestive tract, less than 20 carotenoids with some of their metabolites have been identified in human plasma and tissues. Thus, it is important to evaluate the biological activities of these carotenoids that are detectable in human body.

## 4.2 ANTICARCINOGENIC ACTIVITY OF VITAMIN A, RETINOIDS, AND REXINOIDS

Vitamin A deficiency has been known as a risk factor for various cancers, such as stomach cancer. Thus, vitamin A has been evaluated as a cancer-suppressing agent. However, it has been found that long-term administration of vitamin A is practically difficult due to its hepatic toxicity. In addition, less toxic vitamin A analogs, retinoids (fenretinide, E5166, Am88, KNK41, and others) and rexinoids (LGD1069, LG100268, and others), have been developed and applied for clinical trials to suppress cancer.

Among these vitamin A analogs, differences in potency and mode of action have been found. Therefore, it is important to select the best agents for each individual with different types of cancer. The differences in mode of action may result from differences in binding affinities to receptors. Retinoid receptors are classified into two subfamilies, retinoic acid receptors (RARs) and retinoid X receptors (RXRs). Among the natural vitamin A family, all-*trans*-retinoic acid has affinity for RARs, and 9-*cis*-retinoic acid shows high affinity for both RXRs and RARs.

The RXRs form stable heterodimers with RARs. They also can form homodimers and are capable of acting independently from RARs. Furthermore, RXRs also form heterodimers with the vitamin D receptor, the thyroid hormone receptors, and peroxisome proliferation-activating receptors. In this context, specific analogs for RXRs, which are now called rexinoids, are of particular interest for application to the field of control and regulation for various diseases and biological phenomena, including cancer control.

The first of the rexinoids to be used for this purpose was LGD1069 (Targretin®).[2,3] However, Targretin is not totally specific for binding to RXRs, and new rexinoids, which have essentially no affinity for RARs, such as LG100268, have been synthesized. Interestingly, new rexinoids do not have the classic toxicologic profile of retinoids, and thus seem to be very useful agents for cancer control.

## 4.3 ANTICARCINOGENIC ACTIVITY OF NATURAL AND SYNTHETIC CAROTENOIDS

Among the carotenoids, β-carotene has been expected to be the most promising candidate as a cancer preventive agent. Thus, β-carotene has been tested for cancer-preventive activity in interventional trials; i.e., two Linxian trials (Linxian 1 and Linxian 2), the Alpha-Tocopherol Beta-Carotene (ATBC) cancer prevention study, the β-Carotene and Retinol Efficacy Trial (CARET), the Physicians' Health Study (PHS), and the Skin Cancer Prevention Study (SCPS). In addition to these studies, we have recently completed an intervention trial with supplementation of a mixture of natural carotenoids (lycopene, β-carotene, α-carotene, and others) plus α-tocopherol (Jinno, K., Nishino, H. et al., patent pending: 2002-022958, 2002.1.31; see Section 4.3.8).

### 4.3.1  β-CAROTENE (SYNTHETIC)

In the Linxian 1 study, a protective effect of supplemental β-carotene, vitamin E, and selenium was reported with regard to the incidence and mortality rates of gastric cancer when compared with untreated subjects. In the Linxian 2 study, the relative risk for cancer mortality was 0.97 in men and 0.92 in women (not significant). At the end of follow-up in the ATBC cancer prevention study, 894 cases of lung cancer were reported. The numbers of lung cancer cases by intervention group were 204 in the α-tocopherol group, 242 in the β-carotene group, 240 in the α-tocopherol plus β-carotene group, and 208 in the placebo group. The group receiving β-carotene had a 16% higher incidence of lung cancer than those not given β-carotene. The excess risk associated with β-carotene supplementation was concentrated mainly among people who currently smoked more than 20 cigarettes per day and who drank more than 11 g/day of ethanol.

In the CARET, the relative risk of lung cancer incidence was 1.3 in the group treated with β-carotene and retinal ($p = 0.02$), 1.4 in the current smoker group treated with β-carotene and retinal, and 1.4 in the asbestos-exposed group treated with β-carotene and retinal. In the PHS, no significant modification in risk was found. In the SCPS, the relative risk for skin cancer was 1.4 in the smoker group treated with β-carotene.

### 4.3.2  α-CAROTENE

α-Carotene has been proved to induce $G_1$-arrest of cells in the cell cycle. As various agents that induce $G_1$-arrest have been proved to have cancer preventive activity, we evaluated the anticarcinogenic activity of α-carotene. α-Carotene showed higher activity than β-carotene to suppress the tumorigenesis in skin, lung, liver, and colon.[4]

In the skin tumorigenesis experiment, a two-stage mouse skin carcinogenesis model was used. First, 7-week-old female ICR mice had their backs shaved with electric clipper. From 1 week after initiation by 100 μg of 7,12-dimethyl-benz[a]anthracene (DMBA), 1.0 μg of 12-O-tetradecanoylphorbol-13-acetate (TPA) was applied twice a week. α-Carotene or β-carotene (200 nmol) was applied with each TPA application. The higher potency of α-carotene than β-carotene was observed. The percentage of tumor-bearing mice in the control group was 69%, whereas the percentages of tumor-bearing mice in the groups treated with $\alpha$- and $\beta$-carotene were 25 and 31%, respectively. The average number of tumors per mouse in the control group was 3.7, whereas the $\alpha$-carotene-treated group had 0.3 tumors per mouse ($p < 0.01$, Student's $t$-test). $\beta$-Carotene treatment also decreased the average number of tumors per mouse (2.9 tumors per mouse); however, the difference from the control group was not significant.

The higher potency of $\alpha$-carotene compared to $\beta$-carotene in the suppression of tumor promotion was confirmed by another two-stage carcinogenesis experiment, i.e., 4-nitroquinoline 1-oxide (4NQO)-initiated and glycerol-promoted ddY mouse lung carcinogenesis model. 4NQO (10 mg/kg body weight) was given by a single subcutaneous injection on the first experimental day. Glycerol (10% in drinking water) was given as the tumor promoter from experimental week 5 to week 30 continuously. $\alpha$-Carotene or $\beta$-carotene (at the concentration of 0.05%) or vehicle as a control was mixed as an emulsion into drinking water during the promotion stage. The average number of tumors per mouse in the control group was 4.1, whereas the $\alpha$-carotene-treated group had 1.3 tumors per mouse ($p < 0.001$). $\beta$-Carotene treatment did not show any suppressive effect on the average number of tumors per mouse, but rather induced a slight increase (4.9 tumors per mouse).

In a liver carcinogenesis experiment, a spontaneous liver carcinogenesis model was used. Male C3H/He mice, which have a high incidence of spontaneous liver tumor development, were treated for 40 weeks with $\alpha$- and $\beta$-carotene (at the concentration of 0.05%, mixed as an emulsion into drinking water) or vehicle as a control. The mean number of hepatomas was significantly decreased by $\alpha$-carotene treatment as compared with that in the control group; the control group developed 6.3 tumors per mouse, whereas the $\alpha$-carotene-treated group had 3.0 tumors per mouse ($p < 0.001$). On the other hand, the $\beta$-carotene-treated group did not show a significant difference from the control group, although a tendency toward a decrease was observed (4.7 tumors per mouse).

As a short-term experiment to evaluate the suppressive effect of $\alpha$-carotene on colon carcinogenesis, the effect on colonic aberrant crypt foci formation (ACF) induced by $N$-methylnitrosourea (MNU, three intrarectal administrations of 4 mg in week 1) was examined in Sprague-Dawley (SD) rats. $\alpha$-Carotene or $\beta$-carotene (6 mg, suspended in 0.2 ml of corn oil, intragastric gavage daily) or vehicle as control were administered during weeks 2 and 5. The mean number of colonic ACF in the control group was 63, whereas $\alpha$- or $\beta$-carotene-treated group had 42 (significantly lower than that in the control group, $p < 0.05$) and 56, respectively. Thus, a greater potency of $\alpha$-carotene compared to $\beta$-carotene was again observed.

### 4.3.3 LUTEIN

Lutein is a dihydroxy-form of $\alpha$-carotene, and it is distributed among a large variety of vegetables, such as kale, spinach, and winter squash, and fruits, such as mango, papaya, peaches, prunes, and oranges. An epidemiological study conducted in the Pacific Islands indicated that people with high intakes of the combination of the three carotenoids (β-carotene, α-carotene, and lutein) had the lowest risk of lung cancer.[5]

The effect of lutein on lung carcinogenesis was examined. Lutein showed antitumor-promoting activity in a two-stage carcinogenesis experiment in lung of ddY mice, initiated with 4NQO and promoted with glycerol. Lutein, 0.2 mg in 0.2 ml of mixture of olive oil and Tween 80 (49:1), was given by oral intubation three times a week during tumor promotion stage (25 weeks). Treatment with lutein showed a tendency of a decrease of lung tumor formation: the control group developed 3.1 tumors per mouse, whereas the lutein-treated group had 2.2 tumors per mouse.

The antitumor-promoting activity of lutein was confirmed by another two-stage carcinogenesis experiment. Lutein showed antitumor-promoting activity in a skin carcinogenesis model using ICR mice, initiated with DMBA and promoted with TPA and mezerein. At 1 week after the initiation by 100 μg of DMBA, TPA (10 nmol) was applied once, and then mezerein (3 nmol for 15 weeks, and 6 nmol for subsequent 15 weeks) twice a week. Lutein (1 μmol, molar ratio to TPA = 100) was applied twice (45 min before and 16 h after TPA application). After experimental week 30, the average number of tumors per mouse in the control group was 5.5, whereas the lutein-treated group had 1.9 tumors per mouse ($p < 0.05$).

Lutein also inhibited the development of ACF in SD rat colon induced by MNU (three intrarectal administrations of 4 mg in week 1). Lutein (0.24 mg, suspended in 0.2 ml of corn oil, intragastric gavage daily) or vehicle as control was administered during weeks 2 through 5. The mean number of colonic ACF in the control group at week 5 was 69, whereas the lutein-treated group had 40 (significantly lower than that in the control group: $p < 0.05$).

### 4.3.4 ZEAXANTHIN

Zeaxanthin is a dihydroxy-form of β-carotene. It is distributed in our daily foods, such as corn and various vegetables. Since awareness of zeaxanthin as a beneficial carotenoid has only recently become known, available data for zeaxanthin are few.

Some activities of zeaxanthin have become known. Zeaxanthin suppressed TPA-induced expression of early antigen of Epstein–Barr virus in Raji cells. TPA-enhanced $^{32}$Pi incorporation into phospholipids of cultured cells was also inhibited by zeaxanthin. Anticarcinogenic activity of zeaxanthin *in vivo* has also been examined. It was found that spontaneous liver carcinogenesis in C3H/He male mice was suppressed by treatment with zeaxanthin (at the concentration of 0.005%, mixed as an emulsion into drinking water). Antimetastatic activity of zeaxanthin was also found.

### 4.3.5 LYCOPENE

Lycopene occurs in our diet, predominantly in tomatoes and tomato products. Lycopene is an antioxidant. It has exceptionally high singlet oxygen quenching ability.[6,7] An epidemiological study among elderly Americans indicated that high

**TABLE 4.1**
**Effect of Lycopene on Tumorigenesis in Liver**

| Group | No. of Mice | Tumor-Bearing Mice (%) | Average No. of Tumors per Mouse |
|---|---|---|---|
| Control | 17 | 88 | 7.7 |
| + Lycopene | 13 | 39 | 0.9[a] |

*Note:* Male C3H/He mice at the age of 6 weeks were used. Lycopene, 0.005% in drinking water, was given during the whole period of experiment (40 weeks).

[a] $p < 0.05$.

tomato intake was associated with a 50% reduction of mortality from cancers at all sites.[8] In a case-control study in Italy, high consumption of lycopene from tomatoes was shown to have a potential protective effect against cancers of digestive tract.[9] An inverse association between high intake of tomato products and prostate cancer risk was also reported.[10]

Studies on the anticarcinogenic activity of lycopene in animal models were carried out in mammary gland, liver, lung, skin, and colon.[11] A study in mice with a high rate of spontaneous mammary tumors showed that intake of lycopene delayed and reduced tumor growth.

Lycopene showed antitumor-promoting activity in a two-stage carcinogenesis experiment in lung of ddY mice, initiated with 4NQO and promoted with glycerol. Lycopene, 0.2 mg in 0.2 ml of a mixture of olive oil and Tween 80 (49:1), was given by oral intubation three times a week during tumor promotion stage (25 weeks). Treatment with lycopene resulted in the significant decrease of lung tumor formation: the control group developed 3.1 tumors per mouse, whereas the lycopene-treated group had 1.4 tumors per mouse ($p < 0.05$) (Table 4.1).

The antitumor-promoting activity of lycopene was confirmed by another two-stage carcinogenesis experiment. Lycopene showed antitumor-promoting activity in a skin carcinogenesis with ICR mice, initiated with DMBA and promoted with TPA. Lycopene (160 nmol, molar ratio to TPA = 100) was applied with each TPA application. After experimental week 20, the average number of tumors per mouse in the control group was 8.5, whereas the lycopene-treated group had 2.1 tumors per mouse ($p < 0.05$).

Lycopene also inhibited the development of ACF in SD rat colon induced by MNU (three intrarectal administrations of 4 mg in week 1). Lycopene (0.12 mg, suspended in 0.2 ml of corn oil, intragastric gavage daily) or vehicle as control was administered during weeks 2 through 5. The mean number of colonic ACF in control group at week 5 was 69, whereas the lycopene-treated group had 34 (significantly lower than that in the control group: $p < 0.05$).

Spontaneous liver carcinogenesis in C3H/He male mice was also suppressed. Treatment for 40 weeks with lycopene (at the concentration of 0.005%, mixed as an emulsion into drinking water) resulted in a significant decrease of liver tumor formation as shown in Table 4.1 ($p < 0.005$).

### 4.3.6 β-Cryptoxanthin

β-Cryptoxanthin seems to be a promising carotenoid, since it showed the strongest inhibitory activity in the *in vitro* screening test. β-Cryptoxanthin suppressed TPA-induced expression of early antigen of Epstein–Barr virus in Raji cells at the highest potency among carotenoids tested.[12] TPA-enhanced $^{32}$Pi incorporation into phospholipids of cultured cells was also inhibited by β-cryptoxanthin. β-Cryptoxanthin is distributed in our daily foodstuff, such as oranges, and is one of the major carotenoids detectable in human blood. Thus, it seems worthy to investigate its actions more precisely. In this context, we further examined the anticarcinogenic activity *in vivo*.

β-Cryptoxanthin showed antitumor-promoting activity in a two-stage carcinogenesis experiment in skin of ICR mice, initiated with DMBA and promoted with TPA. β-Cryptoxanthin (160 nmol, molar ratio to TPA = 100) was applied 1 h before each TPA application. At week 20 of promotion, the percentage of tumor-bearing mice in the control group was 64%, whereas the percentage of tumor-bearing mice in the group treated with β-cryptoxanthin was 29%. The average number of tumors per mouse in the control group was 2.7, whereas the β-cryptoxanthin-treated group had 1.6 tumors per mouse ($p < 0.05$).

Effect of β-cryptoxanthin on colon carcinogenesis was also examined. Four groups of F344 rats ($n = 25$ each) received an intrarectal dose of 2 mg MNU, three times a week for 5 weeks, and were fed a diet supplemented with or without β-cryptoxanthin (0.0025%). The colon cancer incidence at week 30 was significantly lower in the β-cryptoxanthin diet group (68%) compared to the control group (96%). The tumor multiplicity was also lower in the β-cryptoxanthin-treated group (1.4 tumors per rat) compared to the control group (1.7 tumors per rat), which was not statistically significant.

### 4.3.7 Other Carotenoids

In addition to the carotenoids mentioned above, fucoxanthin, astaxanthin, capsanthin, crocetin, and phytoene seem to be promising carotenoids, as these carotenoids showed strong inhibitory activity in cancer screening tests. Fucoxanthin is distributed in our daily foodstuff, such as various types of seaweed, and is one of the major carotenoids distributed in marine organisms. Thus, it seems worthy to investigate its actions more precisely.

### 4.3.8 Multicarotenoids

It is now clear that various natural carotenoids are potentially valuable for cancer prevention. These carotenoids may be suitable in combinational use, as well as single use. In fact, we have recently found that multicarotenoids (i.e., a mixture of various carotenoids, such as β-carotene, α-carotene, lutein, lycopene, and so

**TABLE 4.2**
**Composition of Multicarotenoids**

| Carotenoids | % |
|---|---|
| β-Carotene | 45.0 |
| α-Carotene | 24.7 |
| Lutein | 19.0 |
| Lycopene | 10.3 |
| Zeaxanthin | 0.9 |
| β-Cryptoxanthin | 0.1 |
| Total | 100 |

**TABLE 4.3**
**Effect of Oral Administration of Multicarotenoids on the Promotion of Lung Tumor Formation by Glycerol in 4NQO-Initiated Mice**

| Group | (n) | Tumor-Bearing Mice | Average No. of Tumors per Mouse |
|---|---|---|---|
| Control | (15) | 73 | 1.4 |
| +Multicarotenoids | (15) | 27[a] | 0.4[b] |

*Note:* Multicarotenoids (2 mg in 0.2 ml of oil, three times per week) were given during the promotion period.

[a] $p < 0.05$.
[b] $p < 0.01$.

on) showed potent anticarcinogenic activity. For example, administration of a prototype multicarotenoid preparation (Table 4.2) resulted in the suppression of lung tumor promotion, as shown in Table 4.3.

Furthermore, we have recently proved that administration of natural multicarotenoids (a mixture of lycopene, β-carotene, α-carotene, and other natural carotenoids) with α-tocopherol resulted in significant suppression of liver tumor development in liver cirrhosis patients (Jinno, K., Nishino, H. et al., patent pending: 2002-022958, 2002.1.31). Thus, multicarotenoids seem to be promising for clinical use. However, it is important to note that the effectiveness or efficacy of multicarotenoids varied between individuals; i.e., responders and nonresponders were founded in clinical trial. These differences may be explained by single nucleotide polymorphisms (SNPs). Thus, SNPs are now being analyzed in responders and nonresponders.

## 4.4  PRODUCTION OF PHYTOENE IN MAMMALIAN CELLS

### 4.4.1  ESTABLISHMENT OF PHYTOENE-PRODUCING MAMMALIAN CELLS AND ANALYSIS OF THEIR PROPERTIES

Phytoene, which is detectable in human blood, was proved to suppress tumorigenesis in skin cancer models. It has been suggested that the antioxidative activity of phytoene may play an important role in its mechanism of action. To confirm the mechanism, more precise study should be carried out. However, phytoene becomes unstable when it is purified, and thus is very difficult to examine its biological activities. Therefore, stable production of phytoene within target cells was tried. As phytoene synthase encoding gene, *crtB*, has already been cloned from *Erwinia uredovora*,[13] we used it for the expression of the enzyme in animal cells. Plasmids encoding phytoene synthase were transfected into NIH-3T3 cells and expression was determined by Northern blot. These cells expressed a 1.5 kilobases mRNA from the *crtB* gene as a major transcript. That transcript was not present in the cells transfected with the vector alone. Phytoene was detected as a major peak in the HPLC profile in NIH-3T3 cells transfected with pCAcrtB, but not in control cells.

Because lipid peroxidation is considered to play a critical role in tumorigenesis and the antioxidative activity of phytoene may play an important role in its mechanism of anticarcinogenic action, the levels of phospholipid peroxidation induced by oxidative stress in cells transfected with pCAcrtB or vector alone were compared. Oxidative stress was imposed by culturing the cells in a $Fe^{3+}$/adenosine 5´-diphosphate (ADP) containing medium for 4 h. The lipid fraction was examined for peroxidation by HPLC as above. The phospholipid hydroperoxidation level in the cells transfected with pCAcrtB and confirmed to produce phytoene by HPLC was lower than that in the cells transfected with vector alone (Table 4.4). Thus, antioxidative activity of phytoene in animal cells was confirmed.

---

**TABLE 4.4**
**Reduction of Oxidative Stress-Induced Lipid Hydroperoxidation Levels in Cells Producing Phytoene**

| Transfected Plasmid | PCOOH + PEOOH/PC + PE | (% Inhibition) |
|---|---|---|
| Vector | 4.6 | |
| *crtB* | 2.5 | (46) |

*Note:* PCOOH: phosphatidylcholine hydroperoxide, PEOOH: phosphatidylethanolamine hydroperoxide, PC: phosphatidylcholine, PE: phosphatidylethanolamine.

---

**TABLE 4.5**
**Suppression of Transformed Focus Formation Induced by Activated H-*ras* Gene in Cells Producing Phytoene**

| Oncogene | No. of Transformed Foci | |
| | Control | +*crtB* |
| --- | --- | --- |
| *ras*-1 (pNCO102) | 47 | 22 |
| *ras*-2 (pNCO602) | 80 | 15 |

It is of interest to test the effect of the endogenous synthesis of phytoene on the malignant transformation process that is newly triggered in noncancerous cells. Thus, a study was carried out on the NIH-3T3 cells producing phytoene for its possible resistance against oncogenic insult imposed by transfection of the activated H-*ras* oncogene. Plasmids with activated H-*ras* gene were transfected to NIH-3T3 cells with or without phytoene production, and the rate of transformed focus formation in 100-mm-diameter dishes was compared. As a result, it was proved that the rate of transformed focus formation induced by the transfection of activated H-*ras* oncogene was lower in the phytoene-producing cells than in control cells (Table 4.5).

This type of experimental method, using cloned genes for the expression of unstable phytochemicals, may be applied to the evaluation of their anti-carcinogenic and/or antioxidative activities.

### 4.4.2 BIO-CHEMOPREVENTION

Valuable chemopreventive substances, including carotenoids, may be produced in a wide variety of foods by means of biotechnology. This new concept may be appropriately named "bio-chemoprevention." As a prototype experiment, phytoene synthesis in animal cells is demonstrated as described above. Because phytoene produced in animal cells was proved to prevent oxidative damage of cellular lipids, it may become a valuable factor in animal foods to reduce the formation of oxidized oils, which may be carcinogenic and hazardous for health, as well as to keep freshness, resulting in the maintenance of safety and good quality of foods. Furthermore, phytoene-containing foods are valuable in the prevention of cancer, as phytoene is known as an anticarcinogenic substance.

We have also succeeded to produce phytoene in mice (Y. Satomi, H. Nishino et al., 2002, unpublished data), and we are now analyzing their incidence of cancer in these mice. In the next step, we are planning to produce phytoene in pigs and cows.

## 4.5  CONCLUSION

Various vitamin A analogs and natural or synthetic carotenoids seem to be useful for cancer control in humans. Some of them may also be applicable for bio-chemoprevention projects.

## ACKNOWLEDGMENTS

This work was supported in part by grants from the Program for Promotion of Basic Research Activities for Innovative Biosciences (ProBRAIN), the Ministry of Agriculture, Forestry, and Fisheries, the Ministry of Health and Welfare, the Ministry of Education, Science and Culture, and Institute of Free Radical Control (IFRC), Japan. The study was carried out in collaboration with research groups of Kyoto Prefectural University of Medicine, Akita University College of Allied Medical Science, Kyoto Pharmaceutical University, Food Research Institute, Fruit Tree Research Station, National Cancer Center Research Institute, Shikoku Cancer Center, Lion Co., Dainippon Ink & Chemicals, Inc., Kagome Co., Kirin Brewery Co., Koyo Mercantile Co., Japan, Dr. Frederick Khachik, Department of Chemistry and Biochemistry, University of Maryland, U.S.A., and Dr. Zohar Nir, LycoRed Natural Products Industries, Ltd., Israel. The authors are grateful to Dr. Takashi Sugimura, Emeritus President, National Cancer Center, Japan, for his kind encouragement during this study.

## REFERENCES

1. Peto R, Doll R, Buckley JD, Sporn MB. Can dietary beta-carotene materially reduce human cancer rates? *Nature* 1981; 290:201–208.
2. Gottardis MM, Bischoff ED, Shirley MA, Wagoner MA, Lamph WW, Heyman RA. Chemoprevention of mammary carcinoma by LGD1069 (Targretin): an RXR-selective ligand. *Cancer Res* 1996; 56:5566–5570.
3. Bischoff ED, Heyman RA, Lamph WW. Effect of retinoid X receptor-selective ligand LGD1069 on mammary carcinoma after tamoxifen failure. *J Natl Cancer Inst* 1999; 91:2188.
4. Murakoshi M, Nishino H, Satomi Y, Takayasu J, Hasegawa T, Tokuda H, Iwashima A, Okuzumi J, Okabe H, Kitano H, Iwasaki R. Potent preventive action of alpha-carotene against carcinogenesis: spontaneous liver carcinogenesis and promoting stage of lung and skin carcinogenesis in mice are suppressed more effectively by alpha-carotene than by beta-carotene. *Cancer Res* 1992; 52:6583–6587.
5. Le Marchand L, Hankin JH, Kolonel LN, Beecher GR, Wilkens LR, Zhao LP. Intake of specific carotenoids and lung cancer risk. *Cancer Epidemiol Biomarkers Prev* 1993; 2:183–187.
6. Stahl W, Sies H. Physical quenching of singlet oxygen and *cis-trans* isomerization of carotenoids. *Ann NY Acad Sci* 1993; 691:10–19.
7. Ukai N, Lu Y, Etoh H, Yagi A, Ina K, Oshima S, Ojima F, Sakamoto H, Ishiguro Y. Photosensitized oxygenation of lycopene. *Biosci Biotech Biochem* 1994; 58:1718–1719.

8. Colditz GA, Branch LG, Lipnick RJ, Willett WC, Rosner B, Posner BM, Hennekens CH. Increased green and yellow vegetable intake and lowered cancer deaths in an elderly population. *Am J Clin Nutr* 1985; 41:32–36.

9. Franceschi S, Bidoli E, La Veccia C, Talamini R, D'Avanzo B, Negri E. Tomatoes and risk of digestive-tract cancers. *Int J Cancer* 1994; 59:181–184.

10. Giovannucci E, Ascherio A, Rimm EB, Stampfer MJ, Colditz GA, Willet WC. Intake of carotenoids and retinal in relation to risk of prostate cancer. *J Natl Cancer Inst* 1995; 87:1767–1776.

11. Nagasawa K, Mitamura T, Sakamoto S, Yamamoto K. Effects of lycopene on spontaneous tumour development in SHN virgin mice. *Anticancer Res* 1995; 15:1173–1178.

12. Tsushima M, Maoka T, Katsuyama M, Kozuka M, Matsuno T, Tokuda H, Nishino H, Iwashima A. Inhibitory effect of natural carotenoids on Epstein-Barr virus activation activity of a tumor promoter in Raji cells. A screening study for anti-tumor promoters. *Biol Pharm Bull* 1995; 18:227–233.

13. Misawa N, Nakagawa M, Kobayashi K, Yamano S, Izawa Y, Nakamura K, Harashima K. Elucidation of the Erwinian uredovora carotenoid biosynthetic pathway by functional analysis of gene products expressed in *Escherichia coli*. *J Bacteriol* 1990; 172:6704–6712.

# 5 Vitamin D and the Risk of Cancer

*Sujatha Sundaram and David A. Gewirtz*

## CONTENTS

5.1 Introduction..................................................................................................89
5.2 Vitamin D Metabolism.................................................................................90
5.3 Dietary Sources of Vitamin D......................................................................92
5.4 Recommended Intake for Vitamin D............................................................92
5.5 The Vitamin D Receptor...............................................................................94
5.6 Vitamin D and the Cancer Connection.........................................................95
5.7 VDR Polymorphisms and Cancer.................................................................97
    5.7.1 Breast Cancer.....................................................................................97
    5.7.2 Prostate Cancer..................................................................................99
5.8 $1\alpha,25\text{-}(OH)_2D_3$ Analogs in the Treatment of Cancer..........................100
5.9 Conclusion..................................................................................................103
References........................................................................................................103

## 5.1 INTRODUCTION

Vitamin D (calciferol), first discovered by McCollum in 1922, is essential for the proper formation of the skeleton and for mineral homeostasis.[1,2] Following the discovery of vitamin D, two nutritional forms of vitamin D were isolated: vitamin $D_2$ ($D_2$ or ergocalciferol) and vitamin $D_3$ ($D_3$ or cholecalciferol). The chemical structures of $D_2$ and $D_3$ were identified independently by two groups, a British group led by Askew[3] and a German group led by Windaus.[4,5] Windaus's group provided the chemical synthesis of the vitamin D compounds and confirmed their structures. In 1928, Windaus received the Nobel Prize in Chemistry for his contributions. The structures of the nutritional forms of vitamin D are provided in Figure 5.1. Vitamin $D_3$ is synthesized from 7-dehydrocholesterol in the skin upon exposure to ultraviolet (UV) rays from the sun[6–8] while vitamin $D_2$ is produced through irradiation of plant sterols.[3]

The vitamin D requirement of humans can be met if skin is exposed to sufficient amounts of sunlight or artificial UV radiation. The amount of vitamin D synthesis is dependent on the area of skin exposed to sunlight, the time of exposure, and the wavelength of UV radiation impinging on the skin. Some of

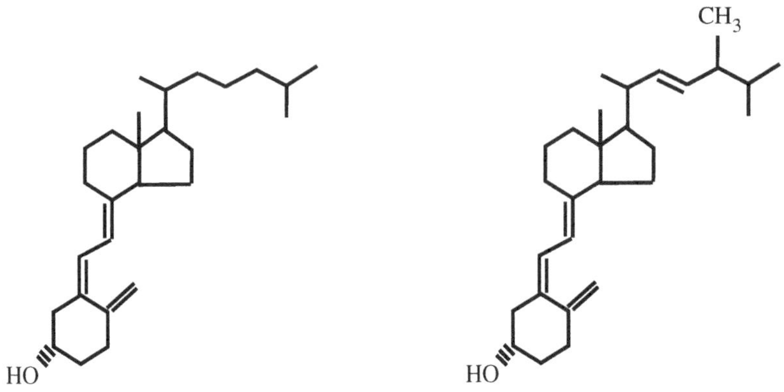

Vitamin D$_3$ or Cholecalciferol                    Vitamin D$_2$ or Ergocalciferol

**FIGURE 5.1** Nutritional forms of vitamin D.

the factors that may influence an individual's vitamin D status are latitude of the residence, customs of dress, and extent of indoor residency and lack of outdoor activity,[9–11] According to Clemens et al.,[12] the extent and efficiency of vitamin D synthesis are dependent on the character of the skin. Skin with high melanin content, such as darker skin, requires much longer exposure to sunlight to achieve the same level of vitamin D synthesis as produced by skin with lower melanin content, such as lighter skin.[10,11]

In addition to the skin color, the capacity of the skin to synthesize vitamin D is influenced by age, with elderly individuals able to synthesize only about half as much vitamin D compared to younger individuals.[10,11] Given the many factors that can influence the extent of UV-dependent vitamin D$_3$ synthesis in an individual, vitamin D should be considered an essential nutrient in the diet. Increasing evidence now indicates that cutaneous vitamin D synthesis is of great importance for the prevention of a variety of diseases, including various malignancies. It has been postulated that cancer mortality could be reduced via careful UV exposure or, more safely, via oral substitution with vitamin D.

## 5.2  VITAMIN D METABOLISM

Vitamin D, as either D$_2$ or D$_3$, does not have significant biological activity. Rather, it must be metabolized within the body to the hormonally active form, 1$\alpha$,25-dihydroxyvitamin D$_3$ (calcitriol or 1$\alpha$,25-(OH)$_2$D$_3$). This transformation occurs in two steps as shown in Figure 5.2. Within the liver, vitamin D$_3$ is hydroxylated to 25-hydroxyvitamin D$_3$ (25-(OH)D$_3$) by the enzyme 25-hydroxylase. The kidney utilizes 25-(OH)D$_3$ as a substrate for 1-alpha-hydroxylase, yielding 1$\alpha$,25-(OH)$_2$D$_3$, the biologically active form of vitamin D. The biochemistry and metabolism of vitamin D have been extensively reviewed by DeLuca[13] and Fraser.[14]

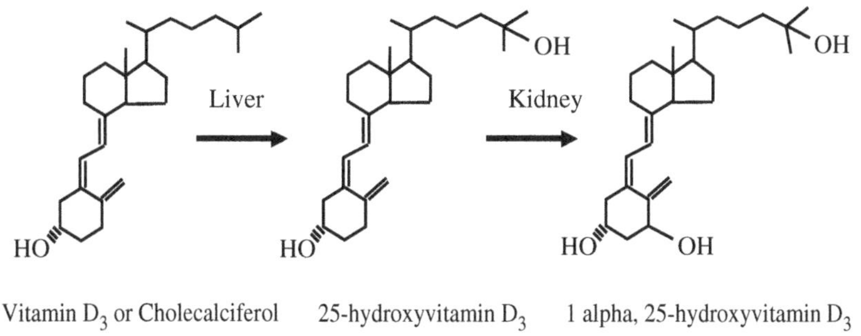

Vitamin $D_3$ or Cholecalciferol     25-hydroxyvitamin $D_3$     1 alpha, 25-hydroxyvitamin $D_3$

**FIGURE 5.2** Activation and metabolism of vitamin $D_3$.

As discussed in detail by DeLuca,[1] 25-$(OH)D_3$ was isolated in its pure form and chemically identified as the first active vitamin D metabolite in 1968.[15–17] However, additional studies conducted with the radiolabeled form of 25-$(OH)D_3$ demonstrated that 25-$(OH)D_3$ was rapidly metabolized to more polar metabolites, suggesting that there were other active metabolites of vitamin D.[18] These findings rekindled interest in studying the metabolic pathway for vitamin D, and several groups[19–22] independently reported on the importance of a polar metabolite, which was modified at the 1 alpha position. The DeLuca group[23–25] successfully isolated this active metabolite, using mass spectrophotometric techniques to demonstrate unequivocally that the active form of vitamin D is $1\alpha,25$-$(OH)_2D_3$.

Subsequent experiments by Fraser and Kodicek[26] identified the organ of synthesis of this active metabolite. They observed that the active metabolite could be produced by homogenates of normal chicken kidneys and was not produced by anephric animals. In the course of identifying the active metabolite of vitamin D, the presence of other metabolites such as 24,25-$(OH)_2D_3$, 25,26-$(OH)_2D_3$ and as many as 30 additional metabolites were reported in the late 1970s and 1980s.[1] In 1985, Brommage and DeLuca[27] made the significant observation with the use of fluoro-derivatives of vitamin D that 25-hydroxylation followed by 1-hydroxylation is the only pathway for vitamin D activation. Further research using other fluoro-derivatives such as 26,27-hexafluoro-25-$(OH)D_3$ and 23-difluoro-25-$(OH)D_3$ substantiated the earlier findings that 26-hydroxylation, 24-hydroxylation, and 23-hydroxylation are not essential to the function of vitamin D.

All of the vitamin D forms mentioned above are hydrophobic and all are transported in blood bound to carrier proteins. The major carrier is called, appropriately, vitamin D-binding protein.[28] The half-life of 25-$(OH)D_3$ is several weeks, while that of $1\alpha,25$-$(OH)_2D_3$ is only a few hours. The biological activity of cholecalciferol is 40 IU/$\mu$g while the activities of 25-$(OH)D_3$ and $1\alpha,25$-$(OH)_2D_3$ are approximately 1.5 and 5 times, respectively, greater than that of vitamin $D_3$.

Typically, an accurate assessment of an individual's vitamin D nutritional status is performed by determining the concentration of 25-$(OH)D_3$ in serum. This is considered to be an accurate integrative measure reflecting an individual's dietary intake and cutaneous production. As mentioned earlier, geographical differences in vitamin D status exist, and a recent studies by Ovesen et al.[29,30] reported that a substantial percentage of the elderly and adolescent population in Europe have low concentrations of 25-(OH)D$_3$. The percentage varied from 10% in the Nordic countries to 40% in France and the average intake of vitamin D in Europe was found to be 2 to 3 μg/day.

When Moore et al.[31] assessed the mean vitamin D intake in the U.S. from data collected from food sources and dietary supplements, and compared these values to the recommended intake, they found that the study population was not meeting the recommended levels. These findings are from the data collected from the Third National Health and Nutritional Survey 1988–1994 (NHANES III) and the 1994–1996 Continuing Survey of Food Intakes by Individuals and its 1998 Supplemental Children Survey (CSFII 1994–1996, 1998) with a sample size of approximately 50,000 individuals. Of particular interest was that the lowest intakes of vitamin D from food were among female teenagers and female adults, while the highest intake was reported among male teenagers. Contrary to this, the European study found that adolescents were among the group that was most likely to consume recommended levels of vitamin D.

## 5.3  DIETARY SOURCES OF VITAMIN D

Milk and dairy products are the main sources of vitamin D in most populations. In the U.S., foods fortified with vitamin D are also major sources of vitamin D. Some of the fortified foods that may contain up to 10 to 15% of the daily value (%DV) include breakfast cereals, bread, pastries, crackers, and cereal bars. Information about selected food sources and their vitamin D values are provided in Table 5.1.

Daily values are reference numbers developed by the Food and Drug Administration (FDA) to help consumers determine specific nutrient content of food. The average DV for vitamin D ranges between 200 and 600 IU depending on age and physical activity, with the biological activity of 1 μg of vitamin D being 40 IU. The %DV of the food sources listed in Table 5.1 is based on a 2000-calorie diet. The %DV denotes what is provided by one serving and is usually listed on the nutrition facts panel of food labels.

## 5.4  RECOMMENDED INTAKE FOR VITAMIN D

Recommended intakes for vitamin D are provided as Dietary Reference Intakes (DRI) developed by the Institute of Medicine (IOM) and the National Academy of Sciences. DRI is the general term for three reference standards used for planning and assessing the nutrient intake for healthy people. These three reference values include Recommended Dietary Allowance (RDA), Adequate Intake (AI), and Tolerable Upper Level Intake (UL). Accordingly:

**TABLE 5.1**
**Food Sources and Their Vitamin D Content**

| Food Sources | International Units (IU) per Serving | Percent Daily Value (% DV) |
|---|---|---|
| Cod liver oil, 1 tablespoon | 1360 | 340 |
| Salmon, cooked, 3.5 ounces | 360 | 90 |
| Mackerel, cooked, 3.5 ounces | 345 | 90 |
| Tuna fish, canned in oil, 3 ounces | 200 | 50 |
| Sardines, canned in oil, drained, 1.75 ounce | 250 | 70 |
| Milk, nonfat, reduced fat, and whole, vitamin D fortified, 1 cup | 98 | 25 |
| Margarine, fortified, 1 tablespoon | 60 | 15 |
| Pudding, prepared from mix and made with vitamin D-fortified milk, 0.5 cup | 50 | 10 |
| Ready-to-eat cereals fortified with 10% of the DV for vitamin D, approximately 1 cup servings (servings vary according to the brand) | 40 | 10 |
| Egg, 1 whole (vitamin D is found in egg yolk) | 20 | 6 |
| Liver, beef, cooked, 3.5 ounces | 15 | 4 |
| Cheese, Swiss, 1 ounce | 12 | 4 |

*Note:* This table was compiled by the Office of Dietary Supplements (ODS) at the National Institutes of Health, Bethesda, MD. Information pertaining to food sources that are not listed can be obtained from http://www.nal.usda.gov/fnic/cgi-bin/nut_search.pl. This table was developed as part of the ODS Supplement's mission to disseminate scientifically accurate research results and to educate the public to promote an enhanced quality of life and health among the U.S. population.

- The RDA recommends the average daily intake that is sufficient to meet the nutrient requirements of nearly all (97 to 98%) healthy individuals in each age and gender group.
- An AI is set when there is insufficient scientific data available to establish a RDA. AIs meet or exceed the amount needed to maintain a nutritional state of adequacy in nearly all members of a specific age and gender group.
- A UL denotes the highest amount that a healthy person can consume without adverse health effects.

As evident from the introductory remarks above, establishing an RDA for vitamin D is a complex issue with multiple variables that affect vitamin D synthesis such as sunlight exposure, coverage of the skin, and skin type. People with adequate sun exposure have no dietary requirement for vitamin D. However, since the U.S. is in the northern latitude, with relatively less sunlight than parts of the world closer to the equator, a dietary supply of vitamin D is essential for this population. According to the 10th edition of RDA published by National

**TABLE 5.2**
**Adequate Intakes for Vitamin D for Different Age Groups (μg/day)**

| Age | Children | Men | Women | Pregnancy | Lactation |
|---|---|---|---|---|---|
| 0–13 years | 5 (= 200 IU) | | | | |
| 14–18 years | | 5 (= 200 IU) | 5 (= 200 IU) | 5 (= 200 IU) | 5 (= 200 IU) |
| 19–50 years | | 5 (= 200 IU) | 5 (= 200 IU) | 5 (= 200 IU) | 5 (= 200 IU) |
| 51–70 years | | 10 (= 400 IU) | 10 (= 400 IU) | | |
| +71 years | | 15 (= 600 IU) | 15 (= 600 IU) | | |

Research Council, the RDA for vitamin D for adults older than 24 years of age was set at 5 μg (200 IU), the same level recommended in 1980. While it has not been determined whether there should be an increased requirement for vitamin D prior to and during pregnancy and lactation, 10 μg (400 IU) per day was originally recommended for this group of individuals. Nevertheless, the IOM recently determined that scientific information available to establish the RDA for vitamin D is insufficient and decided to list recommended intakes as AI, which represents the daily vitamin D intake that should maintain bone health and normal calcium metabolism in healthy people (Table 5.2).

RDA applies only to healthy people and may not be sufficient for individuals with special needs such as metabolic disorders, chronic disease, individuals undergoing drug therapy, people who are under extreme stress, and those who exercise and have a high activity level. Because vitamin D is a lipophilic compound requiring the presence of fat for efficient absorption from the diet, individuals with fat malabsorption also require additional supplements of vitamin D. The Food and Nutrition Board of the IOM has set the tolerable upper level intake (UL) for vitamin D at 25 μg (1000 IU) for infants up to 12 months of age and 50 μg (2000 IU) for children, adults, pregnant, and lactating women.

Calvo and Whiting[32] recently conducted a global perspective of vitamin D intake and found that there was a high prevalence of vitamin D insufficiency worldwide. The authors compared approximately 80 studies conducted over the past 25 years on vitamin D intakes as estimated from food frequency questionnaires, 24-h recall, and multiple day food records. When the data were plotted according to age and classification of the country, it was evident that vitamin D intake was often too low to sustain a healthy circulating levels of 25-$(OH)D_3$ in peoples from countries without mandatory staple food fortification. Dietary supplement use was found to contribute 6 to 47% of the average vitamin D intake. Concern over increased risk of melanoma with unprotected sun exposure has also contributed to vitamin D insufficiency in many populations of the world.

## 5.5  THE VITAMIN D RECEPTOR

From studies performed by Zull and colleagues[33] in which vitamin $D_3$ function was blocked by transcription and protein inhibitors, it became evident that nuclear activity was required for most biological actions of vitamin $D_3$. Following the pioneering studies conducted by Haussler and Norman[34] on the uptake of vitamin $D_3$ into intestinal target tissues in chickens, more definitive evidence began to emerge for the presence of a vitamin D receptor (VDR).

The VDR is a member of the nuclear receptor superfamily. It has been shown that the VDR forms a heterodimeric complex with the retinoic acid receptor (RXR) and binds to vitamin D responsive elements (VDRE) in the DNA consisting of two six-base hexameric motifs in a direct repeated (DR) or inverted palindromic arrangements.[35] Studies by Brumbaugh and Haussler[36,37] indicated that the affinity of the VDR for its radioactively labeled $1\alpha,25\text{-}(OH)_2D_3$ ligand is in the low nanomolar range. Subsequent studies confirmed that VDR could bind to the chromatin fraction in the presence of ligand and that the cytoplasmic VDR translocates to the nucleus upon ligand activation.[38] The VDR contains a characteristic DNA-binding domain (DBD) consisting of 66 amino acids and a C-terminal ligand-binding domain (LBD) of approximately 300 amino acids.[35] The LBD not only binds ligand but also interacts with other nuclear proteins such as corepressors (CoR) and coactivators (CoA). Binding of ligand to the VDR promotes a conformational change within the LBD, thus closing the ligand binding pocket by intramolecular folding,[39] resulting in dissociation from CoRs and association with CoAs. These actions are essential for vitamin D-dependent gene expression.

The known target organs of vitamin $D_3$ include not only the intestine as stated above, but also the kidney, bone, and parathyroid glands. Vitamin $D_3$ and VDR are pivotal regulators of calcium homeostasis and bone mineralization. In addition, recent research using animal tissues, cell lines, and primary cells along with evidence for antiproliferative and pro-differentiating effects of $1\alpha,25\text{-}(OH)_2D_3$ has identified VDR in numerous other tissues and actions of vitamin D in different organs. A list of $1\alpha,25\text{-}(OH)_2D_3$ target tissues and cell types (both tumor and nontumorigenic) along with references is provided in Table 5.3.

## 5.6 VITAMIN D AND THE CANCER CONNECTION

The role of vitamin D in cancer prevention perhaps has been known for more than 50 years. Although excessive sun exposure has been documented to increase the risk of skin cancer, research conducted starting as early as 1936 has proved this population of patients with skin cancer to be at a lower risk for other types of cancer. Sun exposure has been correlated with decreased incidence of certain types of cancer such as cancers of the prostate, breast, and colon. Individuals residing in the U.S., which lies in the northern latitudes, have a risk for cancer incidence which is two to three times higher than the risk of cancer incidence of people living in sunnier, equatorial parts of the world.[40] This intriguing observation by Apperly[40] was followed by several epidemiological studies that demonstrated an inverse relationship between $25\text{-}(OH)D_3$ levels and cancer risk and mortality.[41,42]

## TABLE 5.3
## Tissue Distribution of VDR

| System | Tissue Type |
|---|---|
| Cardiovascular | Cardiac muscle |
| Central nervous system | Neurons |
| Connective tissue | Fibroblasts, stroma |
| Endocrine | Parathyroid gland, thyroid, adrenal, pituitary. Pancreas beta cell |
| Epidermis | Skin, breast, hair follicles |
| Exocrine | Parotid glands, sebaceous gland |
| Gastrointestinal | Esophagus, stomach, small intestine, large intestine, colon |
| Hepatic | Liver parenchyma |
| Immune | Thymus, bone marrow, B cells, T cells |
| Musculoskeletal | Bone osteoblasts, osteocytes, cartilage chondrocytes, striated muscle |
| Renal | Kidney, urethra |
| Reproductive | Testis, ovary, placenta, uterus, endometrium, yolk sac, chorioallontroic membrane |
| Respiratory | Lung alveolar cells |

**Colon Cancer:** With respect to colon cancer, there have been 15 epidemiological studies investigating the association of vitamin D and the risk of colon cancer.[41,43–45] The majority of studies pointed to a higher risk of colon cancer in individuals whose serum 25-$(OH)D_3$ levels were below the median or in the lowest quartile or quintile. In individuals with serum 25-$(OH)D_3$ levels between 27 and 32 ng/ml, the incidence of colon cancer was reduced by 20% compared to individuals with the lowest 25-$(OH)D_3$ levels. Greater reductions in cancer incidence were observed in individuals with serum levels of 25-$(OH)D_3$ above 55 ng/ml. Of the 11 studies evaluating oral vitamin D intake, 6 indicated a 50% decrease in cancer incidence with intakes equal or greater than 650 IU per day. Although the remaining five studies found no association between vitamin D intake and cancer, three of these five studies were performed in areas with relatively high sunlight exposure. Four studies of the geographic association of sunlight intensity with age-adjusted colon cancer mortality rates found markedly lower rates in sunnier areas, further substantiating the association between sunlight-derived vitamin D levels and colon cancer incidence/mortality.

Current U.S. and Canadian adult dietary reference intakes have been formulated based on the assumption that no endogenous vitamin D is available from sunlight exposure. However, no consideration was given to racial differences in vitamin D-synthesizing capacity, despite the well-established effects of differences in skin pigmentation on endogenous vitamin D synthesis. When Calvo and Barton[46] reevaluated the dietary data and serum 25-$(OH)D_3$ levels from the NHANES III study with respect to race (blacks vs. whites), blacks had a significantly higher incidence as well as mortality rates from aggressive cancers compared to that of whites.[46] Mean serum 25-$(OH)D_3$ levels of the white

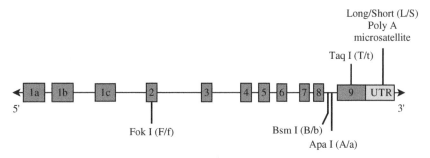

FIGURE 5.3 Structure of human VDR gene. (Adapted from Price et al.[62])

population were 79 ± 0.95 compared to 48.2 ± 1.05 nmol/L in the black population, while average vitamin D intake including food and supplements were 7.92 ± 0.15 and 6.2 ± 0.13 µg/day for white and black populations, respectively.

## 5.7 VDR POLYMORPHISMS AND CANCER

The reported association of VDR polymorphism with bone mineral density was the first study to generate interest in the relationship of receptor polymorphism to cancer. Figure 5.3 presents an illustration of human VDR gene along with the polymorphism sites.

### 5.7.1 BREAST CANCER

In breast cancer, low vitamin D levels in serum have been correlated with disease progression and bone metastases, a situation also noted in prostate cancer and suggesting the involvement of the VDR.[42,47–49] Additionally, the VDR has been detected in several breast tumor cell lines and several groups have investigated the hypothesis that VDR polymorphism might influence the treatment outcomes in women affected by breast cancer in the last decade. Polymorphisms in both the 5′ and the 3′ regions of the VDR gene have been associated with risk of several diseases including breast cancer.

Ruggiero et al.[50] evaluated a total of 88 patients with breast cancer (50 newly diagnosed and 38 women suffering relapse) for individual genetic patterns of VDR by PCR (polymerase change reaction) amplification of genomic DNA followed by digestion with the restriction enzyme Bsm I. While the VDR frequency distribution in the control group comprising 167 healthy women participating in the osteoporosis trial and the primary disease patients in this study did not differ significantly, women who were homozygous (bb) appeared to have almost a four times higher risk of developing metastases than homozygous (BB) women. Similarly, a recent study by Buyru et al.[51] has further shown that the prevalence of both the VDR Taq I and Bsm I alleles and the genotype frequencies were similar in both the normal population and patients with breast cancer.

Because endogenous hormone exposure is known to alter breast cancer susceptibility, genetic variations in VDR along with another nuclear hormone receptor, the androgen receptor (AR), were considered possible candidates for predisposition genes for breast cancer risk in a case-controlled study conducted by Dunning et al.[52] Using two series of Caucasian female breast cancer cases, one incident and one prevalent, and by comparing both cancer case sets with two sets of matched controls from the East Anglican region of Britain, the authors found no association between polymorphism and breast cancer risk. Compared to the individuals with two short alleles (<22 repeats) of the AR polyglutamine tract, the odds ratios (ORs) and 95% confidence intervals (CIs) for individuals with one or two long alleles were 0.82 (95% CI: 0.62 to 1.09) and 1.31 (95% CI: 0.87 to 1.97), respectively. Heterozygotes and homozygotes for the VDR TaqI cutting site had odds ratios of 1.01 (95% CI: 0.81 to 1.27) and 0.97 (95% CI: 0.71 to 1.32). The data suggest that neither the AR nor the VDR polymorphisms had a major effect on the risk of breast cancer.

In contrast to the conclusions of the studies cited above, the results from other controlled studies have suggested a possible association between VDR polymorphism and breast cancer risk.[53–55] Using PCR-RFLP analysis, the allele frequencies of the 3' Taq I polymorphism showed a significant association ($P = 0.0004$, OR: 5.39, CI: 1.81 to 17.20) with breast cancer in a study of Chinese women. The haplotype analysis of Apa I and Taq I showed linkage disequilibrium between the t-allele and A-allele. The frequency of tA haplotype was higher in patients with breast cancer than in controls ($P = 0.001$), indicating that the tA haplotype is associated with increased risk for breast cancer. Studies conducted by Bretherton-Watt et al.[53] and Ingles et al.[55] suggest that both Bsm I and poly-A polymorphisms in the 3' end of the VDR may have an association with increased risk of breast cancer in both the U.K. and U.S. Caucasian population, while the 5' VDR gene variant or the start codon polymorphism, Fok I, had no implications on breast cancer risk. Similarly, Curran et al.[56] have further substantiated these findings in Caucasian populations of Australia. Their results indicate that the allele frequency of the 3' Apa I polymorphism ($p = 0.016$, OR: = 1.56, 95% CI: 1.09 to 2.24) and Taq I RFLP ($p = 0.053$; OR = 1.45; 95% CI: 1.00 to 2.00) showed a similar trend in association with breast cancer while the Fok I polymorphism was not significantly different ($p = 0.97$, OR: 0.99, 95% CI: 0.69 to 1.43).

The apparent discrepancies in the association of VDR polymorphisms and breast cancer risk may be attributed to the variations between different populations based on their ethnicity. It is difficult to equate different polymorphisms between different studies conducted with a heterogeneous population. For example, there could be variations in VDR allele frequencies within the Caucasian population from different parts of the world as shown in the Finnish study on the prevalence of DNA related polymorphism among participants in a large cancer trial.[57] The prevalence of Taq I polymorphism in the control group in the Finnish study was significantly different from the other Caucasian population where there was 99%

concordance between studies.[35] The frequencies of the T allele among Australian,[56] Swedish,[54] and U.K.[53,58] Caucasian control groups ranged from 55 to 57%.

Similarly, differences in VDR polymorphism between different ethnic groups have been documented. With regard to Bsm I polymorphism, the frequency of the b allele in control subjects was reported to be similar: 58%,[58] 57% in non-Latino whites,[55] and 52% in the Italian population.[50] The risk was found to be significantly higher in Latino and in Asian populations with the frequency of 73% and 88 to 95%, respectively.

Although the relationship between VDR polymorphisms and breast cancer is still controversial and has not been confirmed by all studies, there may be some consensus in the limited number of studies reported so far, particularly on the association of VDR polymorphism and breast tumor metastases or disease progression. Schondorf et al.[59] have reported a significant correlation between the absence of both Apa I (AA) (TT) restriction sites in both alleles and the occurrence of bone metastases. Patients with AA genotype had a 1.7-fold increased risk of developing bone metastases, while patients with TT genotype had a 0.5-fold risk. Lundin et al.[60] demonstrated that patients without the Taq I site (TT genotype) were at an increased risk for lymph node metastasis. A tendency toward increased survival was also observed among women who were homozygous for the Taq I site, thus suggesting that VDR polymorphism might influence the tumor progression and treatment response.

## 5.7.2 PROSTATE CANCER

Similar to the studies of breast cancer described above, polymorphisms that occur near the 5' end (FokI and EcoRV) and the 3' end (Bsm I, Taq I, and polyA) of human VDR gene were evaluated to determine their relationship to the relative risk of prostate cancer. Studies by Xu et al.[61] demonstrated that subjects with the ff genotype of Fok I polymorphism had a lower mean percentage of Gleason grade 4/5 cancer (30.3%) than subjects with the FF or Ff genotypes (42.8 and 43.8%, respectively,) which may reflect the outcome after prostatectomy. However, possession of the ff genotype did not translate into improved prostatic specific antigen (PSA) scores or other prognostic markers. More recent data reported by several investigators have indicated no significant relationship between Fok I polymorphisms of the VDR gene start codon and prostate cancer risk in men.[62] However, a threefold increase in prostate cancer risk associated with the less active vitamin D receptor allele (the T allele from VDR TaqI polymorphism at codon 352) among the Southern European population was reported by Ntais et al.[63] It was estimated that almost 50% of cases in men older than 66 years could be attributed to the influence of this risk factor.

A meta-analysis of 14 studies (17 comparisons) with TaqI genotyping (1870 prostate cancer cases; 2843 controls), 6 studies (8 comparisons) with poly (A) repeat genotyping (540 cases; 870 controls), 5 studies with BsmI genotyping (987 cases; 1504 controls), and 3 studies with FokI genotyping (514 cases; 545 controls) showed that the four polymorphisms thus far evaluated are unlikely to be major determinants of susceptibility to prostate cancer on a wide population basis. While these results suggest that polymorphisms in the VDR gene may not be strong predictors of prostate cancer risk among Caucasian men, recent studies conducted by Liu et al.[64] on the Han nationality population in Northern China with a low risk of prostate cancer indicate that there are ethnic differences in the distribution of VDR genotypes. Most notably, the recent study by Tayeb et al.[65] showed that the VDR TaqI polymorphism is associated with a group of Saudi Arabian men with benign prostatic hyperplasia (BPH) who are at an increased risk of prostate cancer, providing a potential tool to assist prediction strategies for this important disease.

Since the first publication on VDR polymorphism was published in 1992, considerable progress has been made on the association of VDR polymorphism and risk of several cancers. However, to this date, molecular and functional consequences of VDR polymorphism are largely unknown. Limited research indicates that Bsm I, Apa I, and Taq I sites present at the 3′ UTR of the gene might be involved in the regulation of VDR expression, particularly through regulation of mRNA stability. It is therefore essential to differentiate between the marker polymorphisms and the truly functional polymorphisms in VDR among patients with cancer. Currently, there is no information available on the correlation of VDR genotypes and VDR mRNA expression, which makes functional and clinical implications of VDR genotypes difficult to interpret. It is however plausible that certain VDR genotypes might alter the ability of VDR to interact with RXR and VDREs, which could ultimately result in differential regulation of VDR target genes that may control cell growth, differentiation, and sensitivity to hormonal levels. Additionally, the interpretation of VDR polymorphisms is also severely limited by the fact that until now, only few polymorphisms in this large gene have been studied and that most of these are anonymous restriction fragment length polymorphisms with unknown functional effects.

## 5.8  1α,25-(OH)$_2$D$_3$ ANALOGS IN THE TREATMENT OF CANCER

In addition to its well-established effects on the regulation of calcium homeostasis, 1α,25-(OH)$_2$D$_3$ has potent regulatory effects on cell growth and differentiation. Experimental evidence suggests a role for 1α,25-(OH)$_2$D$_3$ in tumor cell killing, anti-angiogenesis, and interference with tumor cell invasion, thus making it a potential candidate agent for cancer regulation. 1α,25-(OH)$_2$D$_3$ has been recognized for its regulatory effects on cell cycle checkpoints in several cell types. It has a major inhibitory effect on the G$_1$–S progression by upregulating the cyclin-dependent kinase inhibitors p21 and p27 along with the inhibition of cyclin D1.[66] 1α,25-(OH)$_2$D$_3$ indirectly regulates the cell cycle by increasing the expression of transforming growth factor-beta (TGF-β)[67,68] and decreasing that of epidermal growth factor receptor (EGFR).[69–72] The pro-apoptotic effects observed with vitamin D$_3$ are believed to be mediated either indirectly through insulin-like growth receptor and tumor necrosis factor-$\alpha$ or more directly through BCL-2 family proteins, ceramide pathways, death receptors such as fas, and stress-activated protein kinases (JNK, MAPK, and p38).[66,73,74] Studies demonstrate that 1$\alpha$,25-(OH)$_2$D$_3$ is capable of inhibiting tumor cell invasion, metastasis, and angiogenesis via mechanisms that may include regulation of serine proteinases and metalloproteinases.[66]

Despite the overwhelming evidence that 1$\alpha$,25-(OH)$_2$D$_3$ is not just a nutrient but may be involved in a wide range of activities, its hypercalcemic actions have hindered its potential as a clinically useful anticancer agent. To overcome this effect, several groups have developed analogs of 1$\alpha$,25-(OH)$_2$D$_3$ in an attempt to dissociate its antiproliferative activity from its calcemia-inducing activity. To this date there are at least 2000 1$\alpha$,25-(OH)$_2$D$_3$ analogs, now called deltanoids, that are available for research purpose with a considerable number of analogs at the preclinical/clinical stage of evaluation.

There is extensive literature available on the use of deltanoids as anticancer agents. With VDR being expressed in more than 30 nonclassical target tissues and many cancer-related cells, the deltanoids have been shown to inhibit cell proliferation in many tumor cell types in culture. Initial findings using hemato-poietic-derived tumor cells showed inhibition of cell proliferation. Further evidence indicated the versatile use of deltanoids across several nonhematopoietic malignancies including transformed breast, prostate, skin, lung, colon, ovary, pancreas cells, as well as neuroblastoma and melanoma cells.[66,75–79,80] Although much of the mechanistic data gathered *in vitro* point toward cell cycle arrest, differentiation, and induction of apoptosis, the proposed mechanism of action of deltanoids is likely to differ based on the type of tumor model examined. No unified hypothesis has emerged so far on the basis for the anticancer effects of 1$\alpha$,25-(OH)$_2$D$_3$ and its analogs. In addition, as supraphysiological concentrations are often required to achieve anticancer effects when used alone, recent reports suggest that deltanoids could be more valuable when used in conjunction with other anticancer treatments.

In 1997, Light et al.[81] reported that treatment of murine squamous carcinoma cells with 1$\alpha$,25-(OH)$_2$D$_3$ or its analog Ro23-7553 resulted in a significant growth inhibition, with accumulation of cells in G$_0$–G$_1$ and an accompanying decrease of cells in S phase. The ability to arrest cells in G$_0$–G$_1$ was exploited by combining Ro23-7553 with the cytotoxic agent cisplatin (*cis*-diamminodichloroplatinum; cDDP). Pretreatment with deltanoids for 24 to 48 h significantly enhanced cDDP-mediated tumor cell kill as compared to concurrent treatment with Ro23-7553 and cDDP or cDDP alone.

Deltanoids can be effectively combined with ionizing radiation and chemo-therapeutic agents such as adriamycin to induce apoptosis in breast tumor models both *in vitro* and *in vivo*.[82–86] While the primary response of breast tumor cells to deltanoids such as EB 1089 is growth inhibition, apoptosis has been observed in a fraction of the cell population. The possibility that the combination of deltanoids with radiation might promote cell death (i.e., through a differentiation stimulus plus DNA damage) was investigated by exposing both TP53 wild-type and TP53-mutated breast tumor cells to $1\alpha,25\text{-}(OH)_2D_3$ or EB 1089 for 48 h prior to irradiation. The combination of deltanoids with radiation resulted in enhanced antiproliferative effects in the TP53 wild-type MCF-7 cells based on both a clonogenic assay and the determination of numbers of viable cells. The combination of EB 1089 with radiation increased DNA fragmentation based on both the terminal transferase end-labeling (TUNEL) and bisbenzamide spectrofluorometric assays, suggesting the promotion of apoptosis. Enhancement of local tumor control by deltanoids followed with fractionated radiation was further substantiated *in vivo* with the use of EB 1089, partly through the promotion of apoptotic cell death.

Treatment with EB 1089 was found to block the increase in p21waf1/cip1 levels induced by adriamycin and interfere with induction of MAP kinase activity by ionizing radiation. These effects may be related to the capacity of EB 1089 to promote secretion of insulin-like growth factor binding protein. Similarly, pretreatment with another deltanoid, ILX 23-7553, shifted the dose–response curve for clonogenic survival, increasing sensitivity to adriamycin 2.5-fold and sensitivity to radiation fourfold. Our recent studies demonstrate that EB 1089 delays the accelerated senescence response to fractionated ionizing radiation in the breast tumor cells, promotes cell death in the irradiated cells, and delays proliferative recovery.[82,87] Taken together these findings indicate that deltanoids sensitize breast tumor cells to certain anticancer treatments. These data support the concept that deltanoids could have utility in combination with conventional chemotherapy or radiotherapy in the treatment of cancer.

Trump and Johnson's research groups[88–92] have conducted several studies both *in vitro* and *in vivo* on the various combinations of $1\alpha,25\text{-}(OH)_2D_3$ and other antitumor agents. Yu et al.[93] have shown that $1\alpha,25\text{-}(OH)_2D_3$ increased mitoxantrone/dexamethasone-mediated growth inhibition in prostate cancer PC-3 cells ($p < 0.05$) and that $1\alpha,25\text{-}(OH)_2D_3$ acted synergistically with mitoxantrone. Additionally, such a combination was shown to reduce the surviving fraction per gram tumor compared with mitoxantrone/dexamethasone or untreated controls ($p < 0.03$). The authors have further demonstrated the use of such combination therapy in other tumor models including murine squamous cell carcinoma (SCCVII/SF).[81,91–93] The growth of SCCVII/SF tumors was inhibited in mice treated simultaneously with dexamethasone and $1\alpha,25\text{-}(OH)_2D_3$ when compared to no treatment or single-agent treatment. In this case total VDR content in SCCVII/SF cells was increased after treatment with dexamethasone. Treatment of tumor-bearing animals with dexamethasone (9 µg/day) for 7 days also led to increased VDR-ligand-binding activities in whole-cell extracts from tumor or kidneys and decreased activity in intestinal mucosa. It therefore appears that dexamethasone is capable of enhancing the antitumor effect of $1\alpha,25\text{-}(OH)_2D_3$ by regulating VDR-ligand-binding activity.

The strategy of combining deltanoids with multiple anti-cancer agents is promising. Danilenko and Studzinski[94] have summarized an extensive range of compounds and agents that have been used in combination with deltanoids to increase their differentiation-inducing and antiproliferative activities. They have also discussed in detail the possible mechanistic basis for the observed synergy or additive effect of deltanoids in several different tumor types. Evidence available from the literature on the potentiation of deltanoid effects with other differentiation agents, plant derived compounds, antioxidants, and other agents is presented in the review article by Danilenko and Studzinski.[94]

## 5.9 CONCLUSION

There is accumulating evidence that the vitamin $D_3$/VDR axis is important in multiple cancers. Epidemiological studies on the association of the occurrence and outcome of cancers with serum $1\alpha,25\text{-}(OH)_2D_3$ levels or vitamin $D_3$ status are consistent with vitamin D insufficiency being a factor in the development of certain malignancies, primarily prostate, breast, and colon cancer. Given the direct link between $1\alpha,25\text{-}(OH)_2D_3$ and its nutritional precursor vitamin $D_3$, new frontiers in current research include investigating the physiological role of extrarenal 1-hydroxylases in cells prone to cancer. There is also current emphasis on manipulating $1\alpha,25\text{-}(OH)_2D_3$ levels in patients with cancer as an alternative means of exploiting the anticancer properties of $1\alpha,25\text{-}(OH)_2D_3$. Clinical trials[95–97] are under way examining the safety and efficacy of weekly high dose of $1\alpha,25\text{-}(OH)_2D_3$ in the presence or absence of docetaxel, carboplatin, or dexamethasone in patients with androgen-independent prostate cancer. These studies follow very encouraging phase II trials in the same settings. These trials demonstrated that high intermittent doses of $1\alpha,25\text{-}(OH)_2D_3$ can be administered to patients without toxicity and that $1\alpha,25\text{-}(OH)_2D_3$ has potential as an anticancer agent.

It is important to identify the appropriate recommended dietary allowance for vitamin $D_3$ to achieve normal health or to overcome the occurrence of above-mentioned vitamin $D_3$ insufficiencies in cancer-prone populations. It is advisable to assure adequate vitamin $D_3$ status in relation to carcinomas of the breast, prostate, and colon, especially if sun exposure is curtailed and/or for individuals having a skin type with increased pigmentation. Because $1\alpha,25\text{-}(OH)_2D_3$ and its analogs have the added potential to be used to suppress multiple phases of tumor development such as initiation of carcinogenesis, promotion, and progression, there is definitely a critical need to develop deltanoids as anticancer agents. More experimental approaches are necessary to elucidate the underlying molecular and cellular basis of the anticancer properties of vitamin $D_3$ and its analogs.

## REFERENCES

1. DeLuca HF. Historical overview. In: Feldman D, Glorieux FH, Pike JW, eds. *Vitamin D.* San Diego: Academic Press; 1997:3–11.
2. McCollum EV, Simmonds N, Becker JE, Shipley PG. An experimental demonstration of the existence of a vitamin, which promotes calcium deposition. *J Biol Chem* 1922; 53:293–298.
3. Askew FA, Bourdillon RB, Bruce HM, Jenkins RGC, Webster TA. The distillation of vitamin D. *Proc R Soc* 1931; B107:76–90.

4. Windaus A, Linsert O. Vitamin $D_1$. *Ann Chem* 1928; 468:148.
5. Windaus A, Linsert O, Luttringhaus A, Weidlich G. Crystalline vitamin-$D_2$. *Ann Chem* 1932; 492:226–241.
6. Esvelt RP, DeLuca HF, Wichmann JK, Yoshizawa S, Zurcher J, Sar M, Stumpf WE. $1\alpha$,25-Dihydroxyvitamin $D_3$ stimulated increase of 7,8-didehydrocholesterol levels in rat skin. *Biochemistry* 1980; 19(26):6158–6161.
7. Esvelt RP, Schnoes HK, DeLuca HF. Vitamin $D_3$ from rat skins irradiated in vitro with ultraviolet light. *Arch Biochem Biophys* 1978; 188(2):282–286.
8. Holick MF, MacLaughlin JA, Clark MB, Holick SA, Potts JT Jr, Anderson RR, Blank IH, Parrish JA, Elias P. Photosynthesis of previtamin $D_3$ in human skin and the physiologic consequences. *Science* 1980; 210(4466):203–205.
9. Lawson DEM. Metabolism of vitamin D. In: Norman AW, ed. *Vitamin D: Molecular Biology and Clinical Nutrition*. New York: Marcel Dekker; 1980:93–126.
10. Webb AR, Holick MF. The role of sunlight in the cutaneous production of vitamin $D_3$. *Annu Rev Nutr* 1988; 8:375–399.
11. Webb AR, Kline L, Holick MF. Influence of season and latitude on the cutaneous synthesis of vitamin $D_3$: exposure to winter sunlight in Boston and Edmonton will not promote vitamin $D_3$ synthesis in human skin. *J Clin Endocrinol Metab* 1988; 67(2):373–378.
12. Clemens TL, Adams JS, Henderson SL, Holick MF. Increased skin pigment reduces the capacity of skin to synthesise vitamin D3. *Lancet* 1982; 1(8263):74–76.
13. DeLuca HF. The vitamin D story: a collaborative effort of basic science and clinical medicine. *FASEB J* 1988; 2(3):224–236.
14. Fraser DR. Calcium-regulating hormones: vitamin D. In: Nordin BEC, ed. *Calcium in Human Biology*. London: Springer-Verlag; 1988:27–41.
15. Blunt JW, DeLuca HF, Schnoes HK. 25-hydroxycholecalciferol. A biologically active metabolite of vitamin $D_3$. *Biochemistry* 1968; 7(10):3317–3322.
16. Blunt JW, Tanaka Y, DeLuca HF. The biological activity of 25-hydroxycholecalciferol, a metabolite of vitamin $D_3$. *Proc Natl Acad Sci USA* 1968; 61(4):1503–1506.
17. Blunt JW, Tanaka Y, DeLuca HF. The biological activity of 25-hydroxycholecalciferol, a metabolite of vitamin $D_3$. *Proc Natl Acad Sci USA* 1968; 61(2):717–718.
18. DeLuca HF. Metabolism and function of vitamin D. In: DeLuca HF, Suttie JW, eds. *The Fat-Soluble Vitamins*. Madison: University of Wisconsin Press; 1970:3–20.
19. Haussler MR, Myrtle JF, Norman AW. The association of a metabolite of vitamin $D_3$ with intestinal mucosa chromatin *in vivo*. *J Biol Chem* 1968; 243(15):4055–4064.
20. Lawson DE, Wilson PW, Kodicek E. Metabolism of vitamin D. A new cholecalciferol metabolite, involving loss of hydrogen at C-1, in chick intestinal nuclei. *Biochem J* 1969; 115(2):269–277.
21. Lawson DE, Wilson PW, Kodicek E. New vitamin D metabolite localized in intestinal cell nuclei. *Nature* 1969; 222(189):171–172.
22. Myrtle JF, Haussler MR, Norman AW. Evidence for the biologically active form of cholecalciferol in the intestine. *J Biol Chem* 1970; 245(5):1190–1196.
23. Holick MF, Semmler EJ, Schnoes HK, DeLuca HF. 1-Hydroxy derivative of vitamin $D_3$: a highly potent analog of $1\alpha$,25-dihydroxyvitamin $D_3$. *Science* 1973; 180(82):190–191.

24. Paaren HE, Shnoes HK, Deluca HF. Synthesis of 1β-hydroxyvitamin $D_3$ and 1β-25-dihydroxyvitamin $D_3$. *J Chem Soc Chem Commun* 1977; 890–892.

25. Semmler EJ, Holick MF, Schnoes HK, Deluca HF. The synthesis of 1,25-dihydroxycholecalciferol. A metabolite of vitamin D active in intestine. *Biochemistry* 1972; 10:2799–2804.

26. Fraser DR, Kodicek E. Unique biosynthesis by kidney of a biological active vitamin D metabolite. *Nature* 1970; 228(5273):764–766.

27. Brommage R, DeLuca HF. Evidence that 1α,25-dihydroxyvitamin $D_3$ is the physiologically active metabolite of vitamin $D_3$. *Endocr Rev* 1985; 6(4):491–511.

28. Cooke NE, Haddad JG. Vitamin D binding protein. In: Feldman D, Glorieux FG, Pike JW, eds. *Vitamin D*. San Diego: Academic Press; 1997:87–101.

29. Ovesen L, Andersen R, Jakobsen J. Geographical differences in vitamin D status, with particular reference to European countries. *Proc Nutr Soc* 2003; 62(4):813–821.

30. Ovesen L, Brot C, Jakobsen J. Food contents and biological activity of 25-hydroxyvitamin D: a vitamin D metabolite to be reckoned with? *Ann Nutr Metab* 2003; 47(3–4):107–113.

31. Moore C, Murphy MM, Keast DR, Holick MF. Vitamin D intake in the United States. *J Am Diet Assoc* 2004; 104(6):980–983.

32. Calvo MS, Whiting SJ. A global perspective of vitamin D intake. In: *Cancer Chemoprevention and Cancer Treatment: Is There a Role for Vitamin D, 1α,25 (OH)2-Vitamin $D_3$, or New Analogs (Deltanoids)?* 2004; NIH campus, Bethesda, MD: NIH; 2004:24.

33. Zull JE, Czarnowska-Misztal E, DeLuca HF. On the relationship between vitamin D action and actinomycin-sensitive processes. *Proc Natl Acad Sci USA* 1966; 55(1):177–184.

34. Haussler MR, Norman AW. Chromosomal receptor for a vitamin D metabolite. *Proc Natl Acad Sci USA* 1969; 62(1):155–162.

35. Carlberg C. Current understanding of the function of the nuclear vitamin D receptor in response to its natural and synthetic ligand. In: Reichrath J, Friedrich M, Tilgen W, eds. *Vitamin D Analogs in Cancer Prevention and Therapy*. Berlin: Springer-Verlag; 2003:20–43.

36. Brumbaugh PF, Haussler MR. 1α,25-dihydroxyvitamin $D_3$ receptor: competitive binding of vitamin D analogs. *Life Sci* 1973; 13(12):1737–1746.

37. Brumbaugh PF, Haussler MR. Nuclear and cytoplasmic receptors for 1α,25-dihydroxycholecalciferol in intestinal mucosa. *Biochem Biophys Res Commun* 1973; 51(1):74–80.

38. Brumbaugh PF, Haussler MR. Specific binding of 1α,25-dihydroxycholecalciferol to nuclear components of chick intestine. *J Biol Chem* 1975; 250(4):1588–1594.

39. Moras D, Gronemeyer H. The nuclear receptor ligand-binding domain: structure and function. *Curr Opin Cell Biol* 1998; 10(3):384–391.

40. Apperly FL. The relation of solar radiation to cancer mortality in North America. *Cancer Res* 1941; 1:191–195.

41. Garland CF, Comstock GW, Garland FC, Helsing KJ, Shaw EK, Gorham ED. Serum 25-hydroxyvitamin D and colon cancer: eight-year prospective study. *Lancet* 1989; 2(8673):1176–1178.

42. Garland FC, Garland CF, Gorham ED, Young JF. Geographic variation in breast cancer mortality in the United States: a hypothesis involving exposure to solar radiation. *Prev Med* 1990; 19(6):614–622.

43. Garland C, Shekelle RB, Barrett-Connor E, Criqui MH, Rossof AH, Paul O. Dietary vitamin D and calcium and risk of colorectal cancer: a 19-year prospective study in men. *Lancet* 1985; 1(8424):307–309.

44. Garland CF, Garland FC. Do sunlight and vitamin D reduce the likelihood of colon cancer? *Int J Epidemiol* 1980; 9(3):227–231.

45. Garland CF, Garland FC, Gorham ED. Can colon cancer incidence and death rates be reduced with calcium and vitamin D? *Am J Clin Nutr* 1991; 54(1 Suppl):193S–201S.

46. Calvo MS, Barton CN. Racial differences in vitamin D intake, dietary supplement use and vitamin D status among black and white men and women in the NHANES III survey. In: *Cancer Chemoprevention and Cancer Treatment: Is There a Role for Vitamin D, 1α,25 (OH)2-Vitamin D₃, or New Analogs (Deltanoids)?* 2004; NIH campus, Bethesda, MD: NIH; 2004.

47. Garland CF, Garland FC, Gorham ED. Calcium and vitamin D. Their potential roles in colon and breast cancer prevention. *Ann NY Acad Sci* 1999; 889:107–119.

48. Janowsky EC, Lester GE, Weinberg CR, Millikan RC, Schildkraut JM, Garrett PA, Hulka BS. Association between low levels of 1α,25-dihydroxyvitamin D and breast cancer risk. *Public Health Nutr* 1999; 2(3):283–291.

49. Mawer EB, Walls J, Howell A, Davies M, Ratcliffe WA, Bundred NJ. Serum 1α,25-dihydroxyvitamin D may be related inversely to disease activity in breast cancer patients with bone metastases. *J Clin Endocrinol Metab* 1997; 82(1):118–122.

50. Ruggiero M, Pacini S, Aterini S, Fallai C, Ruggiero C, Pacini P. Vitamin D receptor gene polymorphism is associated with metastatic breast cancer. *Oncol Res* 1998; 10(1):43–46.

51. Buyru N, Tezol A, Yosunkaya-Fenerci E, Dalay N. Vitamin D receptor gene polymorphisms in breast cancer. *Exp Mol Med* 2003; 35(6):550–555.

52. Dunning AM, McBride S, Gregory J, Durocher F, Foster NA, Healey CS, Smith N, Pharoah PD, Luben RN, Easton DF, Ponder BA. No association between androgen or vitamin D receptor gene polymorphisms and risk of breast cancer. *Carcinogenesis* 1999; 20(11):2131–2135.

53. Bretherton-Watt D, Given-Wilson R, Mansi JL, Thomas V, Carter N, Colston KW. Vitamin D receptor gene polymorphisms are associated with breast cancer risk in a UK Caucasian population. *Br J Cancer* 2001; 85(2):171–175.

54. Cui J, Shen K, Shen Z, Jiang F, Shen F. Relationship of vitamin D receptor polymorphism with breast cancer. *Zhonghua Yi Xue Yi Chuan Xue Za Zhi* 2001; 18(4):286–288.

55. Ingles SA, Garcia DG, Wang W, Nieters A, Henderson BE, Kolonel LN, Haile RW, Coetzee GA. Vitamin D receptor genotype and breast cancer in Latinas (United States). *Cancer Causes Control* 2000; 11(1):25–30.

56. Curran JE, Vaughan T, Lea RA, Weinstein SR, Morrison NA, Griffiths LR. Association of A vitamin D receptor polymorphism with sporadic breast cancer development. *Int J Cancer* 1999; 83(6):723–726.

57. Woodson K, Ratnasinghe D, Bhat NK, Stewart C, Tangrea JA, Hartman TJ, Stolzenberg-Solomon R, Virtamo J, Taylor PR, Albanes D. Prevalence of disease-related DNA polymorphisms among participants in a large cancer prevention trial. *Eur J Cancer Prev* 1999; 8(5):441–447.

58. Guy M, Lowe LC, Bretherton-Watt D, Mansi JL, Colston KW. Approaches to evaluating the association of vitamin D receptor gene polymorphisms with breast cancer risk. *Recent Results Cancer Res* 2003; 164:43–54.

59. Schondorf T, Eisberg C, Wassmer G, Warm M, Becker M, Rein DT, Gohring UJ. Association of the vitamin D receptor genotype with bone metastases in breast cancer patients. *Oncology* 2003; 64(2):154–159.

60. Lundin AC, Soderkvist P, Eriksson B, Bergman-Jungestrom M, Wingren S. Association of breast cancer progression with a vitamin D receptor gene polymorphism. South-East Sweden Breast Cancer Group. *Cancer Res* 1999; 59(10):2332–2334.

61. Xu Y, Shibata A, McNeal JE, Stamey TA, Feldman D, Peehl DM. Vitamin D receptor start codon polymorphism (FokI) and prostate cancer progression. *Cancer Epidemiol Biomarkers Prev* 2003; 12(1):23–27.

62. Price DK, Franks ME, Figg WD. Genetic variations in the vitamin D receptor, androgen receptor and enzymes that regulate androgen metabolism. *J Urol* 2004; 171(2 Pt 2):S45–49; discussion S49.

63. Ntais C, Polycarpou A, Ioannidis JP. Vitamin D receptor gene polymorphisms and risk of prostate cancer: a meta-analysis. *Cancer Epidemiol Biomarkers Prev* 2003; 12(12):1395–1402.

64. Liu JH, Li HW, Tong M, Li M, Na YQ. Genetic risk factors of prostate cancer in Han nationality population in Northern China and a preliminary study of the reason of racial difference in prevalence of prostate cancer. *Zhonghua Yi Xue Za Zhi* 2004; 84(5):364–368.

65. Tayeb MT, Clark C, Haites NE, Sharp L, Murray GI, McLeod HL. Vitamin D receptor, HER-2 polymorphisms and risk of prostate cancer in men with benign prostate hyperplasia. *Saudi Med J* 2004; 25(4):447–451.

66. Osborne JE, Hutchinson PE. Vitamin D and systemic cancer: is this relevant to malignant melanoma? *Br J Dermatol* 2002; 147(2):197–213.

67. Park WH, Seol JG, Kim ES, Binderup L, Koeffler HP, Kim BK, Lee YY. The induction of apoptosis by a combined $1\alpha,25(OH)_2D_3$ analog, EB1089 and TGF-$\beta$1 in NCI-H929 multiple myeloma cells. *Int J Oncol* 2002; 20(3):533–542.

68. Yang L, Yang J, Venkateswarlu S, Ko T, Brattain MG. Autocrine TGF-$\beta$ signaling mediates vitamin $D_3$ analog-induced growth inhibition in breast cells. *J Cell Physiol* 2001; 188(3):383–393.

69. Dusso A, Cozzolino M, Lu Y, Sato T, Slatopolsky E. 1$\alpha$,25-Dihydroxyvitamin D downregulation of TGF-$\alpha$/EGFR expression and growth signaling: a mechanism for the antiproliferative actions of the sterol in parathyroid hyperplasia of renal failure. *J Steroid Biochem Mol Biol* 2004; 89–90(1–5):507–511.

70. Fioravanti L, Miodini P, Cappelletti V, DiFronzo G. Synthetic analogs of vitamin $D_3$ have inhibitory effects on breast cancer cell lines. *Anticancer Res* 1998; 18(3A):1703–1708.

71. Garach-Jehoshua O, Ravid A, Liberman UA, Koren R. 1$\alpha$,25-Dihydroxyvitamin D3 increases the growth-promoting activity of autocrine epidermal growth factor receptor ligands in keratinocytes. *Endocrinology* 1999; 140(2):713–721.

72. McGaffin KR, Acktinson LE, Chrysogelos SA. Growth and EGFR regulation in breast cancer cells by vitamin D and retinoid compounds. *Breast Cancer Res Treat* 2004; 86(1):55–73.

73. Ji Y, Kutner A, Verstuyf A, Verlinden L, Studzinski GP. Derivatives of vitamins $D_2$ and $D_3$ activate three MAPK pathways and upregulate pRb expression in differentiating HL60 cells. *Cell Cycle* 2002; 1(6):410–415.

74. Yu W, Liao QY, Hantash FM, Sanders BG, Kline K. Activation of extracellular signal-regulated kinase and c-jun-NH(2)-terminal kinase but not p38 mitogen-activated protein kinases is required for RRR-alpha-tocopheryl succinate-induced apoptosis of human breast cancer cells. *Cancer Res* 2001; 61(17):6569–6576.

75. DeLuca HF, Ostrem VK. Analogs of the hormonal form of vitamin D and their possible use in leukemia. *Prog Clin Biol Res* 1988; 259:41–55.

76. Elstner E, Linker-Israeli M, Le J, Umiel T, Michl P, Said JW, Binderup L, Reed JC, Koeffler HP. Synergistic decrease of clonal proliferation, induction of differentiation, and apoptosis of acute promyelocytic leukemia cells after combined treatment with novel 20-epi vitamin $D_3$ analogs and 9-*cis* retinoic acid. *J Clin Invest* 1997; 99(2):349–360.

77. Inaba M, Okuno S, Nishizawa Y, Yukioka K, Otani S, Matsui-Yuasa I, Morisawa S, DeLuca HF, Morii H. Biological activity of fluorinated vitamin D analogs at C-26 and C-27 on human promyelocytic leukemia cells, HL-60. *Arch Biochem Biophys* 1987; 258(2):421–425.

78. Munker R, Kobayashi T, Elstner E, Norman AW, Uskokovic M, Zhang W, Andreeff M, Koeffler HP. A new series of vitamin D analogs is highly active for clonal inhibition, differentiation, and induction of WAF1 in myeloid leukemia. *Blood* 1996; 88(6):2201–2209.

79. Munker R, Zhang W, Elstner E, Koeffler HP. Vitamin D analogs, leukemia and WAF1. *Leuk Lymphoma* 1998; 31(3–4):279–284.

80. Moore TB, Koeffler HP, Yamashiro JM, Wada RK. Vitamin $D_3$ analogs inhibit growth and induce differentiation in LA-N-5 human neuroblastoma cells. *Clin Exp Metastasis* 1996; 14(3):239–245.

81. Light BW, Yu WD, McElwain MC, Russell DM, Trump DL, Johnson CS. Potentiation of cisplatin antitumor activity using a vitamin D analogue in a murine squamous cell carcinoma model system. *Cancer Res* 1997; 5717:3759–3764.

82. Chaudhry M, Sundaram S, Gennings C, Carter H, Gewirtz DA. The vitamin $D_3$ analog, ILX-23-7553, enhances the response to adriamycin and irradiation in MCF-7 breast tumor cells. *Cancer Chemother Pharmacol* 2001; 47(5):429–436.

83. Gewirtz DA, Gupta MS, Sundaram S. Vitamin $D_3$ and vitamin $D_3$ analogues as an adjunct to cancer chemotherapy and radiotherapy. *Curr Med Chem Anti-Cancer Agents* 2002; 2(6):683–690.

84. Sundaram S, Chaudhry M, Reardon D, Gupta M, Gewirtz DA. The vitamin $D_3$ analog EB 1089 enhances the antiproliferative and apoptotic effects of adriamycin in MCF-7 breast tumor cells. *Breast Cancer Res* Treat 2000; 63(1):1–10.

85. Sundaram S, Gewirtz DA. The vitamin $D_3$ analog EB 1089 enhances the response of human breast tumor cells to radiation. *Radiat Res* 1999; 152(5):479–486.

86. Sundaram S, Sea A, Feldman S, Strawbridge R, Hoopes PJ, Demidenko E, Binderup L, Gewirtz DA. The combination of a potent vitamin $D_3$ analog, EB 1089, with ionizing radiation reduces tumor growth and induces apoptosis of MCF-7 breast tumor xenografts in nude mice. *Clin Cancer Res* 2003; 9(6):2350–2356.

87. DeMasters GA, Gupta MS, Jones KR, Cabot M, Wang H, Gennings C, Park M, Bratland A, Ree AH, Gewirtz DA. Potentiation of cell killing by fractionated radiation and suppression of proliferative recovery in MCF-7 breast tumor cells by the Vitamin D3 analog EB 1089. *J Steroid Biochem Mol Biol* 2004; 92(5):365–374.

88. Ahmed S, Johnson CS, Rueger RM, Trump DL. Calcitriol (1,25-dihydroxychole-calciferol) potentiates activity of mitoxantrone/dexamethasone in an androgen independent prostate cancer model. *J Urol* 2002; 168(2):756–761.

89. Bernardi RJ, Johnson CS, Modzelewski RA, Trump DL. Antiproliferative effects of 1α,25-dihydroxyvitamin D(3) and vitamin D analogs on tumor-derived endothelial cells. *Endocrinology* 2002; 143(7):2508–2514.

90. Bernardi RJ, Trump DL, Yu WD, McGuire TF, Hershberger PA, Johnson CS. Combination of 1α,25-dihydroxyvitamin D(3) with dexamethasone enhances cell cycle arrest and apoptosis: role of nuclear receptor cross-talk and Erk/Akt signaling. *Clin Cancer Res* 2001; 7(12):4164–4173.

91. Hershberger PA, McGuire TF, Yu WD, Zuhowski EG, Schellens JH, Egorin MJ, Trump DL, Johnson CS. Cisplatin potentiates 1α,25-dihydroxyvitamin D₃-induced apoptosis in association with increased mitogen-activated protein kinase kinase 1 (MEKK-1) expression. *Mol Cancer Ther* 2002; 1(10):821–829.

92. Hershberger PA, Yu WD, Modzelewski RA, Rueger RM, Johnson CS, Trump DL. Calcitriol (1,25-dihydroxycholecalciferol) enhances paclitaxel antitumor activity *in vitro* and *in vivo* and accelerates paclitaxel-induced apoptosis. *Clin Cancer Res* 2001; 7(4):1043–1051.

93. Yu WD, McElwain MC, Modzelewski RA, Russell DM, Smith DC, Trump DL, Johnson CS. Enhancement of 1α,25-dihydroxyvitamin D₃-mediated antitumor activity with dexamethasone. *J Natl Cancer Inst* 1998; 90(2):134–141.

94. Danilenko M, Studzinski GP. Enhancement by other compounds of the anti-cancer activity of vitamin D(3) and its analogs. *Exp Cell Res* 2004; 298(2):339–358.

95. Beer TM, Eilers KM, Garzotto M, Hsieh YC, Mori M. Quality of life and pain relief during treatment with calcitriol and docetaxel in symptomatic metastatic androgen-independent prostate carcinoma. *Cancer* 2004; 100(4):758–763.

96. Beer TM, Myrthue A. Calcitriol in cancer treatment: from the lab to the clinic. *Mol Cancer Ther* 2004; 3(3):373–381.

97. Trump DL, Hershberger PA, Bernardi RJ, Ahmed S, Muindi J, Fakih M, Yu WD, Johnson CS. Anti-tumor activity of calcitriol: pre-clinical and clinical studies. *J Steroid Biochem Mol Biol* 2004; 89–90(1–5):519–526.

# 6 Vitamin E Analogs as Anticancer Agents

*Jiri Neuzil, Xiu-Fang Wang, Yan Zhao, and Kun Wu*

## CONTENTS

Abstract .................................................................................................................. 111
6.1    Introduction .................................................................................................. 112
6.2    Vitamin E as an Anticancer Agent — More than an Antioxidant? ........ 113
6.3    Vitamin E Analogs — The Importance of Redox-Silence .................... 116
    6.3.1    Structure–Function Relationship ............................................... 116
    6.3.2    Vitamin E Analogs as Anticancer Agents ................................. 120
    6.3.3    Selectivity of VE Analogs Increases Their Clinical
              Application .................................................................................. 122
    6.3.4    VE Analogs Overcome Resistance of Mutant Cancer Cells
              to Apoptosis, Induce the Mitochondrial Apoptotic Pathway,
              and Cooperate with Immunological Apoptogens ..................... 123
    6.3.5    Vitamin E Analogs as Antitumor Agents: Beyond
              Mitochondria .............................................................................. 126
    6.3.6    Pharmacokinetics of VE Analogs — A Potential Secondary
              Beneficial Bioactivity ............................................................... 127
6.4    Conclusions and Future Directions ........................................................... 128
References ............................................................................................................. 129

### ABSTRACT

Numerous attempts have been made to find antineoplastic dietary supplements. Of the potential food additives, vitamin E (VE) has been a focus of significant research because there are data suggesting its potential effect against cancer, based on the ability of VE to scavenge reactive oxygen species. Although several studies indicated an inverse correlation between VE intake and incidence of cancer, the data are not convincing. As with other epidemiological studies, there has been little outcome, offering no conclusive evidence. On the other hand, recent years have witnessed emergence of novel anticancer agents from the group of VE analogs, epitomized by α-tocopheryl succinate (α-TOS). These agents, unlike VE itself, are redox-silent and, unlike VE, induce apoptosis. Additional data suggest selectivity for malignant cells and their superiority over VE in cancer suppression, at least in preclinical settings. In this chapter, we review the current status of VE and, in particular, its analogs as potential antineoplastic agents and try to suggest future directions so that some of these compounds may prove useful for treatment of multiple malignancies.

## 6.1  INTRODUCTION

Significant efforts have been made to find cures against diseases, of which cancer is, disputably, the greatest challenge. The problem with neoplasia is that the pathology is of clonal origin; therefore, cancer cells are undergoing chromosomal instability and frequent mutations that complicate treatment. Another complication is that many of the established anticancer drugs are nonselective, causing damage not only to the target malignant cells, but also to normal cells and tissues, compromising the treatment outcome.

Focus has been given to dietary supplements as potential anticancer drugs. Thus, agents present in the diet are, generally, nontoxic, so that they may be selective antineoplastic agents, depending on their activities. Of dietary components, vitamin E (VE) has been studied because it is capable of scavenging reactive oxygen species (ROS) that have been implicated in tumorigenesis. Many epidemiological studies have aimed at determining whether dietary VE may inhibit cancer initiation and progression. Despite these investigations, little or no correlation between VE intake and the incidence of a particular neoplastic disease has been found.

Figure 6.1 shows the structure of the biologically most active VE, α-tocopherol (α-TOH) and its analog α-tocopheryl succinate (α-TOS), a redox-silent VE analog with strong anticancer activity.[1] There are three major domains in the structure of the compounds. Domain I (*hydrophobic domain*) is essential for association of the agents with membranes and lipoproteins; Domain II (*signaling domain*) is involved in fine-tuning of the activity of the compounds; and finally, Domain III (*functional domain*) endows the compounds with their overall activity. Thus, the hydroxyl group gives α-TOH its redox activity, while succinate provides α-TOS with its proapoptotic activity. It is now clear that it is the chemistry of the compounds that decide their major biological activity.

Several papers reported superiority of α-TOS over α-TOH in its anticancer effect.[1] This follows from studies mostly using athymic mice with human cancer xenografts. The high anticancer index of α-TOS is linked to its apoptogenic activity. This is a highly intriguing molecule because it not only suppresses cancer by causing apoptosis in malignant cells, but it also inhibits their proliferation and modulates expression of several important genes. Data are now suggesting also an antiangiogenic activity of α-TOS. Importantly, α-TOS is nontoxic to normal cells and tissues.

These notions stipulate that VE analogs hold a promise as selective anticancer agents with clinical use. At present the molecular mechanisms of their activities that translate into their antineoplastic effects are not understood in detail. It is

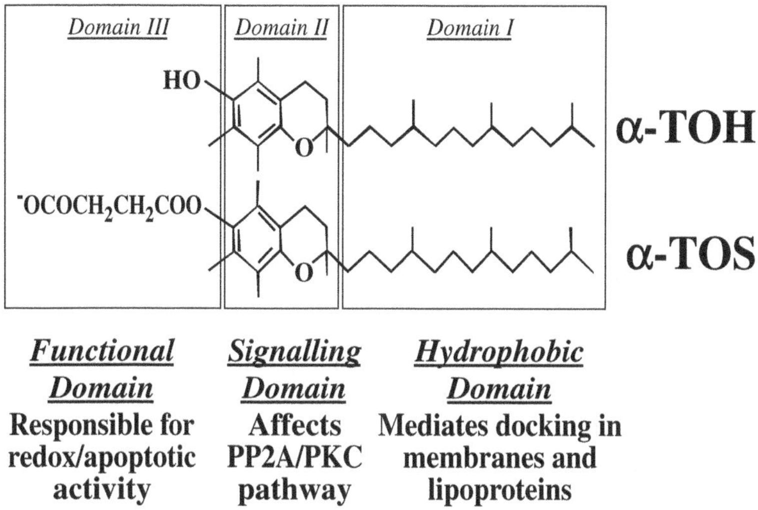

| Domain III | Domain II | Domain I |
|---|---|---|

HO — α-TOH

⁻OCOCH₂CH₂COO — α-TOS

**Functional Domain**
Responsible for redox/apoptotic activity

**Signalling Domain**
Affects PP2A/PKC pathway

**Hydrophobic Domain**
Mediates docking in membranes and lipoproteins

**FIGURE 6.1** Major domains in VE analogs. Shown are the structures of α-TOH and α-TOS with the specification and major function of the three main domains. Domains I and II are identical; Domain III differs. While Domains I and II are important for the extent of the activity, Domain III determines whether the agent does or does not induce apoptosis.

important to enhance our knowledge in this respect, so that clinical trials can commence that will, we hope, lead to generation and use of novel antineoplastic strategies.

## 6.2 VITAMIN E AS AN ANTICANCER AGENT — MORE THAN AN ANTIOXIDANT?

Great interest has been given to the potential use of VE as anticancer drugs. This is rather logical, since VE and other redox-active micronutrients are ingested regularly and their dose can be increased by food fortification. They may be beneficial since they do not exert deleterious effects.

The term VE refers to eight naturally occurring, structurally related agents, four tocopherols (α-, β-, γ-, and δ-TOH), and four tocotrienols (α-, β-, γ-, and δ-T3H). The biological activity of VE has been determined by the rat fetal resorption assay, in which α-TOH exhibits the highest activity among the forms of VE. α-TOH is also the form of VE present at the highest level in serum and dietary supplements. However, the predominant form of VE in a typical Western diet is γ-TOH, which is present in food at levels two to four times higher than those of α-TOH.[2] Plasma as well as tissue concentrations of γ-TOH and α-TOH can be enhanced by supplementation.[2]

Many attempts have been made to find out whether dietary VE has an anticancer activity. Although the best understood function of VE is linked to its redox activity, studies show that VE compounds exhibit antitumor properties. However, the epidemiological evidence supporting a link between α-TOH or other forms of VE and cancer is limited and intervention studies are scarce.

In the Alpha-Tocopherol, Beta-Carotene Cancer Prevention (ATBC) trial, smokers who took α-TOH supplements had a 32% lower incidence of prostate cancer and 41% lower mortality from prostate cancer than the unsupplemented subjects.[3] Higher serum α-TOH was associated with lower lung cancer risk, in particular among those with less cigarette smoke exposure.[4] In contrast, gastric, pancreatic, or colorectal cancers were not affected in the ATBC study.[5-7] In the Linxian trial, subjects who received α-TOH, selenium, and β-carotene, showed a 13% reduced incidence of cancer and 50% reduced mortality from stomach cancer.[8] An ongoing Selenium and Vitamin E Cancer Prevention Trial (SELECT) is the second large-scale study of prevention of prostate cancer with final results anticipated not before the year 2013.[9] The SELECT project offers an opportunity to conduct molecular epidemiologic investigations for assessment of the gene–environment interactions and their role in carcinogenesis. These results may provide much needed evidence about association of VE and cancer.

Observational studies in humans potentially suggesting association between α-TOH and cancer risk have provided inconsistent results. Prediagnostic serum α-TOH levels are inversely associated with lung cancer in some but not all studies, and case-control investigations have been generally supportive of reduced lung cancer risk among persons with higher blood α-TOH levels.[10-12] No association has been found between serum α-TOH and cancer risk in some cohort and case-control studies of prostate, breast, or colon cancers.[13-16] The epidemiological evidence of association of VE with cancer risk is presented in Table 6.1 and Table 6.2.

Attempts to prevent cancer by VE are based on the rationale that tumorigenesis results from free radicals attacking DNA. α-TOH is the major chain-breaking antioxidant in the lipid phase. It is thought to inhibit carcinogenesis at the level of transformation of normal cells into malignant cells, primarily through its antioxidative activity, i.e., by scavenging ROS and reactive nitrogen species. In addition, α-TOH may also inhibit cancer formation through various alternative mechanisms, including inhibition of cell proliferation, cell cycle arrest, prevention of angiogenesis, and enhancement of the immune function. In the prostate cancer lines LNCaP and PC3, α-TOH caused a dramatic reduction of the population of cells in S phase.[17] VE deficiency has been shown to be associated with impairment of the immune system, including both T- and B-cell-mediated functions. Further, VE restored age-related immune dysfunction.[18,19] α-TOH has also been shown to regulate cell growth, probably through its influence on several interconnected pathways. For example, it is thought to increase the level of p27$^{Kip1}$ while decreasing the level of the proliferating cell nuclear antigen,[20] blocking prostaglandin and arachidonic acid metabolism, inhibiting protein kinase C activity, and affecting the expression of hormones and growth factors. Subjects who received α-TOH had significantly lower serum androstenedione and testosterone compared to the placebo group.[21] This finding has been regarded as a possible explanation of the selective reduction in prostate cancer observed in the ATBC

**TABLE 6.1**
**Epidemiological Evidence of Association of Vitamin E with Cancer Risk**

| Country | No. of Subjects | Type of Study | Type of Cancer | RR/OR | 95% CI | Association | Ref. |
|---|---|---|---|---|---|---|---|
| Finland | 29,133 | Cohort | Prostate | 0.32 | 0.12–0.47 | Lower risk | 2 |
| | | | | 0.41 | 0.01–0.65 | | |
| | | | Lung | 0.81 | 0.67–0.97 | Lower risk | 3 |
| | | | Stomach, pancreas, colorectal | ND | ND | No association | 4–6 |
| China | 29,584 | Intervention | Stomach | 0.79 | 0.64–0.99 | Lower risk | 7 |
| USA | 21,116 | Case-control | Prostate | 0.76 | 0.54–1.08 | May be protective | 116 |
| USA | 24-county | Case-control | Breast | 0.75 | 0.49–1.13 | No association for all women and for black women; modest inverse association among white women | 13 |
| USA | 1,045 923 | Cohort | Stomach | 1.02 | 0.82–1.27 | No association | 14 |
| USA | 33-county | Case-control | Colon | 0.9 | 0.6–1.5 | No association for whites | 15 |
| | | | | 0.3 | 0.1–0.6 | Strongly inverse association | |
| Netherlands | 58,279 | Cohort | Prostate | ND | ND | No association | 16 |
| USA | 711,891 | Cohort | Colorectal | 1.08 | 0.85–1.38 | No association | 117 |
| USA | 1,157 | Case-control | Rectal | 2.2 | 1.1–4.3 | Increased risk | 118 |
| | | | | 3.6 for α-TOH | 1.4–9.4 | Stronger increased risk for women aged 60 years | |
| | | | | 5.3 for γ-TOH | 2.11–3.2 | | |
| | | | | 1.9 for β-TOH | 0.9–4.0 | | |
| Italy and Switzerland | 1,826 | Case-control | Laryngeal | 0.4 | 0.3–0.6 | Significant inverse relation | 119 |

*Note:* RR, related risk; OR, odds ratio; CI, confidence interval; ND, no data.

**TABLE 6.2**
**Summary of Epidemiological Evidence of Association of Vitamin E with Cancer Risk**

| Treatment | Type of Cancer | Association of VE with Cancer Risk |
|---|---|---|
| α-TOH, β-carotene | Lung, prostate | Lower cancer risk |
| | Bladder, stomach, pancreas, urinary tract, colorectal | No association |
| α-TOH, β-carotene, lycopene | Rectal | Increased cancer risk |
| VE, selenium, β-carotene | Prostate, stomach | Lower cancer risk |
| VE | Prostate | No association |
| Vitamin A, vitamin C, VE, folate, β-carotene | Prostate, bladder, skin, breast, lymph | No association |
| | Esophagus | Lower cancer risk |
| Vitamin A, vitamin C, VE, carotenoids | Prostate, ovary, lung | Lower cancer risk |
| | Bladder, stomach, breast | No association |
| Vitamin C, VE, β-carotene, calcium | Colon | Lower cancer risk |
| Vitamin C, VE | Bladder, breast, colorectal | No association |
| | Ovary, bladder | Lower cancer risk |
| β-carotene, vitamin C, VE, folate | Stomach, ovary, stomach | Lower cancer risk |
| | Lung | No association |
| Vitamin C/VE/multivitamins | Stomach, breast | No association |

study. Thus, the multiple functions of α-TOH may allow it to inhibit tumorigenesis at various stages, from initiation and promotion to progression and tumor growth; however, this premise awaits experimental verification.

It is now becoming clear that modification of the VE molecule changes, rather dramatically, its anticancer activity, with a recent focus on the proapoptotic effect of the various forms and analogs of VE.[22-24] Table 6.3 documents the relationship between the antioxidant activity of the compounds and their propensity to induce apoptosis in several cell lines. Apparently, there is inverse correlation between the proapoptotic and antioxidant activity of the agents, with the most apoptogenic of them, α-TOS, being completely redox-silent. Recent data reveal that non-antioxidant analogs of VE strongly suppress cancer *in vivo*. The current understanding of this is discussed below.

## 6.3   VITAMIN E ANALOGS — THE IMPORTANCE OF REDOX-SILENCE

### 6.3.1   STRUCTURE–FUNCTION RELATIONSHIP

The superior activity of redox-silent analogs of VE, exemplified by α-TOS, is given by their structure. Figure 6.1 shows the major domains of α-TOS and related compounds. It is the substitution of the phenolic hydroxyl group by the

## TABLE 6.3
## Comparison of Proapoptotic and Antioxidant Activity of Various Vitamin E Compounds

| Vitamin E Analogs | Antioxidant Activity | | Apoptosis, $EC_{50}$ ($\mu$g/ml) | |
| --- | --- | --- | --- | --- |
| | IU/mg | Compared to $\alpha$-TOH | MCF-7 | MDA-MB-435 |
| **Tocopheryl Analogs** | | | | |
| $\alpha$-TOS | | 0 | 7 $\pm$ 1.0 | 8 $\pm$ 1.0 |
| $\alpha$-TOA | | 0 | >200 | >200 |
| **Tocopherols** | | | | |
| $\alpha$-TOH | 1.49 | 100% | >200 | >200 |
| $\beta$-TOH | 0.75 | 50% | >200 | >200 |
| $\gamma$-TOH | 0.15 | 10% | >200 | >200 |
| $\delta$-TOH | 0.05 | 3% | 97 $\pm$ 5.0 | 145 $\pm$ 33 |
| **Tocotrienols** | | | | |
| $\alpha$-T3H | 0.75 | 50% | 14 $\pm$ 2.0 | 176 $\pm$ 23 |
| $\beta$-T3H | 0.08 | 5% | NT | NT |
| $\gamma$-T3H | NT | 0% | 15 $\pm$ 2.0 | 28 $\pm$ 2.6 |
| $\delta$-T3H | NT | 0% | 7 $\pm$ 0.8 | 13 $\pm$ 3.5 |

*Source:* From Yu, W. et al. *Nutr Cancer.* 1999; 33:26–32. With permission.

succinyl moiety that makes $\alpha$-TOS proapoptotic. To understand the importance of the individual domains in the activity of VE analogs, we synthesized compounds in which the various domains were modified or completely removed, and tested the resulting analogs for their efficacy to cause apoptosis in malignant cell types.[25]

The individual analogs studied are shown in Figure 6.2 and their effects on cancer cells are listed in Table 6.4. Compounds derived from $\alpha$-TOH with a lower number of methyl substituents in the signaling domain showed no proapoptotic activity. Esterification of the hydroxyl group with dicarboxylic fatty acids of various lengths revealed that $\alpha$-tocopheryl maleate and $\alpha$-tocopheryl fumarate were the most efficient. Presence of an uncharged fatty acid moiety in the functional domain, as suggested by $\alpha$-tocopheryl acetate, resulted in no apoptotic activity, and methylation of the free carboxylate of the ester group, as shown in case of $\alpha$-TOS or $\delta$-TOS methyl ester completely abrogated the apoptogenic activity.[25] Removal of the hydrophobic domain also wiped out the activity, as exemplified by $\alpha$-Trolox succinate.

An interesting modification to the hydrophobic domain is an exchange of the fully saturated phytyl change by the chain with three double bonds. While $\alpha$-T3H does not cause apoptosis,[25] $\gamma$- and $\delta$-T3H are apoptogenic.[25,26] Reasons for the activity of $\gamma$- and $\delta$-T3H are not known, although the polyunsaturated hydrophobic

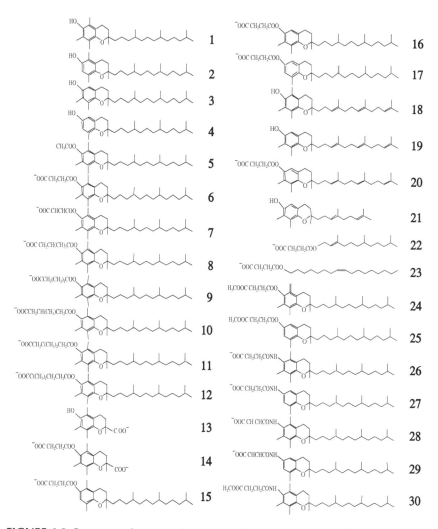

**FIGURE 6.2** Structures of compounds used to understand the structure–function relationship of VE analogs. *(continued)*

domain may act as an inhibitor of farnesyl transferase and geranylgeranyl transferase that modulate apoptosis.[27] Even more efficient than γ-T3H was its succinylated counterpart, γ-T3S.[25] This is an intriguing finding concerning the potential selectivity of the agent. It has been shown that α-TOS is selective for malignant cells.[28] One of the reasons may be that the VE analog is a weak acid with a $pK_a$ of ~5.4.[29] At the neutral pH of normal tissue interstitium, ~98% of the total pool of α-TOS is deprotonated, thus unable to diffuse into the cells. However, at the acidic tumor interstitium (pH 6.2 to 6.5), 10- to 15-fold more α-TOS is protonated; thus the uptake rate of the agent is much higher,[30] as demonstrated for other anticancer agents with acidic $pK_a$.[31] We have shown that the cell "killing rate" for

**FIGURE 6.2 (CONTINUED)**

| No. | Acronym | Name of Analog | No. | Acronym | Name of Analog |
|-----|---------|----------------|-----|---------|----------------|
| 1 | α-TOH | δ-Tocopherol | 16 | γ-TOS | γ-Tocopheryl succinate |
| 2 | β-TOH | β-Tocopherol | 17 | δ-TOS | δ-Tocopheryl succinate |
| 3 | γ-TOH | γ-Tocopherol | 18 | α-T3H | α-Tocotrienol |
| 4 | δ-TOH | δ-Tocopherol | 19 | γ-T3H | γ-Tocotrienol |
| 5 | α-TOA | α-Tocopheryl acetate | 20 | γ-T3S | γ-Tocotrienyl succinate |
| 6 | α-TOS | α-Tocopheryl succinate | 21 | α-T2H | α-2-Geranyl-chromanol |
| 7 | α-TOM | α-Tocopheryl maleate | 22 | PYS | Phytyl succinate |
| 8 | α-TO2MS | α-Tocopheryl 2-methylsuccinate | 23 | OS | Oleyl succinate |
| 9 | α-TOG | α-Tocopheryl glutarate | 24 | α-TOSM | α-Tocopheryl succinyl methyl ester |
| 10 | α-TO3MG | α-Tocopheryl 3-methylglutarate | 25 | δ-TOSM | δ-Tocopheryl succinyl methyl ester |
| 11 | α-TO33DMG | α-Tocopheryl 3,3 dimethylglutarate | 26 | α-TAS | α-Tocopheryl succinyl amide |
| 12 | α-TO22DMG | α-Tocopheryl 2,2-dimethylglutarate | 27 | δ-TAS | δ-Tocopheryl succinyl amide |
| 13 | α-TroH | α-Trolox | 28 | α-TAM | α-Tocopheryl maleyl amide |
| 14 | α-TroS | α-Trolox succinate | 29 | δ-TAM | δ-Tocopheryl maleyl amide |
| 15 | β-TOS | β-Tocopheryl succinate | 30 | α-TASM | α-Tocopheryl succinyl amide methyl ester |

α-TOS increased with low pH while no effect on the apoptotic activity was found for γ-T3H lacking the free carboxyl group,[29] and we have observed that γ-T3H killed cells such as fibroblasts and cardiac myocytes, resistant to α-TOS. Succinylation may thus make agents such as γ-T3H selective for malignant cells.

The ester link between the functional domain and the signaling domain has recently been replaced by an amide bond; the amide analogs are significantly more apoptogenic than their ester counterparts. Of these, α-tocopheryl maleyl amide was most effective, almost 100-fold more active than the prototypic α-TOS.[32] Again, methylation of its free carboxylate completely abrogated its apoptogenic activity.[32]

Collectively, these findings clearly suggest that many modifications are possible within the molecule of α-TOS, modulating the apoptogenic activity of the compound. It is now clear that a VE analog, to be an inducer of apoptosis, needs the hydrophobic chain, the tocopheryl group, and a side group with a free carboxylate. That α-TOS is compatible with these requirements was first suggested by the group of Fariss, who reported that the intact molecule of the VE analog was required for its apoptogenic activity since a similar effect was observed for α-tocopheryl butyrate, a nonhydrolyzable form of α-TOS with an ether link between the functional and the signaling domain.[33] Recently, Kline's group

**TABLE 6.4**
**Apoptotic Activity of Vitamin E Analogs**

| VE Analog[a] | Apoptosis[b] | VE Analog | Apoptosis |
|---|---|---|---|
| None | 9.5 ± 2.1 | δ-TOS (17) | 25.6 ± 3.9 |
| α-TOH (1) | 10.2 ± 2.5 | α-T3H (18) | 9.2 ± 2.1 |
| α-TOA (5) | 10.5 ± 2.9 | γ-T3H (19) | 38.2 ± 5.2 |
| α-TOS (6) | 49.2 ± 6.1 | γ-T3S (20) | 59.8 ± 7.4 |
| α-TOM (7) | 72.1 ± 8.2 | α-T2H (21) | 55.8 ± 6.7 |
| α-TOF | 95.1 ± 4.2 | PYS (22) | 9.1 ± 2.8 |
| α-TO2MS (8) | 36.2 ± 4.3 | OS (23) | 10.2 ± 2.1 |
| α-TOG (9) | 30.2 ± 3.9 | α-TOSM (24) | 12.4 ± 3.1 |
| α-TO3MG (10) | 22.5 ± 3.5 | α-TOSM (25) | 13.9 ± 2.2 |
| α-TO33DMG (11) | 15.1 ± 3.1 | α-TAS (26) | 98.5 ± 7.8 |
| α-TO22DMG (12) | 16.5 ± 2.2 | δ-TAS (27) | 84.1 ± 8.9 |
| α-TroS (14) | 10.2 ± 1.5 | α-TAM (28) | 100 |
| β-TOS (15) | 38.1 ± 4.5 | δ-TAM (29) | 95.6 ± 9.7 |
| γ-TOS (16) | 30.1 ± 4.4 | α-TASM (30) | 15.1 ± 3.1 |

[a] Structures of VE analogs are shown in Figure 6.1, except for α-TOF, which is a geometric isomer of α-TOM.

[b] Apoptosis was assessed in Jurkat cells ($0.5 \times 10^6$ per ml) exposed to individual VE analogs at 50 $\mu M$ for 12 h. The annexin V-FITC binding method was used, and the numbers in the table indicate the percentage of the cells positive for annexin V.

*Source:* Adapted from References 25 and 28.

synthesized a nonhydrolyzable analog of VE more efficient as an inducer of apoptosis in ovarian cancer cells compared to α-TOS, perhaps due to higher stability, which was also efficient against breast cancer and metastasis.[34,35]

### 6.3.2 VITAMIN E ANALOGS AS ANTICANCER AGENTS

The clinical potential of VE analogs follows from reports about their anticancer properties in animal models. These effects can be separated into antitumorigenic and antineoplastic activity. The formed effect has been shown in mice, where α-TOS enhanced breast cancer dormancy.[36] This may be due to inhibition of angiogenesis by the agent, as suggested by downregulation of the vascular endothelial growth factor.[36] We have recently observed that α-TOS also downregulated components of both autocrine and paracrine signaling pathways relevant to tumorigenesis, fibroblast growth factors, and their receptors (J. Neuzil, unpublished data). Suppression of angiogenesis may also be an important factor in inhibition of the onset of melanomas by α-TOS.[37]

Several animal models showed strong efficacy of α-TOS against cancer growth, including colon cancer,[38] melanomas,[39,40] and mesotheliomas[41] (Figure 6.3). α-TOS also suppressed liver metastasis in a colon cancer model.[42]

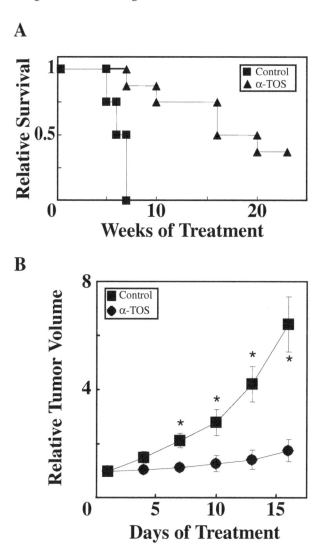

**FIGURE 6.3** Antimesothelioma effects of α-tocopheryl succinate. (A) Immunocompromised mice were injected intraperitoneally (i.p.) with human mesothelioma cells and peritoneal mesotheliomas allowed to established. On week 4 after the animals were injected with the cells, treatment was initiated consisting of i.p. administration of 200 µl of 200 µ*M* α-TOS (in DMSO) every third day for more than 20 weeks. Survival was used as a marker for the effect of α-TOS. (Adapted from Reference 16.) (B) Immunocompromised mice were injected subcutaneously with human mesothelioma cells and tumors allowed to reach 100 mm³ before treatment onset. The mice were then injected i.p. with 200 µl of 200 m*M* α-TOS (in DMSO) every second day for up to 2 weeks. Tumor size was estimated and volume calculated. (Adapted from Reference 96.)

Recently, Kline's group demonstrated anticancer activity of a novel VE analog against breast cancer and lung metastases alone or in combination with celocoxib.[43,44] These data demonstrate the therapeutic promise of α-TOS and are likely to result in clinical application of the agent and design of novel anticancer agents.

A major reason for the anticancer efficacy of VE analogs is their high apoptogenic activity. We observed that while α-TOS significantly suppressed experimental colon cancer, α-TOH showed only marginal, nonsignificant effect.[37] Analysis of the tumor sections revealed that both agents inhibited proliferation, but only α-TOS induced apoptosis.[45,46] Apoptosis as a major mechanism for antitumor activity of VE analogs has also been proposed for its antimelanoma effect[39] and may be expected also in mesotheliomas.[41] Although multiple modes of action may be expected for VE analogs, induction of apoptosis is the major determinant of their anticancer efficacy.

### 6.3.3 SELECTIVITY OF VE ANALOGS INCREASES THEIR CLINICAL APPLICATION

A paradigm rendering VE analogs clinically applicable is their selectivity for neoplastic cells,[1] as shown in many cultured cells.[28,45,47–49] The reasons for the selectivity are not fully understood. Some types of normal cells have the propensity to hydrolyze α-TOS into its redox-active counterpart.[1] Selective hydrolysis of α-TOS may, at least in some cases, explain the selective toxicity of the agent, since the proapoptotic species α-TOS would then accumulate in nonmalignant cells at levels below the toxicity threshold.

Hydrolysis of α-TOS cannot always explain its selectivity. For example, α-TOS is highly toxic to mesothelioma cells but not to nonmalignant mesothelial cells.[41,50] However, in this case, the resistant cells do not hydrolyze α-TOS. It is possible that the selectivity is given here by the resistance of the nonmalignant cells to oxidative stress. It has been published that α-TOS provokes generation of ROS in cancer cells.[51–53] We observed that mesothelioma cells generated ROS as a fast response to α-TOS while nonmalignant mesothelial cells showed very little ROS accumulation (J. Neuzil, unpublished data). It is possible that antioxidant enzymes are more expressed in nonmalignant cells, whereby affording protection from ROS-induced apoptosis. In support of this, it has been published that cells depleted of their mtDNA are resistant to apoptosis,[51,53,54] and a recent paper showed that a reason for this was adaptive upregulation of the mitochondrial superoxide dismutase.[55] It remains to be shown whether this is a mechanism of resistance of nonmalignant cells to apoptosis induced by α-TOS, although there is a report indicating the importance of lack of efficient antioxidant systems to render cancer cells susceptible to the VE analog.[56] A recent report documented a direct correlation between susceptibility of cancer cells to α-TOS and their propensity to respond to this agent by generation of ROS.[57] In support for low ROS accumulation as a mode of resistance to α-TOS, we have observed relatively low accumulation of ROS in α-TOS-resistant differentiated neuroblastoma cells when compared to the α-TOS-susceptible parental cells (J. Neuzil, unpublished data).

There is yet another plausible explanation for selectivity of VE analogs for malignant cells. This is based on the physicochemical nature of these compounds that are weak acids and that are deprotonated at physiological pH but largely protonated at the acidic pH of the tumor interstitium. This allows selective *faster* diffusion of the drug across the plasma membrane of malignant cells. Thus, there are several alternative or parallel mechanisms underlying the selectivity of VE analogs for cancer cells. Because this is one of the most important features of VE analogs, it is important to understand these mechanisms and, consequently, design and synthesize novel agents with higher proapoptotic activity while retaining selectivity.

We have recently studied the effect of α-TOS on neuroblastoma cells and their differentiated counterparts mimicking nonmalignant neurons. While the former were highly susceptible to the VE analog, the latter were relatively resistant.[58] We found two lines of defense against α-TOS in the differentiated cells. First, the cells, unlike the parental neuroblastomas, did not accumulate ROS. Second, their levels of antiapoptotic Bcl-2 family proteins were elevated, in particular that of Mcl-1. These data clearly suggest that mitochondria are important not only in induction of apoptosis, but also in the selectivity of importance VE analogs for malignant cells.

### 6.3.4 VE ANALOGS OVERCOME RESISTANCE OF MUTANT CANCER CELLS TO APOPTOSIS, INDUCE THE MITOCHONDRIAL APOPTOTIC PATHWAY, AND COOPERATE WITH IMMUNOLOGICAL APOPTOGENS

Many cancer cells avoid established therapy by constantly mutating the relevant genes. This is a complicating factor, compromising many successful treatments. Therefore, it is imperative to design novel agents that would overcome these complications. Many anticancer drugs act via induction of apoptosis of malignant cells by causing damage to their genomic DNA, which results in activation of p53 and inhibition of proliferation accompanied by apoptosis. VE analogs show promise for treatment of cancers where such genes are mutated, most likely because they use the mitochondrial apoptogenic route.

It was reported by Coffey's laboratory that Trolox, a water-soluble analog of VE, inhibited proliferation and induced apoptosis in human colon cancer cells by increasing the expression of the cell cycle protein p21$^{Cip1/Waf1}$ in a p53-independent manner.[59] This paper also showed that the agent could efficiently inhibit growth of tumors in athymic mice derived from p53- but not p21$^{Cip1/Waf1}$-deficient colon cancer cells. It was later observed that α-TOS caused efficient apoptosis in both p53- and p21$^{Cip1/Waf1}$-deficient colon cancer cells.[38] These findings place VE analogs among potential anticancer drugs capable of being used instead of or as adjuvants to other drugs whose application may be compromised by mutations in the above genes.

Antiapoptotic/pro-survival consequences of other mutations can also be overcome by VE analogs. For example, overexpression of the receptor tyrosine kinase erbB2/HER2 complicates breast cancer treatment.[60] The reason is that the auto-activated erbB2 activates Akt, a protein kinase phosphorylating multiple substrates, including IκB kinase (IKK), caspase-9, and Bad, resulting in elevated expression of pro-survival genes and inhibition of proapoptotic proteins.[61,62] It has been suggested that VE analogs overcome the erbB2-Akt antiapoptotic signaling. Akazawa et al.[63] showed that α-tocopheryloxybutyric acid suppressed auto-phosphorylation of erbB2, shutting down the whole signaling pathway, although the mechanism is not clear. We have observed that α-TOS caused comparable apoptosis in both erbB2-low and erbB2-high breast cancer cells by a two-tier mechanism[64] that includes cytosolic mobilization of cytochrome c, activating the downstream caspases, as well as that of Smac/Diablo, a protein antagonizing the caspase-inhibitory activity of the inhibition of apoptosis proteins (IAPs) that are elevated due to Akt-dependent activation of nuclear factor-κB (NF-κB).[65,66] α-TOS thus induces apoptosis in cells over-expressing erbB2 on at least three levels (Figure 6.4). We are currently investigating the anticancer activity of VE analogs using transgenic mice overexpressing erbB2 in the mammary epithelial cells, resulting in spontaneous formation of breast carcinomas.[67]

The major apoptogenic pathway induced by VE analogs is linked to mitochondrial destabilization. This is compatible with mitochondria as a novel target for anticancer drugs.[68,69] Mitochondrial proapoptotic signaling has been documented in several papers, and involves activation of the sphingomyelinase pathways, generation of ROS, and mitochondrial translocation of Bax.[51,52,70–73] Conceivably, the ratio between the mitochondrial pro- and antiapoptotic proteins may determine the overall susceptibility of the cells to VE analogs.

Perhaps more importantly, the mode of proapoptotic signaling of VE analogs makes them candidates for adjuvant therapy, that is, synergizing with apoptogens using a different mode of action. α-TOS has been investigated for sensitization of cancer cell to apoptosis induced by the Fas ligand (FasL) and the TNF-related apoptosis-inducing ligand (TRAIL). Kline's group has shown that the VE analog sensitized cancer cells to FasL by mobilizing the latent cytosolic Fas to the plasma membrane,[74,75] as also observed for gastric cancer cells.[76,77] This may suggest a role of α-TOS in cancer surveillance by boosting the immune anticancer/proapoptotic mechanism.

We have explored the possibility that VE analogs synergize/cooperate with TRAIL. In colon cancer cells, α-TOS synergized with TRAIL in apoptosis induction, by utilizing different, convergent pathways. Cooperation between α-TOS and TRAIL was observed in experimental colon cancer.[38] In mesothelioma cells, α-TOS synergized with TRAIL by upregulating the TRAIL death receptor-4 (DR4) and DR5.[50] This report as well as our recent finding that α-TOS extends survival of mice with experimental mesothelioma[41] is important because

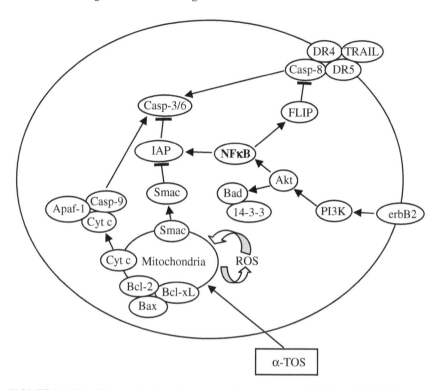

**FIGURE 6.4** Possible mechanism of apoptosis induction by α-TOS in erbB2/HER2 over-expressing cells. α-TOS causes cytosolic mobilization of cytochrome c (Cyt c) and Smac/Diablo. Cyt c forms a ternary complex with Apaf-1 and pro-caspase-9, resulting in activation of the initiator caspase-9 that, in turn, leads to activation of the effector caspases. Smac/Diablo amplifies this process by suppressing the IAP family proteins that are elevated due to Akt-dependent activation of NF-κB. This suggests that α-TOS induces apoptosis in cells overexpressing erbB2 on at least three levels: inhibition of erbB2 activation, induction of the mitochondrial-linked apoptotic pathway, and relocalization of Smac/Diablo, thereby suppressing the caspase-inhibitory IAP activity. Mechanistically, α-TOS induces mitochondrial generation of ROS as well as mitochondrial translocation of Bax. Additional effects of α-TOS include: inhibition of erbB2 and NF-κB activation and suppression of Akt-dependent phosphorylation of Bad (rendering it inactive due to association with the protein 14-3-3) and pro-caspase-9 (suppressing its activity normally leading to activation of effector caspases). These effects of α-TOS not only induce apoptosis in erbB2-overexpressing cells, but also sensitize them to other apoptogens, as shown here for TRAIL.

mesotheliomas are refractory to treatment, largely due to resistance to apoptosis by established drugs.[78] Another mode by which α-TOS can sensitize cancer cells to TRAIL killing is its interference with activation of NF-κB, as shown for Jurkat cells.[79] A possible mechanism of inhibition of the pro-survival transcription factor may be caspase-dependent cleavage of its subunit p65 due to activation of the apoptosis machinery.[80,81]

### 6.3.5 VITAMIN E ANALOGS AS ANTITUMOR AGENTS: BEYOND MITOCHONDRIA

Although the mitochondrial pathway is central to the apoptogenic action of VE analogs, there are other pathways that may play an important role in the effects of the agents. Kline's group reported regulation of the AP-1 and mitogen-activated protein kinase/extracellular-regulated protein kinase pathways as additional signaling routes for apoptosis induced by α-TOS.[82–86] Some but not all papers suggested that α-TOS induces apoptosis by interfering with the tumor necrosis factor-β (TGF-β) signaling, compromising the expression of pro-survival factors.[87–89] These findings may be related to the effect of the VE analog on transition of cell through the cell cycle. Several reports showed that the agent caused arrest in $G_1$ or $G_2$. Turley et al.[90] presented evidence that α-TOS inhibited proliferation of breast cancer cells by interfering with the cyclin A-E2F restriction point machinery. Yeh's group reported that α-TOS inhibited proliferation of cancer cells by modulation of the cell cycle transition[91] as well as cell invasiveness due to inhibition of the activity of matrix metalloproteinase-9.[92] These effects may be more specific for prostate cancer cells, as α-TOS has been reported to inhibit the function of the prostate-specific antigen.[93]

Our results also show inhibitory effects of α-TOS on cell cycle transition, with $G_1$ and/or $G_2$ arrest, depending on the cell type.[94–96] The mode of cell cycle inhibition may be related to the effect of α-TOS on its modulators. The $G_1$ arrest of the osteosarcoma cells may be linked to inhibition of the activity of the cyclin A/cyclin-dependent kinase-2 complex, while the levels of the transcription factor E2F1 were enhanced and were followed by phosphorylation of p53.[94]

Mesothelioma cells undergo a $G_2$ arrest when exposed to low levels of α-TOS.[95,96] This is related to disruption of the FGF-FGFR autocrine proliferation signaling loop by selective downregulation of both FRF2 and its receptor FGFR1 in the mesothelioma but not the nonmalignant mesothelial cells.[95,96] α-TOS exerts its effect on the transcriptional level, downregulating FGFR1 by inhibiting the activity of E2F1,[95] while FGF2 is downregulated via modulating the transcriptional activity of the early-response growth factor-1.[96] The selectivity appears related to the low level of ROS generation by the nonmalignant mesothelial cells while their malignant counterparts respond to α-TOS by early generation of high levels of ROS.[96]

There are reports suggesting the possibility that VE analogs inhibit angiogenesis, which indicates an effect of the agents on tumorigenesis and the metastatic potential. We have observed a reduction in the number of blood vessels in experimental colon cancer xenografts in mice treated with α-TOS (J. Neuzil, unpublished data). Preliminary results also indicate an effect of α-TOS on proangiogenic cytokines in endothelial cells, suggesting a proliferation-suppressive activity of the VE analog. This can be reconciled with findings that α-TOS caused downregulation of VEGF.[36] Another possibility follows from studies indicating that proliferating endothelial cells are highly susceptible to α-TOS while the confluent arrested cells are resistant.[80] This highly intriguing paradigm is supported by comparable results from Hogg's group using a different inducer of apoptosis.[97] Thus, α-TOS may specifically target angiogenic endothelial cells while being nonapoptotic toward normal endothelium. Resistance of endothelial cells suspended in $G_0$ can be explained by high levels of expression of the checkpoint proteins p21[Waf1/Cip1] and p27[Kip1] that prevent reentry of the cells into the cell cycle[98,99] and that inhibit caspase activity.[100]

By virtue of inhibiting angiogenesis, VE analogs would be efficient against cancers irrespective of the frequent mutations in various genes. This area is also worth exploring for novel VE analogs. A recent paper showed a potential antiangiogenic effect of γ-TOH by inhibiting the activity of cyclooxygenase-2,[101] thereby suppressing formation of pro-angiogenic eicosanoids.[102] It is expected that γ-TOS combines an antiangiogenic effect with apoptogenic activity (see Table 6.1).

### 6.3.6 PHARMACOKINETICS OF VE ANALOGS — A POTENTIAL SECONDARY BENEFICIAL BIOACTIVITY

A most intriguing aspect of the potential use of VE analogs as anticancer agents follows from their pharmacokinetics. These agents are esters of VE and, therefore, hydrolyzed upon intestinal intake after ingestion.[103] To overcome the intestinal hydrolysis step, agents such as α-TOS need to be administered intraperitoneally. After reaching the circulation, they associate with lipoproteins[104,105] that carry them to the neoplastic microvasculature. Once in the tumor blood vessels, α-TOS migrates to the malignant tissue where it induces apoptosis, thereby suppressing growth of the tumor. Because the blood components and the peripheral tissue are a dynamic system, there is constant exchange of hydrophobic molecules. α-TOS is thus gradually moved from the tumor and cleared, bound to remnant lipoproteins, via the liver. Here, α-TOS is hydrolyzed by nonspecific esterases. It is then partially disposed of within the bile, partially resecreted into circulation depending on the level of the saturable α-tocopherol-binding protein (α-TTP).[105–108]

The paradigm described above is shown in Figure 6.5. It is clear that, based on this scheme, supported by theoretical considerations and experimental data,[109,110] esters of VE are hydrolyzed in the liver into the redox-active VE that is, in part, returned into circulation. From this, it can be deduced that α-TOS and similar compounds possess at least two bioactivities. In the pro-vitamin form, α-TOS suppresses cancer. After conversion to its vitamin form, it acts as a redox-active compound and as an anti-inflammatory agent.[111–115] Thus, we believe that the novel VE analogs represent agents with thus far unrecognized dual beneficial bioactivity relevant to a variety of highly deleterious pathologies, including cancer and inflammatory diseases.

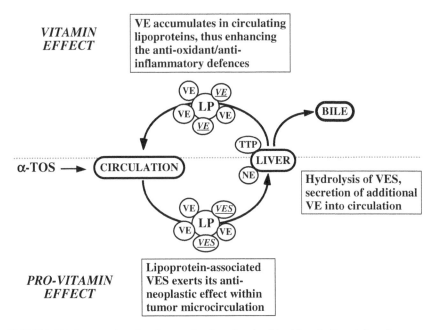

**FIGURE 6.5** Proposed molecular mechanism for the "double-edge" activity of α-tocopheryl succinate. Following entry into the bloodstream, the pro-vitamin α-TOS vitamin E succinate (VES) associates with circulating lipoproteins (LP) that carry the agent to the microvasculature of the neoplastic tissue. Here, VES exerts its antiproliferative/proapoptotic activity toward malignant cells that translates into inhibition of tumor growth. Since there is a constant exchange of hydrophobic molecules between the peripheral tissues and the circulation, α-TOS is gradually removed by virtue of remnant lipoproteins that are endocytosed by hepatocytes that possess high levels of nonspecific esterases (NE). Here, the remnants are dissembled and nascent VLDL formed. α-TOH (VE), both the original and that formed by hydrolysis of VES, is partially shuttled to nascent VLDL bound to the saturable tocopherol-transfer protein (TTP), partially excreted in the bile. Nascent VLDL enriched with VE is then resecreted into circulation, endowing the system with additional VE that promotes the antioxidant and anti-inflammatory defenses.

## 6.4  CONCLUSIONS AND FUTURE DIRECTIONS

The above discussion reveals the exceptional promise of VE analogs as therapeutic agents. There are several features that make these compounds unique: (1) VE analogs induce apoptosis selectively in malignant cells and inhibit tumor growth in experimental models; (2) they overcome resistance to established anticancer drugs due to bypassing mutations in or deletions of critical genes; (3) they synergize with anticancer agents and/or sensitize resistant cells toward them; (4) they cause apoptosis in proliferating endothelial cells, suggesting their anti-angiogenic activity; and (5) they are metabolized into the redox-active VE with secondary beneficial bioactivity.

At this stage, we need more data to understand the exact mechanisms by which these compounds exert their proapoptotic/anticancer activity and, in particular, what makes them selective for malignant cells. Importantly, too, we need to obtain more data from preclinical studies using several experimental models. Thus far, the majority of these data comes from work with athymic mice. Transgenic mice predisposed to develop tumors need to be used because in such animals the role of the immune system, essential for tumor surveillance, is not impaired. It is hoped that, with better understanding of the molecular mechanism underlying the activity of VE analogs, they will be approved for clinical testing. Should they prove successful, the very cheap α-TOS or its derivatives may become drugs of choice against multiple malignancies with a secondary beneficial activity.

## REFERENCES

1. Neuzil J, Tomasetti M, Mellick AS, Alleva R, Salvatore BA, Birringer B, Fariss MW. Vitamin E analogues: a new class of inducers of apoptosis with selective anti-cancer effect. *Curr Cancer Drug Targets* 2004; 4:267–284.
2. Jiang Q, Christen S, Shigenaga MK, Ames BN. γ-Tocopherol, the major form of vitamin E in the US diet, deserves more attention. *Am J Clin Nutr* 2001; 74:714–722.
3. Woodson K, Tangrea JA, Barrett MJ, Virtamo J, Taylor PR, Albanes D. Serum α-tocopherol and subsequent risk of lung cancer among male smokers. *J Natl Cancer Inst* 1999; 91:1738–1743.
4. Heinonen OP, Albanes D, Virtamo J, Taylor PR, Huttunen JK, Hartman AM, Haapakoski J, Malila N, Rautalahti M, Ripatti S, Maenpaa H, Teerenhovi L, Koss L, Virolainen M, Edwards BK. Prostate cancer and supplementation with α-tocopherol and β-carotene: incidence and mortality in a controlled trial. *J Natl Cancer Inst* 1998; 90:440–446.
5. Malila N, Taylor PR, Virtanen MJ, Korhonen P, Huttunen JK, Albanes D, Virtamo J. Effects of α-tocopherol and β-carotene supplementation on gastric cancer incidence in male smokers (ATBC Study, Finland). *Cancer Causes Control* 2002; 13:617–623.
6. Rautalahti MT, Virtamo JR, Taylor PR, Heinonen OP, Albanes D, Haukka JK, Edwards BK, Karkkainen PA, Stolzenberg-Solomon RZ, Huttunen J. The effects of supplementation with α-tocopherol and β-carotene on the incidence and mortality of carcinoma of the pancreas in a randomized, controlled trial. *Cancer* 1999; 86:37–42.
7. Malila N, Virtamo J, Virtanen M, Albanes D, Tangrea JA, Huttunen JK. The effect of α-tocopherol and β-carotene supplementation on colorectal adenomas in middle-aged male smokers. *Cancer Epidemiol Biomarkers Prev* 1999; 8:489–493.
8. Blot WJ, Li JY, Taylor PR, Guo W, Dawsey S, Wang GQ, Yang CS, Zheng SF, Gail M, Li GY. Nutrition intervention trials in Linxian, China: supplementation with specific vitamin/mineral combinations, cancer incidence, and disease-specific mortality in the general population. *J Natl Cancer Inst* 1993; 85:1483–1492.

9. Klein EA, Thompson IM, Lippman SM, Goodman PJ, Albanes D, Taylor PR, Coltman C. SELECT: the next prostate cancer prevention trial. Selenium and Vitamin E Cancer Prevention Trial. *J Urol* 2001; 166:1311–1315.

10. Menkes MS, Comstock GW, Vuilleumier JP, Helsing KJ, Rider AA, Brookmeyer R. Serum β-carotene, vitamins A and E, selenium, and the risk of lung cancer. *N Engl J Med* 1986; 13:1250–1254.

11. Wald NJ, Thompson SG, Densem JW, Boreham J, Bailey A. Serum vitamin E and subsequent risk of cancer. *Br J Cancer* 1987; 56:69–72.

12. Knekt P. Vitamin E and cancer: epidemiology. *Ann NY Acad Sci* 1992; 669:269–279.

13. Moorman PG, Ricciuti MF, Millikan RC, Newman B. Vitamin supplement use and breast cancer in a North Carolina population. *Public Health Nutr* 2001; 4:821–827.

14. Jacobs EJ, Connell CJ, McCullough ML, Chao A, Jonas CR, Rodriguez C, Calle EE, Thun MJ. Vitamin C, vitamin E, and multivitamin supplement use and stomach cancer mortality in the cancer prevention study II cohort. *Cancer Epidemiol Biomarkers Prev* 2002; 11:35–41.

15. Satia-About AJ, Galanko JA, Martin CF, Potter JD, Ammerman A, Sandler RS. Associations of micronutrients with colon cancer risk in African Americans and Whites: results from the North Carolina colon cancer study. *Cancer Epidemiol Biomarkers Prev* 2003; 12:747–754.

16. Schuurman AAG, Goldbohm RA, Brants HA, van den Brandt PA. A prospective cohort study on intake of retinol, vitamins C and E, and carotenoids and prostate cancer risk (Netherlands). *Cancer Causes Control* 2002; 13:573–582.

17. Fleshner N, Fair WR, Huryk R, Heston WDW. Vitamin E inhibits the high-fat diet promoted growth of established human prostate LNCaP tumors in nude mice. *J Urol* 2002; 168:1578–1582.

18. Moriguchi S, Muraga M. Vitamin E and immunity. *Vitam Horm* 2000; 59:305–336.

19. Meydani M, Lipman RD, Han SN, Wu D, Beharka A, Martin KR, Bronson R, Cao G, Smith D, Meydani SN. The effect of long-term dietary supplementation with antioxidants. *Ann NY Acad Sci* 1998; 854:352–360.

20. Venkateswaran V, Fleshner NE, Sugar LM, Klotz LH. Antioxidants block prostate cancer in LADY transgenic mice. *Cancer Res* 2004; 64:5891–5896.

21. Hartman TJ, Dorgan JF, Woodson K, Virtamo J, Tangrea JA, Heinonen OP, Taylor PR, Barrett MJ, Albanes D. Effects of longer α-tocopherol supplementation on serum hormones in older men. *Prostate* 2001; 46:33–38.

22. Kline K, Yu W, Sanders BG. Vitamin E: Mechanisms of action as tumor cell growth inhibitors. In: KN Prasad, WC Cole, eds. *Cancer and Nutrition*. IOS Press; 1998:37–53.

23. Schwartz J, Shklar G. The selective cytotoxic effect of carotenoids and α-tocopherol on human cancer cell lines in vitro. *J Oral Maxillofac Surg* 1992; 50:367–373.

24. Wu K, Shan YJ, Zhao Y, Yu JW, Liu BH. Inhibitory effects of RRR-α-tocopheryl succinate on benzo(a)pyrene-induced forestomach carcinogenesis in female mice. *World J Gastroenterol* 2001; 7:60–65.

25. Birringer M, EyTina JH, Salvatore BA, Neuzil J. Vitamin E analogues as inducers of apoptosis: structure–function relationship. *Br J Cancer* 2003; 88:1948–1955.

26. Yu W, Simmons-Menchaca M, Gapor A, Sanders BG, Kline K. Induction of apoptosis in human breast cancer cells by tocopherols and tocotrienols. *Nutr Cancer.* 1999; 33:26–32.
27. Mo H, Elson CE. Studies of the isoprenoid-mediated inhibition of mevalonate synthesis applied to cancer chemotherapy and chemoprevention. *Exp Biol Med* 2004; 229:567–585.
28. Neuzil J, Weber T, Gellert N, Weber C. Selective cancer cell killing by α-tocopheryl succinate. *Br J Cancer* 2001; 84:87–89.
29. Neuzil J, Zhao M, Ostermann G, Sticha M, Gellert N, Weber C, Eaton JW, Brunk UT. α-Tocopheryl succinate, an agent with *in vivo* anti-tumour activity, induces apoptosis by causing lysosomal instability. *Biochem J* 2002; 362:709–715.
30. Kozin SV, Shkarin P, Gerweck LE. The cell transmembrane pH gradient in tumors enhances cytotoxicity of specific weak acid chemotherapeutics. *Cancer Res* 2001; 61:4740–4743.
31. Neuzil J. Vitamin E succinate and cancer treatment: A vitamin E prototype for selective anti-tumour activity. *Br J Cancer* 2003; 89:1822–1826.
32. Tomic-Vatic A, EyTina JH, Chapmann JM, Mahdavian E, Neuzil J, Salvatore BA. Vitamin E amides, a new class of vitamin E analogues with enhanced proapoptotic activity. *Int J Cancer,* in press.
33. Fariss MW, Fortuna MB, Everett CK, Smith JD, Trent DF, Djuric Z. The selective cytotoxic effect of vitamin E succinate and cholesterol succinate on murine leukemia cells result from the action of the intact molecules. *Cancer Res* 1994; 54:3346–3351.
34. Anderson K, Simmons-Menchaca M, Lawson KA, Atkinson J, Sanders BG, Kline K. Differential response of human ovarian cancer cells to induction of apoptosis by vitamin E succinate and vitamin E analogue, α-TEA. *Cancer Res* 2004; 64:4263–4269.
35. Lawson KA, Anderson K, Simmons-Menchaca M, Atkinson J, Sun L, Saunders BG, Kline K. Comparison of vitamin E derivatives α-TEA and VES in reduction of mouse mammary tumor burden and metastasis. *Exp Biol Med* 2004; 229: 954–963.
36. Malafa MP, Neitzel LT. Vitamin E succinate promotes breast cancer tumor dormancy. *J Surg Res* 2000; 93:163–170.
37. Malafa MP, Fokum FD, Smith L, Louis A. Inhibition of angiogenesis and promotion of melanoma dormancy by vitamin E succinate. *Ann Surg Oncol* 2002; 9:1023–1032.
38. Weber T, Lu M, Andera L, Lahm H, Gellert N, Fariss MW, Korinek V, Sattler W, Ucker DS, Terman A, Schröder A, Erl W, Brunk U, Coffey RJ, Weber C, Neuzil J. Vitamin E succinate is a potent novel anti-neoplastic agent with high tumor selectivity and cooperativity with tumor necrosis factor-related apoptosis-inducing ligand (Apo2 Ligand) *in vivo. Clin Cancer Res* 2002; 8:863–869.
39. Malafa MP, Fokum FD, Mowlavi A, Abusief M, King M. Vitamin E inhibits melanoma growth in mice. *Surgery* 2002; 131:85–91.
40. Kogure K, Manabe S, Hama S, Tokumura A, Fukuzawa K. Potentiation of anticancer effect by intravenous administration of vesiculated α-tocopheryl hemisuccinate on mouse melanoma *in vivo. Cancer Lett* 2003; 192:19–24.
41. Tomasetti M, Gellert N, Procopio A, Neuzil J. A vitamin E analogue suppresses malignant mesothelioma in a pre-clinical model: a prototype of a future drug against a fatal neoplastic disease? *Int J Cancer* 2004; 109:641–642.

42. Barnett KT, Fokum FD, Malafa MP. Vitamin E succinate inhibits colon cancer liver metastases. *J Surg Res* 2002; 106:292–298.

43. Zhang S, Lawson KA, Simmons-Menchaca M, Sun L, Sanders BG, Kline K. Vitamin E analog α-TEA and celecoxib alone and together reduce human MDA-MB-435-FL-GFP breast cancer burden and metastasis in nude mice. *Breast Cancer Res Treat* 2004; 87:111–121.

44. Lawson KA, Anderson K, Snyder RM, Simmons-Menchaca M, Atkinson J, Sun LZ, Bandyopadhyay A, Knight V, Gilbert BE, Sanders BG, Kline K. Novel vitamin E analogue and 9-nitro-camptothecin administered as liposome aerosols decrease syngeneic mouse mammary tumor burden and inhibit metastasis. *Cancer Chemother Pharmacol* 2004; 54:421–431.

45. Neuzil J, Weber T, Schröder A, Lu M, Ostermann G, Gellert N, Mayne GC, Olejnicka B, Nègre-Salvayre A, Sticha M, Coffey RJ, Weber C. Induction of apoptosis in cancer cells by α-tocopheryl succinate: molecular pathways and structural requirements. *FASEB J* 2001; 15:403–415.

46. Tasinato A, Boscoboinik D, Bartoli GM, Maroni P, Azzi A. d-α-Tocopherol inhibition of vascular smooth muscle cell proliferation occurs at physiological concentrations, correlates with protein kinase C inhibition, and is independent of its antioxidant properties. *Proc Natl Acad Sci USA* 1995; 92:12190–12194.

47. Jha MN, Bedford JS, Cole WC, Edward-Prasad J, Prasad KN. Vitamin E (d-α-tocopheryl succinate) decreases mitotic accumulation in γ-irradiated human tumor, but not in normal cells. *Nutr Cancer* 1999; 35:189–194.

48. Kumar B, Jha MN, Cole WC, Bedford JS, Prasad KN. D-α-Tocopheryl succinate (vitamin E) enhances radiation-induced chromosomal damage levels in human cancer cells, but reduces it in normal cells. *J Am Coll Nutr* 2002; 21:339–343.

49. Prasad KN, Kumar B, Yan XD, Hanson AJ, Cole WC. α-Tocopheryl succinate, the most effective form of vitamin E for adjuvant cancer treatment: a review. *J Am Coll Nutr* 2003; 22:108–117.

50. Tomasetti M, Rippo MR, Alleva R, Moretti S, Andera L, Neuzil J, Procopio A. α-Tocopheryl succinate and TRAIL selectively synergise in apoptosis induction in human malignant mesothelioma cells. *Br J Cancer* 2004; 90:1644–1653.

51. Weber T, Dalen H, Andera L, Nègre-Salvayre A, Augé N, Sticha M, Loret A, Terman A, Witting PK, Higuchi M, Plasilova M, Zivny J, Gellert N, Weber C, Neuzil J. Mitochondria play a central role in apoptosis induced by α-tocopheryl succinate, an agent with anticancer activity. Comparison with receptor-mediated proapoptotic signaling. *Biochemistry* 2003; 42:4277–4291.

52. Ottino P, Duncan JR. Effect of α-tocopherol succinate on free radical and lipid peroxidation levels in BL6 melanoma cells. *Free Radical Biol Med* 1997; 22:1145–1151.

53. Higuchi MB, Aggarwal BB, Yeh T. Activation of CPP32-like protease in tumor necrosis factor-induced apoptosis is dependent on mitochondrial function. *J Clin Invest* 1997; 99:1751–1758.

54. Dey R, Moraes CT. Lack of oxidative phosphorylation and low mitochondrial membrane potential decrease susceptibility to apoptosis and do not modulate the protective effect of Bcl-$x_L$ in osteosarcoma cells. *J Biol Chem* 2000; 275:7087–7094.

55. Park SY, Chang I, Kim JY, Kang SW, Park SH, Singh K, Lee MS. mtDNA-depleted cells against cell death: role of mitochondrial superoxide dismutase. *J Biol Chem* 2004; 279:7512–7520.

56. Kogure K, Hama S, Manabe S, Tokumura A, Fukuzawa K. High cytoxicity of α-tocopheryl hemisuccinate to cancer cells is due to failure of their antioxidative defence systems. *Cancer Lett* 2002; 186:151–156.

57. Kang YH, Lee E, Choi MK, Ku JL, Kim SH, Park YG, Lin SJ. Role of reactive oxygen species in the induction of apoptosis by α-tocopheryl succinate. *Int J Cancer* 2004; 112:385–392.

58. Swettenham E, Witting PK, Salvatore, BA, Neuzil J. α-Tocopheryl succinate selectively induces apoptosis in neuroblastoma cells: the role of oxidative stress and Mcl-1. *J Neurochem*, in press.

59. Chinery R, Brockman JA, Peeler MO, Shyr Y, Beauchamp RD, Coffey RJ. Antioxidants enhance the cytotoxicity of chemotherapeutic agents in colorectal cancer: a p53-independent induction of p21$^{WAFI/CIP1}$ via C/EBPβ. *Nat Med* 1997; 3:1233–1241.

60. Zhou BP, Hung MC. Dysregulation of cellular signaling by HER2/neu in breast cancer. *Semin Oncol* 2003; 30:38–48.

61. Vivanco I, Sawyers CL. The phosphatidylinositol 3-kinase-Akt pathway in human cancer. *Natl Rev Cancer* 2002; 2:489–501.

62. Datta SR, Brunet A, Greenberg ME. Cellular survival: a play in three Akts. *Genes Dev* 1999; 15:2905–2927.

63. Akazawa A, Nishikawa K, Suzuki K, Asano R, Kumadaki I, Satoh H, Hagiwara K, Sin SJ. Yano T. Induction of apoptosis in a human breast cancer cell overexpressing erbB2 receptor by α-tocopheryloxybutyric acid. *Jpn J Pharmacol* 2002; 89:417–421.

64. Wang XF, Witting PK, Salvatore BA, Neuzil J. α-Tocopheryl succinate induces apoptosis in HER2/erbB2-overexpressing breast cancer cells by signalling via the mitochondrial pathway. *Biochem Biophys Res Commun* 2005; 326:282–289.

65. LaCasse EC, Baird S, Korneluk RG, MacKenzie AE. The inhibitors of apoptosis (IAPs) and their emerging role in cancer. *Oncogene* 1998; 17:3247–3259.

66. Karin M, Lin A. NF-κB at the crossroads of life and death. *Nat Immunol* 2002; 3:221–227.

67. Guy CT, Webster MA, Schaller M, Parsons TJ, Cardiff RD, Muller WJ. Expression of the neu protooncogene in the mammary epithelium of transgenic mice induces metastatic disease. *Proc Natl Acad Sci USA* 1992; 89:10578–10582.

68. Costantini P, Jacotot E, Decaudin D, Kroemer G. Mitochondrion as a novel target of anticancer chemotherapy. *J Natl Cancer Inst* 2000; 92:1042–1053.

69. Don AS, Hogg PJ. Mitochondria as cancer drug targets. *Trends Mol Med* 2004; 10:372–378.

70. Neuzil J, Svensson I, Weber T, Weber C, Brunk UT. α-Tocopheryl succinate-induced apoptosis in Jurkat T cells involves caspase-3 activation, and both lysosomal and mitochondrial destabilisation. *FEBS Lett* 1999; 445:295–300.

71. Kogure K, Morita M, Nakashima S, Hama S, Tokumura A, Fukuzawa K. Superoxide is responsible for apoptosis in rat vascular smooth muscle cells induced by α-tocopheryl hemisuccinate. *Biochim Biophys Acta* 2001; 1528:25–30.

72. Yamamoto S, Tamai H, Ishisaka R, Kanno T, Arita K, Kobuchi H, Utsumi K. Mechanism of α-tocopheryl succinate-induced apoptosis of promyelocytic leukemia cells. *Free Radical Res* 2000; 33:407–418.

73. Yu W, Sanders BG, Kline K. RRR-α-tocopheryl succinate-induced apoptosis of human breast cancer cells involves Bax translocation to mitochondria. *Cancer Res* 2003; 63:2483–2491.

74. Yu W, Israel K, Liao QY, Aldaz M, Sanders BG, Kline K. Vitamin E succinate (VES) induces Fas sensitivity in human breast cancer cells: Role for $M_r$ 43,000 Fas in VES-triggered apoptosis. *Cancer Res* 1999; 59:953–961.

75. Israel K, Yu W, Sanders BG, Kline K. Vitamin E succinate induces apoptosis in human prostate cancer cells: Role of Fas in vitamin E succinate-triggered apoptosis. *Nutr Cancer* 2000; 36:90–100.

76. Wu K, Li Y, Zhao Y, Shan YJ, Xia W, Yu WP, Zhao L. Roles of Fas signaling pathway in vitamin E succinate-induced apoptosis in human gastric cancer SGC-7901 cells. *World J Gastroenterol* 2002; 8:982–986.

77. Wu K, Zhao L, Li Y, Shan YJ, Wu LJ. Effects of vitamin E succinate on the expression of Fas and PCNA proteins in human gastric carcinoma cells and its clinical significance. *World J Gastroenterol* 2004; 10:945–949.

78. Tomek S, Emri S, Krejcy K, Manegold C. Chemotherapy for malignant pleural mesothelioma: past results and recent developments. *Br J Cancer* 2003; 88:167–174.

79. Dalen H, Neuzil J. α-Tocopheryl succinate sensitises T lymphoma cells to TRAIL killing by suppressing NF-κB activation. *Br J Cancer* 2003; 88:153–158.

80. Neuzil J, Schröder A, von Hundelshausen P, Zernecke A, Weber T, Gellert N, Weber C. Inhibition of inflammatory endothelial responses by a pathway involving caspase activation and p65 cleavage. *Biochemistry* 2001; 40:4686–4692.

81. Levkau B, Scatena M, Giachelli CM, Ross R, Raines EW. Apoptosis overrides survival signals through a caspase-mediated dominant-negative NF-κB loop. *Nat Cell Biol* 1999; 1:227–233.

82. Qian M, Kralova J, Yu W, Bose HR, Dvorak M, Sanders BG, Kline K. c-Jun involvement in vitamin E succinate induced apoptosis of reticuloendotheliosis virus transformed avian lymphoid cells. *Oncogene* 1997; 15:223–230.

83. Zhao B, Yu W, Qian M, Simmons-Menchaca M, Brown P, Birrer MJ, Sanders BG, Kline K. Involvement of activator protein-1 (AP-1) in induction of apoptosis by vitamin E succinate in human breast cancer cells. *Mol Carcinogen* 1997; 19:180–190.

84. Yu W, Simmons-Menchaca M, You H, Brown P, Birrer MJ, Sanders BG, Kline K. RRR-α-tocopheryl succinate induction of prolonged activation of c-jun amino-terminal kinase and c-jun during induction of apoptosis in human MDA-MB-435 breast cancer cells. *Mol Carcinogen* 1998; 22:247–257.

85. Yu W, Liao QY, Hantash FM, Sanders BG, Kline K. Activation of extracellular signal-regulated kinase and c-Jun-NH$_2$-terminal kinase but not p38 mitogen-activated protein kinases is required for RRR-α-tocopheryl succinate-induced apoptosis of human breast cancer cells. *Cancer Res* 2001; 61:6569–6576.

86. Wu K, Zhao Y, Li GC, Yu WP. c-Jun N-terminal kinase is required for vitamin E succinate-induced apoptosis in human gastric cancer cells. *World J Gastroenterol* 2004; 10:1110–1114.

87. You H, Yu W, Munoz-Medellin D, Brown PH, Sanders BG, Kline K. Role of extracellular signal-regulated kinase pathway in RRR-α-tocopheryl succinate-induced differentiation of human MDA-MB-435 breast cancer cells. *Mol Carcinogen* 2002; 33:228–236.

88. Turley JM, Funakoshi S, Ruscetti FW, Kasper J, Murphy WJ, Longo DL, Birchenall-Roberts MC. Growth inhibition and apoptosis of RL human B lymphoma cells by vitamin E succinate and retinoic acid: role for transforming growth factor-β. *Cell Growth Differ* 1995; 6:655–663.

89. Yu W, Sanders BG, Kline K. RRR-α-tocopheryl succinate induction of DNA synthesis arrest of human MDA-MB-435 cells involves TGF-β-independent activation of p21$^{Waf1/Cip1}$. *Nutr Cancer* 2002; 43:227–236.

90. Turley JM, Ruscetti FW, Kim SJ, Fu T, Gou FV, Birchenall-Roberts MC. Vitamin E succinate inhibits proliferation of BT-20 human breast cancer cells: increased binding of cyclin A negatively regulates E2F transactivation activity. *Cancer Res* 1997; 57:2668–2675.

91. Ni J, Chen M, Zhang Y, Li R, Huang J, Yeh S. Vitamin E succinate inhibits human prostate cancer cell growth via modulating cell cycle regulatory machinery. *Biochem Biophys Res Commun* 2003; 300:357–363.

92. Zhang M, Altuwaijri S, Yeh S. RRR-α-tocopheryl succinate inhibits human prostate cancer cell invasiveness. *Oncogene* 2004; 23:3080–3088.

93. Zhang Y, Ni J, Messing EM, Chang E, Yang CR, Yeh S. Vitamin E succinate inhibits the function of androgen receptor and the expression of prostate-specific antigen in prostate cancer cells. *Proc Natl Acad Sci USA* 2002; 99:7408–7413.

94. Alleva R, Benassi MS, Neuzil J, Tomasetti M, Gellert N, Borghi B, Procopio A, Picci P. α-Tocopheryl succinate controls cell growth and apoptosis of osteosarcoma cells by modulation of E2F1 independent of p53. *Biochem Biophys Res Commun* 2005; 331:1515–1521.

95. Stapelberg M, Tomasetti M, Gellert, N, Alleva R, Procopio A, Neuzil J. α-Tocopheryl succinate inhibits proliferation of mesothelioma cells by differential downregulation of fibroblast growth factor receptors. *Biochem Biophys Res Commun* 2004; 318:636–641.

96. Stapelberg M, Gellert N, Swettenham E, Tomasetti M, Witting KP, Procopio A, Neuzil J. α-Tocopheryl succinate inhibits malignant mesothelioma by disruption of the fibroblast growth factor autocrine signaling loop. *J Biol Chem,* in press.

97. Don AS, Kisker O, Dilda P, Donoghue N, Zhao X, Decollogne S, Creighton B, Flynn E, Folkman J, Hogg PJ. A peptide trivalent arsenical inhibits tumor angiogenesis by perturbing mitochondrial function in angiogenic endothelial cells. *Cancer Cell* 2003; 3:497–509.

98. Artwohl M, Roden M, Waldhausl W, Freudenthaler A, Baumgartner-Parzer SM. Free fatty acids trigger apoptosis and inhibit cell cycle progression in human vascular endothelial cells. *FASEB J* 2004; 18:146–148.

99. Chen D, Walsh K, Wang J. Regulation of cdk2 activity in endothelial cells that are inhibited from growth by cell contact. *Arterioscler Thromb Vasc Biol* 2000; 20:629–635.

100. Coqueret O. New roles for p21 and p27 cell-cycle inhibitors: a function for each cell compartment? *Trends Cell Biol* 2003; 13:65–70.

101. Jiang Q, Elson-Schwab I, Courtemanche C, Ames BN. γ-Tocopherol and its major metabolite, in contrast to alpha-tocopherol, inhibit cyclooxygenase activity in macrophages and epithelial cells. *Proc Natl Acad Sci USA* 2000; 97:11494–11499.

102. Jiang Q, Ames BN. γ-tocopherol, but not α-tocopherol, decreases proinflammatory eicosanoids and inflammation damage in rats. *FASEB J* 2003; 17:816–822.

103. Borel P, Pasquier B, Armand M, Tyssandier V, Grolier P, Alexandre-Gouabau MC, Andre M, Senft M, Peyrot J, Jaussan V, Lairon D, Azais-Braesco V. Processing of vitamin A and E in the human gastrointestinal tract. *Am J Physiol* 2001; 280:G95–G103.

104. Pussinen PJ, Lindner H, Glatter O, Reicher H, Kostner GM, Wintersperger A, Malle E, Sattler W. Lipoprotein-associated α-tocopheryl-succinate inhibits cell growth and induces apoptosis in human MCF-7 and HBL-100 breast cancer cells. *Biochim Biophys Acta* 2000; 1485:129–144.

105. Hrzenjak A, Reicher H, Wintersperger A, Steinecker-Frohnwieser B, Sedlmayr P, Schmidt H, Nakamura T, Malle E, Sattler W. Inhibition of lung carcinoma cell growth by high density lipoprotein-associated alpha-tocopheryl-succinate. *Cell Mol Life Sci* 2004; 61:1520–1531.

106. Kayden HJ, Traber MG. Absorption, lipoprotein transport, and regulation of plasma concentrations of vitamin E in humans. *J Lipid Res* 1993; 34:343–358.

107. Traber MG, Ramakrishnan R, Kayden HJ. Human plasma vitamin E kinetics demonstrate rapid recycling of plasma RRR-α-tocopherol. *Proc Natl Acad Sci USA* 1994; 91:10005–10008.

108. Kaempf-Rotzoll DE, Traber MG, Arai H. Vitamin E and transfer proteins. *Curr Opin Lipidol* 2003; 14:249–254.

109. Neuzil J. α-Tocopheryl succinate epitomizes a compound with a shift in biological activity due to pro-vitamin-to-vitamin conversion. *Biochem Biophys Res Commun* 2002; 293:1309–1313.

110. Neuzil J, Massa H. Hepatic processing determines dual activity of vitamin E succinate. *Biochem Biophys Res Commun* 2005; 327:1024–1027.

111. Brigelius-Flohe R, Kelly FJ, Salonen JT, Neuzil J, Zingg JM, Azzi A. The European perspective on vitamin E: current knowledge and future research. *Am J Clin Nutr* 2002; 76:703–716.

112. Neuzil J, Thomas SR, Stocker R. Requirement for, promotion, or inhibition by α-tocopherol of radical-induced initiation of plasma lipoprotein lipid peroxidation. *Free Radical Biol Med* 1997; 22:57–71.

113. Neuzil J, Kontush A, Weber C. Vitamin E in atherosclerosis: Linking the chemical, biological and clinical aspects of the disease. *Atherosclerosis* 2001; 157:257–283.

114. Li-Weber M, Weigand MA, Giaisi M, Suss D, Treiber MK, Baumann S, Ritsou E, Breitkreutz R, Krammer PH. Vitamin E inhibits CD95 ligand expression and protects T cells from activation-induced cell death. *J Clin Invest* 2002; 110:681–690.

115. Li-Weber M, Giaisi M, Treiber MK, Krammer PH. Vitamin E inhibits IL-4 gene expression in peripheral blood T cells. *Eur J Immunol* 2002; 32:2401–2408.

116. Kristal AR, Stanford JL, Cohen JH, Wicklund K, Patterson RE. Vitamin and mineral supplement use is associated with reduced risk of prostate cancer. *Cancer Epidemiol Biomarkers Prev* 1999; 8:887–892.

117. Jacobs EJ, Connell CJ, Patel AV, Chao A, Rodriguez C, Seymour J, McCullough ML, Calle EE, Thun MJ. Vitamin C and vitamin E supplement use and colorectal cancer mortality in a large American cancer society cohort. *Cancer Epidemiol Biomarkers Prev* 2000; 10:17–23.

118. Murtaugh MA, Ma KN, Benson J, Curtin K, Caan B, Slattery ML. Antioxidants, carotenoids, and risk of rectal cancer. *Am J Epidemiol* 2004; 159:32–41.

119. Bidoli E, Bosetti C, La Vecchia C, Levi F, Parpinel M, Talamini R, Negri E, Maso LD, Franceschi S. Micronutrients and laryngeal cancer risk in Italy and Switzerland: a case-control study. *Cancer Causes Control* 2003; 14:477–484.

120. Weiser H, Vecchi M, Schlachter M. Stereoisomers of α-tocopheryl acetate. IV. USP units and α-tocopherol equivalents of all-rac-, 2-ambo- and RRR-α-tocopherol evaluated by simultaneous determination of resorption-gestation, myopathy and liver storage capacity in rats. *Int J Vitamin Nutr Res* 1986; 56:45–56.

121. Leth T, Sondergaard H. Biological activity of vitamin E compounds and natural materials by the resorption-gestation test, and chemical determination of vitamin E activity in foods and feeds. *J Nutr* 1977; 107:2236–2243.

# 7 Vitamin C Blocks Carcinogenic Tumor Formation

*Ki Won Lee, Hyong Joo Lee, and Chang Yong Lee*

## CONTENTS

7.1 Introduction...................................................................................139
7.2 Concepts of Chemoprevention .....................................................140
7.3 Some Major Biomarkers Related to Multistage Carcinogenesis ..........141
7.4 Roles of Oxidative Stress in Multistage Carcinogenesis.......................142
7.5 Underlying Chemopreventive Mechanisms of Vitamin C.....................143
    7.5.1 Antioxidant Effects....................................................................143
    7.5.2 Anti-Inflammatory Activity ......................................................144
    7.5.3 Restoration of Cell-to-Cell Communication..............................145
    7.5.4 Antimetastatic Effects...............................................................146
7.6 Conclusion ....................................................................................146
Acknowledgment....................................................................................147
References ..............................................................................................148

## 7.1 INTRODUCTION

Free radicals induce various cellular injuries (including lipid peroxidation, DNA alteration, and protein inactivation) that may be involved in the etiology of degenerative diseases such as cancer, cardiovascular diseases, and neurodegenerative diseases.[1–3] There is now overwhelming evidence of an inverse relationship between a diet high in antioxidants and the incidence of disease.[4–6] Epidemiological and laboratory studies indicate that high consumption of antioxidant-rich fruits and vegetables can reduce the risk of cancer.[6–9] Currently, the U.S. Department of Agriculture and the National Cancer Institute recommend the consumption of a minimum of five servings of fruits and vegetables per day to prevent cancer.[10] Vitamin C is one of the most prevalent antioxidants in fruits and vegetables, and is considered to exert chemopreventive effects without apparent toxicity at doses substantially higher than the current recommended daily allowance

(RDA) of 60 mg/day.[10] Vitamin C has also been used as a dietary supplement for the prevention of oxidative-stress-mediated chronic diseases such as cancer, cardiovascular disease,[11] hypertension,[12] stroke,[13] and neurodegenerative disorders.[3] In 1997, expert panels at the World Cancer Research Fund and the American Institute for Cancer Research asserted that vitamin C can reduce the risk of stomach, mouth, pharynx, esophagus, lung, pancreas, and cervical cancers.[10]

Vitamin C has been considered primarily as a chemopreventive agent. It can protect cells from oxidative stress by scavenging free radicals and quenching lipid-peroxidation chain reactions, which may cause DNA damage. Thus, vitamin C may block the initiation of carcinogenesis. The carcinogenicity of oxidative stress is primarily attributable to genotoxicities of reactive oxygen species (ROS) and reactive nitrogen species (RNS). However, ROS and RNS can promote cancer through diverse cellular processes. Inflammation, inhibition of gap-junction intercellular communication (GJIC), and activation of matrix metalloproteinase (MMP) play important roles in tumor-promotion and tumor-progression processes, all of which may be mediated by ROS. Therefore, the chemopreventive mechanisms of vitamin C may be associated with the inhibition of these events as well as its protective activity against oxidative DNA damage. This chapter summarizes possible cancer-preventive mechanisms of vitamin C, with an emphasis on its inhibition of epigenetic mechanisms.

## 7.2  CONCEPTS OF CHEMOPREVENTION

There has been an extensive effort over the past three decades to develop effective therapies for cancer. However, according to the current statistics, the overall incidence and mortality of cancer has not decreased.[14,15] Therefore, attention is currently focused on prevention as an alternative strategy for the management of cancer, even though cancer treatment still offers considerable therapeutic benefits to a large group of patients. Recent advances in our understanding of the cellular and molecular events linked to carcinogenesis have led to the development of a new and promising area of cancer-prevention research, termed *chemoprevention*.[16] Chemoprevention is defined as the use of specific chemical substances of either natural or synthetic origin to suppress, retard, or reverse the process of carcinogenesis.

The rational and successful implementation of a chemoprevention strategy relies on a precise understanding of carcinogenesis at the cellular and molecular levels. Carcinogenesis is a multistage process involving a series of discrete steps. Based on experimentally induced models of carcinogenesis, the process of tumorigenesis is generally considered to consist of three distinct steps: initiation, promotion, and progression.[1,17] Throughout these three steps, unique biological and morphological changes occur in cells. *Initiation*, an irreversible and short-term event, has been ascribed to DNA damage leading to mutagenesis. *Promotion*, an interruptible or reversible and long-term process, is believed to be caused by epigenetic mechanisms that result in the expansion of damaged cells to form an actively proliferating multicellular premalignant tumor cell population. *Progres-*

*sion*, an irreversible process, was believed to be caused by genetic instability that leads to mutagenic and epigenetic changes, which are related to the production of new clones of tumor cells with increased proliferative capacity, invasiveness, and metastatic potential. Thus, the development of multistage carcinogenesis may span more than 20 years, suggesting the possibility of reversing or suppressing this disease in its early, premalignant stages. Accordingly, considerable attention has been given to identifying natural chemopreventive substances capable of inhibiting, retarding, or reversing multistage carcinogenesis. There is accumulating evidence that a wide variety of antioxidative substances derived from ordinary foods possess chemopreventive and chemoprotective activities.

## 7.3 SOME MAJOR BIOMARKERS RELATED TO MULTISTAGE CARCINOGENESIS

While numerous antioxidative vitamins and phytochemicals have been found to exert potential cancer chemopreventive activities, the definition of the appropriate biomarkers to quantify their chemopreventive effects remains subjective.[18] The precise understanding of biochemical and molecular mechanisms is the first step to identifying such proper biomarkers and is essential for the successful implementation of chemopreventive strategies.

Cellular enzymes and structural proteins, membranes, simple and complex sugars, and DNA and RNA are all susceptible to oxidative damage that may lead to tumor initiation. The elimination or minimization of exposure to diverse environmental carcinogens is one strategy for preventing the majority of human cancers, but the complete avoidance of exposure to etiologic factors that can initiate cancer may be unrealistic.[1] Therefore, recent chemopreventive strategies have focused more on identifying substances possessing antipromoting or antiprogressive activities that can suppress the transformation of initiated or precancerous cells into malignant ones, rather than searching for anti-initiators.[1]

A promising strategy applicable to the identification and development of chemopreventive agents is the inhibition of inflammation. Cyclooxygenase-2 (COX-2) and inducible nitric oxide synthase (iNOS) are important enzymes that mediate inflammatory processes. Improper upregulation of COX-2 and/or iNOS is associated with the pathophysiology of certain types of human cancers as well as with inflammatory disorders. Tumor promoters and lipopolysaccharide can induce inflammation through the overexpression of COX-2 and iNOS with the concomitant generation of ROS and RNS. Because inflammation is closely linked to tumor promotion, substances with potent anti-inflammatory activities are anticipated to exert chemopreventive effects on carcinogenesis, particularly in the promotion stage.

GJIC is essential for maintaining the homeostatic balance by modulating cell proliferation and differentiation in multicellular organisms.[19] Most normal cells have functional GJIC, while most cancer cells have dysfunctional GJIC.[20] A consistent observation is that tumor promoters[21-24] inhibit GJIC, while antitumor-promoting agents[25,26] and anticancer drugs[27] can reverse the downregulation of GJIC.[20] Because the inhibition of GJIC is strongly related to carcinogenicity, particularly tumor promotion, enhancers of GJIC are also anticipated to prevent cancer.

The inhibition of angiogenesis is considered another prospective strategy in both cancer chemoprevention and therapy, because angiogenesis is an essential process of most cancers. MMPs are enzymes involved in degradation of the extracellular matrix (ECM) and are linked to various steps in the development of metastasis.[28] Therefore, MMPs have been the main target of an increasing number of clinical trials approved for testing the tolerance and therapeutic efficacy of antiangiogenic agents. Although MMPs have long been implicated in cancer-cell invasion and metastasis, recent reports suggest that MMPs are also linked to the tumor promotion process.[29–32] Therefore, the inhibition of MMP production may be associated with antitumor-promoting activities as well as antiangiogenic and antimetastatic activities. Thus, the inhibition of inflammation, enhancement of GJIC, and inactivation of MMP are considered important biomarkers in blocking tumor promotion and tumor progression processes in multistage carcinogenesis.

## 7.4  ROLES OF OXIDATIVE STRESS IN MULTISTAGE CARCINOGENESIS

Oxidation involves the addition or withdrawal of energy by oxygen from reduced carbon-based molecules. The paradox is that this process of free radical oxidation is both deleterious and life sustaining by being coupled to electron transport in the mitochondria of living cells. Cells using oxygen to generate energy represent a source of oxygen radicals and reactive oxygen systems. The action of carcinogens is often accompanied by oxidation reactions acting on DNA. ROS produced in the body include superoxide, hydroxyl, hydroperoxyl, peroxyl, and alkoxyl radicals. RNS include nitric oxide and the peroxynitrite anion. Food and toxicants are also major sources of ROS and RNS.

Investigations of the carcinogenic effects of oxidative stress have been focused primarily on genotoxicity, but ROS are also known to play a significant role in the promotional stage of carcinogenesis. In particular, several oxidants and free radical generators are tumor promoters. A recent theory[1,17,33] on epigenetics also suggests that greater attention must be paid to those multistage processes that do not involve DNA damage. Some reports showed that oxidative stress induced by ROS has been linked to tumor promotion in mouse skin and other tissues.[34–36] Many tumor promoters generate ROS, and the involvement of ROS, particularly hydrogen peroxide, in the tumor promotion is supported by both *in vivo* and *in vitro* studies.[20,34,37] The topical application of tumor promoters to mouse skin results in a distinct increase in the production of hydrogen peroxide in the epidermis, which is correlated with their tumor promoting potential.[38]

Superoxide radicals are also formed in keratinocytes stimulated with the tumor promoters such as 12-$O$-tetradecanoylphorbol-13-acetate.[39]

The generation of oxidative stress is another integral component of the inflammatory response. There is considerable evidence that ROS and RNS are involved in the link between chronic inflammation and cancer.[40] Furthermore, tumor promoters and lipopolysaccharide can induce inflammation through the overexpression of COX-2 and iNOS with the generation of ROS and RNS. It was reported that ROS[41] and RNS[42] also promote cancer through the inhibition of GJIC. As stated above, MMPs have long been implicated in cancer-cell invasion and metastasis, but MMPs are also linked to the tumor promotion process, which may be mediated by ROS.[29–32] Thus, the promotional phase of carcinogenesis is a consequence of epigenetic events involving inflammation,[1] inhibition of GJIC,[22] and activation of MMPs,[43] which could be mediated by ROS.

## 7.5 UNDERLYING CHEMOPREVENTIVE MECHANISMS OF VITAMIN C

Clinical trials involving high dosages of dietary vitamin C supplements do not support a cancer protective role for vitamin C.[44,45] However, there is suggestion for such a role from epidemiological and observational studies based on food intake.[6,46] There was early epidemiologic evidence that a high intake of vitamin C-rich fruits and vegetables as well as a high serum level of vitamin C is inversely associated with the risk of some cancers. In 1991, Henson et al.[46] analyzed 46 epidemiologic studies on the protective effects of vitamin C against various types of cancers, among which 33 found a significant link between vitamin C intake and a reduced incidence of cancers. The more recent analysis by Carr and Frei[47] shows that vitamin C acts as an antioxidant *in vivo*. Of the 44 published *in vivo* studies they examined, 38 showed a reduction in markers of oxidative damage to DNA, lipid, or protein and only 6 showed an increase in oxidative damage after supplementation with vitamin C. Despite the inconsistent findings of previous studies, most of them do support the notion that vitamin C decreases the risk of cancer. The underlying chemopreventive mechanisms are described below.

### 7.5.1 ANTIOXIDANT EFFECTS

Vitamin C is known to stimulate immune function, inhibit nitrosamine formation, and block the metabolic activation of carcinogens, but the cancer-preventive effects of vitamin C may be mainly attributable to its protective effects against oxidative stress. Vitamin C is known to scavenge superoxide anions[48,49] and peroxynitrites,[50,51] as well as to inhibit the formation of superoxide anions and peroxyl radicals.[52] Several studies have revealed that vitamin C has protective effects against DNA damage by ROS and RNS either alone or synergistically[53,54] and exerts preventive effects against DNA damage caused by hydrogen peroxide in human lymphocytes.[55]

Lenton et al.[56] showed a negative correlation between intracellular vitamin C levels and the levels of 8-oxo-deoxyguanosine in lymphocytes from 105 healthy volunteers. In another report, the levels of 8-oxo-deoxyguanosine in mononuclear cell DNA, serum, and urine from subjects undergoing supplementation with 500 mg of vitamin C per day were also decreased, which were strongly correlated with increases in plasma vitamin C concentration.[57] However, the relevance of oxidative modification of DNA bases as a biomarker of carcinogenesis is being questioned because of a frequent artifact in measuring 8-oxo-deoxyguanosine levels in DNA.[58,59] Moreover, the actual level of 8-oxo-deoxyguanosine in human DNA varies widely.[58,59] Taking the above problems into consideration by using a quantitative plasmid-based genetic system, Lutsenko et al.[60] recently demonstrated that vitamin C can prevent hydrogen peroxide-induced mutations in human cells. They suggested that high intracellular concentrations of vitamin C could reduce DNA mutations caused by oxidative stress in humans.[60]

In contrast, vitamin C can also exert pro-oxidant activity under certain conditions, particularly in the presence of transition metal ions or alkali. *In vitro*, vitamin C reduces free ferric iron that generates hydrogen peroxide in the Fenton reaction which results in the production of hydroxyl radicals. The hydroxyl radical reacts rapidly with critical cellular macromolecules, including DNA, which is implicated in the initiation of cancer. However, the amounts of free transition metals *in vivo* are very small because they bind efficiently to proteins. Other studies have indeed demonstrated that the consumption of 500 mg of vitamin C per day did not result in significant oxidative DNA damage[61] and even a daily intake of 5000 mg of vitamin C was shown not to promote cancer or induce DNA damage.[62] Moreover, vitamin C was found predominantly to reduce oxidative damage *in vivo* even in the presence of iron.[47] Therefore, the consensus from *in vitro* and *in vivo* experiments as well as population-based studies reported in the literature is that a high consumption of vitamin C-rich fruits and vegetables is unlikely to be linked with increased oxidative DNA damage or with an elevated risk of cancer.

The intrinsic pro-oxidant potential of vitamin C may also contribute to its chemopreventive properties. A low or baseline level of oxidative stress appears to be essential for the cellular transduction signals that lead to the induction or potentiation of some detoxification/antioxidant enzyme systems. Antioxidant micronutrients may act as mild pro-oxidants to supply limited amounts of ROS when needed for triggering antioxidant signal transduction. If this is the case, it remains to be clarified when and how the pro-oxidant activity of vitamin C is turned on in the intracellular redox milieu while it is fighting, as an antioxidant, against excess oxidative stress.

## 7.5.2 ANTI-INFLAMMATORY ACTIVITY

There is considerable evidence that ROS are somehow involved in chronic inflammation and cancer.[1,2,40,63] The generation of oxidative stress is an integral part of the inflammatory response associated with tumor promotion. Thus, many compounds with antioxidant capability can inhibit tumor promotion and inflammation.[1,2,63] Since several studies have provided strong evidence that gastric cancer is a consequence of chronic inflammation,[64] the inflammatory process caused by the overproduction of ROS could be targeted by vitamin C. Indeed, vitamin C was shown to attenuate gastric cancer by reducing inflammation caused by ROS.[64] A recent human study also showed low levels of vitamin C in gastric juice in the early stages of carcinogenesis.[40] The protective effects of vitamin C against gastric carcinogenesis may be partly related to the scavenging of mucosal oxygen radicals,[65] as well as to inhibiting the formation of carcinogenic nitrosamines. However, pretreatment of endothelial cells with vitamin C in a recent report resulted in the accumulation of a large amount of this antioxidant inside the cells, which consequently decreased both the intracellular oxidant level and iNOS induction.[66] Vitamin C was also shown to inactivate nuclear factor-κB (NF-κB) in endothelial cells during the inflammation process, which was independent of its antioxidant activity.[67] Therefore, the anti-inflammatory activity of vitamin C may be mediated by multifactorial mechanisms, some of which may be unrelated to its intrinsic antioxidant activity.

### 7.5.3 Restoration of Cell-to-Cell Communication

Cell-to-cell communication through gap junction channels is essential for maintaining the homeostatic balance via the modulation of cell proliferation and differentiation in multicellular organisms.[68] Inhibition of cell-to-cell communication is strongly related to carcinogenicity, particularly to tumor promotion.[17,20] Hydrogen peroxide, a well-known tumor promoter, also inhibits GJIC.[38] We reported previously that vitamin C prevented the inhibition of GJIC by hydrogen peroxide.[69] It also protected hyperphosphorylation of connexin 43 protein (Cx43), a protein that regulates GJIC in rat liver epithelial cells. We also found that sustained production of hydrogen peroxide by phenazine methosulfate (PMS) inhibited GJIC in rat liver epithelial cells. The inhibition of GJIC by PMS involved hyperphosphorylation of Cx43 through activation of ERK1/2 (unpublished observation). Vitamin C prevented inhibition of GJIC, hyperphosphorylation of Cx43, and activation of ERK1/2 induced by PMS. In contrast, antioxidants such as propylgallate and Trolox did not prevent the hydrogen peroxide-mediated inhibition of GJIC.[38] Several reports suggest that some antioxidative phenolic substances, such as gallic acid and epigallocatechin gallate, induce DNA damage[70–72] and that their damaging effects are probably due to the generation of hydrogen peroxide. We have found that gallic acid and epigallocatechin gallate generate ROS that contributed to inhibition of GJIC, and that vitamin C protected against these effects (unpublished observation). Thus, the effect of vitamin C on GJIC appears to be a chemopreventive effect different from other antioxidative dietary substances.

A recent analysis by Rosenkranz et al.[73] indicates that inhibition of GJIC is strongly linked to carcinogenicity in rodents possibly by influencing inflammatory processes and developmental effects. Integration of the analysis also suggests that the inhibition of GJIC is involved in the nongenotoxic induction of cancer and in tumor promotion.[73] Therefore, we suggest that the cancer chemopreventive effects of vitamin C are linked to its protective effects against epigenetic mechanisms such as inflammation and the inhibition of GJIC as well as its antioxidant activities.

### 7.5.4 ANTIMETASTATIC EFFECTS

The ECM is a framework of proteins and proteoglycans that provides structural integrity to tissues. It also plays critical roles in cell growth, differentiation, survival, and motility. MMPs are a family of zinc-dependent endopeptidases that can degrade the major components of the ECM. Many studies have shown that ECM-degrading enzymes, including MMPs, play a pivotal role in tumor invasion and metastasis. A recent review suggests that MMP inhibitors exert strong effects at the tumor promotion stage, which may be partly attributable to the inhibition of the expression of enzymes related to inflammation such as COX-2 and iNOS as well as angiogenic factors.[2] Therefore, MMPs may play an important role in tumor promotion as well as in tumor invasion and metastasis.[29,30] Thus, MMPs are considered to be a novel target for noncytotoxic chemoprevention in multistage carcinogenesis.[28]

Vitamin C acts at the transcriptional level to downregulate MMP-2 expression and activity in human amnionic cultured cells.[74] A recent review[43] has provided evidence that ROS are key regulators of MMP production and that these interactions are important in disease pathologies. Sustained production of hydrogen peroxide by PMS-induced activation of pro-MMP-2 through the induction of MT-1 MMP expression in HT1080 fibrosarcoma cells.[75] Vitamin C inhibited activation of pro-MMP-2 by suppressing the activation of MT-1 MMP by PMS, and suppressed PMS-induced motility and invasiveness in HT1080 cells (unpublished observation). The aforementioned generation of ROS by gallic acid, a major dietary phenolic substance, also induced activation of pro-MMP-2 through activation of MT-1 MMP, and this was suppressed by vitamin C (unpublished observation). This demonstrates that vitamin C can protect ROS-mediated activation of MMP, which may contribute to its chemopreventive potential.

The aforementioned putative chemopreventive effects of vitamin C are summarized in Figure 7.1.

## 7.6 CONCLUSION

Vitamin C reportedly exerts substantial cancer chemopreventive effects mainly due to its strong antioxidant activities against DNA damage. This antioxidant has also been used as a dietary supplement to prevent oxidative stress–mediated chronic diseases such as cancer, cardiovascular disease, hypertension, stroke, neurodegenerative disorders, and aging. Several studies have shown that vitamin C has pro-oxidant activity under certain conditions such as in the presence of transition metal ions or alkali.[76] A recent study suggests that even a moderate daily dose of supplementary vitamin C (200 mg) induces the formation of genotoxins from lipid hydroperoxides, which results in DNA damage and the initiation

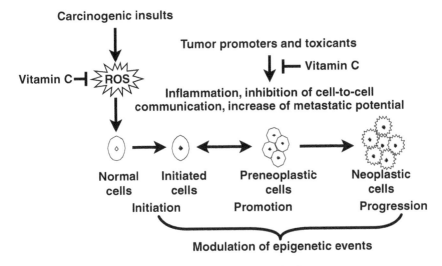

**FIGURE 7.1** Putative chemopreventive effects of vitamin C.

of carcinogenesis.[76] Despite questionable experimental designs and the numerous contradicting reports, the current consensus from epidemiological and human studies is that a low risk of cancer is more strongly related to antioxidant-rich diets than to individual dietary supplement antioxidants.[5]

The elimination or minimization of exposure to diverse environmental carcinogens is one strategy for preventing the majority of human cancers, but the complete avoidance of exposure to etiologic factors that can induce the initiation of cancer may be unrealistic. Since tumor promotion is closely linked to oxidative and inflammatory processes and is a relatively long-term and reversible process, it can be efficiently reversed and suppressed by vitamin C. A recent theory[1,17,33] on epigenetics suggests that greater attention must be paid to multistage carcinogenesis that does not involve DNA damage. Cancer prevention strategies that involve intervention at the tumor-promotion stage (a reversible and long-term process) are more practical than those intervening at the tumor-initiation stage (an irreversible and short-term process). The chemopreventive effects of vitamin C appear to be related to antipromoting or antiprogressive activities such as anti-inflammatory activity, enhancement of cell-to-cell communication, and antiangiogenetic properties as well as antioxidant activity. Taken together, these observations suggest that consumption of five servings of fruits and vegetables (containing 200 to 280 mg of vitamin C) per day can be strongly recommended.

## ACKNOWLEDGMENT

This work was supported by research grants from the Korea Institute of Science and Technology Evaluation and Planning (KISTEP) for functional food research and development, Ministry of Science and Technology.

## REFERENCES

1. Surh Y-J. Molecular mechanisms of chemopreventive effects of selected dietary and medicinal phenolic substances. *Mutat Res* 1999; 428:305–327.
2. Surh Y-J, Chun K-S, Cha H-H, Han SS, Keum YS, Park KK, Lee SS. Molecular mechanisms underlying chemopreventive activities of anti-inflammatory phytochemicals: down-regulation of COX-2 and iNOS through suppression of NF-κB activation. *Mutat Res* 2001; 480–481:243–268.
3. Engelhart MJ, Geerlings MI, Ruitenberg A, Van Sweiten JJ, Hofman A, Witteman JC, Breteler MM. Dietary intake of antioxidants and risk of Alzheimer disease. *J Am Med Assoc* 2002; 287:3223–3229.
4. Surh Y-J. Cancer chemoprevention with dietary phytochemicals. *Natl Rev Cancer* 2003; 3:768–780.
5. Lee KW, Lee HJ, Surh YJ, Lee CY. Vitamin C and cancer chemoprevention: reappraisal. *Am J Clin Nutr* 2003; 78:1074–1078.
6. La C V, Altieri A, Tavani A. Vegetables, fruit, antioxidants and cancer: a review of Italian studies. *Eur J Nutr* 2001; 40:261–267.
7. Doll R, Peto R. The causes of cancer: quantitative estimates of avoidable risks of cancer in the United States today. *J Natl Cancer Inst* 1981; 66:1191–1308.
8. Doll R. An overview of the epidemiological evidence linking diet and cancer. *Proc Nutr Soc* 1990; 49:119–131.
9. Michels KB, Giovannucci E, Joshipura KJ, Rosner BA, Stampfer MJ, Fuchs CS, Colditz GA, Speizer FE, Willett WC. Prospective study of fruit and vegetable consumption and incidence of colon and rectal cancers. *J Natl Cancer Inst* 2000; 92:1740–1752.
10. World Cancer Research Fund/American Institute for Cancer Research. Food research and the prevention of cancer: a global perspective. Washington DC: American Institute for Cancer Research, 1997.
11. Khaw KT, Bingham S, Welch A, Luben R, Wareham N, Oakes S, Day N. Relation between plasma ascorbic acid and mortality in men and women in EPIC-Norfolk prospective study: a prospective population study. European Prospective Investigation into Cancer and Nutrition. *Lancet* 2001; 357:657–663.
12. Duffy, SJ, Gokce N, Holbrook M, Huang A, Frei B, Keaney JFJ, Vita JA. Treatment of hypertension with ascorbic acid. *Lancet* 1999; 354:2048–2049.
13. Kurl S, Tuomainen TP, Laukkanen JA, Nyyssonen K, Lakka T, Sivenius J, Salonen JT. Plasma vitamin C modifies the association between hypertension and risk of stroke. *Stroke* 2002; 33:1568–1573.
14. Jemal A, Thomas A, Murray T, Thun M. Cancer statistics 2002. *CA-Cancer J Clin* 2002; 52:23–47.
15. Howe HL, Wingo PA, Thun MJ, Ries LAG, Rosenberg HM, Feigal EG, Edwards BK. Annual report to the nation on the status of cancer (1973 through 1998), featuring cancers with recent increasing trends. *J Natl Cancer Inst* 2001; 93:824–842.
16. Sporn MB, Suh N. Chemoprevention: an essential approach to controlling cancer. *Nat Rev Cancer* 2002; 2:537–543.
17. Trosko JE. Commentary: is the concept of "tumor promotion" a useful paradigm? *Mol Carcinogen* 2001; 30:131–137.

18. Pezzuto JM. Cancer chemopreventive agents: from plant materials to clinical intervention trials. In: Kinghorn AD, Balandrin MF, eds. *Human Medicinal Agents from Plants*. Washington, DC: American Chemical Society 1990; 204–215.

19. Trosko JE, Ruch RJ. Cell–cell communication in carcinogenesis. *Front Biosci* 1998; 3:208–236.

20. Trosko JE, Chang CC. Modulation of cell–cell communication in the cause and chemoprevention/chemotherapy of cancer. *BioFactors* 2000; 12:259–263.

21. Trosko JE, Chang CC, Upham B, Wilson M. Epigenetic toxicology as toxicant-induced changes in intracellular signalling leading to altered gap junctional intercellular communication. *Toxicol Lett* 1998; 102–103:71–78.

22. Huang RP, Peng A, Golard A, Hossain MZ, Huang R, Liu YG, Boynton AL. Hydrogen peroxide promotes transformation of rat liver non-neoplastic epithelial cells through activation of epidermal growth factor receptor. *Mol Carcinogen* 2001; 30:209–217.

23. Sai K, Upham BL, Kang KS, Hasegawa R, Inoue T, Trosko JE. Inhibitory effect of pentachlorophenol on gap junctional intercellular communication in rat liver epithelial cells *in vitro*. *Cancer Lett* 1998; 130:9–17.

24. Rivedal E, Opsahl H. Role of PKC and MAP kinase in EGF- and TPA-induced connexin43 phosphorylation and inhibition of gap junction intercellular communication in rat liver epithelial cells. *Carcinogenesis* 2001; 22:1543–1550.

25. Nielsen M, Ruch RJ, Vang O. Resveratrol reverses tumor-promoter-induced inhibition of gap-junctional intercellular communication. *Biochem Biophys Res Commun* 2000; 275:804–809.

26. Sai K, Kanno J, Hasegawa R, Trosko JE, Inoue T. Prevention of the down-regulation of gap junctional intercellular communication by green tea in the liver of mice fed pentachlorophenol. *Carcinogenesis* 2000; 21:1671–1676.

27. Na HK, Wilson MR, Kang KS, Chang CC, Grunberger D, Trosko JE. Restoration of gap junctional intercellular communication by caffeic acid phenethyl ester (CAPE) in a ras-transformed rat liver epithelial cell line. *Cancer Lett* 2000; 157:31–38.

28. Birkedal-Hansen H. Proteolytic remodeling of extracellular matrix. *Curr Opin Cell Biol* 1995; 7:728–735.

29. Coussens ML, Fingleton B, Matrisian LM. Matrix metalloproteinase inhibitors and cancer: trials and tribulations. *Science* 2002; 295:2387–2392.

30. Tosetti F, Ferrari N, De Flora S, Albini, A. "Angioprevention": angiogenesis is a common and key target for cancer chemopreventive agents. *FASEB J* 2002; 16:2–14.

31. Egeblad M, Werb Z. New functions for the matrix metalloproteinases in cancer progression. *Nat Rev Cancer* 2002; 2:161–174.

32. Nelson AR, Fingleton B, Rothenberg ML, Matrisian LM. Matrix metalloproteinases: biologic activity and clinical implications. *J Clin Oncol* 2000; 18:1135–1149.

33. Wu CT, Morris JR. Genes, genetics, and epigenetics: a correspondence. *Science* 2001; 293:1103–1105.

34. Cerutti PA. Prooxidant states and tumor promotion. *Science* 1985; 227:375–381.

35. Nishigori C, Hattori Y, Toyokuni S. Role of reactive oxygen species in skin carcinogenesis. *Antioxid Redox Signal* 2004; 6:561–570.

36. Konturek PC, Kania J, Konturek JW, Nikiforuk A, Konturek SJ, Hahn EG. *H. pylori* infection, atrophic gastritis, cytokines, gastrin, COX-2, PPAR gamma and impaired apoptosis in gastric carcinogenesis. *Med Sci Monit* 2003; 9:SR53–66.

37. Upham BL, Kang KS, Cho HY, Trosko JE. Hydrogen peroxide inhibits gap junctional intercellular communication in glutathione sufficient but not glutathione deficient cells. *Carcinogenesis* 1997; 18:37–42.

38. Perchellet EM, Perchellet JP. Characterization of the hydroperoxide response observed in mouse skin treated with tumor promoters *in vivo*. *Cancer Res* 1989; 49:6193–6201.

39. Pence BC, Reiners JJ Jr. Murine epidermal xanthine oxidase activity: correlation with degree of hyperplasia induced by tumor promoters. *Cancer Res* 1987; 47:6388–6392.

40. Wiseman H, Halliwell B. Damage to DNA by reactive oxygen and nitrogen species: role in inflammatory disease and progression to cancer. *Biochem J* 1996; 313:17–29.

41. Kang KS, Wilson MR, Hayashi T, Chang CC, Trosko JE. Inhibition of gap junctional intercellular communication in normal human breast epithelial cells after treatment with pesticides, PCBs, and PBBs, alone or in mixtures. *Environ Health Perspect* 1996; 104:192–200.

42. Sharov VS, Briviba K, Sies H. Peroxynitrite diminishes gap junctional communication: protection by selenite supplementation. *IUBMB Life* 1999; 48:379–384.

43. Nelson KK, Melendez JA. Mitochondrial redox control of matrix metalloproteinases. *Free Radical Biol Med* 2004; 37:768–784.

44. Blot WJ, Li JY, Taylor PR, Guo W, Dawsey S, Wang GQ, Yang CS, Zheng SF, Gail M, Li GY. Nutrition intervention trials in Linxian, China: supplementation with specific vitamin/mineral combinations, cancer incidence, and disease-specific mortality in the general population. *J Natl Cancer Inst* 1993; 85:1483–1492.

45. Yong LC, Brown CC, Schatzkin A, Dresser CM, Slesinski MJ, Cox CS, Taylor PR. Intake of vitamins E, C, and A and risk of lung cancer. The NHANES I epidemiologic followup study. First National Health and Nutrition Examination Survey. *Am J Epidemiol* 1997; 146:231–243.

46. Henson DE, Block G, Levine M. Ascorbic acid: biologic functions and relation to cancer. *J Natl Cancer Inst* 1991; 83:547–550.

47. Carr A, Frei B. Does vitamin C act as a pro-oxidant under physiological conditions? *FASEB J* 1999; 13:1007–1024.

48. Korycka-Dahl MB, Richardson T. Activated oxygen species and oxidation of food constituents. *Crit Rev Food Sci Nutr* 1978; 10:209–241.

49. Lavelli V, Hippeli S, Peri C, Elstner EF. Evaluation of radical scavenging activity of fresh and air-dried tomatoes by three model reactions. *J Agric Food Chem* 1999; 47:3826–3831.

50. Haenen GR, Paquay JB, Korthouwer RE, Bast A. Peroxynitrite scavenging by flavonoids. *Biochem Biophys Res Commun* 1997; 236:591–593.

51. Heijnen CG, Haenen GR, van Acker FA, van der Vijgh WJ, Bast A. Flavonoids as peroxynitrite scavengers: the role of the hydroxyl groups. *Toxicol in Vitro* 2001; 15:3–6.

52. Halliwell B. Drug antioxidant effects. A basis for drug selection? *Drugs* 1991; 42:569–605.

53. Bohm F, Edge R, McGarvey DJ, Truscott TG. Beta-carotene with vitamins E and C offers synergistic cell protection against NOx. *FEBS Lett* 1998; 436:387–389.

54. Green MH, Lowe JE, Waugh AP, Aldridge KE, Cole J, Arlett CF. Effect of diet and vitamin C on DNA strand breakage in freshly-isolated human white blood cells. *Mutat Res* 1994; 316:91–102.

55. Noroozi M, Angerson WJ, Lean MEJ. Effects of flavonoids and vitamin C on oxidative DNA damage to human lymphocytes. *Am J Clin Nutr* 1998; 67:1210–1218.
56. Lenton KJ, Therriault H, Fulop T, Payette H, Wagner JR. Glutathione and ascorbate are negatively correlated with oxidative DNA damage in human lymphocytes. *Carcinogenesis* 1999; 20:607–613.
57. Cooke MS, Evans MD, Podmore ID, Herbert KE, Mistry N, Mistry P, Hickenbotham PT, Hussieni A, Griffiths HR, Lunec J. Novel repair action of vitamin C upon *in vivo* oxidative DNA damage. *FEBS Lett* 1998; 439:363–367.
58. Halliwell B. Why and how should we measure oxidative DNA damage in nutritional studies? How far have we come? *Am J Clin Nutr* 2000; 72:1082–1087.
59. Halliwell B. Effect of diet on cancer development: is oxidative DNA damage a biomarker. *Free Radical Biol Med* 2002; 32:968–974.
60. Lutsenko EA, Carcamo JM, Golde DW. Vitamin C prevents DNA mutation induced by oxidative stress. *J Biol Chem* 2002; 277:16895–16899.
61. Huang HY, Helzlsouer KJ, Appel LJ. The effects of vitamin C and vitamin E on oxidative DNA damage: results from a randomized controlled trial. *Cancer Epidemiol Biomarkers Prev* 2000; 9:647–652.
62. Vojdani A, Bazargan M, Vojdani E, Wright J. New evidence for antioxidant properties of vitamin C. *Cancer Detect Prev* 2000; 24:508–523.
63. Surh Y-J. Anti-tumor promoting potential of selected spice ingredients with antioxidative and anti-inflammatory activities: a short review. *Food Chem Toxicol* 2002; 40:1091–1097.
64. Feiz HR, Mobarhan S. Does vitamin C intake slow the progression of gastric cancer in *Helicobacter pylori*-infected populations? *Nutr Rev* 2002; 60:34–36.
65. Drake IM, Davies MJ, Mapstone NP, Dixon MF, Schorah CJ, White KL, Chalmers DM, Axon AT. Ascorbic acid may protect against human gastric cancer by scavenging mucosal oxygen radicals. *Carcinogenesis* 1996; 17:559–562.
66. Wu F, Tyml K, Wilson JX. Ascorbate inhibits iNOS expression in endotoxin- and IFN gamma-stimulated rat skeletal muscle endothelial cells. *FEBS Lett* 2002; 520:122–126.
67. Bowie AG, O'Neill LAJ. Vitamin C inhibits NF-κB activation by TNF via the activation of p38 mitogen-activated protein kinase. *J Immunol* 2000; 165:7180–7188.
68. Kumar MN, Gilula NB. The gap junction communication channel. *Cell* 1996; 84:381–388.
69. Lee KW, Lee HJ, Kang KS, Lee CY. Preventive effects of vitamin C on carcinogenesis. *Lancet* 2002; 359:172.
70. Shiraki M, Hara Y, Osawa T, Kumon H, Nakayama T, Kawakishi S. Antioxidative and antimutagenic effects of theaflavins from black tea. *Mutat Res* 1994; 323:29–34.
71. Johnson MK, Loo G. Effects of epigallocatechin gallate and quercetin on oxidative damage to cellular DNA. *Mutat Res* 2000; 459:211–218.
72. Yen G-C, Duh P-D, Tsai H-L. Antioxidant and pro-oxidant properties of ascorbic acid and gallic acid. *Food Chem* 2002; 79:307–313.
73. Rosenkranz HS, Pollack N, Cunningham AR. Exploring the relationship between the inhibition of gap junctional intercellular communication and other biological phenomena. *Carcinogenesis* 2000; 21:1007–1011.

74. Pfeffer F, Casanueva E, Kamar J, Guerra A, Perichart O, Vadillo-Ortega F. Modulation of 72-kilodalton type IV collagenase (Matrix metalloproteinase-2) by ascorbic acid in cultured human amnion-derived cells. *Biol Reprod* 1998; 52:326–329.

75. Yoon SO, Park SJ, Yoon SY, Yun CH, Chung AS. Sustained production of $H_2O_2$ activates pro-matrix metalloproteinase-2 through receptor tyrosine kinases/phosphatidylinositol 3-kinase/NF-κB pathway. *J Biol Chem* 2002; 277:30271–30282.

76. Lee SH, Oe T, Blair IA. Vitamin C-induced decomposition of lipid hydroperoxides to endogenous genotoxins. *Science* 2001; 292:2083–2086.

# 8 Folic Acid, Folates, and Cancer

*John J. McGuire*

## CONTENTS

8.1 Folate Metabolism ................................................................................. 153
8.2 Folates in Cancer Therapy ...................................................................... 156
    8.2.1 Dietary Folate Deficiency in Cancer Treatment ......................... 156
    8.2.2 Folate Antagonists (Antifolates) in Cancer Chemotherapy ........ 156
8.3 Folates and Cancer Prevention ............................................................... 156
    8.3.1 Defining Folate Deficiency ......................................................... 157
    8.3.2 Folate Deficiency and DNA Damage ......................................... 158
    8.3.3 Preclinical Data Linking Folate Deficiency and Cancer ........... 159
    8.3.4 Clinical Data Linking Folate Deficiency and Cancer ................ 159
        8.3.4.1 Colon Cancer ............................................................... 160
        8.3.4.2 Childhood Cancer ........................................................ 161
        8.3.4.3 Other Sites ................................................................... 161
    8.3.5 Mechanisms of Carcinogenesis through Folate Deficiency ....... 162
    8.3.6 Other Factors Contributing to Actual or Functional Folate
        Deficiency .................................................................................... 165
    8.3.7 Folate Supplementation .............................................................. 166
References ......................................................................................................... 167

## 8.1 FOLATE METABOLISM

The term folates (pteroylglutamates) denotes a family of essential human vitamins based on the structure of folic acid (pteroylglutamic acid; PteGlu; Figure 8.1). Members of this family differ structurally in three respects:[1,2] (1) oxidation state of the pyrazine ring (fully oxidized, $7,8$-$H_2$, or $5,6,7,8$-$H_4$); (2) substitution at the N5 and/or N10-position(s) by one-carbon units at the oxidation level of methanol, formaldehyde, and formate; and (3) the presence of additional glutamate residues (poly-$\gamma$-glutamates; $H_4PteGlu_n$) attached to the $\gamma$-carboxyl of the single glutamate that is intrinsic to the folate structure. Only $5,6,7,8$-tetrahydrofolates ($H_4PteGlu_n$) carry and transfer one-carbon units and hence are the physiologically active forms of the vitamin; folic acid itself is a provitamin that requires reduction to become active. The various one-carbon units are interconvertible (Figure 8.2), with the exception of the irreversible synthesis of 5-CH$_3$-H$_4$PteGlu. H$_4$PteGlu$_n$ cofactors transfer these one-carbon units in anabolic and catabolic reactions, including the synthesis of serine, glycine, methionine, thymidylate, and purines, and in the degradation of histidine. These reactions occur primarily in the cytosol and mitochondria (Figure 8.2),[3] although there is evidence that nuclei, lysosomes, and the Golgi may also have specialized folate-dependent pathways.[2] Intracellular folates occur almost exclusively as poly($\gamma$-glutamyl) metabolites (Figure 8.1).[4] Monoglutamyl folates (which are transport forms of the vitamin) must be present transiently in the intracellular space, but intracellular levels of monoglutamate are low or undetectable under physiological conditions. A distribution of poly-glutamate lengths generally occurs that is cell lineage-specific; within a given cell lineage, the length distribution is generally identical for folate species con-taining different one-carbon substituents. In human cells, the usual range of lengths is five to eight total glutamates. Poly($\gamma$-glutamylation) of folates serves two primary functions:[2,4] (1) retention of intracellular folates at levels (1 to 10 $\mu M$) far in excess of the extracellular concentration (human plasma is 10 n$M$ in folates[5]) because folylpolyglutamates, especially if more than two glutamates are present, are not substrates for efflux pathways, e.g., the reduced folate carrier (RFC), membrane-bound folate binding proteins (FBPs) and MRP1 and MRP3,[6] while monoglutamates are, and also because passive diffusion out of cells is limited by their high inherent negative charge; and (2) polyglutamyl folates are kinetically preferred (higher $V_{max}/K_m$) over monoglutamyl folates as substrates for most folate-dependent reactions. Catalytic efficiency may also be enhanced by preferential channeling of folylpolyglutamates between active sites in multi-functional folate-dependent enzymes. Although retention is clearly essential at low physiological extracellular folate concentrations, increased catalytic effi-ciency is apparently also essential since a Chinese hamster ovary cell line that transports folates normally, but is unable to synthesize folylpolyglutamates, can-not survive even in the presence of supraphysiological levels of reduced folates.[7] Thus, at least one folate-dependent reaction is insufficiently active with a mono-glutamate substrate to supply required levels of a critical metabolite.

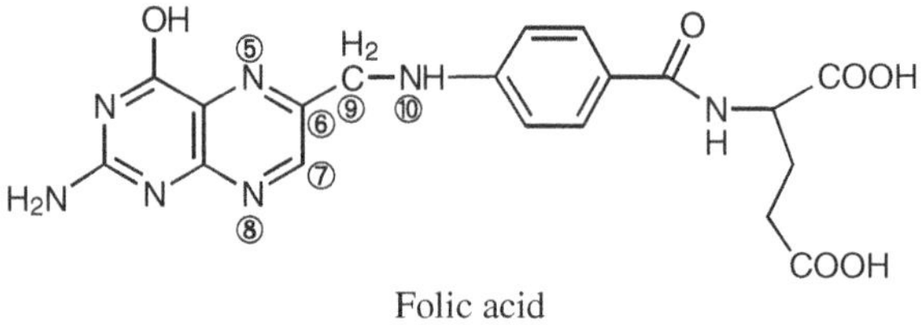

Folic acid

**FIGURE 8.1** Structure of folic acid. The standard numbering of the structure is shown. Only 5,6,7,8-tetrahydrofolates (H$_4$PteGlu$_n$) can carry and transfer one-carbon units. The one-carbon units are attached at N5 and/or N10. The one-carbon units and their attachment positions are: 5-methyl (–CH$_3$), 5-formyl (–HCO), 10-formyl (–HCO), 5-formimino (–CHNH), 5,10-methenyl (=CH$^+$–), and 5,10-methylene (–CH$_2$–). Interconversion of one-carbon forms and the reactions in which they participate are shown in Figure 8.2.

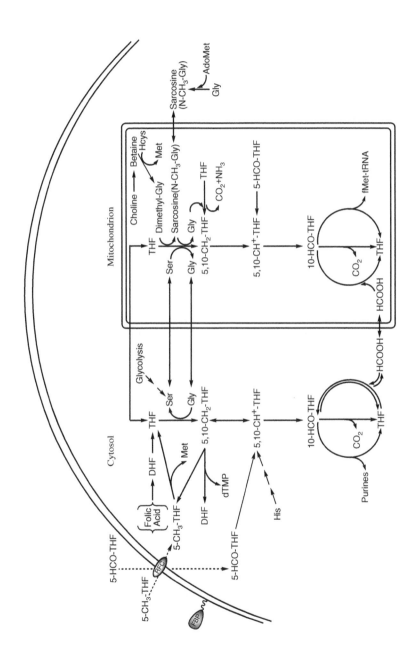

**FIGURE 8.2** Folate-dependent biosynthetic, catabolic, and interconversion reactions in the cytosol and mitochondria of mammalian cells. Some reactions are tissue specific.

## 8.2 FOLATES IN CANCER THERAPY

### 8.2.1 DIETARY FOLATE DEFICIENCY IN CANCER TREATMENT

Even before the key role that folates play in cellular metabolism was fully appreciated, several studies showed that nutritional induction of folate deficiency might be useful in cancer therapy (e.g., Reference 8). These studies were extended in preclinical *in vivo* models and folate deficiency was shown to selectively decrease tumor growth.[9-11] Dietary induction of folate deficiency in humans is not readily achieved,[12] however, and this approach has not been explored further.

### 8.2.2 FOLATE ANTAGONISTS (ANTIFOLATES) IN CANCER CHEMOTHERAPY

Soon after the determination of the structure of folic acid in the 1940s, folic acid analogs were made and their effects on normal animals were noted to be similar to those observed during nutritional folate deficiency.[2] This suggested that pharmacological induction of acute folate deficiency might induce a selective antitumor effect similar to that observed in nutritional folate deficiency. Further efforts to develop folate antagonists (antifolates) culminated in the development of methotrexate (MTX) in the early 1950s. MTX remains the most widely used antifolate for cancer chemotherapy.[2] The most important folate-dependent reactions (Figure 8.2) with respect to cancer chemotherapy are the thymidylate synthase reaction, which provides the only *de novo* source of dTMP, and glycinamide ribonucleotide and 5-aminoimidazole-4-carboxamide ribonucleotide transformylases (Figure 8.2), which both catalyze one-carbon transfer reactions in *de novo* purine synthesis. Both of these pathways are required to provide precursors for DNA synthesis, and it is this requirement that forms the basis for use of antifolates in chemotherapy. Extensive efforts to improve on the efficacy of MTX have led to the recent approval of two new anticancer antifolates, raltitrexed (in Europe only) and pemetrexed, for limited indications.[2]

## 8.3 FOLATES AND CANCER PREVENTION

Folates have been recognized as essential human vitamins since the 1930s[13] when several forms of severe megaloblastic anemia were first linked with deficiency of a dietary factor later identified as folic acid.[14] In recent years, however, occurrence of several pathologic conditions has been found to have previously unrecognized correlations with lower folate status,[15] although not necessarily with clinically defined deficiency, i.e., low plasma or erythrocyte (RBC) folate levels. These pathologic conditions include neural tube defects, neurological diseases (especially of the elderly), heart disease, and cancer. The connection of lower folate status to cancer incidence has been the most difficult to establish, probably because of the multistep nature of carcinogenesis and the multitude of factors in the etiology of this disease.

## 8.3.1 Defining Folate Deficiency

Another important factor contributing to the difficulty in linking low folate status and cancer has been the problem of defining folate deficiency. Initially, required daily folate intake was based on the level sufficient to prevent megaloblastic anemia[16] and normal clinical plasma and RBC ranges were set empirically to achieve this goal; folate deficiency was defined by the occurrence of megaloblastic anemia. As the number of pathologic conditions in which folate status has an impact has increased, however, the definition of folate deficiency has expanded because the pathologic effects (aside from megaloblastosis) may occur despite "normal" laboratory serum or RBC folate levels. This has led to the concept of "functional folate deficiency." Functional folate deficiency could occur in spite of adequate dietary intake of folate and efficient absorption, possibly even when folic acid supplementation is used, for at least two non-exclusive reasons. First is the possibility of localized folate deficiency where folate levels within a particular tissue are subnormal.[17–20] For example, it has been suggested that lung epithelium in smokers has a lower folate level than that of nonsmokers because constituents of tobacco smoke may mediate breakdown or inactivation of folates.[21] A second possibility is that adequate folate may be available in a tissue, but it is not effectively utilized. This could occur if polymorphic forms of folate-dependent enzymes with lower activity hindered overall folate metabolism. A well-studied example is the $5,10\text{-}CH_2\text{-}H_4PteGlu$ reductase (MTHFR) gene that produces the $5\text{-}CH_3\text{-}H_4PteGlu_n$ required for methionine biosynthesis (Figure 8.2). Several polymorphisms that decrease the catalytic efficiency of this enzyme are known that lead to decreased folate utilization (discussed below).

One challenge in this area of study is to identify and validate surrogate markers for functional folate deficiency.[22] Two biomarkers have been of high recent interest. One measure of functional folate deficiency is the occurrence of plasma homocysteine (Hcys). Hcys is produced by hydrolysis of $S$-adenosylhomocysteine (AdoHcys), one product of $S$-adenosylmethionine (AdoMet)-dependent methylation reactions (discussed below). Hcys is normally remethylated by methionine synthase to produce methionine by using $5\text{-}CH_3\text{-}H_4PteGlu_n$ (Figure 8.2). In folate deficiency, Hcys is poorly remethylated and thus increases in plasma. Studies in heart disease have shown that plasma Hcys is a very sensitive indicator of functional folate status.[23] A second surrogate is the presence of deoxyuridine in DNA in whole blood or its isolated cellular components (discussed below). Although helpful for prospective studies, especially if made serially, the present-day level of either surrogate in case-control studies may not be indicative of status at the time when the initial carcinogenic event occurred, given the long lag time in development of cancer. Among other markers that may prove useful are (1) methylation status in lymphocytes or target tissue (either measured globally or in the promoters of specific genes of interest); and (2) presence of micronuclei in peripheral blood lymphocytes.[24]

## 8.3.2 FOLATE DEFICIENCY AND DNA DAMAGE

Carcinogenesis is a multistep process in which an initiating mutation or epigenetic event occurs followed by a promotion phase in which genomic instability is increased by recurring DNA damage until sufficient damage has occurred to allow the cell to break free of normal growth controls.[25,26] Any process that increases DNA damage thus has the potential of contributing to initiation and/or promotion in the development of cancer. Folate deficiency in eukaryotes causes genomic damage that can be observed directly or indirectly. The biochemical mechanisms underlying DNA damage are discussed below. The variety of DNA damage attributed to folate deficiency indicates that it could contribute to carcinogenesis in the initiation and/or promotion phases.

Cytogenetic abnormalities are readily observed in folate deficiency. Bone marrow from clinically folate-deficient patients shows a normal karyotype but the chromosomes display a number of abnormalities including breaks (acentric fragments, gaps, and displaced fragments), incomplete contraction (metaphase chromosomes are qualitatively elongated compared to normal), and broken or widely spread centromeres.[27–29] These abnormalities appear to be randomly distributed and are completely or largely corrected following folate therapy showing a causal relationship. Similar chromosomal abnormalities occur in cell culture models of folate deficiency.[30] Micronuclei are considered secondary manifestations of chromosomal abnormalities.[31] Dietary folate deficiency induces increased levels of micronuclei in peripheral blood red cells in animal models[31] and in human subjects.[32–34] Micronuclei were normalized by folic acid supplementation in those cases where it was evaluated, again arguing for a causal relationship. In preclinical models, occurrence of micronuclei in folate deficiency is further increased by inhibition of DNA repair, again connecting chromosomal damage to their occurrence.[31] Chromosomal fragile sites in humans[35,36] appear to be especially susceptible to folate deficiency. A number of constitutive fragile sites are located in the same regions as breakpoints associated with oncogenesis of leukemias, lymphomas, and solid tumors.[37] Recombination at these breakage sites could lead to oncogene activation,[36] although the importance of fragile sites in oncogenesis has been disputed.[38] Folate deficiency can promote recombination, however, since in yeast starved for thymidylate, which is a major effect of folate deficiency, recombination of nuclear DNA (presumably through double-strand breaks) is increased.[39]

Folate deficiency can also increase mutation frequencies of nuclear genes at least.[40,41] Based on bacterial studies, these mutations should include base substitutions, deletions, duplications, and frame shifts.[42] The importance of folate deficiency in mutation is stressed by the further increase in mutation frequency observed in folate deficiency in the absence of DNA repair.[40]

### 8.3.3 PRECLINICAL DATA LINKING FOLATE DEFICIENCY AND CANCER

A number of preclinical studies have investigated the role of folate deficiency in development of cancer. Interestingly, as of 1995,[43] the carcinogenicity of chronic folate deficiency itself had not been reported; a PubMed search between that date and 2004 also did not yield any such studies. Either what would certainly be very long-term studies have not been performed or the studies were performed but gave inconclusive results. Indirect evidence from studies of chronic MTX treatment, which produces acute folate deficiency,[44] does not support the hypothesis that folate deficiency is carcinogenic.[45] It has been pointed out, however, that nutritional and pharmacologic folate deficiency may not be equivalent.[46] Similarly, methyl-deficient diets (i.e., deficient in methionine and choline) are carcinogenic,[47] but again it is not clear whether this is identical to nutritional folate deficiency, although both lead to decreased methylation (see below). Further support for a role of folate deficiency in carcinogenesis comes from observations that DNA damage caused by a number of known carcinogens is potentiated by prior induction of folate deficiency.[41,48] Also, a number of preclinical studies have demonstrated increased tumor burden in carcinogen-treated folate-deficient animals compared to carcinogen-treated pair-fed controls. These cell culture and *in vivo* studies have been exhaustively reviewed.[36,43,49] Whether folate deficiency initiates or promotes the activity of carcinogens has not been differentiated by studies to date.

### 8.3.4 CLINICAL DATA LINKING FOLATE DEFICIENCY AND CANCER

Epidemiological data are often the only way to establish a cause-and-effect relationship between a particular factor (e.g., folate) and a particular human pathophysiological state (e.g., cancer). The general types of epidemiological studies and their limitations have been well detailed.[49] With regard to folate, epidemiological studies have in general looked for a correlation between folate status and incidence of cancer at a particular site. Folate status is determined by use of dietary questionnaires or direct measurement of plasma and/or RBC folate. It is thought that RBC folate levels are the most accurate and reliable measure of current folate status,[36] but they are also the most difficult to obtain on large populations. The limitations discussed above with regard to functional, as opposed to clinical, folate deficiency must be factored in when examining these data. Because of the large number of nutritional and other variables associated with nutritional epidemiological studies, the problem of confounding variables is particularly acute. The best way, but also the most expensive way, to minimize confounding variables in studies of folates and cancer is the use of folic acid supplementation (intervention studies) to determine its effect. Despite these limitations, there are suggestive data for an inverse correlation between folate status and frequency of occurrence of a number of cancers.[36,49] This inverse correlation is strongest in colon cancer. Similar correlations may exist for cancer at other sites as well, but to date the studies have had too few subjects and/or have not lasted sufficiently long and have thus revealed suggestive trends rather than significant correlations. Some of these data, for example, in childhood leukemia, are of high interest, however.

### 8.3.4.1 Colon Cancer

The association of folate status with occurrence of colorectal cancer has been a topic of continuing interest given the high incidence of this disease (147,000 U.S. cases estimated in 2004) and its poor prognosis if not diagnosed early. Interest was first sparked by the finding[50] that folic acid supplementation significantly reduced, in a concentration-dependent manner, the occurrence of dysplastic foci and colorectal cancer in patients with ulcerative colitis, a chronic inflammation of the colon that predisposes to colon cancer and which currently affects about 1 million people in the U.S. (http://www.ccfa.org/research/info/aboutcd). Studies through 1999 correlating folate status with colorectal adenomas and colorectal cancer have been critically reviewed.[36,49] In general, these studies show a strong inverse relationship between dietary or blood folate status and incidence of adenomas (adenomatous polyps), which are precursors of colorectal cancer, or incidence of colon cancer. One of the largest studies showed that folate deficiency inversely correlated with occurrence of colonic adenomas in the Health Professionals Follow-up Study, a cohort of U.S. male health professionals, and in a large cohort of nurses in the Nurses' Health Study.[51] In a more recent follow-up study, the incidence of colon cancer in the same cohort of 47,931 men was also inversely correlated with dietary folate.[52] Similarly, in male smokers in the 50 to 69 age range, an inverse correlation between dietary folate intake and risk of colon, but not rectal, cancer was observed;[53] serum folate levels did not show this correlation, however. Strong suggestive evidence of an effect of folate on colon cancer risk in women comes from a follow-up prospective cohort study evaluating 88,756 women in the Nurses' Health Study over 14 years.[54] After controlling for other variables, a modestly lower risk for colorectal cancer — relative risk (RR) 0.67 — was noted in women in the quartile of highest folate intake (>400 µg/day) vs. the lowest quartile (<200 µg/day) as assessed in the first year of the study. The protective effect was insignificant in the first 8 years of study, but was highly significant (RR 0.56) in the last 6 years; this time effect is as expected if the folate level is related to causality. Interestingly, among all women who took vitamin supplements that included folic acid (≥100 µg/day; 86% of >400 µg/day group and 13% for <400 µg/day), the data showed only a nonsignificant trend toward less risk of colon cancer for up to 14 years; however, after 15 years an impressive protective effect was observed (RR 0.25). Use of multivitamins did not affect the risk for rectal cancer, however. It was suggested that the folic acid in the multivitamin supplements was responsible for this effect, but the presence of numerous other micronutrients that have anticarcinogenic effects (e.g., carotenoids and vitamins C and E) obviously tempers the strength of this conclusion since multivitamin supplementation decreased risk across all groups of dietary intake. Reliance on dietary folate intake information might have affected the correlation; however, red blood cell folate tracked questionnaire-based folate intake in a limited sampling (188 women) of the population. These data also showed that all women had clinically "normal" blood folate levels (>150 ng/ml) regardless of intake quartile and thus reinforce the concept of functional folate deficiency. Supplements may be beneficial even at high dietary intake because dietary folate may not be as bioavailable as the folic acid in the supplements.[55] The protective effect of folate appeared to be greatest in women whose diet was low in methionine, suggesting that DNA methylation (below) may be involved. Several regional and large national NCI-sponsored folate chemoprevention trials are now ongoing (http://researchportfolio.cancer.gov). Results from these studies should provide solid evidence both for a role of folate deficiency in development of colon cancer and whether the effects of folate deficiency can be reversed at a later date.

### 8.3.4.2 Childhood Cancer

The state of current knowledge about the etiology of childhood cancer, especially acute lymphoblastic leukemia the most common childhood cancer in the U.S., has recently been reviewed.[56] Based on a variety of studies with twins and from newborn screening heel stick cards, the author's overall conclusion is that initiation to a preleukemic state, as evidenced by the presence of specific abnormalities in DNA associated with childhood leukemia (e.g., TEL-AML1 translocation and IgH rearrangements), occurs *in utero* for a significant fraction of childhood leukemia cases. One or more secondary events in the preleukemic cells occurring up to 10 years after birth causes transformation to frank leukemia. Pregnancy is well known to cause maternal (and presumably fetal) vitamin deficiency. Evidence from one case-control study of pregnant women and supplement use suggests that vitamin deficiency could contribute to the initiation event that produces the preleukemic state and that folate deficiency was the primary source of this effect.[57] A second study did not find an effect, however.[58] Finding a correlation between folate deficiency and childhood leukemia would be important because, barring a mutation in the ovum or sperm, the initiating event must occur during the 9-month gestation and this is likely the only case where the timing of a carcinogenic event can be so closely determined.

### 8.3.4.3 Other Sites

Epidemiological studies correlating folate status with the occurrence of cervical dysplasia and cervical cancer, lung dysplasia and lung cancer, esophageal cancer, and brain cancer (e.g., childhood neuroblastoma) have been critically reviewed.[36,49] At this time, the data for these sites generally suggest a trend toward increased incidence in folate deficiency, but all the studies have too little power for their trends to reach significance. Several large prospective studies have indicated an inverse relationship between dietary folate intake and the risk of developing breast cancer (discussed in Reference 59).

Cervical cancer is of special interest because a connection between folate deficiency and cancer was probably first made in cervical cancer when morphological similarities were noted between cervical dysplasia and abnormal cervical cells in folate-deficient patients.[49] Both case-control and intervention epidemiological studies correlating folate status with cervical dysplasia and cervical cancer have been critically reviewed.[36,49] In almost all the case-control studies, an inverse correlation between folate status (established either by dietary questionnaire or direct plasma/RBC assay) and the occurrence of cervical dysplasia was observed. In most cases, the statistical correlation was weak, however. This weak correlation is consistent with the contradictory findings in the two small, perhaps inadequately controlled,[36] intervention trials where one showed a protective effect of folic acid, while a second using high (10 mg/day) folic acid supplementation did not. Folate concentrations vary during the normal estrus cycle, reaching a peak immediately before ovulation.[60] It has been suggested that estrogens present during normal cycling induce turnover of folates after ovulation and may induce localized folate deficiency. Oral contraceptive agents (OCAs) are associated with folate deficiency and the mechanism may be the same as that for estrogens.[60] OCA use is also associated with the appearance of megaloblastic epithelial cells in the cervix,[60] and these changes can be reversed by folic acid even in the absence of other symptoms of folate deficiency. It is unclear whether these abnormal cells can progress to frank cancer. However, folate deficiency causes a greater risk of cervical dysplasia in women infected with human papillomavirus, while high folate levels led to significantly lower risk of dysplasia in this group.[60] Since HPV infection is a known risk factor for cervical cancer, it appears that folic acid is protective in this special case.[60]

### 8.3.5 MECHANISMS OF CARCINOGENESIS THROUGH FOLATE DEFICIENCY

As discussed above, genomic instability is both a cause and effect of cancer. Severe folate deficiency can cause cell death, typically by apoptosis;[40,61] however, those few cells that survive exhibit genomic instability. Genomic instability in folate deficiency is primarily observed as chromosomal damage (strand breaks, recombination, micronucleus formation, etc.), which is thought to occur secondary to single- and double-strand DNA breaks.[39] Two general biochemical mechanisms have been proposed to account for the genomic instability that characterizes folate deficiency and may thus account for the inverse correlation of folate status and incidence of cancer. The first mechanism involves unbalanced nucleotide metabolism, especially involving dTTP, which results in genetic changes (i.e., point mutations and chromosomal damage). The second mechanism involves genetic and epigenetic effects caused by DNA hypomethylation because of a deficiency of the methyl donor AdoMet.

Because folate is required for the *de novo* synthesis of purines and thymidylate, folate deficiency in the absence of adequate salvage of these metabolites from dietary sources leads to alterations in deoxynucleotide (dNTP) pools. These alterations would be further exacerbated by the intricate regulation of dNTP synthesis that is primarily governed by ribonucleotide reductase.[62] Folate deficiency *in vitro*[40] and *in vivo*[63] decreases all dNTP pools (but especially dTTP), causes an imbalance of dNTP pools, and increases dUTP pools. Interestingly, both purine and pyrimidine dNTP pools are unbalanced in folate deficiency *in vivo*;[63] however, it appears that purine depletion is simply lethal, while dTTP depletion leads to genetic changes.[39] Chronically altered dNTP pools are mutagenic[64] and may even lead to a mutator phenotype (high level of spontaneous mutations).[65] In addition, chronically altered dNTP pools cause single- and double-strand breaks.[64] Several biochemical mechanisms have been proposed (discussed in Reference 40) by which imbalanced dNTP pools cause DNA damage. These mechanisms may operate alone, in concert, or may be tissue specific. DNA damage may derive from (1) decreased fidelity in DNA replication with any dNTP in excess prone to misincorporation resulting in transitions and transversions;[64,66,67] (2) DNA repair may be inhibited because of depressed dNTP pools[40,68–70] or exhibit lower fidelity[71] by similar mechanisms (misincorporation of the dNTP in excess, above; or dUTP incorporation, below). Decreased repair may also account for the potentiating effect of folate deficiency on known carcinogens; (3) dTTP depletion leads to DNA synthesis inhibition and damage during the abortive formation of replication complexes; and (4) dUTP is incorporated in place of dTTP and DNA damage occurs as a consequence of a futile cycle of misrepair of dU residues.

Misincorporation of dUTP into DNA has received considerable attention as a primary mechanism of DNA damage in folate deficiency. Although eukaryotic DNA polymerases do not discriminate between dTTP and dUTP,[72] incorporation of dU during replicative DNA synthesis is normally low ($\approx 10^4$ residues/genome). dUTP incorporation is normally low because the dUTP pool is kept low ($<0.3$ n$M$) relative to dTTP (40 $\mu M$) by the action of deoxyuridine 5'-triphosphate nucleotidohydrolase (dUTPase; EC 3.6.1.23; dUTP $\rightarrow$ dUMP + PP$_i$). Incorporated dU residues, as well as those produced by spontaneous hydrolytic deamination of dC,[73] are removed specifically by uracil-DNA glycosylase (UDG) in order to prevent GC $\rightarrow$ AT transitions during replication. Removal of uracil leads to an apyrimidinic (AP) site. The AP site is repaired by a generic system that includes nicking of the AP site by an AP endonuclease, removal of the ribose-phosphate by a deoxyribophosphodiesterase, resynthesis by a DNA polymerase and finally ligation.[73] Analogous to the case with antifolate treatment (i.e., MTX[74]), it is hypothesized that during folate deficiency dUTP synthesis increases to such an extent that dUTPase is overwhelmed and significant dUTP accumulation occurs at the same time that dTTP pools decrease because of insufficient 5,10-CH$_2$-H$_4$PteGlu$_n$ substrates for thymidylate synthase (Figure 8.2). dUTP pools increase because dUMP pools increase dramatically (as a result of decreased utilization in dTMP synthesis and because of dysregulation of dUMP synthesis caused by decreased dTTP) and there is no regulation of phosphorylation of dUMP to dUTP. It is postulated that an increased dUTP/dTTP ratio enhances incorporation of dU into DNA during attempted replication and repair. Since dTTP levels are low, a futile cycle of base excision and misrepair is initiated that results in single-strand breaks. Single-strand breaks on opposite strands that are separated by ≤13 bp can lead to a double-strand break[34,75] that would typically be repaired by recombination. dTTP depletion is known to be very recombinagenic.[39] While some data from folate deficiency (e.g., References 34, 70, and 76 to 78) and antifolate treatment (e.g., Reference 79) support this model, other evidence is not supportive (e.g., References 80 to 82). It is possible that different pathways of lethal damage operate in different tumor types and/or under different treatment conditions or with different agents.

A second biochemical mechanism proposed to account for the genomic instability that characterizes folate deficiency involves genetic and epigenetic effects caused by hypomethylation of DNA at CpG dinucleotides (5-methylcytosine).[26] Under conditions in which methyl donors are limiting, DNA becomes globally hypomethylated.[26] Hypomethylation leads to chromosomal instability including deletions, insertions, large-scale rearrangements, and a mutator phenotype.[26,83,84] In mismatch repair, the strand to be repaired can be discriminated from the parental strand, because the former is undermethylated; hypomethylation could thus lead to poor repair and the fixing of mismatch mutations.[59] In addition, since methylation can regulate transcription by inactivating promoter regions, hypomethylation of specific promoter regions also increases transcription of genes they control.[26] In cancer, genes for growth factors and for oncogenes, such as *c-myc* and *c-ras*, are often hypomethylated, leading to increased expression.[85,86] Methyl donor deficiency increases the incidence of spontaneous and carcinogen-induced tumors.[87] Conditions that lead to hypomethylation would thus be expected to be carcinogenic per se or to promote the action of carcinogens.

Biological methylation reactions, including methylation of CpG dinucleotides in DNA, are generally dependent on AdoMet as the methyl donor. AdoMet is synthesized enzymatically from ATP and methionine. The methionine can be derived from methylation of Hcys by $5\text{-}CH_3\text{-}H_4PteGlu_n$-dependent methionine synthase (Figure 8.2) or from the diet; methionine is considered an essential amino acid[88] because *de novo* synthesis is insufficient to meet metabolic requirements. Folate deficiency decreases the *de novo* synthesis of methionine and, in the absence of sufficient dietary methionine intake, leads to a decrease in cellular AdoMet pools.[89,90] Thus, folate deficiency can result in methyl donor deficiency, consequent hypomethylation of DNA,[89] and may thus increase the incidence of cancer. Despite the global hypomethylation observed in tumor cells, hypermethylation of specific regions occurs;[26] although this is difficult to reconcile with folate deficiency, it may be that hypermethylation is temporally separate from hypomethylation.

## 8.3.6 OTHER FACTORS CONTRIBUTING TO ACTUAL OR FUNCTIONAL FOLATE DEFICIENCY

Intake of folates either in the form of food or as supplements is only one aspect of an individual's folate status. Other factors may play a role, particularly in establishing functional folate status. Methionine intake (above) is one obvious factor. Since vitamin $B_{12}$, as well as folate, is essential for the enzymatic function of methionine synthase (Figure 8.2), vitamin $B_{12}$ status also affects the efficiency of folate metabolism. MTHFR ($5,10\text{-}CH_2\text{-}H_4PteGlu_n$ reductase), which synthesizes $5\text{-}CH_3\text{-}H_4PteGlu_n$ (Figure 8.2), possesses a flavin cofactor and thus riboflavin levels may also affect the functioning of folate metabolism; recently, it was shown that excess riboflavin may actually increase DNA damage in folate deficiency.[91] Vitamin $B_6$ is a cofactor for folate-dependent serine hydroxymethyltransferase (Figure 8.2) adding another possible point of nutrient–nutrient interaction. The interrelationship between dietary folate intake and expression levels of individual or multiple folate-dependent enzymes, and their polymorphic variants, may also affect the functional folate status of the individual.[92] In particular, MTHFR has been examined because its $5,10\text{-}CH_2\text{-}H_4PteGlu_n$ substrates can either be directed to methionine biosynthesis (and hence used for methylation, above) or can be used directly in thymidylate synthesis (Figure 8.2) to support DNA synthesis. It has also been a focus because several polymorphisms exist in MTHFR, including the well-characterized C677T variant that has significantly lower catalytic efficiency (it is also thermolabile, which was its first identified distinguishing characteristic).[93] Phenotypically, this polymorphism is recognized to increase the folate requirement of homozygous individuals; this means that at the same ("normal") folate intake, homozygous C677T individuals may be folate deficient (and also functionally folate deficient). Other low-activity polymorphisms of MTHFR (e.g., A1298C) may also play a role in increased nutritional requirement for folate.[94] The ethnic and sex distribution of the C677T polymorphism tracks with increased risk of common (i.e., excluding T cell and mature B cell) childhood ALL.[57] In contrast, direct studies[93–95] show a protective effect of C677T in some subclasses of childhood ALL. One feature that does not seem to have been addressed sufficiently in childhood ALL is whether the MTHFR genotypes of the mother and the fetus may interact;[95] if both mother and fetus are homozygous for C677T, then perhaps the effect on folate function in the fetus will be more dramatic. Homozygosity for the C677T polymorphism may also protect against colon cancer, but increase risk of endometrial cancer.[54,57] It has been suggested[57,94] that the critical event involving the C677T polymorphism is methylation. With adequate folate intake, both the synthesis dTMP for DNA synthesis and of methyl groups for methylation reactions occur optimally. With inadequate folate and the C677T polymorphism, it is proposed that the lower MTHFR activity shunts more $5,10\text{-}CH_2\text{-}H_4PteGlu_n$ to thymidylate synthase. dTTP (and purine dNTP) pools are preserved (or possibly enhanced) and DNA synthesis occurs with normal fidelity. However, the decreased synthesis of methyl groups leads to decreased DNA methylation, which leads to carcinogenesis. Although this is an interesting hypothesis and is supported by examination of folate pools in red blood cells,[96] no experimental evidence showing the preservation of dNTP pools has been presented. In fact, a recent study[97] suggests that there was no change in genomic instability in lymphocytes from C677T and A1298C homozygous and heterozygous subjects compared to wild-type MTHFR. Further work is clearly needed in this area to evaluate this provocative hypothesis. In addition to factors that directly affect functional folate status, there are factors that can affect the phenotypic effects of that status. One obvious example is DNA repair capability, especially those aspects that relate directly to the damage likely to occur in folate deficiency.[59]

### 8.3.7 FOLATE SUPPLEMENTATION

The above studies suggest that folate supplementation might be beneficial in preventing colon cancer in particular, but other cancers as well. Thus, it would appear that supplementation would be warranted, as long as it is safe. Folic acid is generally perceived as safe even at very high doses.[98] Even doses of 500 mg/day (>1000 times the RDA) are not harmful. It is likely that followers of alternative medicine have used supplements of pure folic acid at high multiples of the RDA for extended periods; no untoward effects have been reported in the literature from this practice. Folate supplementation, especially at high doses can be problematic in several circumstances, however.[98] Of particular concern is the masking of vitamin $B_{12}$ deficiency by large amounts of folic acid and the ultimate occurrence of undetected, irreversible subacute combined degeneration. This is a particular concern in elderly individuals who often have borderline vitamin $B_{12}$ status.[99] A potential danger in folate supplementation is that growth of preexisting, but unrecognized tumors might be accelerated.[8,100,101] On the other hand, in a model system, folate sufficiency decreases the metastatic potential suggesting that folate supplementation may decrease metastasis of established tumors.[102] Of recent interest, it was reported that supplementation of female mice with folate (along with other methyl donors) can lead to unintended epigenetic changes mediated through DNA methylation that are phenotypically apparent in the offspring.[103] Although the changes observed were not necessarily deleterious, similar changes in other genes might well lead to adverse consequences, including the initiation or promotion of cancer.

Should widespread folate supplementation be undertaken? In fact, folate supplementation is currently being done on a nationwide scale in the U.S. and other developed countries. The discovery that neural tube defects were significantly decreased by oral supplementation with folic acid prior to pregnancy (and thus were caused by folate deficiency) led to the U.S. FDA-mandated supplementation of flour, bread, and other cereal grain products with folic acid beginning in January 1998 (http://www.cfsan.fda.gov/~dms/wh-folic.html). The object is to raise folate intake to 0.4 to 1.0 mg folic acid/day, the amount required in women of childbearing age to prevent neural tube defects. Although targeted to reducing birth defects, this supplementation may have the unintended consequence of decreasing functional or localized folate deficiency across the entire population from conception and thus lead to a decrease in other conditions correlated with folate deficiency, including cancer.[104] Prior to supplementation, it was estimated that up to 10% of the U.S. population was borderline folate deficient[36] so a large segment of the U.S. population may benefit from folate supplementation. For cancer incidence, if folate deficiency promotes carcinogenesis, as seems likely based on preclinical studies, then folate supplementation may have an earlier impact on cancer incidence. If the DNA damage dependent on folate status occurs early in life or even *in utero* (above) and functions as an initiating event that requires further promoting events before the development of cancer, it may take decades for the full effects of folate supplementation to become apparent. If this is the case, it may also be that intervention with folate supplementation may not be as useful in the adult population if the later events are less dependent on folate status. To date, the very limited epidemiological data show, in fact, decreased incidence of childhood ALL after the start of mandated supplementation.[95]

Another issue that has not been widely addressed in intervention studies is the form of folate with which to supplement. Folic acid was used in most studies because it is inexpensive, readily available, and (unlike most reduced folates) chemically stable. However, 5-HCO-H$_4$PteGlu (Figure 8.1) is also chemically stable and commercially available as leucovorin (LV), although it is currently expensive. LV has the advantage that it does not require reduction and increases the supply of one-carbon units by one for each molecule absorbed. Commercial sources generally produce LV chemically and the synthetic route produces two diastereomers, *6S* and *6R*; only the *6S* diastereomer is biologically active.[105] Newer separation methods allow industrial production of the pure *6S* diastereomer. It would be worthwhile comparing both the (*6R,S*) diastereomeric mixture and the pure *6S* diastereomer to folic acid itself in intervention trials.

## REFERENCES

1. Shane B. Folylpolyglutamate synthesis and role in the regulation of one-carbon metabolism. *Vitamins Hormones* 1989; 45:263–335.
2. McGuire JJ. Anticancer antifolates: current status and future directions. *Curr. Pharmaceutical Design* 2003; 9:2593–2613.
3. Wagner C. Symposium on the subcellular compartmentation of folate metabolism. *J Nutr* 1996; 126(4 Suppl):1228S–1234S.
4. McGuire JJ, Coward JK. Pteroylpolyglutamates: Biosynthesis, degradation, and function. In: Blakley RL, Benkovic SJ, eds. *Folates and Pterins. Chemistry and Biochemistry of Folates.* Vol. 1. New York: Wiley, 1984:135–190.
5. Cossins EA. Folates in biological materials. In: Blakley RL, Benkovic SJ, eds. *Folates and Pterins. Chemistry and Biochemistry of Folates.* Vol. 1. New York: Wiley, 1984:1–59.

6. Zeng H, Chen ZS, Belinsky MG, Rea PA, Kruh GD. Transport of methotrexate (MTX) and folates by multidrug resistance protein (MRP) 3 and MRP1: effect of polyglutamylation on MTX transport. *Cancer Res* 2001; 61:7225–7232.

7. McBurney MW, Whitmore GF. Isolation and biochemical characterization of folate deficient mutants of Chinese hamster cells. *Cell* 1974; 2:173–182.

8. Heinle RD, Welch AD. Experiments with pteroylglutamic acid and pteroylglutamic acid deficiency in human leukemia. *J Clin Invest.* 1948; 27:539.

9. Potter M, Briggs GM. Inhibition of growth of amethopterin sensitive and amethopterin-resistant pairs of lymphocytic neoplasms by dietary folic-acid deficiency in mice. *J Natl Cancer Inst* 1962; 28:341–351.

10. Rosen F, Nichol CA. Inhibition of the growth of an amethopterin-refractory tumor by dietary restriction of folic acid. *Cancer Res* 1962; 22:495–500.

11. Welch AD. Folic acid: discovery and the exciting first decade. *Perspect Biol Med* 1983; 27:64–75.

12. Herbert V. Experimental nutritional folate deficiency in man. *Trans Assoc Am Phys* 1962; 75:307–320.

13. Wills L. Treatment of "pernicious anemia of pregnancy" and "tropical anemia". With special reference to yeast extract as a curative agent. *Br Med J* 1931; June 20:1059–1064.

14. Mitchell HK, Snell EE, Williams RJ. The concentration of folic acid. *J Am Chem Soc* 1941; 63:2284.

15. Hoffbrand AV, Weir DG. The history of folic acid. *Br J Haematol* 2001; 113:579–589.

16. Herbert V. Minimal daily adult folate requirement. *Arch Intern Med* 1962; 110:649–652.

17. Whitehead N, Reyner F, Lindenbaum J. Megaloblastic changes in the cervical epithelium. Association with oral contraceptive therapy and reversal with folic acid. *J Am Med Assoc* 1973; 226:1421–1424.

18. Heimburger DC. Localized deficiency of folic acid in aerodigestive tissues. *Ann NY Acad Sci* 1992; 669:87–96.

19. Kim YI, Fawaz K, Knox T, Lee YM, Norton R, Arora S, Paiva L, Mason JB. Colonic mucosal concentrations of folate correlate well with blood measurements of folate status in persons with colorectal polyps. *Am J Clin Nutr* 1998; 68:866–872.

20. Meenan J, O'Hallinan E, Scott J, Weir DG. Epithelial cell folate depletion occurs in neoplastic but not adjacent normal colon mucosa. *Gastroenterology* 1997; 112:1163–1168.

21. Abu Khaled M, Watkins CL, Krumdieck CL. Inactivation of $B_{12}$ and folate coenzymes by butyl nitrite as observed by NMR: implications on one-carbon transfer mechanism. *Biochem Biophys Res Commun* 1986; 135:201–207.

22. Mason JB. Biomarkers of nutrient exposure and status in one-carbon (methyl) metabolism. *J Nutr* 2003; 133(Suppl 3):941S–947S.

23. Refsum H, Ueland P, Nygård O, Vollset SE. Homocysteine and cardiovascular disease. *Annu Rev Med* 1998; 49:31–62.

24. MacGregor JT, Wehr CM, Hiatt RA, Peters B, Tucker JD, Langlois RG, Jacob RA, Jensen RH, Yager JW, Shigenaga MK, Frei B, Eynon BP, Ames BN. "Spontaneous" genetic damage in man: evaluation of interindividual variability, relationship among markers of damage, and influence of nutritional status. *Mutat Res* 1997; 377:125–135.

25. Miller EC, Miller JA. Mechanisms of chemical carcinogenesis. *Cancer* 1981; 47:1055–1064.
26. Robertson KD, Jones PA. DNA methylation: past, present and future directions. *Carcinogenesis* 2000; 21:461–467.
27. Heath CW Jr. Cytogenetic observations in vitamin $B_{12}$ and folate deficiency. *Blood* 1966; 27:800–815.
28. Menzies RC, Crossen PE, Fitzgerald PH, Gunz FW. Cytogenetic and cytochemical studies on marrow cells in $B_{12}$ and folate deficiency. *Blood* 1966; 28:581–594.
29. Das KC, Mohanty D, Garewal G. Cytogenetics in nutritional megaloblastic anaemia: prolonged persistence of chromosomal abnormalities in lymphocytes after remission. *Acta Haematol* 1986; 76:146–154.
30. Libbus BL, Borman LS, Ventrone CH, Branda RF. Nutritional folate-deficiency in Chinese hamster ovary cells. Chromosomal abnormalities associated with perturbations in nucleic acid precursors. *Cancer Genet Cytogenet* 1990; 46:231–242.
31. MacGregor JT, Schlegel R, Wehr CM, Alperin P, Ames BN. Cytogenetic damage induced by folate deficiency in mice is enhanced by caffeine. *Proc Natl Acad Sci USA* 1990; 87:9962–9965.
32. Everson RB, Wehr CM, Erexson GL, MacGregor JT. Association of marginal folate depletion with increased human chromosomal damage in vivo: demonstration by analysis of micronucleated erythrocytes. *J Natl Cancer Inst* 1988; 80:525–529.
33. MacGregor JT. Dietary factors affecting spontaneous chromosomal damage in man. *Prog Clin Biol Res* 1990; 347:139–153.
34. Blount BC, Mack MM, Wehr CM, MacGregor JT, Hiatt RA, Wang G, Wickramasinghe SN, Everson RB, Ames BN. Folate deficiency causes uracil misincorporation into human DNA and chromosome breakage: Implications for cancer and neuronal damage. *Proc Natl Acad Sci USA* 1997; 94:3290–3295.
35. Chen AT, Reidy JA, Annest JL, Welty TK, Zhou HG. Increased chromosome fragility as a consequence of blood folate levels, smoking status, and coffee consumption. *Environ Mol Mutagen* 1989; 13:319–324.
36. Glynn SA, Albanes D. Folate and cancer: a review of the literature. *Nutr Cancer* 1994; 22:101–119.
37. Yunis JJ, Soreng AL. Constitutive fragile sites and cancer. *Science* 1984; 226:1199–1204.
38. Sutherland GR, Simmers RN. No statistical association between common fragile sites and nonrandom chromosome breakpoints in cancer cells. *Cancer Genet Cytogenet* 1988; 31:9–15.
39. Barclay BJ, Kunz BA, Little JG, Haynes RH. Genetic and biochemical consequences of thymidylate stress. *Can J Biochem* 1982; 60:172–184.
40. James SJ, Basnakian AG, Miller BJ. *In vitro* folate deficiency induces deoxynucleotide pool imbalance, apoptosis, and mutagenesis in Chinese hamster ovary cells. *Cancer Res* 1994; 54:5075–5080.
41. Branda RF, Hacker M, Lafayette A, Nigels E, Sullivan L, Nicklas JA, O'Neill JP. Nutritional folate deficiency augments the in vivo mutagenic and lymphocytotoxic activities of alkylating agents. *Environ Mol Mutagen* 1998; 32:33–38.
42. Sedwick WD, Brown OE, Glickman BW. Deoxyuridine misincorporation causes site-specific mutational lesions in the lacI gene of *Escherichia coli*. *Mutat Res* 1986; 162:7–20.

43. Jennings E. Folic acid as a cancer-preventing agent. *Med Hypotheses* 1995; 45:297–303.

44. Chu E, Allegra CJ. Antifolates. In: Chabner BA, Longo DL, eds. *Cancer Chemotherapy and Biotherapy.* Philadelphia: Lippincott–Raven, 1996:109–148.

45. Waters MD, Bergman HB, Nesnow S. The genetic toxicology of Gene-Tox noncarcinogens. *Mutat Res* 1988; 205:139–182.

46. Borman LS, Branda RF. Nutritional folate deficiency in Chinese hamster ovary cells. I. Characterization of the pleiotropic response and its modulation by nucleic acid precursors. *J Cell Physiol* 1989; 140:335–343.

47. Henning SM, Swendseid ME. The role of folate, choline, and methionine in carcinogenesis induced by methyl-deficient diets. *Adv Exp Med Biol* 1996; 399:143–155.

48. Branda RF, Blickensderfer DB. Folate deficiency increases genetic damage caused by alkylating agents and gamma-irradiation in Chinese hamster ovary cells. *Cancer Res* 1993; 53:5401–5408.

49. Kim YI. Folate and carcinogenesis: evidence, mechanisms, and implications. *J Nutr Biochem* 1999; 10:66–88.

50. Lashner BA, Heidenreich PA, Su GL, Kane SV, Hanauer SB. Effect of folate supplementation on the incidence of dysplasia and cancer in chronic ulcerative colitis. A case-control study. *Gastroenterology* 1989; 97:255–259.

51. Giovannucci E, Stampfer MJ, Colditz GA, Rimm EB, Trichopoulos D, Rosner BA, Speizer FE, Willett WC. Folate, methionine, and alcohol intake and risk of colorectal adenoma. *J Natl Cancer Inst* 1993; 85:875–884.

52. Giovannucci E, Rimm EB, Ascherio A, Stampfer MJ, Colditz GA, Willett WC. Alcohol, low-methionine-low-folate diets, and risk of colon cancer in men. *J Natl Cancer Inst* 1995; 87:265–273.

53. Glynn SA, Albanes D, Pietinen P, Brown CC, Rautalahti M, Tangrea JA, Gunter EW, Barrett MJ, Virtamo J, Taylor PR. Colorectal cancer and folate status: a nested case-control study among male smokers. *Cancer Epidemiol Biomarkers Prev* 1996; 5:487–494.

54. Giovannucci E, Stampfer MJ, Colditz GA, Hunter DJ, Fuchs C, Rosner BA, Speizer FE, Willett WC. Multivitamin use, folate, and colon cancer in women in the nurses' health study. *Ann Intern Med* 1998; 129:517–524.

55. Cuskelly GJ, McNulty H, Scott JM. Effect of increasing dietary folate on red-cell folate: implications for prevention of neural tube defects. *Lancet* 1996; 347:657–659.

56. Ross JA, Davies SM. Recent report in the etiology of childhood cancer: "greatest hits." *Pediatr Blood Cancer* 2004; 42:3–7.

57. Thompson JR, Gerald PF, Willoughby ML, Armstrong BK. Maternal folate supplementation in pregnancy and protection against acute lymphoblastic leukaemia in childhood: a case-control study. *Lancet* 2001; 358:1935–1940.

58. French AE, Grant R, Weitzman S, Ray JG, Vermeulen MJ, Sung L, Greenberg M, Koren G. Folic acid food fortification is associated with a decline in neuroblastoma. *Clin Pharmacol Ther* 2003; 74:288–294.

59. Han J, Hankinson SE, Zhang SM, De Vivo I, Hunter DJ. Interaction between genetic variations in DNA repair genes and plasma folate on breast cancer risk. *Cancer Epidemiol Biomarkers Prev* 2004; 13:520–524.

60. Butterworth CE Jr. Folate status, women's health, pregnancy outcome, and cancer. *J Am Coll Nutr* 1993; 12:438–441.

61. Koury MJ, Horne DW. Apoptosis mediates and thymidine prevents erythroblast destruction in folate deficiency anemia. *Proc Natl Acad Sci USA* 1994; 91:4067–4071.

62. Reichard P. Interactions between deoxyribonucleotide and DNA synthesis. *Annu Rev Biochem* 1988; 57:349–374.

63. James SJ, Cross DR, Miller BJ. Alterations in nucleotide pools in rats fed diets deficient in choline, methionine and/or folic acid. *Carcinogenesis* 1992; 13:2471–2474.

64. Kunz BA, Kohalmi SE, Kunkel TA, Mathews CA, McIntosh EM, Reidy JA. Deoxyribonucleoside triphosphate levels: A critical factor for maintenance of genetic stability. *Mutat Res* 1994; 318:1–64.

65. Weinberg G, Ullman B, Martin DW Jr. Mutator phenotypes in mammalian cell mutants with distinct biochemical defects and abnormal deoxyribonucleoside triphosphate pools. *Proc Natl Acad Sci USA* 1981; 78:2447–2451.

66. Phear G, Meuth M. The genetic consequences of DNA precursor pool imbalance: sequence analysis of mutations induced by excess thymidine at the hamster aprt locus. *Mutat Res* 1989; 214:201–206.

67. Das SK, Kunkel TA, Loeb LA. Effects of altered nucleotide concentrations on the fidelity of DNA replication. *Basic Life Sci* 1985; 31:117–126.

68. Snyder RD. Consequences of the depletion of cellular deoxynucleoside triphosphate pools on the excision-repair process in cultured human fibroblasts. *Mutat Res* 1988; 200:193–199.

69. Choi SW, Kim YI, Weitzel JN, Mason JB. Folate depletion impairs DNA excision repair in the colon of the rat. *Gut* 1998; 43:93–99.

70. Duthie SJ, Hawdon A. DNA instability (strand breakage, uracil misincorporation, and defective repair) is increased by folic acid depletion in human lymphocytes in vitro. *FASEB J* 1998; 12:1491–1497.

71. Holliday R. Aspects of DNA repair and nucleotide pool imbalance. *Basic Life Sci* 1985; 31:453–460.

72. Mosbaugh DW, Bennett SE. Uracil-excision DNA repair. *Prog Nucleic Acids Res Mol Biol* 1994; 48:315–370.

73. Friedberg EC, Walker GC, Siede W. *DNA Repair and Mutagenesis*. Washington, DC: ASM Press; 1995.

74. Curtin NJ, Harris AL, Aherne GW. Mechanism of cell death following thymidylate synthase inhibition: 2'-deoxyuridine-5'-triphosphate accumulation, DNA damage, and growth inhibition following exposure to CB3717 and dipyridamole. *Cancer Res* 1991; 51:2346–2352.

75. Dianov GL, Timchenko TV, Sinitsina OI, Kuzminov AV, Medvedev OA, Salganik RI. Repair of uracil residues closely spaced on the opposite strands of plasmid DNA results in double-strand break and deletion formation. *Mol Gen Genet* 1991; 225:448–452.

76. Luzzatto L, Falusi AO, Joju EA. Uracil in DNA in megaloblastic anemia. *N Engl J Med* 1981; 305:1156–1157.

77. Wickramasinghe SN, Fida S. Misincorporation of uracil into the DNA of folate- and $B_{12}$-deficient HL60 cells. *Eur J Haematol* 1993; 30:127–132.

78. Wickramasinghe SN, Fida S. Bone marrow cells from vitamin $B_{12}$- and folate-deficient patients misincorporate uracil into DNA. *Blood* 1994; 83:1656–1661.

79. Goulian M, Bleile B, Tseng BY. Methotrexate-induced incorporation of uracil into DNA. *Proc Natl Acad Sci USA* 1980; 77:1956–1960.

80. Bestwick RK, Moffett GL, Spiro C, Mathews CK. Differential effects of methotrexate or fluorodeoxyuridine upon mitochondrial and cellular nucleotide pools. In: Blair JA, ed. *Chemistry and Biology of Pteridines*. Berlin: Walter de Gruyter; 1983:311–315.

81. Brown SD, Ladner R, Maybaum J, Aherne GW. Deoxyuridine triphosphate (dUTP) accumulation: relevance to the cytotoxic effects of thymidylate synthase (TS) inhibitors. *Proc Am Assoc Cancer Res* 1997; 38:477.

82. Sundseth R, Singer S, Yates B, Smith G, Ferone R, Dev I. Thymineless apoptotic death induced by 1843U89 in human tumor cell lines is independent of dUTP accumulation and misincorporation of dUMP into DNA. *Proc Am Assoc Cancer Res* 1997; 38:476.

83. Pogribny IP, Basnakian AG, Miller BJ, Lopatina NG, Poirier LA, James SJ. Breaks in genomic DNA and within the p53 gene are associated with hypomethylation in livers of folate/methyl-deficient rats. *Cancer Res* 1995; 55:1894–1901.

84. Chen RZ, Pettersson U, Beard C, Jackson-Grusby L, Jaenisch R. DNA hypomethylation leads to elevated mutation rates. *Nature* 1998; 395:89–93.

85. Feinberg AP, Vogelstein B. Hypomethylation distinguishes genes of some human cancers from their normal counterparts. *Nature* 1983; 301:89–92.

86. Wainfan E, Poirier LA. Methyl groups in carcinogenesis: effects on DNA methylation and gene expression. *Cancer Res* 1992; 52:2071s–2077s.

87. Lombardi B, Chandar N, Locker J. Nutritional model of hepatocarcinogenesis. Rats fed choline-devoid diet. *Digest Dis Sci* 1991; 36:979–984.

88. Shaw GM, Velie EM, Schaffer DM. Is dietary intake of methionine associated with a reduction in risk for neural tube defect-affected pregnancies? *Teratology* 1997; 56:295–299.

89. Balaghi M, Wagner C. DNA methylation in folate deficiency: use of CpG methylase. *Biochem Biophys Res Commun* 1993; 193:1184–1190.

90. Miller JW, Nadeau MR, Smith J, Smith D, Selhub J. Folate-deficiency-induced homocysteinaemia in rats: disruption of *S*-adenosylmethionine's coordinate regulation of homocysteine metabolism. *Biochem J* 1994; 298:415–419.

91. Kimura M, Umegaki K, Higuchi M, Thomas P, Fenech M. Methylenetetrahydrofolate reductase C677T polymorphism, folic acid and riboflavin are important determinants of genome stability in cultured human lymphocytes. *J Nutr* 2004; 134:48–56.

92. Ulrich CM, Robien K, Sparks R. Pharmacogenetics and folate metabolism — a promising direction. *Pharmacogenomics* 2002; 3:299–313.

93. Robien K, Ulrich CM. 5,10-Methylenetetrahydrofolate reductase polymorphisms and leukemia risk: a HuGE minireview. *Am J Epidemiol* 2003; 157:571–582.

94. Wiemels JL, Smith RN, Taylor GM, Eden OB, Alexander FE, Greaves MF. Methylenetetrahydrofolate reductase (MTHFR) polymorphisms and risk of molecularly defined subtypes of childhood acute leukemia. *Proc Natl Acad Sci USA* 2001; 98:4004–4009.

95. Krajinovic M, Lamothe S, Labuda D, Lemieux-Blanchard E, Theoret Y, Moghrabi A, Sinnett D. Role of MTHFR genetic polymorphisms in the susceptibility to childhood acute lymphoblastic leukemia. *Blood* 2004; 103:252–257.

96. Bagley PJ, Selhub J. A common mutation in the methylenetetrahydrofolate reductase gene is associated with an accumulation of formylated tetrahydrofolates in red blood cells. *Proc Natl Acad Sci USA* 1998; 95:13217–13220.

97. Narayanan S, McConnell J, Little J, Sharp L, Piyathilake CJ, Powers H, Basten G, Duthie SJ. Associations between two common variants C677T and A1298C in the methylenetetrahydrofolate reductase gene and measures of folate metabolism and DNA stability (strand breaks, misincorporated uracil, and DNA methylation status) in human lymphocytes *in vivo*. *Cancer Epidemiol Biomarkers Prev* 2004; 13:1436–1443.

98. Campbell NRC. How safe are folic acid supplements? *Arch Intern Med* 1996; 156:1638–1644.

99. Pietrzik K, Brönstrup A. Folate in preventive medicine: a new role in cardiovascular disease, neural tube defects and cancer. *Ann Nutr Metab* 1997; 41:331–343.

100. Farber S, Diamond LK, Mercer RD, Sylvester RF, Wolff JA. Temporary remissions in acute leukemia in children produced by folic acid antagonist, 4-aminopteroylglutamic acid (aminopterin). *N Engl J Med* 1948; 238:787–793.

101. Lewisohn R, Leuchtenberger C, Leuchtenberger R, Keresztesy JC. The influence of liver *L. casei* factor on spontaneous breast cancer in mice. *Science* 1946; 104:436–437.

102. Branda RF, McCormack JJ, Perlmutter CA, Mathews LA, Robison SH. Effects of folate deficiency on the metastatic potential of murine melanoma cells. *Cancer Res* 1988; 48:4529–4534.

103. Waterland RA, Jirtle RL. Transposable elements: targets for early nutritional effects on epigenetic gene regulation. *Mol Cell Biol* 2003; 23:5293–5300.

104. Weir DG, Scott JM. Colonic mucosal folate concentrations and their association with colorectal cancer. *Am J Clin Nutr* 1998; 68:763–764.

105. McGuire JJ, Russell CA. Biological and biochemical properties of the natural (6S) and unnatural (6R) isomers of leucovorin and their racemic (6R,S) mixture. *J Cell Pharmacol* 1991; 2:317–323.

# Part III

Dietary Components That
Protect from Cancer: Minerals

# 9 Calcium and Chemoprevention of Colon Cancer

*Subhas Chakrabarty*

## CONTENTS

9.1 Introduction...................................................................................................177
9.2 Induction of Differentiation ..................................................................178
9.3 Cell Adhesions and Differentiation......................................................178
9.4 Calcium and the Calcium-Sensing Receptor.........................................180
9.5 Cell Cycle Control and the Induction of Differentiation ....................180
9.6 Calcium and CaSR Function in Colon ..................................................181
9.7 Perspectives and Conclusion..................................................................181
References .......................................................................................................183

## 9.1 INTRODUCTION

The malignant phenotype is not irreversible. Many agents are known to induce or restore a more differentiated or "normal" phenotype to malignant cells.[1-7] Agents that can induce a differentiated phenotype in malignant cells are called differentiation-inducing agents. The action of many of these differentiation-inducing agents in a variety of cancer cell types *in vitro* has been reported.[1-7] How differentiation-inducing agents act to restore a "normal" phenotype to malignant cells has been under intense investigation over the past two to three decades. The goal of such investigation has been to identify differentiation-inducing agents with therapeutic potential and/or differentiation associated cellular mechanisms with potential for therapeutic intervention.

Chemoprevention of cancer may be operationally defined as the use of agents to prevent, delay, or reverse the carcinogenic process *in vivo*. Because differentiation-inducing agents can reverse the malignant phenotype or restore a more normal phenotype to malignant cells, many differentiation-inducing agents possess chemopreventive properties. A good example of such agents is the retinoids.[7-10] Of the major epithelial cancers such as breast, prostate, and colon, colon cancer appears to be most susceptible to chemoprevention. Animal studies, epidemiological studies, and clinical trials strongly suggest that $Ca^{2+}$ (or in combination with vitamin D) is a good chemopreventive agent for colon cancer.[11–14] How $Ca^{2+}$ acts at the molecular level in the chemoprevention of colon cancer, however, is not understood. Recent studies suggest that the actions of $Ca^{2+}$ at the cellular and molecular level are diverse and that $Ca^{2+}$ and the calcium-sensing receptor (CaSR) function as a ligand receptor system in controlling the proliferation and differentiation of colon epithelial cells. The focus of this chapter is on the cellular and molecular mechanisms of this ligand receptor system and on linking together its diverse action into unifying concepts in order to better understand its function in the colon.

## 9.2 INDUCTION OF DIFFERENTIATION

Early work has shown that the biological effects of many differentiation-inducing agents are diverse. In colon carcinoma, most of these agents have a growth inhibitory effect and alter the expression of cellular proteins, the expression and secretion of extracellular matrix (ECM) adhesion proteins and receptors for these ECM adhesion proteins.[1–6,15–18] The significance of these biological effects is now understood in view of recent advances in our understanding of the biological function of cellular adhesion molecules and their associated signal transduction processes, in terms of their mechanisms controlling cell cycle progression. Therefore, in order to truly appreciate the function of $Ca^{2+}$ and the CaSR, a discussion of cellular adhesion and cell cycle control in regulating the differentiation process is warranted.

## 9.3 CELL ADHESIONS AND DIFFERENTIATION

There are predominantly two types of cell adhesions: cell adhesion to the ECM and cell–cell adhesion. The ECM is composed of a myriad of glycoproteins and glycosoaminoglycans.[19] Cell adhesion to the ECM activates intracellular signal transduction mechanisms that control gene expression (in a tissue-dependent manner) and regulate the differentiated function of epithelial cells.[20–22]

Adhesion to the ECM is mediated through specific cell-surface adhesion receptors that span the plasma membrane and communicate with the cytoskeleton.[22–25] The integrin superfamily of adhesion receptors is composed of noncovalently linked heterodimers, which mediate cell adhesion to the ECM.[23–26] At least 15 different heterodimers are formed from different combinations of 11-$\alpha$ and 6-$\beta$-integrin chains, and each of these integrins has unique structural and functional properties and characteristic tissue distribution.[27,28] Integrins have small cytoplasmic regions that bind to the elements of the actin cytoskeleton and colocalize in focal adhesion contacts (cell attachment points to the ECM) with adhesion plaque proteins such as talin and $\alpha$-actinin to form a signal transduction complex.[29] Integrin-mediated adhesions are intimately involved in regulating cell growth, differentiation, cell-to-cell recognition, intercellular communication, and cytotoxic T-lymphocyte killing of target cells.[22,27,28] Thus, it is not surprising that abnormal expression of integrins underlies many pathological processes, including malignant transformation.[24,26,30,31] For example, the ECM adhesion protein fibronectin and its $\alpha5\beta1$ integrin receptor possess tumor-suppressing properties.[1-3,31-35] Disruption of fibronectin binding to the $\alpha5\beta1$ integrin abrogates cellular quiescence and induces DNA synthesis.[36] The induction of differentiation in transformed cells, on the other hand, has been shown to restore a normal profile of ECM adhesion protein production and integrin expression.[1-3]

Cell–cell adhesion is mediated by adhesion molecules. The cadherin family of homophilic cell–cell adhesion molecules is expressed in all epithelial tissues.[37,38] E-Cadherin, a 120-kDa transmembrane glycoprotein localized at the adherens junctions, is a prominent cell–cell adhesion molecule and plays a major role in epithelial cell–cell adhesion.[37] In the presence of $Ca^{2+}$, the E-cadherin extracellular domain interacts homotypically with the E-cadherin molecules of neighboring cells to maintain intercellular adhesion and epithelial integrity, while its cytoplasmic carboxyl end interacts with a group of closely related but distinct membrane undercoat proteins, termed $\alpha$-, $\beta$-, and $\gamma$-catenins.[37-39] $\beta$-Catenin complexes with APC (adenomatous polyposis coli) tumor-suppressor protein and functions as a downstream component of the Wnt/wingless signal transduction pathway.[40,41]

E-Cadherin-mediated cell–cell adhesion has been shown to be intimately associated with the normal function and cell physiology of the colon epithelium, including cell growth and invasion in response to tissue injury.[42,43] E-Cadherin is considered to be a tumor suppressor, and reduced E-cadherin expression is associated with increased malignancy not only in colon carcinoma, but also in other epithelium-derived tumors.[44-49] Defective E-cadherin-mediated adhesion is found in poorly differentiated and highly invasive colon tumors, and correction of this defect reduces invasive behavior.[50] Exactly how E-cadherin mediates its tumor-suppressive function is not well understood. It has been reported that the E-cadherin-mediated adhesion is essential not only for structural organization of epithelial cells, but also for control of cell growth.[46,51]

$\beta$-Catenin may be activated through cell adhesion processes or through Wnt1 signaling.[37] The Wnt gene family encodes a family of secreted glycoproteins that modulate cell fate and behavior in embryos through activation of receptor-mediated signaling pathways.[40,41,52] Activation of Wnt1 leads to inactivation of glycogen synthase kinase $3\beta$ (GSK$3\beta$) and accumulation of $\beta$-catenin in the cytosol. If $\beta$-catenin is not degraded, it accumulates in the nucleus and interacts with transcription factors of the lymphoid enhancer factor–T-cell factor family in modulating gene expression and driving malignant cell behavior.[53] The tumor-suppressive protein APC complexes with $\beta$-catenin, which leads to the $\beta$-catenin degradation. Thus, the loss of APC function through mutations has been implicated as a crucial event in the early transformation of the colon epithelium.[54]

## 9.4  CALCIUM AND THE CALCIUM-SENSING RECEPTOR

The functions of $Ca^{2+}$ in cell physiology are diverse. Intracellular $Ca^{2+}$ has long been regarded as a "second messenger" in many signal transduction processes.[55,56] The characterization and cloning of the cell-surface calcium-sensing receptor (CaSR) from the human parathyroid gland, however, has shown that extracellular $Ca^{2+}$ and the CaSR constitute a first messenger system in controlling physiologic function.[57] It is now known that the CaSR is a member of the superfamily of G protein–coupled receptors, which can sense minute changes in extracellular $Ca^{2+}$ concentration and coordinate the secretion of endocrine hormones in the control and regulation of systemic $Ca^{2+}$ homeostasis.[58–62] Recent studies, however, suggest that the CaSR possesses diverse functions that are quite different from the systemic control of $Ca^{2+}$ homeostasis and that it may regulate diverse cellular processes in different cell types.[63–68] For example, the CaSR is implicated in inhibiting proliferation and promoting the differentiation of keratinocytes in the skin as these cells migrate up the epidermis.[65,66] Kallay and colleagues[67,68] reported in 1997 and 2000 that the Caco-2 human adenocarcinoma cell line expressed the CaSR and that the CaSR and extracellular $Ca^{2+}$ function to inhibit Caco-2 cell proliferation. The expression of CaSR in rat intestinal epithelium was reported in 1997.[69] The expression of CaSR in human gastric mucosa and rat colon epithelial cells was subsequently reported by other investigators.[70,71]

## 9.5  CELL CYCLE CONTROL AND THE INDUCTION OF DIFFERENTIATION

Inhibition of proliferation is tightly linked to proper cellular differentiation while abnormal proliferation (escape from normal growth control) is implicated in circumventing the normal differentiation pathway and in driving malignant progression.[72] Cell proliferation at the molecular level is regulated by sets of positive regulators such as the cyclins and cyclin-dependent kinases. These molecules interact in concert to drive cell cycle progression while a set of negative regulators, such as the inhibitors of cyclin-dependent kinases, function to inhibit or "put a brake" on cell cycle progression.[73] P21/Waf1 is a prominent member of cyclin-dependent kinase inhibitors and increased expression of p21/Waf1 is linked to inhibition of proliferation and induction of differentiation in keratinocytes and colon cancer cells.[74–76]

Induction of differentiation of malignant cells is associated with the restoration of normal growth control and the suppression of malignant properties. While normal cells do not grow in semisolid soft agarose (anchorage-independent growth), a hallmark of malignant transformation is the ability to grow in soft agarose. Malignant cells treated with differentiation-inducing agents are unable to grow in soft agarose.[4–6] In addition, the ability of malignant cells to invade a matrigel matrix is significantly reduced when treated with differentiation-inducing agents.[4–6]

## 9.6 CALCIUM AND CaSR FUNCTION IN COLON

Normal human colon crypt epithelial cells express the CaSR, whereas cells of differentiated tumors express significantly lower amounts of CaSR, and in cells of undifferentiated tumors, CaSR expression is lost completely.[77] The expression of CaSR is restricted to epithelial cells; stromal cells do not express CaSR. This finding leads to the hypothesis that the CaSR functions to regulate proliferation and differentiation of the colon epithelial cells and that loss of CaSR expression is associated with loss of growth control and malignant transformation. This hypothesis may be tested using human colon carcinoma cell lines that were developed from differentiated primary human colon tumors that express the CaSR. These cell lines respond to receptor stimulation by $Ca^{2+}$ and by $Gd^{3+}$, a CaSR agonist that does not pass through the plasma membranes.[77] Stimulation of CaSR in these cells induces a more "normal" phenotype and results in many alterations at the cellular and molecular levels.[77] At the cellular level, there is an inhibition of proliferation and suppression of anchorage-independent growth and the propensity to invade matrigel. At the molecular level, many changes occur. These changes include the induction of E-cadherin (a tumor suppressor), p21/Waf1 (functions to block cell cycle progression), and γ-catenin (may function to suppress wnt signaling) expression. Changes also include the suppression of the constitutive T-cell factor (TCF) transcriptional activation activity and suppression of β-catenin/TCF4 complex formation (which functions to drive malignant cell behavior). Thus, taken together, these data suggest that the $Ca^{2+}$/CaSR ligand receptor system functions to promote differentiation and suppress malignant transformation. These data also suggest that loss of CaSR expression or function or both may undermine the proper differentiation pathway and promote a pathway in the direction of malignant transformation. Figure 9.1 summarizes how the $Ca^{2+}$/CaSR ligand receptor system may function to regulate differentiation in colon cells, and how disrupted CaSR function may promote malignant transformation, a hypothetical model.

## 9.7 PERSPECTIVES AND CONCLUSION

It is generally accepted that $Ca^{2+}$ is a chemopreventive agent for colon cancer, albeit its mechanisms of action are not understood. This chapter presents some potential mechanisms through which $Ca^{2+}$ may act to prevent, delay, or reverse the carcinogenic process. The functional involvement of CaSR in the action of $Ca^{2+}$ is novel and many unanswered questions remain regarding the physiologic role of this ligand/receptor system in the colon. The stem cells of the colon crypts continuously migrate from the bottom of the crypts upward in the direction of the lumen. As these cells migrate upward, proliferation slows and the cells differentiate into functionally matured epithelial cells. Intricate mechanisms, though poorly understood, are involved in regulating the proper differentiation of these cells. The $Ca^{2+}$/CaSR may constitute an important ligand receptor system in controlling proper differentiation through its effects on regulating cell–cell adhesion, cell cycle

### A. Functional Ca²⁺/CaSR

Robust E-Cadherin expression, robust epithelial integrity and robust γ-catenin expression

γ-Catenin, accumulates in nucleus and down-regulates activation of T cell factors

Up-regulation of p21/Waf1, cell cycle arrest and down-regulation of cellular proliferation

### Proper Differentiation Pathway

### B. Disrupted Ca²⁺/CaSR Function

Loss of E-Cadherin, loss of epithelial integrity with down-regulated γ-catenin expression

β-Catenin accumulates in nucleus and activates T cell factors

Down-regulated γ-Catenin expression, promotes the activation of T cell factors

Down-regulated p21/Waf1 expression, promotes cellular proliferation

### Abnormal Differentiation Pathway and Malignant Progression

**FIGURE 9.1** (A) Hypothetical model of how the Ca²⁺/CaSR system functions to promote proper differentiation; (B) how disrupted Ca²⁺/CaSR function promotes abnormal differentiation and malignant transformation.

progression, and the β-catenin associated wnt pathways. Recent studies suggest that this system may also mediate its action by regulating cell adhesion to the ECM (unpublished results). How cell-ECM adhesion is regulated by the CaSR and how cell–ECM adhesion modulates differentiation is currently under investigation. The proliferating crypt stem cells do not express the CaSR but acquire CaSR expression as they migrate upward in the direction of the lumen (unpublished results).

How the expression of the CaSR is regulated at the molecular level is not known and poses an intriguing question.

## REFERENCES

1. Varani J, Chakrabarty S. Modulation of fibronectin synthesis and fibronectin binding during transformation and differentiation of mouse AKR fibroblasts. *J Cell Physiol* 1990; 143:445–454.
2. Varani J, Chakrabarty S. Changes in the extracellular matrix during transformation and differentiation. In: FW Orr, MR Buchanan, L Weiss, eds. *Microcirculation in Cancer Metastasis.* Boca Raton, FL: CRC Press; 1991:1–22.
3. Harris H. The role of differentiation in the suppression of malignancy. *J Cell Sci* 1990; 97:5–10.
4. Reynolds S, Rajagopal S, Chakrabarty S. Differentiation-inducing effect of retinoic acid, difluoromethylornithine, sodium butyrate and sodium suramin in human colon cancer cells. *Cancer Lett* 1998; 134:53–60.
5. Wang H, Rajagopal S, Reynolds S, Cederberg H, Chakrabarty, S. Differentiation-promoting effect of 1-O(2 methoxy) hexadecyl glycerol in human colon cancer cells. *J Cell Physiol* 1999; 178:173–178.
6. Wang H, Chakrabarty S. Platelet-activating factor activates mitogen-activated protein kinases, inhibits proliferation, induces differentiation and suppresses the malignant phenotype of human colon carcinoma cells. *Oncogene* 2003; 22:2186–2191.
7. Varani J, Fligiel SEG, Schuger L, Perone P, Inman D, Griffiths CEM, Voorhees JJ. Effects of all-*trans*-retinoic acid and Ca++ on human kin in organ culture. *Am J Pathol* 1993; 142:189–198.
8. Takatsuka J, Takahashi N, Luigi MDL. Retinoic acid metabolism and inhibition of cell proliferation: an unexpected liaison. *Cancer Res* 1996; 56:675–678.
9. Fisher GJ, Datta, SC, Talwar HS, Wang ZQ, Varani J, Kang S, Voorhees JJ. Molecular basis of sun-induced premature skin ageing and retinoid antagonism. *Nature* 1996; 335–339.
10. McCormick DL, Rao KVN, Steele VE, Lubet RA, Kellof GJ, Bosland MC. Chemoprevention of rat prostate carcinogenesis by 9-*cis*-retinoic acid. *Cancer Res* 1999; 59:521–524.
11. Lipkin M. Preclinical and early human studies of calcium and colon cancer prevention. *Ann NY Acad Sci* 1999; 889:120–127.
12. Wargovich MJ, Jimenez A, McKee K, Steele VE, Velasco M, Woods J, Price R, Gray K, Kelloff GJ. Efficacy of potential chemopreventive agents on rat colon aberrant crypt formation and progression. *Carcinogenesis* 2000; 21:1149–1155.
13. Garland CF, Garland FC, Gorham ED. Calcium and vitamin D. Their potential roles in colon and breast cancer prevention. *Ann N Y Acad Sci* 1999; 889:107–119.
14. Dalberg J, Jacobsen O, Nielsen NH, Steig BA, Storm HH. Colorectal cancer in the Faroe Islands — a setting for the study of the role of diet. *J Epidemiol Biostat* 1999; 4(1):31–36.

15. Chakrabarty S, Tobon A, Varani J, Brattain MG. Induction of carcinoembryonic antigen secretion and modulation of protein secretion/expression and fibronectin/laminin expression in human colon carcinoma cells by transforming growth factor-β. *Cancer Res* 1988; 48:4059–4064.

16. Chakrabarty S. Regulation of human colon carcinoma cell adhesion to extracellular matrix by transforming growth factor-β1. *Int J Cancer* 1992; 50:968–973.

17. Huang S, Chakrabarty S. Regulation of fibronectin and laminin receptor expression, fibronectin and laminin secretion in human colon cancer cells by transforming growth factor-β1. *Int J Cancer* 1994; 57:742–746.

18. Wang H, Radjendirane V, Wary KK, Chakrabarty S. Transforming growth factorβ regulates cell–cell adhesion through extracellular matrix remodeling and activation of focal adhesion kinase. *Oncogene* 2004; 23:5558–5561.

19. Hay ED. Extracellular matrix. *J Cell Biol* 1981; 91:205s–223s.

20. Lin CQ, Bissel MJ. Multi-faceted regulation of cell differentiation by extracellular matrix. *FASEB J* 1993; 7:737–741.

21. Roskelley CD, Desprez PY, Bissell MJ. Extracellular matrix-dependent tissue-specific gene expression in mammary epithelial cells required both physical and biochemical signal transduction. *Proc Natl Acad Sci USA* 1994; 91:12378–12382.

22. Clark EA, Brugge JS. Integrins and signal transduction pathway: the road taken. *Science* 1995; 268:233–238.

23. Ruoslahti E, Pierschbacher MD. New perspectives in cell adhesion: RGD and integrins. *Science* 1987; 238:491–497.

24. Kramer RH, Enenstein J, Ramos DM, Vu MP, Cheng YF. The role of integrin receptors in tumor cell adhesion to the microvasculature. In: MR Buchanan, L Weiss, eds. *Microcirculation in Cancer Metastasis.* Boca Raton, FL: CRC Press; 1991.

25. Heidemann SR. A new twist on integrins and the cytoskeleton. *Science* 1993; 260:1080–1081.

26. Schwartz MA, Ingber DE. Integrating with integrins. *Mol Biol Cell* 1994; 5:389–393.

27. Mcintyre BW, Bednarczyk JL, Passini CA, Szabo MC, Udagawa T, Wygant JN. Integrins: cell adhesion receptors in health and disease. *Cancer Bull* 1991; 43:51–57.

28. Hynes RO. Integrins: versatility, modulation and signaling and cell adhesion. *Cell* 1992; 69:11–25.

29. Yamada KM, Miyamoto S. Integrin membrane signaling and cytoskeletal control. *Curr Opin Cell Biol* 1995; 7:681–689.

30. Juliano RL. Signal transduction by integrins and its role in the regulation of tumor growth. *Cancer Metab Rev* 1994; 13:25–30.

31. Schwartz MA. Integrins, oncogenes, and anchorage independence. *J Cell Biol* 1997; 139:575–578.

32. Giancotti FG, Ruoslahti E. Elevated levels of the α5β1 fibronectin receptor suppress the transformed phenotype of Chinese hamster ovary cells. *Cell* 1990; 60:849–859.

33. Schreiner C, Fisher M, Hussein S, Juliano RL. Increased tumorigenicity of fibronectin receptor deficient Chinese hamster ovary cell variants. *Cancer Res* 1991; 51:1738–1740.

34. Akamatsu H, Tanaka KI, Ozono K, Kamiike W, Matsuda H, Sekiguchi K. Suppression of transformed phenotypes of human fibrosarcoma cells by overexpression of recombinant fibronectin. *Cancer Res* 1996; 56:4541–4546.

35. Kondo M, Watanabe M, Amanuma K, Oka S, Ishida N. Overexpression of MP41 gene in a transformed endothelial cell line correlates with the increase fibronectin expression and a decreased incidence of tumorigenicity. *Biochem Biophys Res Commun* 1996; 219:398–404.

36. Gong J, Ko TC, Brattain MG. Disruption of fibronectin binding to alpha 5 beta 1 integrin stimulates the expression of cyclin-dependent kinases and DNA synthesis through activation of extracellular signal-regulated kinase. *J Biol Chem* 1998; 273(3):1662–1669.

37. Takeichi M. Cadherin cell adhesion receptors as a morphogenetic regulator. *Science* 1991; 251:1451–1455.

38. Gumbiner BM, McCrea PD. Catenins as mediators of the cytoplasmic functions of cadherins. *J Cell Sci* 1993; 17:155–158.

39. Valizadeh A, Karayiannakis AJ, El-Hariry I, Kmiot W, Pignatelli M. Expression of E-cadherin-associated molecules (α-, β, and ϒ-catenins and p120) in colorectal polyps. *Am J Pathol* 1997; 150:1977–1984.

40. Peifer M, Wieschaus E. The segment polarity gene armadillo encodes a functionally modular protein that is the *Drosophila* homolog of human plakoglobin. *Cell* 1990; 63:1167–1178.

41. Peifer, M. Cell adhesion and signal transduction: the Armadillo connection. *Trends Cell Biol* 1995; 5:224–229.

42. Hanby AM, Chinery R, Poulsom R, Playford RJ, Pignatelli M. Downregulation of E-cadherin in the reparative epithelium of the human gastrointestinal tract. *Am J Pathol* 1995; 148:723–729.

43. Pollack AL, Barth IM, Altschuler Y, Nelson WJ, Mostov KE. Dynamics of β-catenin interactions with APC protein regulate epithelial tubulogenesis. *J Cell Biol* 1997; 137:1651–1662.

44. Kinsella AR, Lepts GC, Hill CL, Jones M. Reduced E-cadherin expression correlates with increased invasiveness in colorectal carcinoma cell lines. *Clin Exp Metastasis* 1994; 12:335–342.

45. MacCalman CD, Brodt P, Doublet JD, Jednak R, Elkilali MM, Bazinet M, Blaschuk OW. The loss of E-cadherin transcripts in rat prostate tumors is accompanied by increased expression of mRNA transcripts encoding fibronectin and its receptor. *Clin Exp Metastasis* 1994; 12:101–107.

46. Watabe M, Nagafuchi A, Tsukita S, Takeichi M. Induction of polarized cell–cell association and retardation of growth by activation of the E-cadherin–catenin adhesion system in a dispersed carcinoma line. *J Cell Biol* 1994; 127:247–256.

47. Dorudi S, Hanby AM, Poulsom R, Northover J, Hart IR. Level of expression of E-cadherin mRNA in colorectal cancer correlates with clinical outcome. *Br J Cancer* 1995; 71:614–616.

48. Jawhari A, Farthing M, Pignatelli M. The importance of E-cadherin–catenin complex in the maintenance of intestinal epithelial homeostasis: more than intercellular glue? *Gut* 1997; 41:581–584.

49. Hiraguri S, Godfrey T, Nakamura H, Graff J, Collins C, Shayesteh L, Doggett N, Johnson K, Wheelock M, Herman J, Baylin S, Pinkel D, Gray J. Mechanisms of inactivation of E-cadherin in breast cancer cell lines. *Cancer Res* 1998; 58:1972–1977.

50. Breen E, Steele G, Mercurio AM. Role of the E-cadherin/α-catenin complex in modulating cell-cell and cell-matrix adhesive properties of invasive colon carcinoma cells. *Ann Surg Oncol* 1995; 2:378–385.

51. Croix BS, Sheehan C, Rak JW, Florenes VA, Slingerland JM, Kerbel RS. E-cadherin-dependent growth suppression is mediated by the cyclin-dependent kinase p27KIPI. *J Cell Biol* 1998; 142:557–571.

52. Moon RT, Brown JD, Torres M. WNTs modulate cell fate and behavior during vertebrate development. *Trends Genet* 1997; 13:157–162.

53. Behrens J, Jerchow B.-A, Wurtele M, Grimm J, Asbrand C, Wirtz R, Uhl M, Wedlich D, Birchmeier W. Functional interaction of an axin homolog, conductin, with β-catenin, APC and GSK3β. *Science* 1998; 280:596–599.

54. Korinek V, Barker N, Morin PJ, Wichen D, Weger RD, Kinzler KW, Vogelstein B, Clevers H. Constitutive transcriptional activation by a β-catenin–Tcf complex in APC-/-colon carcinoma. *Science* 1997; 275:1784–1787.

55. Schaller MD, Borgman CA, Cobb BS, Vines RI, Reynolds AB, Parsons JT. pp125FAK, a structurally distinctive protein-tyrosine kinase associated with focal adhesions. *Proc Natl Acad Sci USA* 1992; 89:5192–5196.

56. Berridge MJ, Lipp P, Bootman MD. The versatility and universality of calcium signalling. *Nat Rev Mol Cell Biol* 2000; 1:11–21.

57. Garrett JE, Capuano IV, Hammerland LG, Hung BCP, Brown EM, Hebert SC, Nemeth EF, Fuller F. Molecular cloning and functional expression of human parathyroid calcium receptor cDNAs. *J Biol Chem* 1995; 270:12919–12925.

58. Hebert SC, Brown EM. The extracellular calcium receptor. *Curr Opin Cell Biol* 1995; 7:484–492.

59. Hory B, Roussanne MC, Drueke TB, Bourdeau A. The calcium receptor in health and disease. *Exp Nephrol* 1998; 6:171–179.

60. Chattopadhyay N. Biochemistry, physiology and pathophysiology of the extracellular calcium-sensing receptor. *Int J Biochem Cell Biol* 2000; 32:789–804.

61. Brown EM. Principles and practice of endocrinology and metabolism. In: Becker KL, ed. 3rd ed. Philadelphia: J.B. Lippincott, 2001:478–489.

62. Jiang YF, Zhang Z, Kifor O, Lane CR, Quinn SJ, Bai M. Protein kinase C (PKC) phosphorylation of the $Ca^{2+}$-sensing receptor (CaR) modulates functional interaction of G proteins with the CaR cytoplasmic tail. *J Biol Chem* 2002; 277:50543–50549.

63. McNeil SE, Hobson SA, Nipper V, Rodland K. Functional calcium-sensing receptors in rat fibroblasts are required for activation of src kinase and mitogen-activated protein kinase in response to extracellular calcium. *J Biol Chem* 1998; 273:1114–1120.

64. Rutten MJ, Bacon KD, Marlink KL, Stoney M, Meichsner CL, Lee FP, Hobson SA, Rodland KD, Sheppard BC, Trunkey DD, Deveney KE, Deveney CW. $Ca^{2+}$-sensing receptor in normal human gastric mucous epithelial cells. *Am J Physiol* 1999; 277:G662–G670.

65. Tu C-L, Oda Y, Bikle DD. Effects of a calcium receptor activator on the cellular response to calcium in human keratinocytes. *J Invest Dermatol* 1999; 113:340–345.

66. Tu CL, Chang W, Bikle DD. The extracellular calcium-sensing receptor is required for calcium-induced differentiation in human keratinocytes. *J Biol Chem* 2001; 276:41079–41085.

67. Kallay E, Kifor O, Chattopadhyay N, Brown EM, Bischof MG, Peterlik M, Cross HS. Calcium-dependent c-myc proto-oncogene expression and proliferation of CACO-2 cells: a role for luminal extracellular calcium-sensing receptor. *Biochem Biophys Res Commun* 1997; 232:80–83.

68. Kallay E, Bajna E, Wrba F, Kriwanek S, Peterlik M, Cross HS. Dietary calcium and growth modulation of human colon cancer cells: role of the extracellular calcium-sensing receptor. *Cancer Detect Prevent* 2000; 24:127–136.

69. Gama L, Baxendale-Cox LM, Breitwieser GE. Ca$^{2+}$-sensing receptors in intestinal epithelium. *Am J Physiol* 1997; 273:C1168–C1175.

70. Rutten MJ, Bacon KD, Marlink KL, Stoney M, Meichsner CL, Lee FP, Hobson SA, Rodland KD, Sheppard BC, Trunkey DD, Deveney KE. CASR function in colon carcinoma. *Am J Physiol* 1999; 277:G662–G670.

71. Cheng SX, Okuda M, Hall AE, Geibel JP, Hebert SC. Expression of calcium-sensing receptor in rat colonic epithelium: evidence of modulation of fluid secretion. *Am J Physiol* 2002; 283:G240–G250.

72. Assoian RK. Anchorage-dependent cell cycle progression. *J Cell Biol* 1997; 136:1–4.

73. Jacks T, Weinberg RA. The expanding role of cell cycle regulators. *Science* 1998; 280:1035–1037.

74. Steinman RA, Hoffman B, Iro A, Guillouf C, Liebermann DA, El-Houseini ME. Induction of p21(WAF-1/CIP1) during differentiation. *Oncogene* 1994; 9:3389–3396.

75. Di Cunto F, Topley G, Calautti E, Hsiao J, Ong L, Seth PK, Dotto GP. Inhibitory function of p21[Cip1/WAF1] in differentiation of primary mouse keratinocytes independent of cell cycle control. *Science* 1998; 280:1069–1072.

76. Hunt KK, Fleming JB, Abramian A, Zhang L, Evans DB, Chiao PJ. Overexpression of the tumor suppressor gene Smad4/DPC4 induces p21[waf1] expression and growth inhibition in human carcinoma cells. *Cancer Res* 1998; 58:5636–5661.

77. Chakrabarty S, Radjendirane V, Appelman H, Varani J. Extracellular calcium and calcium sensing receptor function in human colon carcinomas: promotion of E-cadherin expression and suppression of β-catenin/TCF activation. *Cancer Res* 2003; 63:67–71.

# 10 Relationship of Selenium Intake to Cancer

*P. D. Whanger*

## CONTENTS

10.1   Introduction .................................................................................................189
10.2   Selenium ....................................................................................................190
10.3   Selenocompounds in Plants and Animals ............................................191
10.4   Epidemiological Studies ..........................................................................192
10.5   Human Trials ............................................................................................193
10.6   Selenium and Tumors in Small Animals................................................196
10.7   Selenium Metabolism in Tissue Culture Models..................................197
10.8   Mechanisms of Cancer Reduction by Selenium ..................................198
        10.8.1   Role of Selenoenzymes .............................................................198
        10.8.2   Effects on Carcinogen Metabolism ..........................................199
        10.8.3   Effects on Immunity...................................................................200
        10.8.4   Antitumorigenic Selenium Metabolites ....................................200
        10.8.5   Selenium and Apoptosis ............................................................201
        10.8.6   Selenium and DNA Repair.........................................................203
        10.8.7   Selenium as an Antiangiogenic Agent ......................................204
10.9   Forms of Selenium in Foods and Supplements ....................................204
10.10 Levels of Selenium Necessary for Nutritive Benefit ..........................207
10.11 Conclusions and Future Research ..........................................................208
References .............................................................................................................208

## 10.1   INTRODUCTION

The selenocompounds in plants can have a profound effect on the health of animals and humans. Selenomethionine (Semet) is the major selenocompound in cereal grains and enriched yeast, whereas Se-methylselenocysteine (SeMCYS) is the major selenocompound in selenium accumulator plants and some plants of economic importance such as garlic and broccoli exposed to excess selenium. Epidemiological studies indicate an inverse relationship between selenium intake and the incidence of certain cancers. Usually blood or plasma levels of selenium are lower in patients with cancer than those without this disorder, but inconsistent results have been found with toenail selenium values and the incidence of cancer.

There have been eight human trials conducted on the influence of selenium on cancer incidence or biomarkers, and, except for one, all of them showed a positive benefit of selenium on cancer reduction or biomarkers of this disorder. This is consistent with more than 100 small-animal studies where selenium was shown to reduce tumors in the majority of these trials. Selenium-enriched yeast is the major form of selenium used in the human trials, but animal data indicate that selenium-enriched garlic and broccoli are also beneficial in reduction of tumors. In the mammary tumor model, SeMCYS was shown to be the most effective selenocompound identified so far in reduction of tumors. Based on animal data, selenium-enriched plants such as garlic and broccoli may be more effective in mammary tumor reduction than enriched yeast. Several mechanisms have been proposed on the mechanism whereby selenium reduces tumors, but there is no universal agreement by researchers on which one or ones are involved in tumor reductions. Even though SeMCYS was shown to be the most effective selenocompound in reduction of mammary tumors, it may not be the most effective selenocompound for reduction of colon tumors. This suggests that various tissue tumors may not respond to the same extent to different selenocompounds.

Selenium has come full circle in two aspects. Initially the only concern for this element was its toxicity.[1] It is now recognized as an important essential element. It was once thought to promote cancer, but it is now realized that this element will prevent certain types of cancer. A discussion of the anticarcinogenic function of selenium is the purpose of this chapter.

## 10.2  SELENIUM

The concentration of selenium in the Earth's crust is less than that of gold. The chemical and physical properties of selenium are very similar to those of sulfur.[1] Selenium and sulfur have similar outer-valence shell electronic configurations and atomic sizes and their bond energies, ionization potentials, and electron affinities are virtually the same. Despite these similarities, the biochemistry of selenium and sulfur differ in at least two respects that distinguish them in biological systems. First, selenium compounds are metabolized to more reduced states, whereas sulfur compounds are metabolized to more oxidized states. Second, these compounds differ in the acid strengths of their hydrides. The hydride, $H_2Se$, is much more acidic than is $H_2S$. This difference in acidic strengths is reflected in the dissociation behaviors of the selenohydryl groups of selenocysteine and the sulfhydryl groups on cysteine. Hence, while thiols such as cysteine are predominantly protonated at physiological pHs, the selenohydryl groups of selenols such as selenocysteine are predominantly dissociated under the same conditions. These chemical differences between selenium and sulfur are the reasons selenocompounds are usually 600 times more effective than their sulfur analogs against tumors.[2]

## 10.3 SELENOCOMPOUNDS IN PLANTS AND ANIMALS

The metabolism of selenocompounds and distribution of selenium on a worldwide basis have been presented.[3–7] As much as 80% of the total selenium in some accumulator plants is present as SeMCYS, which until recently was thought to be absent in nonaccumulator plants. Selenocompounds present in plants may have a profound effect on the health of animals and humans. The total selenium content cannot be used as an indication of its efficacy but the knowledge of individual selenocompounds is critical for proper interpretation of the results. Thus, speciation of the selenocompounds has moved to the forefront. Because animals and humans are dependent on plants for their nutritional requirements, this makes the types of selenocompounds in plants even more critical.

When rats are injected with selenite, the majority of the selenium is present in tissues in the form of selenocysteine.[8,9] As expected, no Semet was found under the conditions of these studies. In contrast to plants, there is no known pathway in animals for synthesis of Semet from inorganic selenium, and thus they must depend on plant or microbial sources for this selenoamino acid. However, animals can convert Semet to selenocysteine. One day after injection of Semet there is about three times as much Semet as selenocysteine in tissues, but 5 or more days afterward the majority (46 to 57%) of the selenium is present as selenocysteine.[9,10]

Selenium exists in the form of selenoproteins. A total of 25 selenoproteins have been identified in eukaryotes.[11,12] These selenoproteins have been subdivided into groups based on the location of the selenocysteine. The first group (including glutathione peroxidase, GPX) is the most abundant and includes proteins in which selenocysteine is located in the N-terminal portion of a relatively short functional domain. This group includes the four GPXs, selenoproteins P, Pb, W, W2, T, T2, and BthD (from *Drosophila*). The second group of eukaryotic selenoproteins is characterized by the presence of selenocysteine in C-terminal sequences. These include the three thioredoxin reductases and the G-rich protein from *Drosophila*. Other eukaryotic selenoproteins are currently placed in the third group that consists of the three deiodinase isozymes, selenoproteins R and N, the 15-kDa selenoprotein and selenophosphate synthetase.

The four GPXs are located in different parts of tissues and all detoxify hydrogen peroxide and fatty acid–derived hydroperoxides and thus are considered antioxidant selenoenzymes. The three deiodinases convert thyroxine to triiodothyronine, thus regulating thyroid hormone metabolism. The thioredoxin reductases reduce intramolecular disulfide bonds and, among other reactions, regenerate vitamin C from its oxidized state. These reductases can also affect the redox regulation of a variety of factors, including ribonucleotide reductase, the glucocorticoid receptor, and the transcription factors.[13] Selenophosphate synthetase synthesizes selenophosphate, which is a precursor for the synthesis of selenocysteine.[14] The functions of the other selenoproteins have not been definitely identified.

Selenium is present in all eukaryotic selenoproteins as selenocysteine.[11] Semet is incorporated randomly in animal proteins in place of methionine. By contrast, the incorporation of selenocysteine into proteins known as selenoproteins is not random. Thus, in contrast to Semet, selenocysteine does not randomly substitute for cysteine. In fact, selenocysteine has it own triplet code (UGA) and is considered to be the 21st genetically coded amino acid. Interestingly, UGA has a dual role in the genetic code, serving as a signal for termination and also a codon for selenocysteine insertion. Whether it serves as a stop codon or encodes selenocysteine depends on the location of what is called the selenocysteine insertion sequence.[14] The selenocysteine insertion sequences (seven so far) for the various selenoproteins have been presented.[12]

## 10.4  EPIDEMIOLOGICAL STUDIES

There have been a number of epidemiological studies in the U.S. and throughout the world on the relationship between selenium and cancer. Shamberger and Frost[15] reported that the selenium status of humans might be inversely related to the risk of some kinds of cancer. Two years later,[16] more extensive studies indicated that the mortality due to lymphomas and cancers of the gastrointestinal tract, peritoneum, lung, and breast were lower for men and women residing in areas of the U.S. that have high concentrations of selenium in forage crops than those residing in areas with low selenium content in the forages. Those studies were supported by a later analysis of colorectal cancer mortality using the same forage data.[17] A 27-country comparison revealed that total cancer mortality rate and age-corrected mortality due to leukemia and cancers of the colon, rectum, breast, ovary, and lung varied inversely with estimated per capita selenium intake.[18] Similar results were also reported in China, a country where selenium intakes range from deficient to toxic levels.[19]

Lower selenium levels were found in serum collected from American subjects 1 to 5 years prior to diagnosis of cancer as compared to those who remained cancer free during this time.[20] This association was strongest for gastrointestinal and prostatic cancers. Evidence that low serum selenium is a prediagnostic indicator of higher cancer risk was subsequently shown in studies conducted in Finland[21] and Japan.[22] In further case-control studies, low serum or plasma selenium were found to be associated with increased risk of thyroid cancer,[23] malignant oral cavity lesions,[24] prostate cancer,[25] esophageal and gastric cancers,[26] cervical cancer mortality rates,[27] and colorectal adenomas.[28] A decade-long prospective study of selenium status and cancer incidences indicated that initial plasma selenium concentration was inversely related to subsequent risks of both nonmelanoma skin cancer and colonic adenomatous polyps.[29] Patients with plasma selenium levels less than 128 ng/ml (the average normal value) were four times more likely to have one or more adenomatous polyps.

An 8-year retrospective case control study in Maryland revealed no significant association of serum selenium level and cancer risk at sites other than the bladder,[30] but those with low plasma selenium levels had a twofold greater risk of bladder cancer than those with high plasma selenium. In a study with Dutch patients the mean selenium levels were significantly less than that of controls in men, but no differences were found in plasma selenium levels between healthy control women and those with cancer.[31] No significant associations in three other studies were found between serum selenium concentration and risk of total cancers[32] or cancers of the lungs, stomach, or rectum.[33,34] In other work, significant increases of urinary selenium excretion were found in Mexican women with cervical uterine cancer as compared to controls.[35] Selenium was beneficial as a supportive element in chemotherapy in women with ovarian cancer.[36] In other research there appeared to be a relationship between the loss of hMLH1 and improved survival in advanced ovarian cancer.[37] Additional work needs to be conducted on the relationship of DNA mismatch repair and ovarian cancer.

Toenail selenium appears to be a useful biomarker of long-term exposure to this element.[38] Five studies indicated that low toenail selenium values were associated with higher risks of developing cancers of the lung,[39] stomach,[40] breast,[41] and prostate.[42,43] In contrast, five other studies showed no significant difference between cancer cases and controls.[44–48] It has been suggested that the reason for those not showing a relationship is because the selenium intakes of most of the subjects tested were below that necessary for protection.[49] Obviously, these results indicate that many factors must be taken into consideration when evaluating plasma and toenail selenium concentrations in relation to cancer incidence.

## 10.5 HUMAN TRIALS

There have been eight trials conducted on the association of selenium supplementation and the incidence of cancer or cancer biomarkers in humans and all of them have shown cancer protective effects of selenium. Five of these were conducted in China and one each in India, Italy, and in the United States.

The first human intervention trial was conducted in Qidong, a region north of Shanghai, China, where there is a high incidence of primary liver cancer (PLC). Subjects were given table salt fortified with 15 µg selenium per gram as sodium selenite, which provided about 30 to 50 µg selenium daily for 8 years.[49a,50] This resulted in a drop of the PLC incidence to almost one half (27.2 per 100,000 populations vs. 50.4 per 100,000 populations consuming ordinary salt). Upon withdrawal of selenium from the treated group, the PLC incidence began to rise. In a separate study, risk populations receiving selenite salt as a source of selenium also showed a significant reduction in the incidence of viral infectious hepatitis, a major predisposing PLC risk factor in this region.[51] The selenium-fortified salt was distributed to a general population of 20,800 persons. People in six neighboring townships served as controls and were given normal table salt.

In a second trial, members of families at risk of PLC were either given 200 µg of selenium daily in the form of high-selenium yeast or a placebo.[50] During the 2-year study period, 1.26% of the controls developed PLC vs. 0.69% in those given selenium-enriched yeast. This decrease was significantly different ($P < 0.05$). Furthermore, of 226 hepatitis B surface antigen carriers, 7 of 113 subjects in the placebo group developed PLC during 4 years as opposed to no cases in those taking selenium-enriched yeast.

A third human trial on the effects of selenium on cancer was conducted in China with 3698 subjects. This intervention trial was conducted from 1984 to 1991 in Linxian, China, a rural county in Henan Province, where the mortalities from esophageal cancer are among the highest in the world.[52] The results indicated that a treatment containing selenium (50 µg Se/day as Se-enriched yeast plus vitamin E and β-carotene) produced a modest protective effect against esophageal and stomach cancer mortality among subjects in the general population.[52,53] Probably the reason for only a modest reduction of cancer by selenium is because only 50 µg were given daily in contrast to other studies where up to 200 µg were given per day.

In the fourth trial, a total of 29,584 adults in China were used to evaluate the effects of vitamins and minerals on cancer.[54] Four combinations of nutrients were evaluated in a factorial design: (1) retinal and zinc, (2) riboflavin and niacin, (3) vitamin C and molybdenum, and (4) β-carotene, vitamin A, and selenium (50 µg selenium daily as enriched yeast). No significant effects were associated with the first three supplement regimens but total mortality and cancer mortality were significantly lower (relative risk [RR] 0.87; 95% confidence interval [CI] 0.75 to 1.00) among those who received the combination of β-carotene, vitamin E, and selenium. The reduction was slightly greater for stomach cancer compared to esophageal cancers and began to be apparent about 2 years into the supplementation.[55] Rates of lung cancer, the third most common cancer, were only about half as high among those receiving vs. those not receiving β-carotene, vitamin E, and selenium.

In the fifth human study, 3318 persons with cytologic evidence of esophageal dysplasia were randomly assigned to receive daily supplements of 14 vitamins and 12 minerals with 50 µg selenium as selenate or placebo for 6 years.[56] Doses of vitamins and minerals were two to three times the U.S. recommended daily allowances. Cumulative esophageal/gastric and cardiac death rates were 8% lower (RR = 0.92; 95% CI = 0.67 to 1.28) among individuals receiving supplements rather than the placebos, which was not statistically significant. Risk of total mortality was 7% lower (RR = 0.93; 95% CI = 0.75 to 1.16). There are probably at least two reasons a greater difference was not obtained between the supplemented and placebo groups. Animal studies indicate that selenium is much more effective in the prevention of tumors rather than in reversing them,[57] and thus the selection of subjects with evidence of esophageal dysplasia may not have been the best choice. Second, as noted in the above study, 50 µg selenium per day may not be sufficient to provide maximum protection.

In the study conducted in India, 298 subjects were used. One half of the subjects with precancerous lesions in the oral cavity were supplemented with a mixture of four nutrients — vitamin A, riboflavin, zinc and selenium (100 µg daily for 6 months and 50 µg the final 6 months as selenium-enriched yeast) — and compared to the other one half who served as control patients and received placebos.[58] The frequency of micronuclei and DNA adducts were significantly reduced in the supplemented groups at the end of the 1-year study. The adducts were decreased by 95% in subjects taking selenium with all categories of lesions and by 72% in subjects without lesions. No such effects were noted in the placebo group.

In the Italian study subjects were given a mixture called "Bio-selenium," which provided 200 µg selenium as L-Semet daily plus zinc and vitamins A, C, and E for 5 years, and compared to those taking a placebo.[59] A total of 304 patients participated in this study and the incidence of metachronous adenomas of the large bowel was evaluated. Patients with prior resected adenomatous polyps were used in a randomized trial in which new adenomatous polyps were noted. The observed incidence of metachronous adenomas was 5.6% in the group given the "Bio-selenium" mixture vs. 11% in the placebo group, which was statistically significant ($P < 0.05$).

One of the most exciting clinical trials on selenium and cancer in humans was conducted in the U.S. A simple experimental design in a double-blind, placebo-controlled trial with 1312 older Americans with histories of basal and/or squamous cell carcinomas of the skin was used.[60,61] The use of daily oral supplements of selenium-enriched yeast (200 µg Se/day) did not affect the risk of recurrent skin cancers. However, such supplementation for a mean of 4.5 years significantly reduced the incidence of lung, colon, and prostate cancers by 46, 58, and 64%, respectively. There were significant reductions in total cancer (RR = 0.63; 95% CI = 0.47 to 0.85) in the supplemented patients vs. controls.

There were also significant decreases in lung cancer incidence (hazard ratio [HR] = 0.56; 95% CI = 0.31 to 1.01, $P = 0.5$); prostate cancer incidence (HR = 0.35, 95% CI = 0.18 to 0.65), and colorectal cancer incidence (HR = 0.61, 95% CI = 0.17 to 0.90, $P = 0.03$). Restricting the analysis to the 843 patients with initially normal levels of prostate-specific antigen, only four cases were diagnosed with cancer in the selenium treated group but 16 cases were diagnosed in the placebo group (HR = 0.26; P = 0.009) after a 2-year treatment lag.[61] Even though Clark et al.[60] did not observe any effect of selenium on skin cancer in their study, the results strongly indicated that other types of skin disorders may be reduced by selenium.

After 10 years of the trial, the trends were similar; prostate, lung, and colorectal cancers were reduced by 48, 29, and 53%, respectively.[62] Selenium supplementation reduced total (HR = 0.75; 95% CI = 0.58 to 0.97) and prostate (HR = 0.48, 95% CI = 0.28 to 0.80) cancer incidence but was not significantly associated with lung (HR = 0.74, 95% CI = 0.44 to 1.24) and colorectal (HR = 0.46; 95% CI = 0.21 to 1.02) cancer incidence. The protective effect of selenium was confined to males (HR = 0.67, 95% CI = 0.50 to 0.89) and was most pronounced in former smokers. Even though prostate cancer was the only cancer that was statistically reduced, this is probably due to the small number of patients remaining, particularly those with colorectal cancer (only 9 in the selenium treatment group vs. 19 in the placebo group).

The cancer incidence was evaluated according to the baseline plasma selenium levels at the beginning of the study. The subjects with the lower tertile of plasma selenium (less than 105 and 105 to 122 ng Se/ml) had significantly lower incidences of cancer when supplemented with this selenium-enriched yeast. However, those in the highest tertile of plasma selenium (122 ng Se/ml and greater) showed no effect of selenium supplementation on the cancer incidence. This is in direct contrast to the epidemiological studies where an inverse relationship in the incidence of cancer was observed with plasma selenium levels, and thus further evaluation of the data is paramount. However, an explanation could be that there is a threshold in plasma level above which further benefits would not be seen and thresholds may be near or above the plasma level achieved in most populations in the epidemiological studies.

The author is aware of at least two human trials — two in the U.S. (University of Arizona, and the SELECT trial at NCI; Reference 63) and one in Europe (PRECISE, Reference 64), which is planned. With use of HPLC and ion channel plasma mass spectrometry, Semet was detected in the majority of prostate tissues.[65] These patients had total selenium levels in serum and in prostate tissue in a range expected for normal selenium intake. This is the first time Semet has been detected in prostate tissue.

Finally, in another trial, topical application of Semet was effective in protecting against acute ultraviolet irradiation damage to skin of humans.[66] Maximal protection appeared to be attained at concentrations between 0.02 and 0.05%. These results are consistent with some animal data. Hairless mice treated by topical application of Semet (0.02%) or given drinking water with 1.5 μg selenium/ml as Semet had significantly less skin damage due to ultraviolet irradiation.[67] This is consistent with an earlier study that indicated that dietary selenium (1 μg/g) fed to mice significantly reduced the number of skin tumors induced by two carcinogenic chemicals plus croton oil.[68] In other animal work, the influence of dietary selenium as either selenate, Semet, SEMCYS, and selenized yeast at two different concentrations (0.3 and 3 ppm) were studied on established orthotopic PC3 tumors in the prostates of 6-week-old male nude mice.[69] Interestingly, selenate was most effective in retarding the growth of primary prostatic tumors and the development of retroperitoneal lymph node metastases. This was associated with a decrease in angiogenesis. It was concluded that inorganic selenium inhibits the progression of hormone refractory prostate cancer, which is due at least in part to a decrease in angiogenesis.

## 10.6   SELENIUM AND TUMORS IN SMALL ANIMALS

There have been more than 100 trials conducted with small animals on the relationship of tumor incidences to selenium status.[70,71] Interestingly, the first evidence that selenium may counteract tumors was presented in 1949 in a study that reported that the addition of selenium to a diet for rats significantly reduced tumors caused by ingestion of an azo dye.[72] Even these researchers, because of the negative image selenium held at that time, ignored these results. The first evidence of the essentiality of selenium was presented in 1957,[73] at which time selenium was still considered a carcinogenic element.

A number of reviews on selenium and carcinogenesis in animals have been presented, including those by Milner,[74] Ip and Medina,[75] Medina and Morrison,[76] and Whanger.[77] Two thirds of the animal studies showed significant reductions by selenium in the tumor incidence with one half showing reductions of 50% or more.[71] In the majority of those studies selenium as selenite was used, but that may not have been the most effective form (as noted later) to use. Those results with animals and the epidemiological surveys showing a positive relationship between selenium and cancer incidence were the main motivating factors for conducting human trials.

## 10.7  SELENIUM METABOLISM IN TISSUE CULTURE MODELS

Present research efforts are primarily focused on the mechanism of cancer reduction by selenium, and tissue cultures have been used advantageously to study how tumors are reduced by this element. Research with mouse mammary epithelial cells indicate that the beta-lyase mediated production of a monomethylated selenium metabolite, namely, methylselenol, from SeMCYS is a key step in cancer chemoprevention by this agent.[78] In order for SeMCYS to be effective, cells must possess this beta-lyase. One way to get around this is to use methylselenenic acid, which is even effective in cells without this lyase. Apparently, mouse mammary epithelial cells have low levels of the beta-lyase. Interestingly, the distinction between these two compounds disappears *in vivo* where their cancer chemopreventive efficacies were found to be very similar. The reason for this is that the beta-lyase enzyme is abundant in many tissues and thus the animal has ample capacity to convert SeMCYS to methylselenol.

Further work with these mammary cells using methylselenenic acid produced similar results, providing additional support that monomethylated forms of selenium are the critical effector molecules in selenium-mediated growth inhibition *in vitro*.[79] Further research is needed to identify why a monomethylated form of selenium is required, whereas other forms of selenium cannot fulfill this effect. SeMCYS was shown to induce apoptosis through caspase activation in human promyelocytic leukemia cells.[80] Moreover, SeMYCS increased both the apoptotic cleavage of poly (ADP-ribose) polymerase and caspase-3 activity, whereas selenite did not, indicating specific effects of various selenocompounds.

In other research, selenium was shown to significantly downregulate the expression of prostate-specific antigen transcript and protein within hours in the androgen-responsive cells.[81] Selenium also suppressed the binding of androgen receptor to the androgen responsive element site, as shown by electrophoretic mobility shift assay of the androgen receptor–androgen responsive element complex. In further work from this laboratory, exposure to sub-apoptotic concentration of methylseleninic acid specifically inhibited prostate specific antigen expression in the androgen-responsive LNCaP prostate cancer cell model.[82] Interestingly, selenite and Semet lacked this inhibitory effect. Work from another laboratory indicated that the use of the recombinant enzyme methioninase, methylselenol-generating chemiluminescence by superoxide was shown to be catalytically produced from Semet, selenoethionine but not from methionine or SeMYCS. It was concluded that methylselenol can be produced from other sources in addition to the action of beta lyase upon SeMYCS.[83]

As prostate cancer is the most common cancer diagnosed and the second leading cause of cancer-related deaths in men in the U.S.,[84] obviously any research to reduce the incidence of this cancer has significant implications. With the use of the H520 and H522 human lung cancer cell lines, methylseleninic acid was shown to inhibit cell growth, arrested cell cycle progression, and induced apoptosis as a late event.[85]

## 10.8  MECHANISMS OF CANCER REDUCTION BY SELENIUM

A number of reviews have been written on the chemopreventive effects of selenium including most recently those by Combs and Gray,[71] Ganther,[86] Ip,[57] Schrauzer,[49] El-Bayoumy,[87] and Fleming et al.[88] An entire volume of *Nutrition and Cancer* was devoted to selenium and cancer in honor of the late Larry Clark.[89] The mechanism for selenium as an anticarcinogenic element is not known but several speculations have been advanced. It is well established that the most effective dose of selenium for cancer protection is at elevated levels, often called supranutritional or pharmacological levels. The suggested mechanisms for cancer prevention by selenium include its effects on programmed cell death, effects on DNA repair, its role in selenoenzymes, its effects on carcinogen metabolism, its effects on the immune system, selenium as an antiangiogenic agent, and its specific inhibition of tumor cell growth by certain selenium metabolites. Detailed discussions have been devoted to the role of selenium in selenoenzymes, effects on carcinogen metabolism, effects on the immune system, specific inhibition of tumor cell growth and apoptosis,[71] and thus these are discussed only briefly here.

### 10.8.1  ROLE OF SELENOENZYMES

Because GPXs act to convert peroxides to less harmful compounds and because peroxidative damage is associated with cancer, it was reasonable to assume that these peroxidases would be involved in the reduction of tumors. However, there is little information to support this possibility. The greatest protection of selenium against tumors is at high intakes, but the activities of GPXs reach a plateau at nutritional levels with no further increase at higher levels in most tissues.

Interestingly, protection by selenium as selenite against skin tumors induced in rats either by ultraviolet-B (UV-B) light[90] or phorbol esters[91] correlated with the activity of GPX in skin. The hypothesis was advanced that thioredoxin reductase may be involved in reduction of tumors,[86] but experimental data did not support this possibility.[92] Thioredoxin reductase activity was not affected by high dietary levels of SeMCYS or methylseleninic acid, precursors of methylselenol, in rat liver.

The findings that antitumorigenic amounts of selenium (1.5 mg/kg or above) reduced tissue lipid peroxidation potential only slightly[93] or not at all[94] suggest that those effects are independent of the function of the GPXs. Therefore, at present it is probable that antitumorigenic effects of high levels of selenium involve mechanisms unrelated to the activities of GPXs. The 15 kDa (sep 15) selenoprotein has been suggested to be involved in the reduction of tumors. The sep 15 selenoprotein is localized on chromosome 1p31, a genetic locus commonly mutated or deleted in human cancers.[95,96] The sep 15 selenoprotein genes are manifested at highest levels in prostate, liver, kidney, testis, and brain in humans and mice; these levels of this selenoprotein are reduced substantially in malignant prostate cell line and in hepatocarcinoma. Because there is loss of heterozygosity at the sep 15 locus in certain human tumor types, it was suggested that this selenoprotein may be involved in cancer development, risk, or both.[95] It is interesting to note that a 15-kDa protein was found in the prostatic epithelium where it accounted for about two thirds of the protein-bound 75Se.[97] Unless the levels of sep 15 can be shown to be elevated with high intakes of selenium, the likelihood of its significant involvement in tumor reduction does not appear likely. However, it could still be involved in tumor reduction with nutritional intakes of selenium because the tumor suppressor gene and p53 were altered in mice where the selenocysteine (Sec) tRNA [Ser Sec] gene was deleted in transgenic mice carrying the Cre recombinase gene. This recombinase gene is under control of the mouse tumor virus, suggesting greater susceptibility of these mice to cancer.[98]

## 10.8.2 Effects on Carcinogen Metabolism

Studies of carcinogen metabolism have yielded varying results. One study yielded comparable dietary levels of selenium to reduce the formation of covalent DNA adducts of aflatoxin in the chick[99] but to increase that process in the rat.[100] In rats, treatment with selenium increased the hydroxylation and subsequent oxidation of azoxymethane[101] and reduced DMBA–DNA adduct formation,[102] thus reducing the effect of these carcinogens. Selenium supplementation of rats was shown to reduce the hepatic microsomal production of mutagenic metabolites of several carcinogens, including $N,N$-dimethylaniline,[103] DMBA,[104] 2-acetylaminofluorene,[105] and benzo($a$)pyrene.[106] These publications indicate that while the effect may not be universal with respect of either carcinogen or host species, high-level selenium supplementation can affect carcinogen metabolism by methods that would be expected to inhibit the initiation stage of carcinogenesis.

### 10.8.3 EFFECTS ON IMMUNITY

Since the immunity of patients with cancer is reduced and selenium has been shown to boost the immune system, it is logical to conclude that selenium could reduce tumors by this method. Several studies found that supranutritional levels of selenium will stimulate the cytotoxic activities of natural killer cells[107–109] and lymphokine-activated killer cells.[110] Two intervention human studies with the same level of selenium intake (200 μg/day) were shown to reduce cancer risks and improved the immunity.[111,112] The enhancement by selenium of the expression of the high-affinity interleukin-2 receptor resulted in an increased capacity to produce cytotoxic lymphocytes and macrophages that can destroy tumor cells.[109] Upregulation of the receptor is expected to enhance the clonal expansion of cytotoxic effector cells and thereby modulating T-cell-mediated responses in response to signals generated by interleukin-2. Other roles of selenium in the immune system are suggested by recent findings that the mRNAs of several T-cell-associated genes have open reading frames resembling that of selenoprotein P and potential stem-loop RNA structures with consensus SeCys-insertion sequences,[53] suggesting the possibility that they may encode functional seleno-proteins yet to be identified. Along this line, because plasma selenium levels, glutathione concentrations, and GPX activity are subnormal in HIV-infected individuals,[113] selenium studies were conducted to investigate any relationships. By using 75Se-labeled human Jurkat T cells it was shown that the levels of four 75Se containing proteins (57, 26, 21, and 15 kDa species) are lower in HIV-infected cell populations than in uninfected cells.[114] SDS/PAGE gels indicated that these selenium containing proteins are subunits of thioredoxin reductase, cellular GPX, phospholipid hydroperoxide GPX, and the 15-kDa selenoprotein. There appeared to be greater levels of low-molecular-mass 75Se compounds in HIV-infected cells than in normal ones. While these results are intriguing, further research is needed on the relationships of selenoproteins to HIV.

### 10.8.4 ANTITUMORIGENIC SELENIUM METABOLITES

It is possible that selenium can lead to the formation of selenotrisulfides involving protein sulfhydryl groups that could inhibit sulfhydryl-sensitive enzymes to impair tumor cell metabolism. Selenium was shown to inhibit bovine pancreatic ribonuclease by forming an intramolecular selenotrisulfide bridge in place of the normal one,[115] and the formation of selenotrisulfides involving the sulfhydryl groups of chick hepatic fatty acid synthase resulted in inhibition of that enzyme activity.[116] The selenotrisulfide produced by the thiol-dependent reaction of selenite, GSSeSG, can be active in inhibiting protein synthesis and enhancing apoptosis.[117,118] It should be pointed out, however, that these selenotrisulfides are rather short lived and somewhat unstable, raising some questions of their long-term effects.

As noted elsewhere, the antitumorigenic effects of selenium are mediated by the methylated metabolite, methylselenol. Arsenic, which inhibits the methylation of selenide, greatly reduced the antitumorigenic effects of selenite while it enhanced the efficacy of several synthetic selenium compounds that are metabolized to methylselenol.[119,120] Several synthetic alkyl and aryl selenocyanates have been evaluated in animal models. The more effective of these are benzylselenocyanate (BSC) and 1,4-phenylene-bis(methylene) selenocyanate (p-XSC).[121,122] In comparisons with other selenium compounds p-XSC was shown to be more effective against tumorigenesis, but less effective as a source of selenium in supporting the expression of GPX and relatively less toxic.[123] This further suggests that GPXs do not play a significant role in counteraction of tumors. Another synthetic selenium compound, triphenylselenonium chloride (TPSC), has also been found to be antitumorigenic[124] but had only minimum effects in the induction GPX activity. In mice, TPSC has the greatest safety margin yet observed for any chemopreventive selenocompounds. The chemopreventive effects of such synthetic selenocompounds as BCS, p-XSC, and TPSC, which release their selenium only very slowly to the general metabolism of the element, may involve more direct effects, perhaps as effective analogs of the anticarcinogenic metabolites of natural forms of the element.[71]

### 10.8.5 SELENIUM AND APOPTOSIS

The evidence indicates that one possible mechanism by which selenium reduces tumors is through its effects on apoptosis.[125–127] Methylselenenic acid produced a more robust response at one tenth the concentration of SeMCYS in the inhibition of cell proliferation and the induction of apoptosis in mouse mammary epithelial cells.[78] Work with mouse mammary epithelial tumor cells indicates that SeMCYS mediates apoptosis by activating one or more caspases.[128] Of the caspases, caspase-3 activity appeared to be activated to the greatest extent. Apparently these cells have ample lyases to convert SeMCYS to methylselenol.

There are some other factors that should be considered concerning selenium and apoptosis. The feeding of high levels of dietary selenium as selenite to rats increased hepatic concentrations of both reduced (GSH) and oxidized (GSSG) glutathiones with a decreased GSH:GSSG ratio.[129] Similar changes were seen in cultured hepatoma cells treated with high levels of selenite, and selenium treatment was found to retard cell-doubling time, increasing the duration of various phases of the cell cycle. Selenium-induced increases in GSSG may affect protein synthesis because this oxidized form is known to activate a protein kinase that inactivates through phosphorylation eukaryotic initiation factor 2.[130] This has also been found to be inactivated by selenite[131] or its selenotrisulfide derivative, GSSeSG.[132] This selenotrisulfide was found to be more effective in inhibiting the growth of Ehrlich ascites tumors in mice than either the inorganic or amino acid forms of selenium.[133] Apoptotic responses have been demonstrated for cells treated with high levels of selenite,[134] GSSeSG,[135] p-XSC,[136] or TPSC.[134]

The influence of selenocompounds on transcription factor-DNA binding has been summarized.[137] The influence of p-XSC on the binding activities of the transcription factors nuclear factor-κB (NF-κB), activator protein-1 (AP-1), SP-1, and SP3 were evaluated both *in vitro* and *in vivo*. p-XSC and selenite reduced the consensus site binding activity of NF-κB in a concentration-dependent manner when nuclear extracts from cells (HCT-116, a human colorectal adenocarcinoma) stimulated with tumor necrosis factor-α were incubated with either selenocompound. However, only p-XSC inhibited NF-κB consensus recognition site binding when the cells were pretreated with either compound and were then stimulated with tumor necrosis factor-α. In contrast, the consensus site binding activity of AP-1 was inhibited only with selenite but not with p-XSC *in vitro* or *in vivo*. p-XSC or selenite reduced the consensus site binding of transcription factors SP-1 and SP-3 in concentration- and time-dependent manners when nuclear extracts from cells treated with either compound *in vivo* were assayed by electrophoretic mobility shift assay. Interestingly, the sulfur analog of p-XSC, which is inactive in chemoprevention, had no effect on the oligonucleotide binding of SP-1 and SP-3. Certain genes involved in the inhibition of apoptosis also contain SP-1 binding sites in their promoter regions.[138] Therefore, it is likely that SP-1 plays an important role not only in the regulation of cell growth and proliferation but also in programmed cell death. Another selenocompound, GSSG, will increase the induction and translocation of NF-κB, but decreases its binding to DNA.[139] Although these findings show that very high levels of selenium can impair cellular proliferation by enhancing programmed cell death, it is not all that clear whether they can be extrapolated to living systems in which tissue selenium levels tend to be several orders of magnitude less.

The regulation of protein kinase C (PKC) by selenium may be involved in cancer prevention. PKC is a receptor for certain tumor promoters.[140] Oxidant tumor promoters activate PKC by reacting with zinc-thiolates present within the regulatory domain, but in contrast some selenocompounds such as methylseleneninic acid selectively inactivates PKC.[141] Interestingly, thioredoxin reductase reverses selenium-induced inactivation of PKC. However, this effect was eliminated when the selenocysteine in thioredoxin reductase was either selectively alkylated or removed by carboxypeptidase treatment.[140] Similarly, *Escherichia coli* thioredoxin reductase, which is not a selenoprotein, was also not effective, indicating a specific effect of the selenoenzyme. Other studies indicate that the PKC pathway is involved in induction of the selenoproteins, thioredoxin reductase, and GPX,[142,143] further suggesting the influence of this pathway on selenoenzymes.

The induction of apoptosis has been attributed to changes in genes such as cyclin-dependent kinase 2 (cdk2) and gadd45.[125,144] The cdk2 and DNA damage-inducible gadd genes are related to cell cycle arrest. *In vitro*, SeMCYS has been reported to arrest mouse mammary tumor epithelial cells at a phase that coincided with a specific block of cdk2 kinase and an elevated expression of gadd34, gadd45, and gadd153.[143] The alterations in cdk2 and gadd45 suggest that the effect of selenium in these cells may be related to the P53-mediated apoptosis. The P53 protein is a factor that enhances transcription of several genes, including gadd45. In work with LNCaP human prostate cancer cells, selenite treatment led to a significant increase in P53 phosphorylation on Ser-15.[145] In contrast to this apoptotic sensitivity, these cells were rather resistant to similar concentrations of the methylselenol precursor, methylseleninic acid.

In general, there is a correlation between the effectiveness of selenocompounds as chemopreventive agents *in vivo* and their ability to inhibit cell growth and induce apoptosis *in vitro*.[146] The influence of GSSeSG and p-XSC on normal human oral mucosa cells and human oral squamous carcinoma cells (SCCs) were investigated. SCCs were significantly more sensitive to induction to apoptosis by GSSeSG than normal human oral mucosa cells, but the differences were marginal with p-XSC. Both selenocompounds induced the expression of Fas ligand in oral cells to a degree that correlated with the extent of apoptosis induction. Also, both selenocompounds induced the stress pathway kinases, Jun NH2-terminal kinase and p38 kinases at concentrations causing apoptosis. In work with the LNCaP human prostate cancer cell line after acute exposure to selenite, they exhibited mitochondrial injury and cell death, mainly apoptosis.[147] Upregulation by selenite of the cyclin-dependent kinase inhibitor p21 correlated with cell growth inhibitions.

## 10.8.6 Selenium and DNA Repair

It was shown that Semet can activate p53 by a redox mechanism independent of DNA damage.[148] By using a peptide containing only p53 cysteine residues 275 and 277, the importance of these residues in the Semet-induced response was demonstrated. Mouse embryo fibroblasts wild-type or null for p53 genes were used to obtain evidence that the DNA repair branch of the p53 pathway was activated. In further work, Semet was shown to induce a DNA repair response in normal human fibroblasts *in vitro* and protects cells from DNA damage.[149] It has been estimated that each cell sustains approximately 10,000 potentially mutagenic lesions per day due to endogenous DNA damage and the potential of selenium inducing DNA repair hold great value. Because SeMCYS has been shown to be the most effective selenocompound against mammary tumorigenesis, it will be interesting to determine if this compound is more effective than Semet in activation of the p53 tumor suppressor protein and thus DNA repair.

Work by other researchers indicated that thioredoxin reductase was induced but GPX was repressed in malignancies relative to controls in transgenic mice and prostate cell lines.[113] In the colon cell line, p53 expression resulted in elevated GPX but repressed thioredoxin reductase. The data indicated that thioredoxin reductase and GPX are regulated in a contrasting manner in the cancer systems tested and reveal the p53-dependent regulation of selenoprotein expression. If selenium activates p53 as indicated above,[148] then this could be a mechanism whereby selenium induces apoptosis because p53 is involved in this program cell death. Thus, further investigations into the involvement of selenium in DNA repair appear to be an extremely fruitful avenue to pursue.

### 10.8.7 SELENIUM AS AN ANTIANGIOGENIC AGENT

Angiogenesis, which is the process of formation of new microvessels from existing vessels, is a critical and obligatory component of promotion, progression, and metastasis of solid cancers. The chemopreventive effect of increased selenium intake against chemically induced mammary carcinogenesis is associated with reduced intratumoral microvessel density and an inhibition of the expression of vascular endothelial growth factor.[150] The results suggest a methylselenol specific inhibition of the angiogenic switch mechanism through multiple processes.

The evidence indicates that selenium exerts its cancer chemopreventive activity through an anti-angiogenic mechanism.[151] The mammary carcinomas in rats fed diets with either selenium-enriched garlic or selenite were 24 to 34% lower than in those animals fed the control diet. The reduction of small vessels by selenium treatment indicated that mechanisms governing the genesis of new vessels were inhibited by this element. Based on data from several laboratories it was concluded that selenocompounds that feed into the hydrogen selenide pool will be less desirable as chemopreventive agents for humans and, conversely, those that enter the methylselenol pool would be more desirable selenium forms for human application.[151]

## 10.9 FORMS OF SELENIUM IN FOODS AND SUPPLEMENTS

The efficacy of various selenocompounds using the mammary tumor model has been summarized in Table 10.1. The incidence of breast cancer is greatest of all cancers in women, but it is the third highest cause of all cancer deaths in the U.S.,[152] probably reflecting the improved methods for detecting and treatment of breast cancer compared to other cancers. Although usually not mentioned, a small number of men develop breast cancer with even some deaths. About 400 men die of breast cancer each year compared to 43,300 breast cancer deaths in women in the U.S.

SeMCYS and selenobetaine are the most effective selenocompounds identified thus far against mammary tumorigenesis in animals (Table 10.1). Although selenobetaine is just as effective, SeMCYS is considered the most interesting selenocompound because it is the predominant one present in selenium-enriched plants such as garlic,[153] broccoli florets,[153] onions,[154] sprouts,[155] and wild leeks.[156] In contrast, most of the selenium in enriched wheat grain,[157] corn and rice,[158] soybeans,[159] and selenium-enriched yeast[153] is Semet. Selenium-enriched yeast is the most common source of selenium available commercially.[49] The selenoamino acid, Semet, is also available to the public. Selenobetaine has never been detected in selenium-enriched plants. Therefore, SeMCYS has received the most recent attention as possibly the most useful compound for cancer reduction. Except for Semet and selenocystine, the other selenocompounds listed in Table 10.1 are not present in plants and thus are mostly of academic interest. However, some of them are of therapeutic interest.

**TABLE 10.1**
**Anticarcinogenic Efficacy of Different Selenium Compounds for Reduction of Mammary Tumors in Rats**

| Compound | Dietary Selenium (µg/g) for 50% Inhibition |
|---|---|
| Se-methylselenocysteine | 2 |
| Selenobetaine | 2 |
| Selenobetaine methyl ester | 2–3 |
| Selenite | 3 |
| Selenomethionine | 4–5 |
| Selenocystine | 4–5 |
| PXSC[a] | 8–10 |
| Triphenylselenonium | 10–12 |
| Dimethylselenoxide | >10 |
| Trimethylselenonium | (No effect at 80 µg/g) |

[a] 1,4-Phenylene bis (methylene) selenocyanate.

*Source*: Data from References 160–162.

Selenobetaine and SeMCYS are good precursors for generating monomethylated selenium.[57,160] Selenobetaine tends to lose a methyl group before scission of the Se-methylene carbon bond to form methylselenol. SeMCYS is converted to methylselenol directly when cleaved by beta-lyase, and unlike Semet it cannot be incorporated nonspecifically into proteins. That these selenocompounds can be converted directly to methylselenol is presumably the reason they are more efficacious than other forms of selenium. Dimethylselenoxide and selenobetaine methyl ester are converted to dimethylselenide but are less effective for reduction of tumors.[57] Trimethylselenonium is essentially not effective in tumor reduction. Thus, there is a negative correlation between the effectiveness of these selenocompounds and the degree of methylation.

Even though Semet is effective against mammary tumors, one disadvantage as noted above is that it can be incorporated directly into general proteins instead of converted to compounds that most effectively reduce tumors.[57] When this occurs, its efficacy for tumor reduction is reduced. For example, when a low-methionine diet is fed, there is significant reduction in the protective effect of Semet even though the tissue selenium was actually higher in animals as compared to those given an adequate amount of methionine.[163] When methionine is limiting, a greater percentage of Semet is incorporated nonspecifically into body proteins in place of methionine because the methionine-tRNA cannot distinguish between methionine and Semet. Feeding diets with Semet to animals as the main selenium source will result in greater tissue accumulation of selenium than other forms of selenium.[164,165] It is not known whether this stored selenium can serve as a reserved pool of this element, but the evidence indicates that it is metabolically active.[166]

With the knowledge of the effects of these selenocompounds as anticarcinogenic agents, it was of interest to investigate the most appropriate methods for delivery to the general population. One obvious approach was to investigate additional methods for expeditious ways to deliver these protective agents through the food system. This appears to be a logical approach because it is estimated that an intake of five servings of fruits and vegetables per day would reduce cancer by as much as 20%,[167] and the enrichment with selenium should make them more effective. One strategy in this direction was the investigation of enriching garlic with selenium.[168] The addition of selenium-enriched garlic to yield 3 μg selenium/g diet significantly reduced the mammary tumor incidence in rats from 83 to 33%. Similar to garlic, selenium-enriched broccoli also reduced mammary tumors from 90 to 37%.[155]

Selenium-enriched garlic was shown to be twice as effective as selenium-enriched yeast in the reduction of mammary tumors.[153] Chemical analysis of selenium in these two products indicated that Semet was the predominant form of selenium in enriched yeast, whereas SeMCYS (as the glutamyl derivative) was the predominant form of selenium in enriched garlic.[153] The glutamyl derivative is considered a carrier of SeMCYS and both of these compounds were shown to be equally effective in the reduction of mammary tumors.[169] These results are consistent with those in Table 10.1, where SeMCYS was more effective than Semet for reduction of mammary tumors. The chemical composition of selenocompounds in these two sources of selenium is apparently responsible for this difference in efficacy. However, it is not known whether doubling the amount of selenium as selenium-enriched yeast will be as effective as enriched garlic. Neither is it known whether the combination of enriched yeast and enriched garlic would be more effective than either alone.

Even though Semet was shown to be the major selenocompound in enriched yeast,[153] this has not always been the observation. As low as 30% of the selenium as Semet was found in enriched yeast that had been stored for several years.[57] The relative amounts of selenocompounds in enriched yeast from several sources varied markedly, ranging from 27 to 60% for Semet.[169a] In one source, Semet (together with three unidentified selenium compounds) was predominant in the sample hydrolysates. One batch of yeast that had been stored for 10 years contained only 27% of the selenium as Semet. Thus, it is concluded that the speciation of selenium changes with storage, even when kept at cool temperatures. Loss of selenium has been noted in selenium-enriched broccoli powder even though it was stored at −10°C (P.D. Whanger, unpublished data). The total selenium decreased by 60% in this enriched broccoli powder over a period of 4 years at −10°C, and thus the forms of selenium are likely to have changed. It is suggested that this also happens with enriched yeast stored for extended periods of time even at very low temperatures.

Using another model, selenium enriched broccoli florets,[155,170,171] as well as enriched broccoli sprouts,[155] significantly reduced colon tumors in rats. This is intriguing because colon cancer is the third most common newly diagnosed cancer in the U.S., resulting in about 55,000 deaths per year due to this type of cancer,[152] which is the second leading cause of cancer-related deaths in men in the U.S.[84]

Selenium-enriched broccoli was more effective than selenite, selenate, or Semet in the reduction of induced colon carcinogenesis.[171–173] In contrast, selenite, selenate, and Semet were more effective for induction of GPX activity than selenium-enriched broccoli.[171] This indicates that the plant converts the selenium to more effective forms for reduction of these tumors and these results emphasize the need to study the effects of selenium in food forms. Similar to chemically induced colon tumors, there were significantly fewer intestinal tumors when mice with a genetic defect for development of intestinal tumors were fed selenium-enriched broccoli.[174] These results along with previous data indicate that selenium-enriched broccoli is effective against both chemically and genetically induced intestinal tumors. Data from work with another strain of mice that develop spontaneous intestinal tumors is consistent with these results where selenium deficiency resulted in activation of genes involved in DNA damage.[175]

## 10.10 LEVELS OF SELENIUM NECESSARY FOR NUTRITIVE BENEFIT

The Chinese data have been used almost exclusively to establish the required levels of selenium for nutritive benefit as well as to establish the safe levels for protecting human health.[176–178] It is fortunate to have a country like China where areas vary from deficient to toxic levels of selenium, and this has made it convenient to collect critical information on the metabolism and effects of various levels of selenium in humans. Significant correlations have been found between daily selenium intake and selenium content of whole blood, plasma, breast milk, and 24-hour urine.[176] Highly significant correlations were also found between levels of whole blood selenium and hair selenium, fingernail selenium and toenail selenium, hair selenium and fingernail or toenail selenium, and whole blood selenium and toenail or fingernail selenium. Morphological changes in fingernails were used as the main criterion for clinical diagnosis of selenosis.[178] The fingernail changes and loss of hair are the main signs of excess selenium intakes. With excess selenium intakes, the fingernails become brittle and are easily cracked.

A daily intake of nearly 5 mg of selenium resulted in definite occurrence of selenosis, characterized by hair and nail losses. One suggested reason the subjects were able to tolerate this high level of selenium is because they consumed a high-fiber diet. The low adverse effect level of dietary selenium was calculated to range between 1540 and 1600 µg daily. However, some effects were noted in individuals with a daily intake of 900 µg. The maximum safe dietary selenium intake was calculated to be about 800 µg/day, but there were some individuals where an amount of 600 µg/day was the maximum safe intake. To provide a safety factor, the maximum safe dietary selenium intake was suggested as 400 µg/day. A level of about 40 µg daily was suggested as the minimum requirement while an intake of less than 11 µg daily will definitely result in deficiency problems. Deficiency of selenium in humans results in a cardiac and muscular disorder called Keshan disease, and deficiency of selenium is thought to be one of the contributing factors to a joint disorder called Kaschin Beck disease.

## 10.11   CONCLUSIONS AND FUTURE RESEARCH

Daily doses of 100 to 200 µg selenium inhibit genetic damage and cancer development in humans. About 400 µg selenium per day is considered an upper safe limit. The recommended daily allowance (RDA) for selenium is 55 µg for both men and women,[179] and the FAO/WHO has set 26 and 34 µg selenium daily for women and men, respectively.[180] Clearly, doses above the RDA or FAO/WHO levels are needed to inhibit genetic damage and prevent cancer. Despite concerns about the toxicity of higher dietary levels of selenium, humans consuming up to 600 µg of selenium daily appear to have no adverse clinical symptoms.

Available information from both animal and human research indicate that more than 100 and up to 200 µg of additional selenium daily are necessary for greatest reduction of cancer. This is because a methylated form of selenium is necessary for maximum reduction of mammary cancer, and this methylated form is present at highest levels with elevated intakes of this element. In most human trials, the subjects were supplemented with 200 µg selenium per day, and in trials where only 50 µg were supplemented there was not as much reduction of cancer. Therefore, it is concluded that the selenium requirement for maximum reduction of cancer appears to be at least four times the RDA. However, because only 50 to 200 µg additional selenium has been used, it is not possible to indicate which level will give maximum protection. For example, it is not known whether supplemental levels of selenium above 200 µg daily in addition to the dietary intake of selenium will provide any additional protection against cancer.

## REFERENCES

1. Combs GF, Combs SB. Chemical aspects of selenium. In: *The Role of Selenium in Nutrition*. San Diego, CA: Academic Press; 1986:1–8.
2. Ip C, Ganther HE. Comparison of selenium and sulfur analogs in cancer prevention. *Carcinogenesis* 1992; 13:1167–1170.
3. Whanger PD. Selenium and its relationship to cancer: An update. *Br J Nutr* 2004; 91:11–28.
4. Whanger PD. Selenocompounds in plants and their effects on animals. In: *Toxicants of Plant Origin. Vol. III, Proteins and Amino Acids*, PR Cheeke, ed. Boca Raton, FL: CRC Press; 1989:141–167.
5. Whanger PD. Selenocompounds in plants and animals and their biological significance. *J Am Coll Nutr* 2002; 21:223–232.

6. Whanger PD. Metabolic pathways of selenium in plants and animals and their nutritional significance. In: *Nutritional Biotechnology in the Feed and Food Industries*. Lyons TP, Jacques KA, eds. Proceedings of Allteck's 19th Annual Symposium. Nottingham, U.K.: Nottingham University Press; 2003:51–58.

7. Terry N, Zayed AM, deSouza MP, Tarun AS. Selenium in higher plants. *Annu Rev Plant Physiol Plant Mol Biol* 2000; 51:401–432.

8. Olson OE, Palmer IS. Selenoamino acids in tissues of rats administered inorganic selenium. *Metabolism* 1976; 25:299–306.

9. Beilstein MA, Whanger PD. Glutathione peroxidase activity and chemical forms of selenium in tissues of rats given selenite or selenomethionine. *J Inorgan Biochem* 1988; 33:31–46.

10. Beilstein MA, Whanger PD. Chemical forms of selenium in rat tissues after administration of selenite or selenomethionine. *J Nutr* 1986; 116:1711–1719.

11. Gladyshev VN. Identity, evolution and function of selenoproteins and selenoprotein genes. In: *Selenium, Its Molecular Biology and Role in Human Health*. Hatfield DL, ed. Boston: Kluwer Academic; 2001:99–114.

12. Kryukov GV, Castellano S, Novoselov SV, et al. Characterization of mammalian selenoproteins. *Science* 2003; 300:1439–1443.

13. Holmgren A. Selenoproteins of the thioredoxin system. In: *Selenium, Its Molecular Biology and Role in Human Health*. Hatfield DL, ed. Boston: Kluwer Academic; 2001:179–189.

14. Mansell JB, Berry MJ. Towards a mechanism for selenocysteine incorporation in eukaryotes. In: *Selenium, Its Molecular Biology and Role in Human Health*. Hatfield DL, ed. Boston: Kluwer Academic; 2001:69–81.

15. Shamberger RJ, Frost DV. Possible protective effect of selenium against human cancer. *Can Med Assoc J* 1969; 104:82–84.

16. Shamberger RJ, Willis CE. Selenium distribution of human cancer mortality. *CRC Crit Rev Clin Lab Sci* 1971; 2:211–219.

17. Clark LC, Cantor KP, Allaway WH. Selenium in forage crops and cancer mortality in U.S. counties. *Arch Environ Health* 1981; 46:37–42.

18. Schrauzer GN, White DA, Schneider CJ. Mortality correlation studies. III. Statistical association with dietary selenium intakes. *Bioinorg Chem* 1977; 7:23–31.

19. Yu SY, Chu YJ, Gong XL, et al. Regional variation of cancer mortality incidence and its relation to selenium levels in China. *Biol Trace Element Res* 1985; 7:21–29.

20. Willett WC, Polk BF, Morris JS, et al. Prediagnostic serum selenium and risk of cancer. *Lancet* 1983; 2:130–134.

21. Salonen JT, Alfthan G, Huttunen JK, Puska P. Association between serum selenium and the risk of cancer. *Am J Epidemiol* 1984; 120:342–349.

22. Ujiie S, Itoh Y, Kukuchi H. Serum selenium contents and the risk of cancer. *Gan To Kogaku Ryoho* 1988; 12:1891–1897 [translated from Japanese].

23. Glattre EY, Thomassen SO, Thoresen T, Haldorsen PG, Lund-Larsen LF. Prediagnostic serum selenium in a case-control study of thyroid cancer. *Int J Epidemiol* 1989; 18:45–49.

24. Toma S, Micheletti A, Giacchero A, et al. Selenium therapy in patients with precancerous and malignant oral cavity lesions; preliminary results. *Cancer Detect Prev* 1991; 15:491–494.

25. Brooks JD, Metter BEJ, Chan DW, et al. Plasma selenium level before diagnosis and the risk of prostate cancer development. *J Urol* 2001; 166:2034–2038.

26. Mark SD, Qiao Y-L, Dawsey SM, et al. Prospective study of serum selenium levels and incident of esophageal and gastric cancers. *J Natl Cancer Inst* 2000; 92:1753–1763.

27. Guo W-D, Hsing AW, Li J-Y, Chen J-S, Chow W-H, Blot WJ. Correlation of cervical cancer mortality with reproductive and dietary factors, and serum markers in China. *Int J Epidemiol* 1994; 23:1127–1132.

28. Russo MW, Murray SC, Wurzelmann JI, Woosley JT, Sandler SR. Plasma selenium and the risk of colorectal adenomas. *Nutr Cancer* 1997; 28:125–129.

29. Clark L, Hixson LJ, Combs GF, Reid ME, Turnabull BW, Sampliner RE. Plasma selenium concentration predicts the prevalence of colorectal adenomatous polyps. *Cancer Epidemiol Biomarkers Prev* 1993; 2:41–46.

30. Helzlsouer KJ, Comstock WG, Morris JS. Selenium, lycopene, alpha-tocopherol, beta-carotene, retinol and subsequent bladder cancer. *Cancer Res* 1989; 49:6144–6148.

31. Kok FJ, de Bruijn AM, Hofman A, Vermeeren R, Valkenburg HA. Is serum selenium a risk factor for cancer in men only? *Am J Epidemiol* 1987; 125:12–16.

32. Coates RJ, Weiss NS, Daling JR, Morris JS, Labbe RF. Serum levels of selenium and retinol and the subsequent risk of cancer. *Am J Epidemiol* 1988; 128:515–523.

33. Nomura A, Heilbrun LK, Morris JS, Stemmermann GN. Serum selenium and the risk of cancer by specific sites: case-control analysis of prospective data. *J Natl Cancer Inst* 1987; 79:103–108.

34. Kabuto M, Imai H, Yonezawa C, et al. Prediagnostic serum selenium and zinc levels and subsequent risk of lung and stomach cancer in Japan. *Cancer Epidemiol Biomarkers Prev* 1994; 13:465–469.

35. Navarrete M, Gaudry A, Revel G, Martinez T, Cabrera L. Urinary selenium excretion in patients with cervical uterine cancer. *Biol Trace Element Res* 2001; 79:97–105.

36. Sieja K, Talerczyk M. Selenium as an element in the treatment of ovarian cancer in women receiving chemotherapy. *Gynecol Oncol* 2004; 93:320–327.

37. Scartozzi M, De Nictolis M, Galizia E, et al. Loss of hMLH1 expression correlates with improved survival in stage III-IV ovarian cancer patients. *Eur J Cancer* 2003; 39:1144–1149.

38. Krogh V, Pala V, Vinceti M, et al. Toenail selenium as biomarker: reproducibility over a one-year period and factor influencing reproducibility. *J Trace Element Med Biol* 2003; 17:31–36.

39. van den Brandt PA, Goldbohm RA, van't Veer P, Bode P, Dorant E. A prospective cohort study on selenium status and risk of lung cancer. *Cancer Res* 1993; 53: 4860–4865.

40. van den Brandt PA, Goldbohm RA, van't Veer P, et al. A prospective cohort study of toenail selenium levels and risk of gastrointestinal cancer. *J Natl Cancer Inst* 1993; 85:224–229.

41. Garland M, Morris JS, Stampfer MJ, Colditz GA, Spate VL, et al. Prospective study of toenail selenium levels and cancer among women. *J Natl Cancer Inst* 1995; 87:497–505.

42. Yoshizawa K, Willett WC, Morris SJ, et al. Study of prediagnostic selenium level in toenails and the risk of advanced prostate cancer. *J Natl Cancer Inst* 1998; 90:1219–1224.

43. van den Brandt PA, Zeegers MP, Bode P, Goldbohm RA. Toenail selenium levels and the subsequent risk of prostate cancer: a prospective cohort study. *Cancer Epidemiol Biomarkers Prev* 2003; 12:866–871.

44. Noord PA van, Collette HJ, Maas MJ, de Waard F. Selenium levels in nails of premenopausal breast cancer patients assessed prediagnostically in a cohort-nested case-referent study among women screened in the DOM project. *Int J Epidemiol* 1987; 16:318–322.

45. Rogers MA, Thomas DB, Davis S, Weiss NS, Vaughan TL, Nevissi AL. A case-control study of oral cancer and pre-diagnostic concentrations of selenium and zinc in nail tissue. *Int J Cancer Res* 1991; 48:182–188.

46. Van't Veer P, van der, Wielen RP, Kok FJ, Hermus RJ, Sturmans F. Selenium in diet, blood, and toenails in relation to breast cancer: a case control study. *Am J Epidemiol* 1990; 131:987–994.

47. Hunter DJ, Morris JS, Stampfer MJ, Colditz GA, Speizer FE, Willet WC. A prospective study of selenium status and breast cancer risk. *J Am Med Assoc* 1990; 264:1128–1131.

48. Allen NE, Morris JS, Ngwenyama RA, Key TJ. A case-control study of selenium in nails and prostate cancer risk in British men. *Br J Cancer* 2004; 90:1392–1396.

49. Schrauzer GN. Anticarcinogenic effects of selenium. *Cell Mol Life Sci* 2000; 57:1864–1874.

49a. Yu Sh-Y, Zhu Y-J, Huang Q-S, Zhi-Huang C, Zhang QN. A preliminary report of the intervention trials of primary liver cancer in high risk populations with nutritional supplementation of selenium in China. *Biol Trace Element Res* 1991; 29:289–294.

50. Yu Sh-Y, Zhu YJ, Li WG. Protective role of selenium against hepatitis B virus and primary liver cancer in Qidong. *Biol Trace Element Res* 1997; 56:117–124.

51. Yu Sh-Y, Li W-G, Zhu Y-J, Yu WP, Hou C. Chemoprevention trial of human hepatitis with selenium supplementation in China. *Biol Trace Element Res* 1989; 20:15–22.

52. Blot WJ, Li J-Y, Taylor PR, Guo W, Dawsey SM, Li B. Linxian trials: mortality rates by vitamin-mineral intervention group. *Am J Clin Nutr* 1995; 62:1424S–1426S.

53. Taylor PR, Li B, Dawsey SM, et al. Prevention of esophageal cancer: the nutrition intervention trials in Linxian, China. *Cancer Res* 994; 54:2029s–2031s.

54. Blot WJ, Li J-Y, Taylor JR, et al. Nutrition intervention trials in Linxian, China: Supplementation with specific vitamin/mineral combinations, cancer incidence, and disease-specific mortality in the general population. *J Natl Cancer Inst* 1993; 85:1483–1490.

55. Blot WJ. Vitamin/mineral supplementation and cancer risk: international chemoprevention trials. *PSEBM* 1997; 216:291–296.

56. Li JY, Taylor PR, Li B, et al. Nutrition intervention trials in Linxian, China. *J Natl Cancer Inst* 1993; 85:1492–1498.

57. Ip C. Lessons from basic research in selenium and cancer prevention. *J Nutr* 1998; 128:1845–1854.

58. Prasad MP, Mukunda MA, Krishnaswamy K. Micronuclei and carcinogen DNA adducts as intermediate end points in nutrient intervention trial of precancerous lesions in the oral cavity. *Eur J Cancer B Oral Oncol* 1995; 31B:155–159.

59. Bonelli L, Camoriano A, Ravelli P, Missale G, Bruzzi P, Aste H. Reduction of the incidence of metachronous adenomas of the large bowel by means of antioxidants. In: *Proceedings of International Selenium Tellurium Development Association*, Palmieri Y, ed. Scottsdale, AZ; 1998:91–94.
60. Clark LC, Combs GF, Turnbull BW, Slate E, Alberts D. The nutritional prevention of cancer with selenium 1983–1993; a randomized clinical trial. *J Am Med Assoc* 1996; 276:1957–1963.
61. Clark LC, Dalkin B, Krongrad A, Combs GF, Turnbull W. Decreased incidence of prostate cancer with selenium supplementation: results of a double-blind cancer prevention trial. *Br J Urol* 1998; 81:730–734.
62. Duffield-Lillico AJ, Reid ME, Turnbull BW, et al. Baseline characteristics and the effect of selenium supplementation on cancer incidence in a randomized clinical trial: a summary report of the nutritional prevention of cancer trial. *Cancer Epidemiol Biomarker Prev* 2002; 11:630–639.
63. Klein EA, Thompson LM, Lippman SM, et al. SELECT: The next prostate cancer prevention trial. *J Urol* 2001; 166:1311–1315.
64. Rayman MP. The importance of selenium in human health. *Lancet* 2000; 356:233–241.
65. Nyman DW, Stratton S, Kopplin MJ, et al. Selenium and selenomethionine levels in prostate cancer patients. *Cancer Detect Prev* 2004; 28:8–16.
66. Burke KE, Burford RG, Combs GF, French IW, Skeffington DR. The effect of topical L-selenomethionine on minimal erythema dose of ultraviolet irradiation in humans. *Photodermatol Photoimmunol Photomed* 1992; 9:52–57.
67. Burke KE, Combs GF, Gross EG, Bhuyan KC, Abu-Libdeh H. The effects of topical and oral L-selenomethionine on pigmentation and skin cancer induced by ultraviolet irradiation. *Nutr Cancer* 1992; 17:123–137.
68. Shamberger RJ. Relationship of selenium to cancer. I. Inhibitory effect of selenium on carcinogenesis. *J Natl Cancer Inst* 1970; 44:931–936.
69. Corcoran NM, Najdovska M, Costello AJ. Inorganic selenium retards progression of experimental hormone refractory prostate cancer. *J Urol* 2004; 171:907–910.
70. Combs GF, Combs SB. Selenium and cancer. In: *The Role of Selenium in Nutrition*. San Diego, CA: Academic Press; 1986:413–462.
71. Combs GF, Gray WP. Chemopreventive agents: *Selenium. Pharmacol Ther* 1998; 79:179–192.
72. Clayton CC, Bauman CA. Diet and azo dye tumors: effect of diet during a period when the dye is not fed. *Cancer Res* 1949; 9:575–580.
73. Schwarz K, Foltz CM. Selenium as an integral part of factor 3 against dietary necrotic liver degeneration. *J Am Chem Soc* 1957; 79:3292–3293.
74. Milner JA. Effect of selenium on virally induced and transplanted tumor models. *Fed Proc* 1985; 44:2568–2572.
75. Ip C, Medina D. Current concepts of selenium and mammary tumorigenesis. In: *Cellular and Molecular Biology of Breast Cancer*. Medina D, Kidwell W, Heppner G, Anderson EP, eds. New York: Plenum Press; 1987:479–494.
76. Medina D, Morrison DG. Current ideas on selenium as a chemopreventive agent. *Pathol Immunopathol Res* 1998; 7:187–199.
77. Whanger PD. Selenium in the treatment of heavy metal poisoning and chemical carcinogenesis. *J Trace Element Electrolytes Health Dis* 1992; 6:209–221.

78. Ip C, Thompson HJ, Zhu Z, Ganther HE. *In vitro* and *in vivo* studies of methylse-leninic acid: evidence that a monomethylated selenium metabolite is critical for cancer chemoprevention. *Cancer Res* 2000; 60:2882–2886.

79. Sinha R, Kiley SC, Ju JX, et al. Effects of methylselenocysteine on PKC, edk 2 phosphorylation and gad gene expression in synchronized mouse mammary epi-thelial tumor cells. *Cancer Lett* 1999; 146:135–145.

80. Kim T, Jung U, Cho D-Y, Chung A-S. Se-methylselenocysteine induces apoptosis through caspase activation in HL-60 cells. *Carcinogenesis* 2001; 22:559–565.

81. Dong Y, Lee SO, Zhang H, et al. Prostate specific antigen expression is down-regulated by selenium through disruption of androgen receptor signaling. *Cancer Res* 2004; 64:19–22.

82. Cho SD, Jiang C, Malewicz B, et al. Methyl selenium metabolites decrease prostate-specific antigen expression by inducing protein degradation and suppress-ing androgen-stimulated transcription. *Mol Cancer Ther* 2004; 3:605–611.

83. Spallholz JE, Palace VP, Reid TW. Methioninase and selenomethionine but not Se-methylselenocysteine generate methylselenol and superoxide in an *in vitro* chemiluminescent assay: Implications for the nutritional carcinostatic activity of selenoamino acids. *Biochem Pharmacol* 2004; 67:547–554.

84. Meuillet E, Stratton S, Prasad CD, et al. Chemoprevention of prostate cancer with selenium: an update on current clinical trials and preclinical findings. *J Cell Biochem* 2004; 91:443–458.

85. Swede H, Dong Y, Reid M, et al. Cell cycle arrest biomarkers in human lung cancer cells after treatment with selenium in culture. *Cancer Epidemiol Biomar-kers Prev* 2003; 12:1248–1252.

86. Ganther HE. Selenium metabolism, selenoproteins and mechanisms of cancer prevention: complexities with thioredoxin reductase. *Carcinogenesis* 1999; 20:1657–1666.

87. El-Bayoumy K. The protective role of selenium on genetic damage and on cancer. *Mutat Res* 2001; 475:123–139.

88. Fleming J, Ghose A, Harrison PR. Molecular mechanisms of cancer prevention by selenium compounds. *Nutr Cancer* 2001; 40:42–49.

89. Cohen LA, Ed. Larry Clark, In memoriam. *Nutr Cancer* 2001; 40:1–77.

90. Pence BC, Pelier E, Dunn CG. Effects of dietary selenium on UVB-induced skin carcinogenesis and epidermal antioxidant status. *J Invest Dermatol* 1994; 102:759–761.

91. Perchellet JP, Abney NL, Thomas RM, Guislan YL, Perchellet EM. Effects of combined treatments with selenium, glutathione and vitamin E on glutathione peroxidase activity, ornithine decarboxylase induction and complete and multi-stage carcinogenesis in mouse skin. *Cancer Res* 1987; 47:477–485.

92. Ganther HE, Ip C. Thioredoxin reductase activity in rat liver is not affected by supranutritional levels of monomethylated selenium in vivo and is inhibited only by high levels of selenium in vitro. *J Nutr* 2001; 131:301–304.

93. Lane HW, Medina D. Mode of action of selenium inhibition of 7,12-dimethy-lobenz(a)-induced mouse mammary tumorigenesis. *J Natl Cancer Inst* 2001; 75:675–679.

94. Horvath PM, Ip C. Synergistic effect of vitamin E and selenium in the chemo-prevention of mammary carcinogenesis in rats. *Cancer Res* 1983; 43:5335–5341.

95. Kumaraswamy E, Malykh A, Korothov KV, et al. Structure-expression relationships of the 15-kDa selenoprotein gene. Possible role of the protein in cancer etiology. *J Biol Chem* 2000; 275:35540–35547.

96. Hu YJ, Korothov KV, Mehta R, et al. Distribution and functional consequences of nucleotide polymorphisms in the 3′ untranslated region of the human Sep 15 gene. *Cancer Res* 2001; 61:2307–2310.

97. Behne D, Kyriakopoulos A, Kalchlosch M, et al. Two new selenoproteins found in the prostatic glandular epithelium and in the spermatid nuclei. *Biomed Environ Sci* 1997; 10:340–345.

98. Kumaraswamy E, Carlson, BA, Morgan F, et al. Selective removal of the selenocysteine tRNA [Ser] Sec gene (Trsp) in mouse mammary epithelium. *Mol Cell Biol* 2003; 23:1477–1488.

99. Chen J, Goetchius MP, Combs GF, Campbell TC. Effects of dietary selenium and vitamin E on covalent binding of aflatoxin to chick liver cell macromolecules. *J Nutr* 1982; 112:350–355.

100. Chen J, Goetchius MP, Campbell TC, Combs GF. Effects of dietary selenium and vitamin E on hepatic mixed-function oxidase activities and in vivo covalent binding of aflatoxin B1 in rats. *J Nutr* 1982; 112:324–349.

101. Fiala ES, Joseph C, Sohn OS, El-Bayoumy K, Reddy BS. Mechanism of benzylselenocyanate inhibition of azoxymethane-induced colon carcinogenesis in F344 rats. *Cancer Res* 1991; 54:2826–2830.

102. Liu J, Gilbert K, Parker H, Haschek W, Milner JA. Inhibition of 7,12-dimethylbena(a)anthracene-induced mammary tumors and DNA adducts by dietary selenite. *Cancer Res* 1991; 51:4613–4617.

103. Olsson U, Onfelt A, Beije B. Dietary selenium deficiency causes decreased N-oxygenation of N,N-diethylaniline and increased mutagenicity of dimethylnitrosamine in the isolated rat liver/cell culture system. *Mutat Res* 1984; 126:73–80.

104. Martin SE, Schillaci M. Inhibitory effects of selenium on mutagenicity. *J Agric Food Chem* 1984; 32:426–433.

105. Chow CK, Gairola GC. Influence of dietary vitamin E and selenium on metabolic activation of chemicals to mutagens. *J Agric Food Chem* 1984; 32:443–447.

106. Teel RW, Kain RS. Selenium modified mutagenicity and metabolism of benzo(a)pyrene in an S9-dependent system. *Mutat Res* 1984; 127:9–14.

107. Koller LD, Exon JH, Talcott PA, Osborne CA, Henningsen GM. Immune responses in rats supplemented with selenium. *Clin Exp Immunol* 1986; 63:570–576.

108. Peatrie HT, Klassen LW, Klassen PS, O'Dell JR, Kay HD. Selenium and the immune response. 2. Enhancement of murine cytotoxic T-lymphocyte and natural killer cell cytotoxicity *in vivo*. *J Leukocyte Biol* 1989; 45:215–220.

109. Kiremidjian-Schumacher L, Roy M, Wishe HI, Cohen MW, Stotzky G. Supplementation with selenium augments the functions of natural killer and lymphokine-activated killer cells. *Biol Trace Element Res* 1996; 52:227–239.

110. Roy M, Kiremidjian-Schumacher L, Wishe HI, Cohen MW, Stotzky G. Supplementation with selenium and human immune cell functions. 1. Effect of lymphocyte proliferation and interleukin 2 receptor expression. *Biol Trace Element Res* 1994; 41:103–113.

111. Kiremidjian-Schumacher L, Roy M, Wishe HI, Cohen MW, Stotzky G. Supplementation of selenium and human immune cell functions. II. Effect on cytoxic lymphocytes and natural killer cells. *Biol Trace Element Res* 1994; 41:115–126.

112. Taylor EW. Selenium and cellular immunity. Evidence that selenoproteins may be coded in the +1 reading frame overlapping the human CD4, CD8 and HLA-DR genes. *Biol Trace Element Res* 1995; 49:85–95.

113. Diamond AM, Hu YJ, Mansur DB. Glutathione peroxidase and viral replications: implications for viral evolution and chemoprevention. *BioFactors* 2001; 14:205–210.

114. Gladyshev VN, Stadtman TC, Hatfield DL, Jeang KT. Levels of major selenoproteins in T cells decrease during HIV infection and low molecular mass selenium compounds increase. *Proc Natl Acad Sci USA* 1999; 96:835–839.

115. Ganther HE, Corcoran C. Selenotrisulfides II. Cross-linking of reduced pancreatic ribonuclease with selenium. *Biochemistry* 1969; 8:2557–2563.

116. Donaldson WE. Selenium inhibition of avian fatty acid synthase complex. *Chem Biol Interact* 1977; 17:313–320.

117. Harrison PR, Lanfear J, Wu L, Fleming J, Blower L. Mechanisms of chemoprevention and growth inhibition by selenium compounds. In: *Proceedings of the 6th International Symposium on Selenium in Biology and Medicine*, Beijing. 1996:74–82.

118. Pence BC, Stewart M, Walsh L, Cameron G. Modulation of oxidative damage in DNA by sodium selenite via the mechanism of apoptosis. In: *Proceedings of the 6th International Symposium on Selenium in Biology and Medicine*, Beijing. 1996:82–88.

119. Ip C, Ganther HE. Activity of methylated forms of selenium in cancer prevention. *Cancer Res* 1990; 50:1206–1211.

120. Ip C, Ganther HE. Biological activities of trimethylselenonium as influenced by arsenite. *J Inorg Biochem* 1992; 46:215–222.

121. El-Bayoumy K. Effects of organoselenium compounds on induction of mouse forestomach tumors by benzo(a)pyrene. *Cancer Res* 1985; 45:3631–3635.

122. Nayini J, El-Bayoumy K, Sugie S, Cohen LA, Reddy BS. Chemopreventive of experimental mammary carcinogenesis by the synthetic organoselenium compound, benzylselenocyanate, in rats. *Carcinogenesis* 1989; 10:509–512.

123. Ip C, Ganther HE. Novel strategies in selenium cancer chemoprevention research. In: *Selenium in Biology and Human Health*, Burk RF, ed. New York: Springer-Verlag; 1993:171–180.

124. Lu J, Jiang C, Kaech M, Ganther H E, Ip C, Thompson H. Cellular and metabolic effects of triphenylselenonium chloride in a mammary cell cultured model. *Carcinogenesis* 1995; 16:513–516.

125. Sinha RS, Kiley C, Jui JX et al. Effects of methylselenocysteine on PKC, cdk2 phosphorylation and gadd gene expression in synchronized mouse mammary epithelial tumor cells. *Cancer Lett* 1999; 146:135–145.

126. Ip C, Dong Y. Methylselenocysteine modulates proliferation and apoptosis biomarkers in premalignant lesions of the rat mammary gland. *Anticancer Res* 2001; 21:863–867.

127. Wang Z, Jiang C, Ganther HE, Lu J. Antimitogenic and proapoptotic activities of methylseleninic acid in vascular endothelial cells and associated effects on PI3K-AKT, ERK, JNK and P38 MAPK signaling. *Cancer Res* 2001; 61:7171–7178.

128. Unni E, Singh U, Ganther HE, Sinha R. Se-methylselenocysteine activates caspase-3 in mouse mammary epithelial tumor cells *in vitro*. *BioFactors* 2001; 14:169–177.

129. Le Boeuf RA, Hoekstra WG. Adaptive changes in hepatic glutathione metabolism in response to excess dietary selenium. *J Nutr* 1983; 113:845–854.

130. Jacobs MM, Matney JA, Griffin AC. Inhibitory effects of selenium on the mutagenicity of 2-acetylaminofluorene (AAF) and AAF derivatives. *Cancer Lett* 1977; 2: 319–322.

131. Safer B, Jagaus B, Crouch D. Indirect inactivation of eukaryotic initiation factor 2 in reticulocyte lysates by selenite. *J Biol Chem* 1980; 2545:6913–6917.

132. Vernie LN, Hamburg CJ, Bont WS. Inhibition of the growth of malignant mouse lymphoid cells by selenodiglutathione and selenocystine. *Cancer Lett* 1981; 14:303–308.

133. Poirier KA, Milner JA. Factors influencing the antitumorigenic properties of selenium in mice. *J Nutr* 1983; 113:2147–2154.

134. Lu J, Jiang C, Kaeck M, Ganther HE, Ip C, Thompson H. Cellular and metabolic effects of triphenhylselenonium chloride in a mammary cell cultured model. *Carcinogenesis* 1995; 16:513–516.

135. Lanfear J, Flemming JJ, Wu L, Webster G, Harrison PR. The selenium metabolite selenodiglutathione induces p53 and apoptosis: relevance to the chemopreventive effects of selenium? *Carcinogenesis* 1994; 15:1387–1392.

136. El-Bayoumy K, Chen YH, Upadhyaya P, Mescher C, Cohen LA, Reddy BS. Selenium in chemoprevention of carcinogenesis II. Inhibition of 7, 12-dimethyl-benz(a)-anthracene-induced tumors and DNA adduct formation in the mammary glands of female Sprague-Dawley rats by the synthetic organoselenium compound 1, 4-phenylenebis-(methylene) selenocyanate. *Cancer Res* 1992; 52:2402–2407.

137. Youn BW, Fiala ES, Sohn OS. Mechanisms of organoselenium compounds in chemoprevention: Effects of transcription factor-DNA binding. *Nutr Cancer*, 2001; 40:28–33.

138. Dong L, Wang W, Wang F, Stoner M, Reed JC. Mechanism of transcriptional activation of bcl-2 gene expression by 17β-estradiol in breast cancer cells. *J Biol Chem* 1999; 274:32099–32107.

139. Galter D, Mihm S, Droge W. Distinct effect of glutathione disulfide on the nuclear transcription factor kB and the activator protein-1. *Eur J Biochem* 1994; 221:639–648.

140. Gopalakrishna R, Gundimeda U. Protein kinase C as a molecular target for cancer prevention by selenocompounds. *Nutr Cancer* 2002; 40:55–63.

141. Gopalakrishna R, Gundimeda U. Antioxidant regulation of protein kinase C in cancer prevention. *J Nutr* 2002; 132:3819S–3823S.

142. Kumar S, Holmgren A. Induction of thioredoxin, thioredoxin reductase and glutaredoxin activity in mouse skin by TPA, a calcium ionophore and other tumor promoters. *Carcinogenesis* 1999; 20:1761–1767.

143. Jornot I, Junod AF. Hyperoxia, unlike phorbol ester, induces glutathione peroxidase through a protein kinase C-independent mechanism. *Biochem J* 1997; 326:117–123.

144. Kaeck M, Lu J, Strange R, Ip C, Ganther HE. Differential induction of growth arrest inducible genes by selenium compounds. *Biochem Pharmacol* 1997; 53:921–926.

145. Jiang C, Hu H, Malewicz B, Lu J. Selenite-induced p53 Ser-15 phosphorylation and caspase-media apoptosis in LNCaP human prostate cancer cells. *Mol Cancer Ther* 2004; 3:877–884.

146. Ghose A, Fleming J, El-Bayoumy K, Harrison PR. Enhanced sensitivity of human oral carcinomas to induction of apoptosis by selenium compounds: involvement of mitogen-activated protein kinase and Fas pathways. *Cancer Res* 2001; 61:7479–7487.

147. Zhong W, Oberley TD. Redox-mediated effects of selenium on apoptosis and cell cycle in the LNCaP human prostate cancer cell line. *Cancer Res* 2001; 61:7071–7078.

148. Seo YR, Kelley MR, Smith ML. Selenomethionine regulation of p53 by a ref1-dependent redox mechanism. *Proc Natl Acad Sci USA* 2002; 99:14548–14553.

149. Seo YR, Sweency C, Smith ML. Selenomethionine induction of DNA repair response in human fibroblasts. *Oncogene* 2002; 21:3663–3669.

150. Lu J, Jiang C. Antiangiogenic activity of selenium in cancer chemoprevention: metabolite-specific effects. *Nutr Cancer* 2001; 40:64–73.

151. Lu J. Apoptosis and angiogenesis in cancer prevention by selenium. *Nutrition and Cancer Prevention*, edited under the auspices of AICR. New York: Kluwer Academic/Plenum Press; 2000:131–145.

152. American Cancer Society. *Cancer Facts & Figures*. Atlanta, GA: American Cancer Society; 2000.

153. Ip C, Birringer M, Block E, et al. Chemical speciation influences comparative activity of selenium-enriched garlic and yeast in mammary cancer prevention. *J Agric Food Chem* 2000; 48:2062–2070.

154. Cai X-J, Block E, Uden PC, Zhang X, Quimby BD, Sullivan JJ. Allium chemistry: identification of selenoamino acids in ordinary and selenium-enriched garlic, onion and broccoli using gas chromatography with atomic emission detection. *J Agric Food Chem* 1995; 43:1754–1757.

155. Finley JW, Ip C, Lisk DJ, Davis CD, Hintze K, Whanger PD. Investigations on the cancer protective properties of high selenium broccoli. *J Agric Food Chem* 2001; 49:2679–2683.

156. Whanger PD, Ip C, Polan CE, Uden PC, Wilbaum G. Tumorigenesis, metabolism, speciation, bioavailability and tissue deposition of selenium in selenium-enriched ramps (*Allium tricoccum*). *J Agric Food Chem* 2000; 48:5723–5730.

157. Olson OE, Novacek EJ, Whitehead EI, Palmer IS. Investigation of selenium in wheat. *Phytochemistry* 1970; 9:1181–1188.

158. Beilstein MA, Whanger PD, Yang GQ. Chemical forms of selenium in corn and rice grown in a high selenium area of China. *Biomedical Environ Sci* 1991; 4:392–398.

159. Yasumoto K, Iwami K, Yoshida M. Nutritional efficiency and chemical form of selenium, an essential trace element, contained in soybean protein. *Se-Te Abstr* 1984; 25:73150.

160. Ip C, Ganther HE. Novel strategies in selenium cancer chemoprevention research. In: *Selenium in Biology and Human Health*. Burk RF, ed. New York: Springer-Verlag; 1993:170–180.

161. Ip C, El-Bayoumy K, Upadhyaya P, Ganther HE, Vadhanavikit S, Thompson H. Comparative effect of inorganic and organic selenocyanate derivatives in mammary cancer chemoprevention. *Carcinogenesis* 1994; 15:187–192.

162. Ip C, Thompson HJ, Ganther HE. Activity of triphenylselenonium chloride in mammary cancer prevention. *Carcinogenesis* 1994; 15:2879–2882.

163. Ip C. Differential effects of dietary methionine on the biopotency of selenome-thionine and selenite in cancer chemoprevention. *J Natl Cancer Inst* 1988; 80:258–262.

164. Ip C, Lisk DJ. Characterization of tissue selenium profiles and anticarcinogenic responses in rats fed natural sources of selenium-rich products. *Carcinogenesis* 1994; 15:573–576.

165. Whanger PD, Butler JA. Effects of various dietary levels of selenium as selenite or selenomethionine on tissue selenium levels and glutathione peroxidase activity in rats. *J Nutr* 1988; 118:846–852.

166. Waschulewski IH, Sunde RA. Effect of dietary methionine on utilization of tissue selenium from dietary selenomethionine for glutathione peroxidase in the rat. *J Nutr* 1988; 118:367–374.

167. Keck AS, Finley JW. Cruciferous vegetables: cancer protective mechanisms of glucosinolate hydrolysis products and selenium. *Integr Cancer Ther* 2004; 3:5–12.

168. Ip C, Lisk DJ, Stoewsand GS. Mammary cancer prevention by regular garlic and selenium-enriched garlic. *Nutr Cancer* 1992; 17:279–286.

169. Dong Y, Lisk DJ, Block E, Ip C. Characterization of the biological activity of (γ-glutamyl-Se-methylselenocysteine: a novel, naturally occurring anticancer agent from garlic. *Cancer Res* 2001; 61:2923–2928.

169a. Larsen EH, Hansen M, Paulin H, et al. Speciation and bioavailability of selenium in yeast-based intervention agents used in cancer chemoprevention studies. *J AOAC Int* 2004; 87:225–232.

170. Finley JW, Davis C, Feng Y. Selenium from high-selenium broccoli is protective against colon cancer in rats. *J Nutr* 2000; 130:2384–2389.

171. Finley JW, Davis CD. Selenium (Se) from high-selenium broccoli is utilized differently than selenite, selenate and selenomethionine, but is more effective in inhibiting colon carcinogenesis. *BioFactors* 2001; 14:191–196.

172. Feng Y, Finley JW, Davis CD, Becker WK, Fretland AJ, Hein DW. Dietary selenium reduces the formation of aberrant crypts in rats administered 3,2′-dimethyl-4-aminobiphenyl. *Toxicol Appl Pharmacol* 1999; 157:36–42.

173. Davis CD, Feng Y, Hein DW, Finley JW. The chemical form of selenium influences 3, 2′-dimethyl-4-aminobiphenyl-DNA adduct formation in rat colon. *J Nutr* 1999; 29:63–69.

174. Davis C, Zeng H, Finley JW. Selenium-enriched broccoli decreases intestinal tumorigenesis in multiple intestinal neoplasia mice. *J Nutr* 2002; 132:307–309.

175. Rao L, Puschner B, Prolla TA. Gene expression profiling of low selenium status in the mouse intestine: transcriptional activation of genes linked to DNA damage, cell cycle control and oxidative stress. *J Nutr* 2001; 131:3175–3181.

176. Yang GQ, Yin S, Zhou R. Studies on safe maximal daily dietary Se-intake in a seleniferous area in China, Part I. Relationship between selenium intake and tissue levels. *J Trace Element Electrolytes Health Dis* 1989; 3:77–87.

177. Yang GQ, Yin S, Zhou R, et al. Studies on safe maximal daily dietary Se-intake in a seleniferous area in China. Part II. Relation between selenium intake and manifestations of clinical signs and certain biological altercations. *J Trace Element Electrolytes Health Dis* 1989; 3:123–130.

178. Yang G, Zhou R. Further observations on the human maximum safe dietary selenium intake in a seleniferous area of China. *J Trace Element Electrolytes Health Dis* 1994; 8:159–165.

179. Food and Nutrition Board, Institute of Medicine. *Selenium. Dietary Reference Intakes for vitamin C, vitamin E, Selenium and Carotenoids.* Washington, DC: National Academy Press; 2000:284–324.
180. Human vitamin and mineral requirements: Report of a joint FAO/WHO expert consultation, Bangkok, Thailand; 2002.

# Part IV

Dietary Components That
Protect from Cancer:
Phytosterols

# 11 Phytosterols: Sources and Metabolism

*Elke A. Trautwein and Guus S.M.J.E. Duchateau**

## CONTENTS

11.1 Introduction .................................................................................223
11.2 Sterol Nomenclature .....................................................................224
11.3 Phytosterol Sources.......................................................................226
    11.3.1 Occurrence of Phytosterols in Plants......................................226
    11.3.2 Food Sources of Phytosterols.................................................228
    11.3.3 Commercial Sources..............................................................228
11.4 Dietary Intake of Phytosterols......................................................230
11.5 Health Benefits of Phytosterols ....................................................230
    11.5.1 Plasma Cholesterol-Lowering Effect .....................................230
    11.5.2 Anti-Atherogenic Effects of Phytosterols ...............................231
    11.5.3 Anti-Inflammatory Effects and Effects on the Immune
          System........................................................................232
    11.5.4 Antioxidant Activity ..............................................................232
    11.5.5 Beneficial Effects on Prostatic Hyperplasia...........................232
    11.5.6 Possible Health Concerns and Safety Aspects........................233
11.6 Metabolism of Phytosterols..........................................................235
    11.6.1 Absorption of Phytosterols.....................................................235
    11.6.2 Effect of Phytosterols on Cholesterol Absorption ..................237
    11.6.3 Distribution and Metabolism: Post-Absorptive Fate of
          Phytosterols...............................................................238
    11.6.4 Excretion................................................................................239
11.7 Conclusion ...................................................................................239
References ..............................................................................................241

## 11.1 INTRODUCTION

Phytosterols (plant sterols and stanols) are like cholesterol steroid alcohols (triterpenes). They are the equivalent of cholesterol in mammalian species and resemble cholesterol both in structure and biological function. They are essential

---

* Both authors contributed equally to this work.

structural components of the cell membrane, where they regulate membrane fluidity and permeability as well as membrane-associated metabolic processes.

Phytosterols present a diverse group of more than 200 different compounds found in various plants and marine sources. They have a steroid nucleus, a 3β-hydroxyl group, a double bond in the steroid nucleus, most commonly located between the C-atoms five and six, and an alkyl side chain. Major differences are found in their side chain substitution and saturation. Phytostanols (plant stanols) are the saturated forms of plant sterols, lacking the double bond in the steroid nucleus, and in the alkyl side chain.

In this chapter the term *phytosterols* refers to both plant sterols and their saturated counterparts, plant stanols. Phytosterols are known to have various bioactive properties, which may have an impact on human health, and as such boosted interest in phytosterols in the past decade. The most important function is their plasma cholesterol-lowering effect via inhibition of intestinal cholesterol absorption. Other claimed benefits of phytosterols are possible antioxidant activity, anti-inflammatory activity, and an anti-atherogenic effect. It is not clear whether mechanisms other than their cholesterol-lowering action as such also contribute to an anti-atherogenic action, i.e., effects independent from the reduction in plasma cholesterol concentration. Furthermore, there is accumulating evidence that phytosterols, in particular plant sterols, have beneficial effects in the development of different types of cancers. The potential anticancer effects and possible underlying mechanisms are the focus of another chapter of this book (see Chapter 12).

This chapter aims to provide an overview of the structural diversity of phytosterols, their occurrence in nature, and summarizes aspects regarding their metabolism as well as their established and potential health benefits. Because of their beneficial health effects, phytosterols are considered a functional ingredient and already a limited number of phytosterol-enriched food products and dietary supplements are commercially available.

## 11.2   STEROL NOMENCLATURE

Phytosterols are products of the isoprenoid biosynthesis pathway and like cholesterol are synthesized from acetyl coenzyme A via squalene involving more than 30 enzyme-catalyzed reactions all taking place in plant cell membranes.[1] Similar to cholesterol, phytosterols serve as precursors for plant steroid hormones, so called brassinosteroids.[2]

Phytosterols are found in various plants and marine sources.[3] They all have a steroid nucleus, a hydroxyl group at carbon 3 in the β-position and a double bond most commonly located between the C-atoms five and six in the B-ring (Figure 11.1 and Figure 11.2). Major differences are found in the alkyl side chain, which can vary in the absence or presence of a methyl or ethyl group on C24, saturation and position of a double bound, and geometry of the substitution at C24. Phytostanols are the saturated forms of plant sterols, lacking the double bonds in the steroid nucleus and the alkyl side chain.

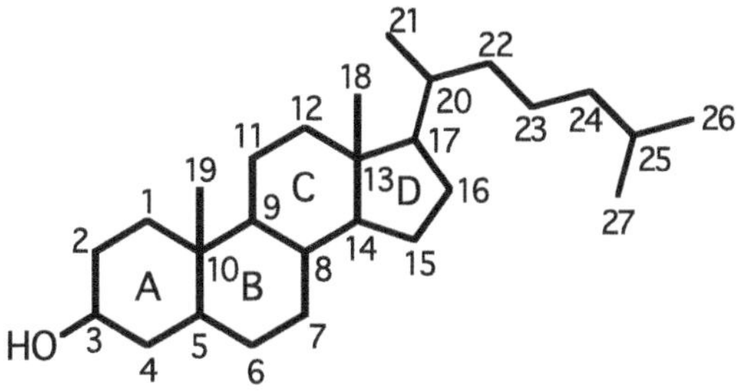

FIGURE 11.1 Basic sterol skeleton with ring and carbon identification.

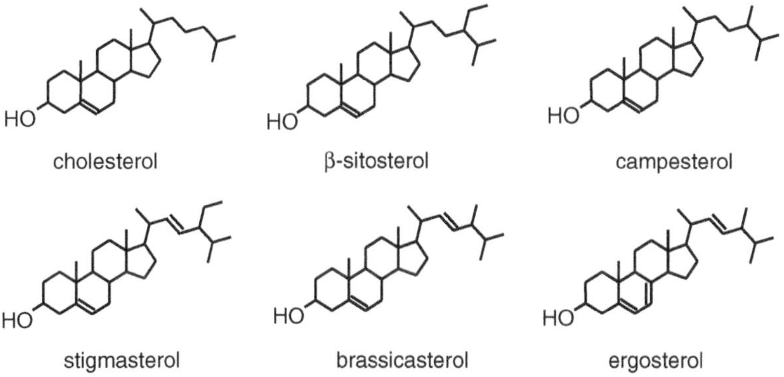

FIGURE 11.2 Main sterols of the 4-desmethyl class.

Phytosterols are divided based on structural and biosynthetic aspects into so-called classes mainly based on their different polarity related to the presence or absence of methyl groups on C4 (two, one, or none). This has resulted in the past in significantly different behavior in the early analytical techniques such as thin layer chromatography (TLC). Separation of sterols in such polarity-based techniques resulted in three distinct TLC bands or classes consisting of 4,4-dimethylsterols (least polar), 4-monomethylsterols, and 4-desmethylsterols (most polar).

Most of the biologically relevant phytosterols belong to the 4-desmethylsterol class. These include cholesterol (C27), and the common 28 and 29 C-atoms phytosterols such as sitosterol (C29), campesterol (C28), stigmasterol (C29), brassicasterol (C28), and ergosterol (C28) (Figure 11.2). The two plant stanols, sitostanol and campestanol, are 5,6-saturated analogs of the main 4-desmethylsterols, sitosterol and campesterol (Figure 11.3).

The 4-monomethylsterols and 4,4-dimethylsterols are metabolic intermediates in the biosynthesis pathway leading to 4-desmethylsterols, but are usually only minor compounds found in some plant materials. Compared to 4-desmethylsterols, the number of different 4-monomethylsterol compounds is rather small. One example of a 4-monomethylsterol is gramisterol. Cycloartenol and 24-methylenecycloartanal found in rice bran oil are the major examples of

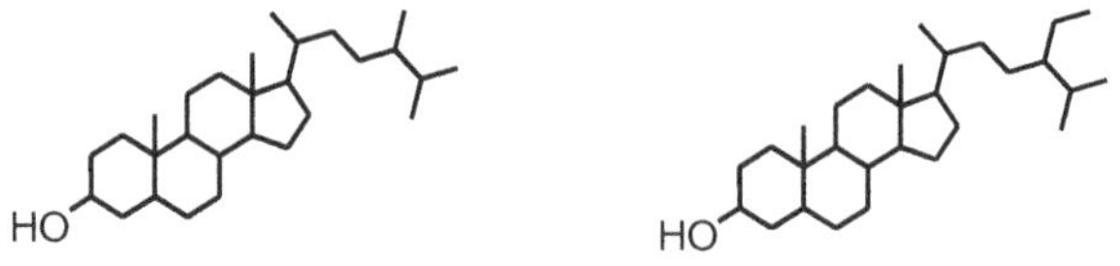

campestanol sitostanol

**FIGURE 11.3** Structure of sitostanol and campestanol.

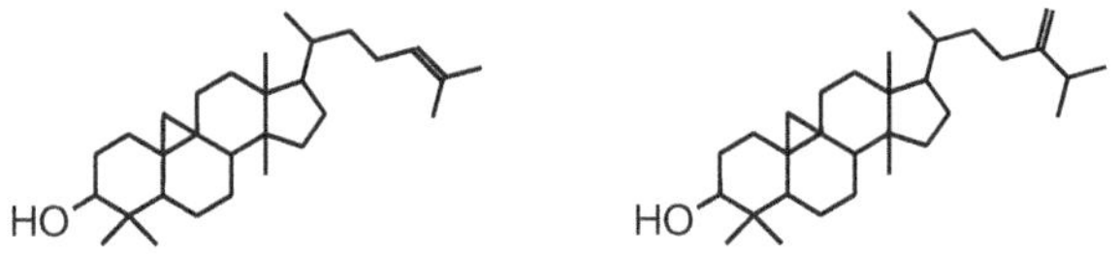

cycloartenol 24-Methylene cycloartanal

**FIGURE 11.4** Examples of 4,4-dimethylsterols.

4,4-dimethylsterols (Figure 11.4). The structure of triterpene alcohols resembles partly those of 4,4-dimethylsterols, but in contrast to the tetracyclic ring structure, triterpene alcohols usually have a five-ring structure. Triterpene alcohols like β-amyrin, α-amyrin, or lupeol are found in higher concentrations in shea nut oil.

## 11.3 PHYTOSTEROL SOURCES

### 11.3.1 Occurrence of Phytosterols in Plants

Plant sterols occur naturally in all foods of plant origin where they are found in the lipid-rich and fiber-rich fractions. Plant sterols exist in various forms, such as free sterols, sterol esters esterified to fatty acids or other organic acids (e.g., ferulic acid for oryzanol in rice bran oil or coumaric acid), plant steryl glycosides, and acylated plant steryl glycosides.[1,3,4] Sterol fatty acid esters and sterol glycosides are also referred to as phytosterol conjugates having another component being covalently bound to the 3β-hydroxyl group of the A-ring in the steroid nucleus. In case of phytosterol ester, the 3β-hydroxyl group is ester-linked with a fatty acid or an organic acid and in the case of glycosides the link is via a 1-O-β-glycosidic bond with glucose or another hexose.

The different forms of phytosterols are assumed to exist in different parts of the plant cells. While free plant sterols are a structural part of the cell membrane, phytosterol esters are located intracellularly and represent storage products. In vegetable oil, plant sterols occur mainly as free sterols and esters of linoleic and oleic acids. The proportions of free and esterified plant sterols vary greatly between different vegetable oils.[1,5,6] Steryl glycosides as well as steryl esters of phenolic acids are commonly found in cereals and grain products.

Because of the relatively low concentrations in edible oils and due to the lack of sensitive analytical techniques available in the past, a clear differentiation of

**TABLE 11.1**
**Relative Distribution of Different Free and Esterified Sterols in Some Vegetable Oil Sources**

| Source | 4-Desmethyl-sterols | 4-Monomethyl-sterols | 4,4-Dimethyl-sterols | Ratio Free/Esterified Sterols |
|---|---|---|---|---|
| Palm | ++ | − | − | ~1 to >1 |
| Rapeseed | +++ | − | − | <1 |
| Soybean | ++ | + | − | >1 |
| Sunflower seed | ++ | + | − | >1 |
| Corn | +++ | − | − | <1 |
| Shea nut | − | + | ++ | — |
| Rice bran | +++ | + | ++ | <<1 |
| Tall oil | ++ | | | a |
| Olive oil | ++ | | | ~1 to >1 |

Esters are fatty acid, ferulic or cinnamic acid type

[a] Due to the nature of the process, tall oil contains only free sterols and free fatty acids.

the concentrations of free sterols and esterified sterols was not available in full detail until recently. The level of esterification, mostly with common fatty acids, for sterols in most edible oil sources is on average about 40 to 50% but ranges from as low as a few percent to 60 to 70%.[5–7] An indicative overview of the presence, concentrations, and degree of esterification is presented in Table 11.1.

In general, there is good agreement between data from different authors, but for some oils the ratios may vary. This could be related to limited sample numbers analyzed or samples from different harvest. Most data are available on processed oils, but during refinement the free-to-esterified sterol ratio drops due to a somewhat more selective removal of the free sterols. In general, the total level of sterols is not dramatically lowered.[3,7] Comparison of crude and refined oils from the same batch confirms this.[6]

Although cholesterol is the major sterol in mammalian cells and ergosterol in yeast and fungal cells, a complex mixture of different sterols characterizes plant cells.

The principal sterols are β-sitosterol, which comprises 45 to 95% of the total sterols in most plants.[8] Campesterol and stigmasterol are present at significant, but lower concentrations. Brassicasterol, another 4-desmethylsterol, is typically found in *Brassicaceae* species such as rapeseed and generally accounts for up to 5 to 10% of total plant sterols. Distribution of the main sterols in some plant sources is indicated in Figure 11.5. These data are derived from the literature and our own analyses.

Typical concentration ranges for food-grade sterols can be found in the *Food Chemical Codex* monograph for sterols.[9] The most common plant sterol profile consists of β-sitosterol 30 to 65%, stigmasterol 0 to 35%, campesterol 10 to 40%,

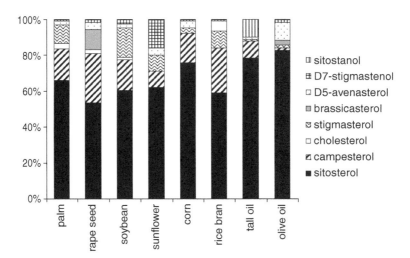

**FIGURE 11.5** Distribution of the main desmethylsterols in some oils. Average values are indicated but may vary.

and a few percent of brassicasterol. The most recent European Novel Foods Specification describes a profile with upper limits for β-sitosterol at 80%, β-sitostanol at 15%, campesterol at 40%, campestanol at 5%, stigmasterol at 30%, brassicasterol at 3%, and a maximum of 3% other sterols/stanols.[10]

### 11.3.2 FOOD SOURCES OF PHYTOSTEROLS

A comprehensive review of important food sources of phytosterols including aspects of ripening, post-harvest, and processing changes in phytosterol contents was published in 2003.[11] All plant foods contain appreciable amounts of phytosterols. In particular, vegetable oils and products made from oils such as spreads and margarine are good sources of plant sterols.[1,8,12] The concentrations found in a recent survey of edible commercially available oils and fats ranges from about 0.05 to 1%.[6] Other foods that contribute to the daily intake of plant sterols are cereal grains, cereal-based products, nuts, legumes, vegetables, and fruits.[13,14] Table 11.2 gives an overview of typical foods sources of plant sterols.

Plant stanols are also found in some foods, but at much lower concentrations. They are found in some cereal grains such as rye, corn, and wheat and in nonhydrogenated vegetable oils.[15,16] They are also found in plant material from coniferous trees such as pine and spruce.

### 11.3.3 COMMERCIAL SOURCES

On commercial scale, plant sterols are mainly derived from edible vegetable oils, such as sunflower, rapeseed, or soybean, as well as from tall oil, which is a product obtained in the wood pulping industry. The term *tall oil* is derived from the Swedish "tallolja" meaning pine oil. Tall oil sterols typically contain up to

**TABLE 11.2**
**Phytosterol Contents of Typical Foods**

| Food | Total Plant Sterols, mg/100 g |
|---|---|
| **Fats and Oil** | |
| Corn oil (refined) | 715–952 |
| Rapeseed oil (refined) | 250–731 |
| Soybean oil (refined) | 221–328 |
| Olive oil (extra virgin) | 144–150 |
| Palm oil (refined) | 49–61 |
| Vegetable oil margarine, full-fat | 310 |
| Vegetable oil margarine, half-fat | 140 |
| **Nuts** | |
| Almonds | 143 |
| Peanuts | 220 |
| Walnuts | 108 |
| **Grain and Cereal Products** | |
| Corn | 178 |
| Rye | 91–110 |
| Barley | 59–83 |
| Wheat | 60–69 |
| Wheat germs | 344 |
| Cornflakes | 26 |
| Bran flakes | 65 |
| Oat bran | 46 |
| Wheat bran | 200 |
| Rye bread | 51 |
| Wheat bread | 54 |
| **Fruits** | |
| Apples, banana, grapefruit, melons, kiwi, orange, peach, pear, pineapple | 1.3–44 |
| **Vegetables** | 4–50 |
| Broccoli | 39 |
| Carrots | 16 |
| Cauliflower | 40 |
| Mushrooms | 18 |
| Olives, green and black | 35/50 |
| Tomato | 5 |
| White cabbage | 13 |

*Source:* Data from References 8, 11, 13, and 14.

85% β-sitosterol, about 8 to 15% sitostanol, 5 to 10% campesterol, and a number of minor sterols and stanols at low concentrations (<1.5% each). Stanols are obtained by hydrogenation of plant sterols.

## 11.4  DIETARY INTAKE OF PHYTOSTEROLS

The average daily intake of plant sterols varies between 150 mg/day with a typical Western European diet to 400 mg/day for a Japanese and Mexican diet.[17–21] Data from a more recent Dutch cohort showed that the daily intake of plant sterols was 307 ± 104 mg/day for men and 263 ± 84 mg/day for women.[22] The major plant sterols were β-sitosterol with 64% of the total sterol intake followed by campesterol with 18%. The main food sources contributing to the daily plant sterol intake were bread, in particular fiber-rich bread and vegetable oils and fats with 36 and 26% of the total plant sterol intake. For vegetarians the intake of plant sterols is in the range of 500 mg to 1 g.[23,24] The daily intake of plant stanols has been less well studied. Available data report an intake in the magnitude of about 25 mg/day.[22,25] The dietary intake of plant stanols comes mainly from the consumption of fiber-rich breads and cereal-based products.

## 11.5  HEALTH BENEFITS OF PHYTOSTEROLS

### 11.5.1  PLASMA CHOLESTEROL-LOWERING EFFECT

The most important physiological effect of phytosterols relates to their cholesterol-lowering action. The cholesterol-lowering properties of plant sterols were discovered in the early 1950s, when Peterson et al.[26–28] observed that soybean sterols prevented the expected increase in plasma cholesterol normally seen in cholesterol-fed chicken. Later it was shown that plant sterols could significantly reduce plasma cholesterol concentrations in humans.[29] Since then, numerous studies both in animals and humans have demonstrated the total- and LDL-cholesterol-lowering effect of plant sterols. The early studies with normo- and hyperlipidemic subjects and with children having familial hypercholesterolemia used pharmacological treatments of mainly pure sitosterol preparations of different origin in doses up to 50 g/day.[30,31]

The interest in the pharmacological treatment with plant sterols peaked during the 1970s and declined later due to the high doses required to achieve a significant cholesterol-lowering effect from the poorly soluble plant sterol preparations. The high doses were related to the less-optimal crystal form in the early pharmaceutical formulations. Interest in phytosterols was regained in the 1980s when it was shown that the physical properties and thus the handling of phytosterols could be improved by esterification with fatty acids. The esterification resulted in both better efficacy and food formulation properties; plant sterol and stanol esters are very similar in behavior to vegetable oils, thus allowing easy incorporation into different food products and uptake in the dietary mixed micelles in the gut.

Numerous studies over the recent years have shown that food products enriched with plant sterol and stanol esters can effectively lower plasma total and LDL cholesterol concentrations. Several reviews have summarized the wealth of evidence that administration of plant sterols and stanols in the form of conventional food products are effective in lowering cholesterol in humans.[32–36] There is no difference in the inhibition of intestinal cholesterol absorption, and thus there is no difference in the cholesterol-lowering efficacy between plant sterol and stanol esters.[36] Although esterification of plant sterols and stanols eases their incorporation into a food matrix due to increased solubility in the fat phase of the product, recent studies suggest that properly formulated free phytosterols may be as effective as sterol and stanol esters in lowering total and LDL cholesterol.[3,36–38] However, further studies with a direct head-to-head comparison of free vs. esterified phytosterols would be useful to fully clarify this aspect.

Recently, in a meta-analysis of 41 studies with various plant sterol or stanol enriched foods it was concluded that the optimal daily dose of phytosterols is 2 g/day, which results in a 10% reduction in LDL cholesterol. Higher doses add only little additional effect.[35] Long-term efficacy studies lasting up to 1 year have shown that phytosterol ester intake consistently lowered total and LDL cholesterol, demonstrating that the effect is sustained when phytosterol-enriched foods are regularly ingested.[39,40]

## 11.5.2 Anti-Atherogenic Effects of Phytosterols

So far, no long-term studies on the effect of phytosterols on atherosclerosis and thus coronary heart disease (CHD) risk reduction in humans are available. Animal studies, however, have convincingly shown beneficial, anti-atherogenic effects. More than 30 studies have investigated the effect of plant sterols on experimental atherosclerosis models in different animals, such as rabbits, knockout mice, and hamsters.[41–46] These studies have shown clear protective effects, e.g., reduction in arterial lipid accumulation, plaque development, and/or lesion size due to the cholesterol-lowering action of plant sterols. Although one study found no regression of established atherosclerotic lesions, the lesion-size increase was smaller in the plant sterol–fed group compared to control.[47]

*In vitro* studies utilizing vascular smooth muscle cells (VSMC) isolated from rats have found that plant sterols stimulated prostacyclin release from VSMC suggesting that natural plant sterols may prevent VSMC hyperproliferation, which could play a beneficial role in atherosclerosis development.[48] A more recent *in vitro* study with macrophages found a reduced release of prostaglandins possibly offering protection from atheroma development via affecting platelet aggregation or vasodilatation of blood vessels.[49]

Human studies have yet not demonstrated clear possible benefits of phytosterols on other risk factors related to the development of atherosclerosis besides the substantial reduction of total and LDL cholesterol. For example, coagulation and fibrinolytic parameters as well as endothelial markers such as vascular cell adhesion molecule 1 (VCAM) and intercellular adhesion molecule 1 (ICAM) and inflammation markers, i.e., C-reactive protein (CRP), were not significantly affected after plant sterol or stanol intake.[50,51] In a study with children with familial hypercholesterolemia, short-term phytosterol intake did not improve endothelial dysfunction as measured by flow-mediated dilation despite the clear reduction in LDL cholesterol.[52] Therefore, it is still uncertain whether plant sterols contribute to the anti-atherosclerotic effect with other possible effects next to lowering LDL cholesterol.

### 11.5.3 ANTI-INFLAMMATORY EFFECTS AND EFFECTS ON THE IMMUNE SYSTEM

Some evidence suggests that phytosterols, particularly plant sterols, may have anti-inflammatory activity. Suggested mechanisms for such an activity are possibly via inhibition of secretion of inflammatory markers such as interleukin-6 (IL-6) or tumor necrosis factor alpha (TNF-$\alpha$) by monocytes.[53] Furthermore, some beneficial effects of doses of plant sterols and sterolins ($\beta$-sitosterol glucosides) as low as 60 mg/day on immune function and virological markers have been suggested.[53] These benefits of phytosterols are believed to play a preventive role in various diseases such as pulmonary tuberculosis, HIV, stress-induced immune suppression, allergic reactions, and rheumatoid arthritis; however, the available evidence is weak and inconclusive. Considering that the normal dietary plant sterol intake is around 150 to 400 mg/day, it seems doubtful whether such an additional low intake of phytosterols could result in distinct effects on the immune function.

### 11.5.4 ANTIOXIDANT ACTIVITY

There is some evidence suggesting that plant sterols have a possible antioxidant activity.[54] For example, delta-5 avenasterol found in high concentrations in oats may have antioxidant activity.[55] Under *in vitro* conditions, sitosterol and sitosterol glucosides were found to decrease lipid peroxidation of platelet membranes.[56] In a human study, the intake of plant stanols not only lowered LDL cholesterol, but also decreased oxidized LDL, an atherogenic lipoprotein, suggesting that plant sterols may be beneficial in protecting LDL oxidation.[57] Whether phytosterols indeed have distinct antioxidant properties and whether these have any relevance to human health await further investigation.

### 11.5.5 BENEFICIAL EFFECTS ON PROSTATIC HYPERPLASIA

Symptomatic benign prostatic hyperplasia is a common medical condition in older men.[58] Clinical symptoms of benign hyperplasia have been shown to be improved by dietary supplementation of small doses (60 to 130 mg/day) of $\beta$-sitosterol.[59]

An increased urinary flow rate and a decreased residual urinary volume was demonstrated after sitosterol treatment.[60] These beneficial effects of $\beta$-sitosterol were seen after 6 months in the treated men, and were maintained for 18 months.[59]

However, data on long-term safety and ability to prevent complications related to benign prostatic hyperplasia are lacking.

The mechanisms responsible for such an effect on the prostate remain unclear, but may be related to an altered testosterone metabolism.[61,62] Androgens play a major role in human prostatic carcinogenesis, but the precise mechanisms by which they affect this process are yet unknown. As plant sterols might interfere with the testosterone metabolism, they might not only favor a preventive effect on the development of benign hyperplasia, but also of prostatic cancer. Several studies indicate that plant sterols may have a beneficial effect against various forms of cancer.[63,64] These aspects are addressed in another part of this book (Chapter 12).

## 11.5.6 POSSIBLE HEALTH CONCERNS AND SAFETY ASPECTS

Phytosterols have been used for their cholesterol-lowering properties for the last half century, originally as pharmaceutical formulations and lately in the form of enriched foods. They have been found to be efficacious and safe. A series of safety studies have been conducted for both pharmaceutical formulations such as Cytellin® as well as for plant sterol and stanol esters added to foods.[65–76] These studies have shown no evidence of genotoxicity, no effect on the reproductive system including estrogenicity, no toxicity in animal studies, and no indication of adverse effects in human studies. Safety of phytosterols has been reviewed by several regulatory agencies. The U.S. Food and Drug Administration has concluded that phytosterol esters are asserted to be generally recognized as safe (GRAS). It was further confirmed that the absorption of plant sterols and stanols is low. Regular intake of plant sterols results in an increase in plasma concentrations of $\beta$-sitosterol and campesterol by 20 to 40% and 40 to 70%, respectively.[40,77–80] In contrast, plant stanols lower plasma plant sterol concentrations by 15 to 45%, while causing an increase in plasma stanol concentrations by 45 to 120%.[81]

In absolute terms, the increase in plasma plant sterols is in the magnitude of 0.02 mmol/L, that of plant stanols is about 0.0005 mmol/L, as compared to a reduction in LDL cholesterol of on average 0.4 to 0.5 mmol/L. In view of the other possible health benefits, e.g., anticancer and antioxidant activities of natural plant sterols, one could argue whether a specific plasma concentration range could be desirable, while consumption of a dietary component that lowers those concentrations might perhaps be unfavorable.[3]

Epidemiological studies, both cross-sectional and case-control studies, suggested that even slightly elevated plasma concentrations of plant sterols, similar to pathologically high plasma concentrations as seen in sitosterolemia, might be associated with an increased risk of CHD.[82–84] Sitosterolemia is a rare inherited disease characterized by hyperabsorption of plant sterols. These findings do not, however, reveal a consistent positive association between plasma plant sterol concentrations and CHD risk independent of plasma cholesterol. Hence, the validity of this association remains hypothetical. At the low concentrations of serum plant sterols found in healthy subjects, it is unlikely that plant sterols are more atherogenic than cholesterol itself. Vegetarians have a higher dietary intake of plant sterols resulting in an approximate doubling of the concentrations of sitosterol and campesterol in their plasma. However, vegetarians have a lower risk of CHD compared to the general population.[23]

Plasma plant sterol concentrations, in particular sitosterol, are influenced by dietary intakes. In a study with postmenopausal hyperandrogenic women it was shown that adopting a plant-based diet rich in nuts, seeds, and soy foods led to higher plasma concentrations of plant sterols, with plasma sitosterol and campesterol increased by 20 to 22%.[85]

In a recent study the intriguing question about the potential atherogenic properties of phytosterols was approached by studying different types of transgenic mice: ABC G5/8 knockout mice with 30- to 100-fold increases in plasma plant sterol concentrations as well as hypercholesterolemic mice lacking both ABC G5/8 and the LDL receptor.[86] Despite the elevated plasma plant sterol concentrations (~12 to 30% of the circulating plasma sterols) in these knockout models, few or no atherosclerotic lesions were found. Even in the severely hypercholesterolemic mice (ABC G5/8, LDLr double knockout) with significant atherosclerosis, the increase in plasma plant sterols did not lead to more aortic lesions. These data suggest that plant sterols are not more atherogenic than cholesterol at least in mice.[86]

Interestingly, plasma plant sterol concentrations measured in subjects from the Dallas Heart Study did not show any association with CHD; whereas plasma cholesterol concentrations were significantly higher in subjects with a family history of CHD. Moreover, coronary calcium scores, a marker of the degree of atherosclerosis, were also not related to plasma plant sterol concentrations in this large cohort of subjects at risk of CHD. These data provide strong evidence that in humans an elevated plasma concentration of plant sterols is not associated with atherosclerosis.[86]

As plant sterols interfere with intestinal cholesterol absorption, a potential concern relates to their effects on the absorption of fat-soluble vitamins and carotenoids. Several studies have shown that regular intake of foods enriched in plant sterols and stanols does not affect plasma concentrations of retinol, vitamin D and K, but significantly lowers the plasma concentrations of carotenoids and vitamin E.[35,36] As carotenoids and vitamin E are transported by lipoproteins, usually their concentrations are standardized for plasma lipid concentrations. After such lipid standardization, plasma concentrations of tocopherols generally remain unaltered, whereas the concentrations for alpha- and beta-carotene and lycopene are decreased by up to 20%. In these studies, carotenoid concentrations remained still within the normal inter-individual range and typical seasonal variations.[87] Whether this reduction in plasma carotenoids is of clinical importance remains to be established. Moreover, the phytosterol-induced decrease in plasma carotenoid concentrations can be counterbalanced by consuming more fruits and vegetables.[88]

Phytosterols are incorporated into cellular membranes similar to cholesterol and may influence membrane properties.[89] Specific changes in membrane properties have been observed *in vitro*, but these may not translate to *in vivo* situations.[90] Ratnayake et al.[91] studied the effects of phytosterols in stroke-prone spontaneously hypertensive (SHRSP) rats and observed that increased incorporations of plant sterols led to deformity of red blood cell membranes. In addition, the survival time of these SHRSP rats was shortened after plant sterol and stanol intake, perhaps because phytosterols replace cholesterol in the erythrocyte membranes, which may make them less deformable and more fragile.[92] SHRSP rats may have at least two relevant defects, which lead to these abnormal reactions to dietary plant sterols/stanols. First, they express a defect in the *ABC g5* gene, which results in an increased accumulation of plant sterols/stanols in tissues.[93] Second, they may have a defect in cell membrane cholesterol metabolism. Whether these effects are relevant for humans is questionable. In fact, after long-term intake of plant sterols, no adverse effects on red blood cell membrane fragility in normo- and hypercholesterolemic subjects were reported.[40] Also, other studies did not show changes in osmotic fragility in red blood cells, as measured by hemolysis, after plant sterol or stanol intake.[94]

## 11.6 METABOLISM OF PHYTOSTEROLS

### 11.6.1 ABSORPTION OF PHYTOSTEROLS

Despite the structural similarity between cholesterol and the major phytosterols, their absorption by mammalian intestine is low. Salen et al.[95] have demonstrated that the absorption rate of β-sitosterol in hypercholesterolemic subjects was 5%, while that of cholesterol ranged from 45 to 54%. Using an intestinal perfusion technique, the intestinal sterol absorption as measured in ten healthy males averaged 33% for cholesterol, 10% for campesterol, 5% for stigmasterol, and 4% for β-sitosterol.[96] More recently, Ostlund et al.[97] found absorption of 0.5% for sitosterol, 1.9% for campesterol and of 0.04% for sitostanol and 0.16% for campestanol. Like cholesterol, phytosterols are solubilized in mixed micelles. Phytosterol esters from the diet appear to be hydrolyzed by pancreatic ester hydroxylase (cholesterol esterase).

Sterol absorption was, for a long time, believed to be by passive diffusion. It is now believed that sterol absorption is a protein-mediated process involving specific transporters. Several receptors and transporters seem involved in facilitating sterol influx into enterocytes and efflux back into the intestinal lumen although exact details of the mechanism or mechanisms are still not fully elucidated.[98,99] Given the small structural differences between cholesterol and phytosterols, this process must be a very selective mechanism. The ABC transporter proteins, ABC G5 and ABC G8, are involved in the excretion or efflux of phytosterols and to a lesser degree of cholesterol out of the enterocytes back into the intestinal lumen.[100] Effectively, this means that the majority of noncholesterol sterols entering the intestinal cells is pumped back into the lumen, and hence limits their absorption. This knowledge was triggered by an increased nonselective sterol hyper-absorption and accumulation of plant sterols in tissues in sitosterolemia (also known as phytosterolemia), a rare autosomal recessive disorder characterized by defects and thus reduced efficacy of these efflux transporters.[101,102]

These ABC G5/G8 half-transporters are genetically controlled with highest expression levels in liver and intestine. Expression levels are upregulated by cholesterol feeding in mice. Moreover, upregulation of these transporters is dependent on activation of nuclear hormone receptors. Many regular food constituents can act as ligands for these receptors.[103] Recent work has identified both *ABCG5* and *ABCG8* in the intestine as target genes of the oxysterol nuclear hormone receptors: liver X receptor LXRα and LXRβ.[104] Cholesterol as well as phytosterol oxidation products may act as such ligands with a high potency.[105,106] The same transporters also act in the liver to remove sterols from the blood compartment into the bile. The concerted action of these transporters and the inherent selectivity toward cholesterol result in low phytosterol absorption at the gut level and high excretion level at the liver; the net result is a low plasma noncholesterol sterol concentration.

While the selective removal of phytosterols from the intestinal cells or from the plasma compartment is now clearly linked to the activity of these efflux transporters, recently a new transporter involved in the receptor-mediated entry or influx into enterocytes has been identified. The uptake of cholesterol and/or phytosterols from the dietary mixed micelles requires active transport. Several enterocyte membrane proteins, for example, the scavenger receptor class B member I (SR-BI), have been suggested to facilitate intestinal sterol influx;[107] however, animal studies investigating their role in sterol absorption were not able to support this hypothesis.[108] Whether the SR-BI receptor is located at the apical or basolateral side of the enterocyte, as well as the direction of transport of cholesterol, is still under discussion. The current level of understanding is that this transporter is present at both sides of the enterocytes, but expression levels vary over the gut length underlining the hypothesis that SR-BI is involved with both cholesterol uptake (proximal small intestine) and excretion (more distal).[109]

Recently, again via understanding the molecular mechanism of a rare disease by reproducing the phenotype in a knockout model, the responsible transporter has been identified and named Niemann-Pick C1 like 1 (NPC1L1) protein. It has been postulated that this influx-transporter imports cholesterol and other sterols into the intestinal cells and thus plays a critical role in the cholesterol absorption process.[110] A new class of cholesterol absorption blockers interferes with this transporter and as such reduces cholesterol concentration in plasma.[111,112] Another ABC transporter, ABCA1, located at the basolateral side of the enterocyte has also been suggested to play a role in sterol absorption[113] by promoting efflux of sterols out of the enterocyte. Within the enterocyte, cholesterol and a fraction of phytosterols are esterified by Acyl CoA: cholesterol acyltransferase 2 (ACAT2). The intestinal esterification of sterols by ACAT2 is, however, less efficient for phytosterol than for cholesterol,[114] perhaps contributing to the lower absorbability of phytosterols.

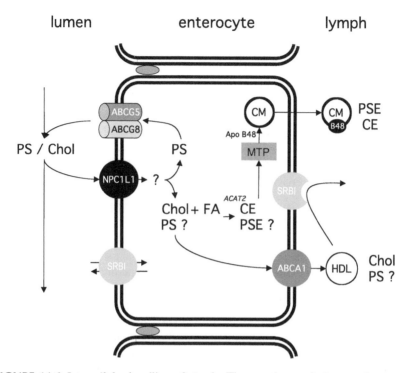

**FIGURE 11.6** Intracellular handling of sterols. The question mark denotes the not-yet-understood sorting mechanism that differentiates between sterols and noncholesterol sterols. ABC = adenosine triphosphate binding cassette, ACAT = acyl-coenzyme A:cholesterol acyltransferase, CM = chylomicrons, ApoB48 = apolipoprotein B48, MTP = microsomal triacylglycerol transfer protein, HDL = high-density lipoprotein, NPC1L1 = Niemann Pick like protein C 1, SRBI = scavenger receptor class B member I.

The overall description of the sterol influx and efflux process is shown in Figure 11.6. As the uptake and efflux for cholesterol and noncholesterol sterols follow the same pattern on the luminal apical side of the enterocyte, the question that now arises is about the sorting mechanism in the cell between cholesterol and noncholesterol sterols.[115]

## 11.6.2 EFFECT OF PHYTOSTEROLS ON CHOLESTEROL ABSORPTION

Phytosterols lower plasma cholesterol concentrations by inhibiting intestinal cholesterol absorption, with a consequential increase in fecal excretion of cholesterol and its intestinal breakdown products. Several studies have directly measured the effect of increased dietary phytosterol intake on cholesterol absorption. Both plant sterols and stanols reduce intestinal cholesterol absorption to a similar extent. Intakes of 0.7 to 9.0 g/day of plant sterols or stanols resulted in a reduction in cholesterol absorption in the range of 7 to 69%.[36] An intake of 2 g/day of plant sterols or stanols reduces cholesterol absorption by 30 to 40%, leading to a 10%

lowering of LDL cholesterol. Whether the physical state, i.e., free vs. esterified phytosterols, has any impact on the cholesterol absorption efficacy is debated and depends highly on their solubilization in the gut. Regarding the mechanisms of action of inhibiting cholesterol absorption, different mechanisms such as competition with cholesterol for solubilization in dietary mixed micelles, co-crystallization with cholesterol to form insoluble mixed crystals, interference with the hydrolysis process by lipases and cholesterol esterase, as well as transport-mediated processes of cholesterol uptake contribute to the cholesterol-lowering action.[107]

### 11.6.3 DISTRIBUTION AND METABOLISM: POST-ABSORPTIVE FATE OF PHYTOSTEROLS

Similar to cholesterol, absorbed phytosterols are carried in plasma by chylomicrons (CM), mainly as unesterified, free sterols.[114] Despite the different distribution of cholesterol and phytosterols in CM particles, plant sterols appear not to influence CM metabolism.[116] Similar to cholesterol, plant sterols are taken up by the liver in the form of CM remnants and these plant sterols are secreted into the blood as a lipid constituent of VLDL particles.[101]

Because of their low absorption and effective biliary secretion, the total phytosterol concentration in plasma is less than 1 mg/dl = 0.025 mmol/l[116] and represents less than 0.4% of total plasma sterols in healthy subjects. Data on the distribution of phytosterols in different lipoproteins in humans are scarce. The concentrations of plant sterols seem to parallel those of cholesterol with LDL and HDL as the major transporters of phytosterols. In a fasting state following a normal consumption of phytosterols, about 70% are found in LDL, 24% in HDL, and 6% in VLDL.[117] In contrast to CM, the percent of esterified phytosterol in VLDL and LDL is identical to that of cholesterol in the corresponding lipoprotein fractions.[118] The biochemical properties of phytosterol-rich VLDL and LDL are not different from phytosterol-poor VLDL and LDL. In humans, the relative proportion of phytosterols in peripheral tissues, in blood, and in monocytes matched that of plasma VLDL and LDL, indicating that phytosterols and cholesterol are taken up equally by tissues.[119,120] Phytosterols carried in HDL were also shown to be selectively secreted into bile.[118] This observation concurs with the fact that the phytosterol/cholesterol ratio in bile is usually higher than that in plasma. Taken together, these data indicate that HDL plays an important role in the elimination of phytosterols from the body.

Phytosterols taken up by cells can be stored in the cytoplasm or incorporated into the cell membranes. So far, no data have shown that plant sterols influence physical or biological properties of cell membranes such as red blood cell deformability or fragility. No evidence has shown that phytosterols might be different from cholesterol with regard to the regulation of the activities of LDL receptor, cholesteryl ester-transfer protein, or lecithin-cholesterol acyl transferase (LCAT). Some reports show that phytosterols have a lesser capacity to suppress HMG-CoA reductase activity when compared with cholesterol. In cultured human macrophages incubated with 100 μg/ml of sitosterol, HMG-CoA reductase activity was not affected, whereas cholesterol under the identical experimental conditions suppressed the activity of this enzyme by 53%.[121] In rats fed or infused with phytosterols, HMG-CoA reductase activity was not decreased.[122,123] These findings indicate that the cholesterol-lowering action of phytosterols is not via suppressing endogenous cholesterol synthesis. Labeled sitosterol and campesterol were found in adrenal glands, ovary, and testis of animals, providing evidence that plant sterols follow similar metabolic pathways to that of cholesterol.[74]

### 11.6.4 EXCRETION

Phytosterol elimination by excretion into bile has been shown to be similar to that of cholesterol and takes place primarily via the biliary route[124] with a minor fraction excreted through the skin.[118,125] The endogenous phytosterol pool size is low compared to cholesterol due to the lesser absorption in the intestine and the faster excretion via the bile.[95,126,127] Sterols have varying half-lives, reflecting the different types of body pools. The short initial $t_{1/2\alpha}$ reflects the fast distribution into the various body tissues with a rapid excretion, while the second and longer $t_{1/2\beta}$ reflects elimination from tissue with storage function. The $t_{1/2\alpha}$ for campesterol and sitosterol are estimated at $4.1 \pm 0.3$ and $2.9 \pm 0.2$ days, respectively, compared to those of sitostanol and campestanol at $1.8 \pm 0.2$ and $1.7 \pm 0.1$ days, respectively.[97] The slow mixing pool consists of approximately 35% of the total sitosterol pool[128] and has a $t_{1/2\beta}$ of 12.7 days.[95]

In contrast to cholesterol from which $C_{24}$ bile acids are formed, it is not established whether plant sterols are the precursor for $C_{24}$ bile acid synthesis and results are conflicting. Salen et al.[95] reported that intravenously administered 22,23-$^3$H-sitosterol was efficiently transformed into cholic and chenodeoxycholic acid in humans. In contrast, no significant conversion into labeled $C_{24}$ bile acids was found after administration of 4-$^{14}$C sitosterol.[129] In rats a conversion of plant sterols into bile acids could also not be shown.[130] Moreover, the end products of plant sterol hydroxylation appear not to be conventional $C_{24}$ bile acids but rather more polar $C_{21}$ bile acids. Recent evidence indicates that plant sterols that lose their side chain end up catabolized like cholesterol in the different organs.[74]

Data on the metabolic fate of plant stanols are lacking and it is not certain whether they are catabolized in a similar manner as plant sterols and cholesterol.

The differentiation made by the body into cholesterol and noncholesterol sterols seems to be dependent on the similarity (or lack of similarity) with cholesterol. Absorption and excretion rates are inversely related to the similarity with cholesterol. The combined effect of this is a low-plasma concentration for noncholesterol sterols. A schematic presentation of the combined effect of absorption and excretion rate on the plasma concentration is shown in Figure 11.7.

## 11.7 CONCLUSION

Phytosterols refer to a class of naturally occurring compounds found in plants that include the plant sterols sitosterol, campesterol, and stigmasterol as well as

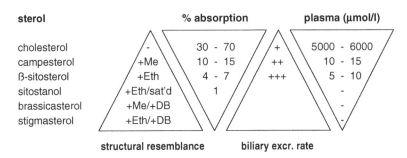

**FIGURE 11.7**  Schematic presentation of the effect of absorption and biliary excretion on the plasma concentration. Me = methyl group on C24; Eth = ethyl group at C24; sat'd = fully saturated phytosterol = stanol; +DB = presence of an additional double bond in the sterol structure.

some other minor sterols. Plant stanols, i.e., sitostanol and campestanol, are the fully saturated forms of plant sterols. While plant sterols are natural dietary components that occur abundantly in many foods, plant stanols are found in much smaller concentrations in food sources, such as cereal grains and are present in material from coniferous trees such as pine.

Phytosterols have been used because of their cholesterol-lowering properties for the past half-century. They have been shown be to safe and effective in lowering plasma total and LDL cholesterol concentrations. The importance of their cholesterol-lowering effect has been acknowledged in recent dietary recommendations, e.g., the recent National Cholesterol Education Program (NCEP III) guidelines.[131] The underlying mechanisms of the cholesterol-lowering action relate to the inhibition of intestinal cholesterol absorption and more in-depth insight into the molecular actions on how phytosterols inhibit cholesterol absorption have been elucidated in recent years. In addition to their well-established cholesterol-lowering effect, other potential health benefits are described. However, evidence for such promising effects, e.g., antioxidant and anti-inflammatory actions, as well as benefits on the immune system are still in a rudimentary stage and more research is clearly needed to draw firm conclusions.

Being present in a normal diet at levels up to a few hundred milligrams, the absorption and excretion of phytosterols are regulated in a way very similar, but not identical to cholesterol. Nature has evolved the human body genetically to handle noncholesterol sterols in an efficient way.[132] In fact, for phytosterols, for which no established human physiological role exists, the absorption and excretion processes are optimized to minimize circulating levels. At the same time, no harmful side effects are described for phytosterols upon normal dietary or even increased dietary intakes. Their safety upon increased intake levels has been reviewed by many regulatory bodies resulting in approvals for their use in foods for normal consumption. Recently, an expert panel concluded that their positive health effects outweigh a potential risk, if any.[35] Even at extreme testing conditions, with respect to intake levels, in both animal and human studies no indication could be obtained for any toxicological or harmful effects. More importantly, no adverse effects have been reported since their introduction as functional food ingredients.

## REFERENCES

1. Piironen V, Lindsay DG, Miettinen TA, Toivo J, Lampi AM. Plant sterols: biosynthesis, biological function and their importance to human nutrition. *J Sci Food Agric* 2000; 80:939–966.
2. Clouse SD. Brassinosteroids — plant counterparts to animal steroid hormones? *Vitam Horm* 2002; 65:195–223.
3. Moreau RA, Whitaker BD, Hicks KB. Phytosterols, phytostanols, and their conjugates in foods: structural diversity, quantitative analysis, and health-promoting uses. *Prog Lipid Res* 2002; 41:457–500.
4. Wojciechowski ZA. Biochemistry of phytosterol conjugates. In: *Physiology and Biochemistry of Sterols*. Patterson GW, Nes WD, eds. Champaign, IL: American Oil Chemists' Society; 1991:361–394.
5. Verleyen T, Forcades M, Verhe R, Dewettinck K, Huyghebaert A, De Greyt W. Analysis of free and esterified sterols in vegetable oils. *J Am Oil Chem Soc* 2002; 79:117–122.
6. Phillips KM, Ruggio DM, Toivo JI, Swank MA, Simpkins AH. Free and esterified sterol composition of edible oils and fats. *J Food Compost Anal* 2002; 15:123–142.
7. Kochhar SP. Influence of processing on sterols of edible vegetable-oils. *Prog Lipid Res* 1983; 22:161–188.
8. Weihrauch JL, Gardner JM. Sterol content of foods of plant origin. *J Am Diet Assoc* 1978; 73:39–47.
9. Anonymous. Vegetable oil phytosterol esters. In: *Committee on Food Chemicals Codex*, Food Chemicals Codex. Washington DC: The National Academic Press, 2004:492–494.
10. Commission of the European Communities. Commission Decision 31 March 2004. *Official Journal of the European Commission* 2004; 105:46–47.
11. Piironen V, Toivo J, Puupponen-Pimia R, Lampi AM. Plant sterols in vegetables, fruits and berries. *J Sci Food Agric* 2003; 83:330–337.
12. Itoh T, Tamura T, Matsumoto T. Sterol composition of 19 vegetable oils. *J Am Oil Chem Soc* 1973; 50:122–125.
13. Normén L, Johnsson M, Andersson H, van Gameren Y, Dutta P. Plant sterols in vegetables and fruits commonly consumed in Sweden. *Eur J Nutr* 1999; 38:84–89.
14. Normén L, Bryngelsson S, Johnsson M, Evheden P, Ellegard L, Brants H, Andersson H, Dutta P. The phytosterol content of some cereal foods commonly consumed in Sweden and in the Netherlands. *J Food Compost Anal* 2002; 15:693–704.
15. MacMurry TA, Morrison WR. Composition of wheat-flour lipids. *J Agric Food Chem* 1970; 21:520–528.
16. Barnes PJ. Non-saponifiable lipids in cereals. *Lipids in Cereal Technology*. London: Academic Press; 1983:33–55.
17. Cerqueira MT, Fry MM, Connor WE. Food and nutrient intakes of the Tarahumara Indians of Mexico. *Am J Clin Nutr* 1979; 32:905–915.

18. Hirai K, Shimazu C, Takezoe R, Ozeki Y. Cholesterol, phytosterol and poly-unsaturated fatty-acid levels in 1982 and 1957 Japanese diets. *J Nutr Sci Vitaminol (Tokyo)* 1986; 32:363–372.

19. Morton GM, Lee SM, Buss DH, Lawrance P. Intakes and major dietary sources of cholesterol and phytosterols in the British diet. *J Hum Nutr Diet* 1995; 8:429–440.

20. Phillips KM, Tarrago-Trani MT, Stewart KK. Phytosterol content of experimental diets differing in fatty acid composition. *Food Chem* 1999; 64:415–422.

21. Schothorst RC, Jekel AA. Oral sterol intake in the Netherlands: evaluation of the results obtained by GC analysis of duplicate 24-h diet samples collected in 1994. *Food Chem* 1999; 64:561–566.

22. Normen AL, Brants HAM, Voorrips LE, Andersson NA, van den Brandt PA, Goldbohm RA. Plant sterol intakes and colorectal cancer risk in the Netherlands Cohort Study on Diet and Cancer. *Am J Clin Nutr* 2001; 74:141–148.

23. Vuoristo M, Miettinen TA. Absorption, metabolism, and serum concentrations of cholesterol in vegetarians — effects of cholesterol feeding. *Am J Clin Nutr* 1994; 59:1325–1331.

24. Jenkins DJA, Kendall CWC, Popovich DG, Vidgen E, Mehling CC, Vuksan V, Ransom TPP, Rao AV, Rosenberg-Zand R, Tariq N, Corey P, Jones PJH, Raeini M, Story JA, Furumoto EJ, Illingworth DR, Pappu AS, Connelly PW. Effect of a very-high-fiber vegetable, fruit, and nut diet on serum lipids and colonic function. *Metabolism* 2001; 50:494–503.

25. Czubayko F, Beumers B, Lammsfuss S, Lutjohann D, Vonbergmann K. A simpli-fied micromethod for quantification of fecal excretion of neutral and acidic sterols for outpatient studies in humans. *J Lipid Res* 1991; 32:1861–1867.

26. Peterson DW. Effect of soybean sterols in the diet on plasma and liver cholesterol in chicks. *Proc Soc Exp Biol Med* 1951; 78:143–147.

27. Peterson DW, Nichols CW. Some relationships among dietary sterols, plasma and liver cholesterol levels, and atherosclerosis in chicks. *J Nutr* 1952; 47:57–65.

28. Peterson DW, Shneour EA, Peek NF, Gaffey HW. Dietary constituents affecting plasma and liver cholesterol in cholesterol-fed chicken. *J Nutr* 1953; 50:191–201.

29. Pollak OJ. Reduction of blood cholesterol in man. *Circulation* 1953; 7:696–701.

30. Lees AM, Mok HYI, Lees RS, McCluskey MA, Grundy SM. Plant sterols as cholesterol-lowering agents — clinical trials in patients with hypercholesterolemia and studies of sterol balance. *Atherosclerosis* 1977; 28:325–338.

31. Pollak OJ, Kritchevsky D. Sitosterol. *Monogr Atheroscler* Basel: Karger; 1981.

32. Jones PJH, MacDougall DE, Ntanios F, Vanstone CA. Dietary phytosterols as cholesterol-lowering agents in humans. *Can J Physiol Pharmacol* 1997; 75:217–227.

33. Law M. Plant sterol and stanol margarines and health. *Br Med J* 2000; 320:861–864.

34. Moghadasian MH, Frohlich JJ. Effects of dietary phytosterols on cholesterol metabolism and atherosclerosis: clinical and experimental evidence. *Am J Med* 1999; 107:588–594.

35. Katan MB, Grundy SM, Jones P, Law M, Miettinen T, Paoletti R. Efficacy and safety of plant stanols and sterols in the management of blood cholesterol levels. *Mayo Clin Proc* 2003; 78:965–978.

36. Normén L, Frohlich JJ, Trautwein EA. Role of plant sterols in cholesterol lowering. In: *Dutta PC, ed. Plant Sterols: Analytical, Nutritional, and Safety Aspects as Functional Food.* New York: Marcel Dekker; 2004:243–315.

37. Ostlund REJ, Spilburg CA, Stenson WF. Sitostanol administered in lecithin micelles potently reduces cholesterol absorption in humans. *Am J Clin Nutr* 1999; 70:826–831.

38. Plat J, Kerckhoffs DAJM, Mensink RP. Therapeutic potential of plant sterols and stanols. *Curr Opin Lipidol* 2000; 11:571–576.

39. Miettinen TA, Puska P, Gylling H, Vanhanen H, Vartainen E. Reduction of serum cholesterol with sitostanol-ester margarine in a mildly hypercholesterolemic population. *N Engl J Med* 1995; 333:1308–1312.

40. Hendriks HFJ, Brink EJ, Meijer GW, Princen HMG, Ntanios FY. Safety of long-term consumption of plant sterol esters-enriched spread. *Eur J Clin Nutr* 2003; 57:681–692.

41. Ikeda I, Kawasaki A, Samezima K, Sugano M. Anti-hypercholesterolemic activity of beta-sitostanol in rabbits. *J Nutr Sci Vitaminol (Tokyo)* 1981; 27:243–251.

42. Moghadasian MH, McManus BM, Pritchard PH, Frohlich JJ. "Tall oil"-derived phytosterols reduce atherosclerosis in ApoE-deficient mice. *Arterioscler Throm Vasc Biol* 1997; 17:119–126.

43. Ntanios FY, Jones PJH. Effects of variable dietary sitostanol concentrations on plasma lipid profile and phytosterol metabolism in hamsters. *Biochim Biophys Acta* 1998; 1390:237–244.

44. Moghadasian MH, McManus BM, Godin DV, Rodrigues B, Frohlich JJ. Pro-atherogenic and antiatherogenic effects of probucol and phytosterols in apolipoprotein E-deficient mice — possible mechanisms of action. *Circulation* 1999; 99:1733–1739.

45. Volger OL, Mensink RP, Plat J, Hornstra G, Havekes LM, Princen HMG. Dietary vegetable oil and wood derived plant stanol esters reduce atherosclerotic lesion size and severity in apoE*3-Leiden transgenic mice. *Atherosclerosis* 2001; 157:375–381.

46. Ntanios FY, van der Kooij A, de Deckere AM, Duchateau GSMJE, Trautwein EA. Effects of various amounts of dietary plant sterol esters on plasma and hepatic sterol concentration and aortic foam cell formation of cholesterol-fed hamsters. *Atherosclerosis* 2003; 169:41–50.

47. Moghadasian MH. Pharmacological properties of plant sterols — *in vivo* and *in vitro* observations. *Life Sci* 2000; 67:605–615.

48. Awad AB, Smith AJ, Fink CS. Plant sterols regulate rat vascular smooth muscle cell growth and prostacyclin release in culture. *Prostag Leukotr Ess Fatty Acids* 2001; 64:323–330.

49. Awad AB, Toczek J, Fink CS. Phytosterols decrease prostaglandin release in cultured P388D¹/MAB macrophages. *Prostag Leukotr Ess Fatty Acids* 2004; 70:511–520.

50. Plat J, de Jong A, Bragt M, Mensink R. Plant sterol and stanol esters do not influence markers for endothelial function and inflammation in subjects on statin treatment despite a significant reduction in LDL cholesterol. *Atheroscler Suppl* 2004; 5:34.

51. Plat J, Mensink RP. Vegetable oil based versus wood based stanol ester mixtures: effects on serum lipids and hemostatic factors in non-hypercholesterolemic subjects. *Atherosclerosis* 2000; 148:101–112.

52. de Jongh S, Vissers MN, Rol P, Bakker HD, Kastelein JJP, Stroes ESG. Plant sterols lower LDL cholesterol without improving endothelial function in prepubertal children with familial hypercholesterolaemia. *J Inherit Metab Dis* 2003; 26:343–351.

53. Bouic PJD. The role of phytosterols and phytosterolins in immune modulation: a review of the past 10 years. *Curr Opin Clin Nutr Metab Care* 2001; 4:471–475.

54. Wang T, Hicks KB, Moreau R. Antioxidant activity of phytosterols, oryzanol, and other phytosterol conjugates. *J Am Oil Chem Soc* 2002; 79:1201–1206.

55. White PJ, Armstrong LS. Effect of selected oat sterols on the deterioration of heated soybean oil. *J Am Oil Chem Soc* 1986; 63:525–529.

56. van Rensburg SJ, Daniels WMU, van Zyl JM, Taljaard JJF. A comparative study of the effects of cholesterol, beta- sitosterol, beta-sitosterol glucoside, dehydroepiandrosterone sulphate and melatonin on *in vitro* lipid peroxidation. *Metab Brain Dis* 2000; 15:257–265.

57. Homma Y, Ikeda I, Ishikawa T, Tateno M, Sugano M, Nakamura H. Decrease in plasma low-density lipoprotein cholesterol, apolipoprotein B, cholesteryl ester transfer protein, and oxidized low-density lipoprotein by plant stanol ester-containing spread: a randomized, placebo-controlled trial. *Nutrition* 2003; 19:369–374.

58. Berry SJ, Coffey DS, Walsh PC, Ewing LL. The development of human benign prostatic hyperplasia with age. *J Urol* 1984; 132:474–479.

59. Berges RR, Kassen A, Senge T. Treatment of symptomatic benign prostatic hyperplasia with beta-sitosterol: an 18-month follow-up. *BJU Int* 2000; 85:842–846.

60. Klippel KF, Hiltl DM, Schipp B. A multicentric, placebo-controlled, double-blind clinical trial of beta-sitosterol (phytosterol) for the treatment of benign prostatic hyperplasia. *Br J Urol* 1997; 80:427–432.

61. Awad AB, Garcia MD, Fink CS. Effect of dietary phytosterols on rat tissue lipids. *Nutr Cancer* 1997; 29:212–216.

62. Awad AB, Hartati MS, Fink CS. Phytosterol feeding induces alteration in testosterone metabolism in rat tissues. *J Nutr Biochem* 1998; 9:712–717.

63. Awad AB, Fink CS. Phytosterols as anticancer dietary components: evidence and mechanism of action. *J Nutr* 2000; 130:2127–2130.

64. Normén L, Anderson SW. Does phytosterol intake affect the development of cancer. In: Dutta PC, eds. *Plant Sterols: Analytical, Nutritional, and Safety Aspects as Functional Food.* New York: Marcel Dekker, 2004:191–242.

65. Baker VA, Hepburn PA, Kennedy SJ, Jones PA, Lea LJ, Sumpter JP, Ashby J. Safety evaluation of phytosterol esters. Part 1. Assessment of oestrogenicity using a combination of in vivo and in vitro assays. *Food Chem Toxicol* 1999; 37:13–22.

66. Hepburn PA, Horner SA, Smith M. Safety evaluation of phytosterol esters. Part 2. Subchronic 90-day oral toxicity study on phytosterol esters-a novel functional food. *Food Chem Toxicol* 1999; 37:521–532.

67. Ayesh R, Weststrate JA, Drewitt PN, Hepburn PA. Safety evaluation of phytosterol esters. Part 5. Faecal short-chain fatty acid and microflora content, faecal bacterial enzyme activity and serum female sex hormones in healthy normolipidaemic volunteers consuming a controlled diet either with or without a phytosterol ester-enriched margarine. *Food Chem Toxicol* 1999; 37:1127–1138.

68. Weststrate JA, Ayesh R, Bauer-Plank C, Drewitt PN. Safety evaluation of phytosterol esters. Part 4. Faecal concentrations of bile acids and neutral sterols in healthy normolipidaemic volunteers consuming a controlled diet either with or without a phytosterol ester-enriched margarine. *Food Chem Toxicol* 1999; 37:1063–1071.

69. Waalkens-Berendsen DH, Wolterbeek APM, Wijnands MVW, Richold M, Hepburn PA. Safety evaluation of phytosterol esters. Part 3. Two-generation reproduction study in rats with phytosterol esters — a novel functional food. *Food Chem Toxicol* 1999; 37:683–696.

70. Whittaker MH, Frankos VH, Wolterbeek APM, Waalkens-Berendsen DH. Two-generation reproductive toxicity study of plant stanol esters in rats. *Regul Toxicol Pharmacol* 1999; 29:196–204.

71. Turnbull D, Frankos VH, van Delft JHM, DeVogel N. Genotoxicity evaluation of wood-derived and vegetable oil-derived stanol esters. *Regul Toxicol Pharmacol* 1999; 29:205–210.

72. Turnbull D, Frankos VH, Leeman WR, Jonker D. Short-term tests of estrogenic potential of plant stanols and plant stanol esters. *Regul Toxicol Pharmacol* 1999; 29:211–215.

73. Turnbull D, Whittaker MH, Frankos VH, Jonker D. 13-week oral toxicity study with stanol esters in rats. *Regul Toxicol Pharmacol* 1999; 29:216–226.

74. Sanders DJ, Minter HJ, Howes D, Hepburn PA. The safety evaluation of phytosterol esters. Part 6. The comparative absorption and tissue distribution of phytosterols in the rat. *Food Chem Toxicol* 2000; 38:485–491.

75. Wolfreys AM, Hepburn PA. Safety evaluation of phytosterol esters. Part 7. Assessment of mutagenic activity of phytosterols, phytosterol esters and the cholesterol derivative, 4-cholesten-3-one. *Food Chem Toxicol* 2002; 40:461–470.

76. Lea LJ, Hepburn PA, Wolfreys AM, Baldrick P. Safety evaluation of phytosterol esters. Part 8. Lack of genotoxicity and subchronic toxicity with phytosterol oxides. *Food Chem Toxicol* 2004; 42:771–783.

77. Weststrate JA, Meijer GW. Plant sterol-enriched margarines and reduction of plasma total- and LDL-cholesterol concentrations in normocholesterolaemic and mildly hypercholesterolaemic subjects. *Eur J Clin Nutr* 1998; 52:334–343.

78. Jones PJ, Raeini-Sarjaz M, Ntanios FY, Vanstone CA, Feng JY, Parsons WE. Modulation of plasma lipid levels and cholesterol kinetics by phytosterol versus phytostanol esters. *J Lipid Res* 2000; 41:697–705.

79. Maki KC, Davidson MH, Umporowicz DM, Schaefer EJ, Dicklin MR, Ingram KA, Chen S, McNamara JR, Gebhart BW, Ribaya-Mercado JD, Perrone G, Robins SJ, Franke WC. Lipid responses to plant-sterol-enriched reduced-fat spreads incorporated into a National Cholesterol Education Program Step I diet. *Am J Clin Nutr* 2001; 74:33–43.

80. Mussner MJ, Parhofer KG, von Bergmann K, Schwandt P, Otto C. Effects of phytosterol ester-enriched margarine on plasma lipoproteins in mild to moderate hypercholesterolemia are related to basal cholesterol and fat intake. *Metabolism* 2002; 51:189–194.

81. Hallikainen MA, Sarkkinen ES, Uusitupa MIJ. Plant stanol esters affect serum cholesterol concentrations of hypercholesterolemic men and women in a dose-dependent manner. *J Nutr* 2000; 130:767–776.

82. Glueck CJ, Speirs J, Tracy T, Streicher P, Illig E, Vandegrift J. Relationships of serum plant sterols (phytosterols) and cholesterol in 595 hypercholesterolemic subjects, and familial aggregation of phytosterols, cholesterol, and premature coronary heart-disease in hyperphytosterolemic probands and their 1st-degree relatives. *Metabolism* 1991; 40:842–848.

83. Sutherland WHF, Williams MJA, Nye ER, Restieaux NJ, De Jong SA, Walker HL. Associations of plasma noncholesterol sterol levels with severity of coronary artery disease. *Nutr Metab Cardiovasc Dis* 1998; 8:386–391.

84. Sudhop T, Gottwald BM, von Bergmann K. Serum plant sterols as a potential risk factor for coronary heart disease. *Metabolism* 2002; 51:1519–1521.

85. Muti P, Awad AB, Schunemann H, Fink CS, Hovey K, Freudenheim JL, Wu YWB, Bellati C, Pala V, Berrino F. A plant food-based diet modifies the serum beta-sitosterol concentration in hyperandrogenic postmenopausal women. *J Nutr* 2003; 133:4252–4255.

86. Wilund KR, Yu L, Xu F, Vega G, Grundy S, Cohen JC, Hobbs H. Plant sterol levels are not associated with atherosclerosis in mice and men. *Arterioscler Throm Vasc Biol* 2004; 24:1–7.

87. Ntanios FY, Duchateau GSMJE. A healthy diet rich in carotenoids is effective in maintaining normal blood carotenoid levels during the daily use of plant sterol-enriched spreads. *Int J Vitam Nutr Res* 2002; 72:32–39.

88. Noakes M, Clifton P, Ntanios F, Shrapnel W, Record I, McInerney J. An increase in dietary carotenoids when consuming plant sterols or stanols is effective in maintaining plasma carotenoid concentrations. *Am J Clin Nutr* 2002; 75:79–86.

89. Child P, Kuksis A. Differential uptake of cholesterol and plant sterols by rat erythrocytes *in vitro*. *Lipids* 1982; 17:748–754.

90. Halling KK, Slotte JP. Membrane properties of plant sterols in phospholipid bilayers as determined by differential scanning calorimetry, resonance energy transfer and detergent-induced solubilization. *Biochim Biophys Acta* 2004; 1664:161–171.

91. Ratnayake WMN, L'Abbe MR, Mueller R, Hayward S, Plouffe L, Hollywood R, Trick K. Vegetable oils high in phytosterols make erythrocytes less deformable and shorten the life span of stroke-prone spontaneously hypertensive rats. *J Nutr* 2000; 130:1166–1178.

92. Ratnayake WMN, Plouffe L, L'Abbe MR, Trick K, Mueller R, Hayward S. Comparative health effects of margarines fortified with plant sterols and stanols on a rat model for hemorrhagic stroke. *Lipids* 2003; 38:1237–1247.

93. Scoggan KA, Gruber H, Lariviere K. A missense mutation in the Abcg5 gene causes phytosterolemia in SHR, stroke-prone SHR, and WKY rats. *J Lipid Res* 2003; 44:911–916.

94. de Jong A, Plat J, Mensink R. Plant sterol or stanol consumption does not change osmotic fragility of the erythrocytes. *Proceedings 7th EAS Congress*, Seville, Spain, April 2004; 2004:115.

95. Salen G, Ahrens EH, Grundy SM. Metabolism of β-sitosterol in man. *J Clin Invest* 1970; 49:952–967.

96. Heinemann T, Axtmann G, Vonbergmann K. Comparison of intestinal absorption of cholesterol with different plant sterols in man. *Eur J Clin Invest* 1993; 23:827–831.

97. Ostlund RE Jr, Mcgill JB, Zeng CM, Covey DF, Stearns J, Stenson WF, Spilburg CA. Gastrointestinal absorption and plasma kinetics of soy delta(5)-phytosterols and phytostanols in humans. *Am J Physiol Endocrinol Metab* 2002; 282:E911–E916.

98. Chen HC. Molecular mechanisms of sterol absorption. *J Nutr* 2001; 131:2603–2605.

99. Allayee H, Laffitte BA, Lusis AJ. Biochemistry — an absorbing study of cholesterol. *Science* 2000; 290:1709–1711.

100. Berge KE, Tian H, Graf GA, Yu LQ, Grishin NV, Schultz J, Kwiterovich P, Shan B, Barnes R, Hobbs HH. Accumulation of dietary cholesterol in sitosterolemia caused by mutations in adjacent ABC transporters. *Science* 2000; 290:1771–1775.

101. Bhattacharyya AK, Connor WE. Beta-sitosterolemia and xanthomatosis. A newly described lipid storage disease in two sisters. *J Clin Invest* 1974; 53:1033–1043.

102. Gregg RE, Connor WE, Lin DS, Brewer HB. Abnormal metabolism of shellfish sterols in a patient with sitosterolemia and xanthomatosis. *J Clin Invest* 1986; 77:1864–1872.

103. Chawla A, Repa JJ, Evans RM, Mangelsdorf DJ. Nuclear receptors and lipid physiology: opening the X-files. *Science* 2001; 294:1866–1870.

104. Repa JJ, Berge KE, Pomajzl C, Richardson JA, Hobbs H, Mangelsdorf DJ. Regulation of ATP-binding cassette sterol transporters ABCG5 and ABCG8 by the liver X receptors alpha and beta. *J Biol Chem* 2002; 277:18793–18800.

105. Bjorkhem I, Meaney S, Diczfalusy U. Oxysterols in human circulation: which role do they have? *Curr Opin Lipidol* 2002; 13:247–253.

106. Kaneko E, Matsuda M, Yamada Y, Tachibana Y, Shimomura I, Makishima M. Induction of intestinal ATP-binding cassette transporters by a phytosterol-derived liver-X receptor agonist. *J Biol Chem* 2003; 278:36091–36098.

107. Trautwein EA, Duchateau GSMJE, Lin Y, Mel'nikov SM, Molhuizen HOF, Ntanios FY. Proposed mechanisms of cholesterol-lowering action of plant sterols. *Eur J Lipid Sci Technol* 2003; 105:171–185.

108. Voshol PJ, Schwarz M, Rigotti A, Krieger M, Groen AK, Kuipers F. Downregulation of intestinal scavenger receptor class B, type I (SR-BI) expression in rodents under conditions of deficient bile delivery to the intestine. *Biochem J* 2001; 356:317–325.

109. Cai SF, Kirby RJ, Howles PN, Hui DY. Differentiation-dependent expression and localization of the class B type I scavenger receptor in intestine. *J Lipid Res* 2001; 42:902–909.

110. Altmann SG, Davis HR, Zhu LJ, Yao X, Hoos LM, Tetzloff G, Iyer SPN, Maguire M, Golovko A, Zeng M, Wang L, Murgolo N, Graziano MP. Niemann-Pick C1 like protein is critical for intestinal cholesterol absorption. *Science* 2004; 303:1201–1204.

111. van Heek M, Farley C, Compton DS, Hoos L, Davis HR. Ezetimibe selectively inhibits intestinal cholesterol absorption in rodents in the presence and absence of exocrine pancreatic function. *Br J Pharmacol* 2001; 134:409–417.

112. van Heek M, Compton DS, Davis HR. The cholesterol absorption inhibitor, ezetimibe, decreases diet-induced hypercholesterolemia in monkeys. *Eur J Pharmacol* 2001; 415:79–84.

113. Repa JJ, Turley SD, Lobaccaro JMA, Medina J, Li L, Lustig K, Shan B, Heyman RA, Dietschy JM, Mangelsdorf DJ. Regulation of absorption and ABC1-mediated efflux of cholesterol by RXR heterodimers. *Science* 2000; 289:1524–1529.

114. Ikeda I, Tanaka K, Sugano M, Vahouny GV, Gallo LL. Discrimination between cholesterol and sitosterol for absorption in rats. *J Lipid Res* 1988; 29:1583–1591.

115. Klett EL, Patel SB. Will the real cholesterol transporter please stand up. *Science* 2004; 303:1149–1150.

116. Salen G, Shefer S, Nguyen L, Ness GC, Tint GS, Shore V. Sitosterolemia. *J Lipid Res* 1992; 33:945–955.

117. Tilvis RS, Miettinen TA. Serum plant sterols and their relation to cholesterol. *Am J Clin Nutr* 1986; 43:92–97.

118. Robins SJ, Fasulo JM. High density lipoproteins, but not other lipoproteins, provide a vehicle for sterol transport to bile. *J Clin Invest* 1997; 99:380–384.

119. Nguyen LB, Shefer S, Salen G, Horak I, Tint GS, McNamara DJ. The effect of abnormal plasma and cellular sterol content and composition on low density lipoprotein uptake and degradation by monocytes and lymphocytes in sitosterolemia with xanthomatosis. *Metabolism* 1988; 37:346–351.

120. Salen G, Horak I, Rothkopf M, Cohen JL, Speck J, Tint GS, Shore V, Dayal B, Chen T, Shefer S. Lethal atherosclerosis associated with abnormal plasma and tissue sterol composition in sitosterolemia with xanthomatosis. *J Lipid Res* 1985; 26:1126–1133.

121. Nguyen LB, Salen G, Shefer S, Tint GS, Ruiz F. Macrophage 3-hydroxy-3-methylglutaryl coenzyme a reductase activity in sitosterolemia: effects of increased cellular cholesterol and sitosterol concentrations. *Metabolism* 2001; 50:1224–1229.

122. Ide T, Gotoh Y, Sugano M. Dietary regulation of hepatic 3-hydroxy-3-methyl-glutaryl-CoA reductase and cholesterol synthetic activities in fasted-refed rats. *J Nutr* 1980; 110:158–168.

123. Boberg KM, Akerlund JE, Bjorkhem I. Effect of sitosterol on the rate-limiting enzymes in cholesterol synthesis and degradation. *Lipids* 1989; 24:9–12.

124. Robins SJ, Fasulo JM, Pritzker CR, Patton GM. Hepatic transport and secretion of unesterified cholesterol in the rat is traced by the plant sterol, sitosterol. *J Lipid Res* 1996; 37:15–21.

125. Bhattacharyya AK, Connor WE, Lin DS. The origin of plant sterols in the skin surface in humans: from diet to plasma to skin. *J Invest Dermatol* 1983; 80:294–296.

126. Grundy SM, Ahrens EH, Jr, Salen G. Dietary beta-sitosterol as an internal standard to correct for cholesterol losses in sterol balance studies. *J Lipid Res* 1968; 9:374–387.

127. Lin DS, Connor WE, Phillipson BE. Sterol composition of normal human bile. Effects of feeding shellfish (marine) sterols. *Gastroenterology* 1984; 86:611–617.

128. Ostlund RE, Mcgill JB, Zeng CM, Covey DF, Stearns J, Stenson WF, Spilburg CA. Gastrointestinal absorption and plasma kinetics of soy delta(5)-phytosterols and phytostanols in humans. *Am J Physiol Endocrinol Metab* 2002; 282:E911–E916.

129. Boberg KM, Einarsson K, Bjorkhem I. Apparent lack of conversion of sitosterol into C24-bile acids in humans. *J Lipid Res* 1990; 31:1083–1088.

130. Subbiah MT, Kuksis A. Differences in metabolism of cholesterol and sitosterol following intravenous injection in rats. *Biochim Biophys Acta* 1973; 306:95–105.

131. Cleeman JI, Grundy SM, Becker D, Clark LT, Cooper RS, Denke MA, Howard WJ, Hunninghake DB, Illingworth DR, Luepker RV, McBride P, McKenney JM, Pasternak RC, Stone NJ, Van Horn L, Brewer HB, Ernst ND, Gordon D, Levy D, Rifkind B, Rossouw JE, Savage P, Haffner SM, Orloff DG, Proschan MA, Schwartz JS, Sempos CT, Shero ST, Murray EZ. Executive summary of the third report of the National Cholesterol Education Program (NCEP) expert panel on detection, evaluation, and treatment of high blood cholesterol in adults (Adult Treatment Panel III). *J Am Med Assoc* 2001; 285:2486–2497.
132. Klett EL, Patel S. Genetic defences against noncholesterol sterols. *Curr Opin Lipidol* 2003; 14:341–345.

# 12 Phytosterols: Bioactivity on Cancer

*Peter G. Bradford and Atif B. Awad*

## CONTENTS

12.1 Dietary Phytosterols: Introduction ........................................................251
12.2 Dietary Phytosterols and Cancer: Epidemiological Studies ................253
12.3 Dietary Phytosterols and Cancer: Animal Experimentation Studies ....255
    12.3.1 Colon Cancer ........................................................................255
    12.3.2 Breast and Prostate Cancer ....................................................257
12.4 Dietary Phytosterols and Cancer: Mechanisms of Action ..................258
    12.4.1 Effects on Apoptosis ..............................................................258
    12.4.2 Effects on Cholesterol Biosynthesis .......................................261
    12.4.3 Effects on Cell Cycle .............................................................261
    12.4.4 Effects on Membrane-Bound Enzymes ..................................262
    12.4.5 Effects on Models of Tumor Metastasis ................................262
    12.4.6 Effects on Immune Function ..................................................263
    12.4.7 Estrogenic Actions .................................................................263
    12.4.8 Effects on Membrane Structure .............................................264
12.5 Conclusions ........................................................................................265
References ......................................................................................................266

## 12.1 DIETARY PHYTOSTEROLS: INTRODUCTION

Phytosterols are plant sterols. The most abundant dietary phytosterols are beta-sitosterol, campesterol, and stigmasterol (Figure 12.1). These are structurally related to cholesterol, but are not made by humans. In humans, the only source of phytosterols is diet and there is only limited absorption of dietary phytosterols. Whereas approximately 50% of dietary cholesterol is absorbed, less than 20% of dietary campesterol and less than 7% of dietary beta-sitosterol are absorbed. The limited absorption of dietary phytosterols is mediated by the cholesterol transporter in the proximal jejunum localized on the surface of the absorptive enterocytes.[1] This common transporter has been identified as Niemann-Pick C1 like 1 protein.[1] The transporter is selectively inhibited by ezetimibe, a drug marketed as Zetia for the reduction of cholesterol absorption and for the treatment of sitosterolemia.[2] Despite the fact that the bulk of phytosterols is transported by

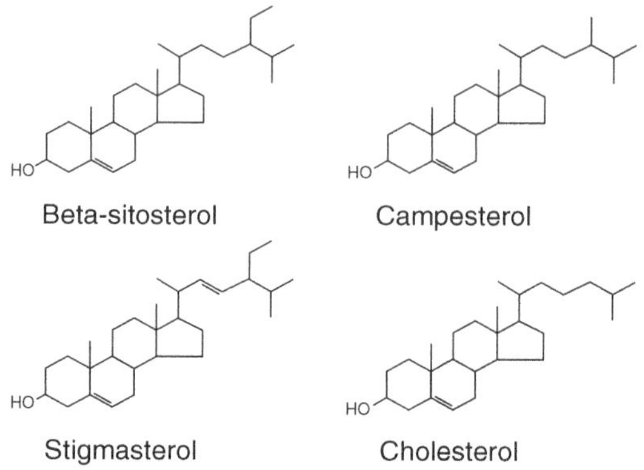

FIGURE 12.1 Structures of common sterols.

the same transporter as cholesterol, the normal low net absorption of phytosterols is the result of selective rapid efflux of phytosterols into the bile and intestinal lumen via the ATP binding cassette co-transporters ABCG5 and ABCG8, expressed on the apical surface of enterocytes as well as hepatocytes.[3–5] Experimental support for this model comes in part from the observation that ABCG5-null mice have significantly elevated levels of beta-sitosterol (37-fold) and campesterol (7.7-fold) compared to wild-type controls.[6] Furthermore, there is clear evidence for a strong founder effect for a novel *ABCG8* mutation in dyslipidemic individuals on the Micronesian island of Kosrae.[7] Heterozygotes and homozygotes for the mutated ABCG8 allele exhibit increased plasma phytosterol levels.[7] However, despite the mechanisms for rapid efflux of absorbed dietary phytosterols, significant levels of phytosterols circulate in the blood of normal, healthy individuals. The concentration of plasma beta-sitosterol in humans ranges from 0.005 to 0.024 mmol/L, depending on diet; whereas in sitosterolemic patients the mean baseline circulating levels of beta-sitosterol and campesterol average 0.50 and 0.27 mmol/L, respectively.[2,7]

Phytosterols from breads and cereals are bioavailable. In a study of 35 healthy subjects that was designed to measure the effects on serum lipids of diets containing high phytosterol, plasma concentrations of beta-sitosterol and campesterol increased significantly while subjects were on a defined diet.[8] The study design monitored sterol levels during a 2-week baseline period during which subjects consumed diets of phytosterol-free foods and then a 12-week period during which subjects consumed phytosterol-enriched foods, averaging 6.6 g phytosterol intake/day. Plasma levels of beta-sitosterol and campesterol were 3.32 ± 1.47 and 3.14 ± 1.53 mg/L at baseline and increased to 5.00 ± 1.86 and 6.62 ± 2.48 mg/L, respectively, after 12 weeks of a diet high in phytosterols. In a separate study, Muti et al.[9] evaluated whether plant food-based diets might increase serum phytosterol levels in postmenopausal women. In this study, subjects consuming diets high in nuts, seeds, and soy for 11 to 16 weeks, without caloric changes, exhibited increases in serum beta-sitosterol up to 20%, confirming the bioavailability of phytosterols from these dietary sources.

**TABLE 12.1**
**Dietary Phytosterols: Effects on the Incidence of Cancers and Hyperproliferative Disorders — Epidemiological Studies**

| Clinical Study Design | Cancer or Disease | Phytosterol Effect | Ref. |
|---|---|---|---|
| Case control | Colorectal | Inhibitory | 10 |
| Randomized, placebo-control | Prostate BPH | Inhibitory | 13 |
| Randomized, placebo-control | Prostate BPH | Inhibitory | 14 |
| Case control | Lung | Inhibitory | 17 |
| Case control | Breast | Inhibitory | 18 |
| Case control | Stomach | Inhibitory | 19 |
| Case control | Esophageal | Inhibitory | 20 |
| Cohort study | Colorectal | No association | 21 |
| Case control | Ovarian | Inhibitory | 24 |

*Note:* Study designs can be found in the text and in the individual references.

## 12.2 DIETARY PHYTOSTEROLS AND CANCER: EPIDEMIOLOGICAL STUDIES

Epidemiological studies suggest that dietary phytosterols confer protection against specific cancers (Table 12.1).

A protective role of dietary phytosterols in colon carcinogenesis had been suggested from early association studies. Seventh-day Adventists, whose principles promote an ovolactovegetarian diet, have relatively high dietary intakes of phytosterols. The estimated average intake of beta-sitosterol and stigmasterol in the Seventh-day Adventists is 344 mg/day, compared to an average intake of 78 mg/day for the general American population.[10] Of significance, is that Seventh-day Adventists experience a lower rate of colorectal cancer, as well as other cancers compared to the general population.[10] This select population also has been determined to have relatively low rates of bile acid excretion. Because bile acids have been reported to function as tumor promoters in colon carcinogenesis, the decreased bile acid secretion in phytosterol-consuming individuals has been proposed to be a physiological mechanism underlying the observed lower colorectal cancer rates in Seventh-day Adventists.[11,12]

A potential therapeutic role for dietary beta-sitosterol has also been reported in patients with benign prostatic hypertrophy (BPH).[13,14] BPH is not prostatic cancer, but rather an enlargement of the central area of the prostate, associated with excessive cellular proliferation in both the glandular and stromal elements. The studies of Berges et al.[13] and of Klippel et al.[14] were multicentered, randomized, double-blind, placebo-controlled clinical trials lasting at least 6 months. Patients with BPH in the active arm of the studies were given either 20 mg beta-sitosterol three times a day[13] or 65 mg of beta-sitosterol twice a day.[14] The Berges et al. study used beta-sitosterol (Harzol, Hoyer, Germany), a phytopharmacological preparation containing mainly beta-sitosterol with smaller amounts of campesterol, stigmasterol, and other sterols along with their glucosides. The Klippel et al. study used beta-sitosterol containing only defined compositions of free phytosterolic compounds (aglycons) produced by current manufacturing processes.

Both the Berges and the Klippel studies showed that supplemental phytosterols were associated with significant symptomatic improvements in prostate function compared to placebo. In the Berges et al.[13] study, all clinical end points including modified Boyarsky scores, International Prostate Symptoms scores, and urinary flow parameters were significantly improved in the beta-sitosterol group without any relevant adverse side effects. Improvements compared favorably to those seen in clinical studies with alpha-receptor-blocking agents or finasteride.[15,16] However, no reduction in prostate volume was detected. Despite this, the Berges study clearly established the efficacy, safety, and benefits of beta-sitosterol therapy in the treatment of BPH. In the Klippel et al.[14] study, patients taking 65 mg free beta-sitosterol twice a day for 6 months showed statistically significant improvements in International Prostate Symptoms scores, peak urinary flow rates, and post-void residual urinary volumes. Prostate volume was not assessed by transabdominal ultrasonography or by any other means. Overall, these two controlled studies suggested that beta-sitosterol affects the enlarged prostate producing symptomatic relief and offers an effective option in the treatment of BPH.

Other case control studies have investigated the role of dietary phytosterols in the risk of specific cancers.[17-20] These studies addressed the question of whether or not phytosterols in the diet offers a potentially protective role in lung cancer, breast cancer, stomach cancer, or esophageal cancer. These case control studies included from 100 to 500 newly diagnosed and histologically verified cases of specific cancers at major hospitals and one to three times as many controls who were frequency-matched on age, gender, residence, and urban/rural status. All patients were interviewed using food frequency questionnaires based on 64 food items considered representative of local diet. Published food composition data were used to assess specific intakes of beta-sitosterol, campesterol, stigmasterol, and total phytosterol. Food groups and relative phytosterol intake were categorized into terciles or quartiles, and the relative risks, approximated by odds ratios (OR), for specific cancers were determined. After controlling for major confounding factors, a potential protective role of dietary phytosterol was observed for the major cancers that were studied: lung cancer, breast cancer, stomach cancer, and esophageal cancer. Total phytosterol intake was associated with specific protective effects in adenocarcinoma of the lung (OR = 0.29, 95% CI = 0.14 to 0.63), breast cancer (OR = 0.41, 95% CI = 0.26 to 0.65), stomach cancer (OR = 0.33, 95% CI = 0.17 to 0.65), and esophageal cancer (OR = 0.21, 95% CI = 0.10 to 0.50).[17-20]

In 2001, the results of a prospective cohort study on plant sterol intake and colorectal cancer were published as an extension of the Netherlands Cohort Study on Diet and Cancer.[21] After 6.3 years of follow-up, 620 colon cancer and 344 rectal cancer cases were detected in the cohort of more than 120,000 subjects. Semiquantitative food frequency questionnaires that included 150 food items were obtained and intakes of plant dietary sterols were determined from responses to questions on fruit, vegetables, potatoes, bread, grains, grain products, cakes, cookies, chocolate, nuts, seeds, peanut butter, and vegetable fats. The questionnaire was validated and tested for reproducibility, concluding that it ranked subjects adequately according to phytosterol intake.[22,23] Total intake of phytosterols in the cohort was calculated as 307.3 ± 103.9 mg/day for men and 262.9 ± 83.7 mg/day for women. The study concluded that in men and women there was no clear association between either plant sterol or stanol intake and colon cancer risk. The exception was for men with high intake of stigmasterol for which there was a negative statistical association with the risk of colon cancer (relative risk = 0.68, 95% CI = 0.46 to 0.99).

McCann et al.[24] examined the relationship between dietary phytochemical intake, including phytosterols, and the risk of ovarian cancer. This case control study included 124 women with incident, primary, histologically confirmed cases of ovarian carcinoma and 696 women serving as case controls frequency-matched for age (40 to 85 years). The investigators used food frequency questionnaires and published food composition data to assess beta-sitosterol, campesterol, stigmasterol, and total phytosterol dietary intake. In the rank analysis, the study found reduced ovarian cancer risk observed for the highest vs. lowest quintile intakes of stigmasterol (OR = 0.42, $p < 0.05$, 95% CI = 0.20 to 0.87). Despite no reduction in ovarian cancer risk related to intake of other phytosterols or total phytosterols, the odds ratios for the highest two quintiles of total phytosterol intake were 0.70 and 0.92, demonstrating a trend toward cancer protection. However, these odds ratios did not achieve levels of significance in this study.

Perhaps because of the limited number of controlled studies, a clear conclusion cannot be made regarding dietary phytosterols and cancer prevention. Epidemiologic analyses and specific controlled studies have demonstrated a cancer protective effect of phytosterols, but other studies of diet and cancer have not supported these conclusions. One must look at the types of studies that were performed: case-control studies, cohort studies, and randomized placebo-controlled trials. Case-control studies are less reliable than either cohort studies or randomized placebo-controlled trials. The determination of a statistical relationship between dietary phytosterol and a lower incidence of specific cancer as seen in most published case-control studies does not necessarily mean that the former caused that latter. However, support for such a conclusion is strengthened by animal experimentation studies discussed below.

## 12.3  DIETARY PHYTOSTEROLS AND CANCER: ANIMAL EXPERIMENTATION STUDIES

### 12.3.1  COLON CANCER

Animal studies have been designed to determine whether or not dietary phytosterols provide protection against colon cancer. These studies assessed the effects of defined dietary intakes of phytosterols on the incidence of colon cancer induced

**TABLE 12.2**
**Dietary Phytosterols: Effects on Animal Experimental Cancer Models**

| Experimental Model | Phytosterol Effect | Ref. |
|---|---|---|
| Colon Cancer | | |
| Rat intracolonic MNU administration | Inhibitory | 25 |
| Rat intracolonic MNU administration | Inhibitory | 26 |
| Rat intracolonic MNU administration | Inhibitory | 27 |
| Rat dietary cholic acid administration | Inhibitory | 29 |
| Rat azoxymethane injection | No effect | 30 |
| Mouse dietary cholic acid administration | Inhibitory | 28 |
| Breast Cancer | | |
| SCID mouse MDA-MB-231 cell injection | Inhibitory | 32 |
| Athymic mouse MCF7 cell injection | Inhibitory | 34 |
| Prostate Cancer | | |
| SCID Mouse PC-3 cell injection | Inhibitory | 33 |

*Note:* Individual experimental details can be found in the text and in the individual references.
MNU = *N*-methyl-*N*-nitrosourea.

by chemical carcinogens or indirectly on any changes in risk factors associated with the development of colon cancer (Table 12.2).

Early studies by Raicht et al.[25] demonstrated that dietary beta-sitosterol protects from colon cancer that was chemically induced by intracolonic administration of *N*-methyl-*N*-nitrosourea (MNU). Rats fed a 2% beta-sitosterol mixture (made up of 95% beta-sitosterol, 4% campesterol, and 1% stigmasterol) in the diet had only one third the number of tumors compared to the control: 0.4 tumors/animal in the beta-sitosterol dietary group vs. 1.3 tumors/animal in the control group. Furthermore, the phytosterol-supplemented diet resulted in a significant reduction in the proportion of animals carrying tumors, 33 vs. 54%, respectively.

Three subsequent studies assessed the effect of dietary phytosterols on cell proliferation of colonic mucosa. The basis of these studies is the proposition that increased colonic mucosal cell proliferation underlies the development of colon cancer and thus is considered a risk factor.[26,27] Using intracolonic administration of MNU to rats on chronic diets containing 0.2% beta-sitosterol, Deschner et al.[27] observed both a reduction in the size of the proliferative compartment as well as in the labeling index of colonocytes in the crypt columns. Janezic and Rao[28] studied the effect of dietary phytosterols on colonic epithelium proliferation in mice. Feeding mice a diet supplemented with 0.3 to 2% phytosterols, along with 0.1% cholic acid, which increases both sterol absorption and baseline cell proliferation, resulted in a dose-dependent reduction in cell proliferation. Phytosterol feeding reduced the number of mucosal cells in the S phase as measured by labeling index assessment. Using rats, Awad et al.[29] confirmed Janezic and Rao's findings on mice. A total of 18 Sprague-Dawley rats were fed one of three diets for 22 days: a control diet, a diet containing 0.2% cholic acid, or a diet containing 0.2% cholic acid plus a 2% phytosterol mixture. The phytosterol mixture contained, by weight, 56% beta-sitosterol, 28% campesterol, 10% stigmasterol, and 6% dihydrobrassicasterol. Cell proliferation in the proximal colon was measured by the bromodeoxyuridine DNA incorporation method. Animals fed the diet containing 0.2% cholic acid had a 65% higher labeling index than the control animals, whereas those fed phytosterols plus cholic acid had labeling index similar to that of the control. With the cholic acid alone diet, there was a 37% expansion of the proliferative zone of the colonic mucosa compared to that in animals on the control or phytosterol diet. This study demonstrates that phytosterols in the diet are associated with reduced colonic cell division after challenge with a proliferative stimulus.

Contrary to these studies, Wargovich et al.[30] reported a lack of effect of dietary beta-sitosterol on the development of aberrant crypt foci in Fisher 344 male rats following injection of the carcinogen azoxymethane. Aberrant crypt foci are preneoplastic lesions in the colon that are induced by administering chemical carcinogens and are an accepted animal model to assess colon cancer.[31] The difference between the results of Wargovich et al. and those from other studies that demonstrated antiproliferative, cancer-protective properties of beta-sitosterol could be due to several factors including the length of the feeding period, the level of beta-sitosterol in the diet, the strain of rodents, or the type of the chemical carcinogen used.

## 12.3.2 BREAST AND PROSTATE CANCER

There have been three reports of animal experiments testing the efficacy of dietary phytosterols in inhibiting the proliferation and development of explanted human breast and prostate cancer cells. The studies involved immune deficient mice lacking either both B and T cells (SCID mice) or just T cells (nude or athymic mice). Awad et al.[32] fed SCID mice semisynthetic diets supplemented with a 2% phytosterol mixture plus 0.2% cholic acid, 2% cholesterol plus 0.2% cholic acid, or 0.2% cholic acid alone. After 2 weeks, animals were injected with MDA-MB-231 estrogen-independent human breast cancer cells into their inguinal mammary fat pads. Mice were maintained on the respective diets for 8 weeks. The phytosterol diet resulted in a 40% decrease in serum cholesterol but a 20-fold increase in serum beta-sitosterol and a 30-fold increase in campesterol concentrations. After 8 weeks, the tumor sizes in the animals fed the phytosterol diet were 33% smaller than those in animals fed the cholesterol diet. Pathological analysis indicated that the tumor cells had metastasized to lymph nodes and lungs in 71% of the cholesterol-fed animals compared to only 57% of the phytosterol-fed animals.

In similar studies using the same protocol, Awad et al.[33] examined the potential protective effect of phytosterols against proliferation and metastasis of PC-3 human prostate cancer cells in male SCID mice. At the end of the 8-week feeding period, there was a 40 to 43% reduction in tumor size in animals fed the

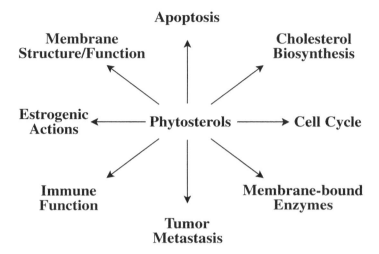

**FIGURE 12.2** Mechanisms of action of dietary phytosterols.

phytosterol diet vs. the cholesterol diet. Animals fed the phytosterol diet had only approximately half the rate of cell metastasis to lung, liver, and lymph nodes compared to those fed the cholesterol diet. In similar human tumor cell explant experiments, Ju et al.[34] reported a 32 to 42% decrease in human breast cancer (MCF7) tumor size in ovariectomized nude or athymic mice fed a diet rich in beta-sitosterol vs. a control, low phytosterol diet.

Results from these experiments using animal models of colon, breast, and prostate cancer support the hypothesis that dietary phytosterols are protective against cancer cell growth and metastasis.

## 12.4 DIETARY PHYTOSTEROLS AND CANCER: MECHANISMS OF ACTION

Phytosterols exert an impact on several cellular systems that could affect cancer initiation or progression (Figure 12.2).

### 12.4.1 EFFECTS ON APOPTOSIS

Programmed cell death or apoptosis is a physiological cell suicide response essential for mammalian homeostasis. Apoptosis is initiated by the activation of a cascade of apoptosis-related cysteine proteases also called cytosolic aspartate-specific proteases or caspases.[35] Depending on the triggers of apoptosis and which initiator caspases are involved, apoptotic pathways are termed either extrinsic or intrinsic.

The extrinsic pathway is triggered by external signals and is mediated by cell surface death receptors. Death receptors belong to the tumor necrosis factor receptor superfamily of receptors, which consist of more than 20 distinct proteins.[36] Upon binding their cognate ligands, death receptors such as Fas, tumor necrosis factor receptor-1, and tumor necrosis-related apoptosis-inducing ligand receptor (TRAILR) aggregate and recruit adaptor molecules such as Fas-associated death domain (FADD) and TRAIL-associated death domain inside the cell. The aggregated death domains in turn recruit, oligomerize, and activate the initiator caspase procaspase-8 through their homologous death effector domains. Activated caspase-8 cleaves the precursor forms of the effector or executioner caspases-3, -6, and -7. Thus activated, the effector caspases cleave specific substrates leading to proteolysis of structural proteins, cleavage and degradation of chromosomal DNA, and ultimately cell death.

The intrinsic pathway is triggered by stresses detected within the cell including growth factor withdrawal, hypoxia, ionizing radiation, and other initiators of cellular damage.[37] The intrinsic pathway involves the mitochondria and the release from the mitochondria of proapoptotic regulators. This mitochondrial checkpoint involves the antiapoptotic protein BCL-2 and the proapoptotic BAX and BAK proteins. Cellular stresses or damage lead to inhibition of BCL-2 and activation of BAX. The resultant mitochondrial damage allows leakage of cytochrome c and the scaffold protein apoptotic protease activating factor-1 (Apaf-1). The conformational change in Apaf-1 induced by its binding cytochrome c allows it to recruit procaspase-9 and oligomerize into a large, ~1-megadalton "apoptosome." Activated caspase-9 subsequently cleaves and activates downstream caspase-3 and caspase-7, leading to apoptosis by mechanisms common to the extrinsic pathway.

Ceramide is a biologically active sphingolipid and functions as an endogenous cancer suppressor.[38] Ceramide is also a strong inducer of apoptosis, particularly through the activation of the intrinsic pathway.[39] Increases in ceramide levels precede the activation of apoptosis mediated by the mitochondrial pathway.[40] Ceramide itself has been shown to increase the permeability of the mitochondrial outer membrane to small proteins.[41] In addition, ceramide-induced apoptosis can be inhibited by the overexpression of the antiapoptotic proteins of the BCL-2 family.[42] Furthermore, BAX regulates the mitochondrial release of cytochrome c and is an activator for ceramide-mediated apoptosis.[43] Other studies have demonstrated the lack of effect of ceramide on the extrinsic apoptotic pathway and on Fas activation in the prostatic carcinoma cell lines PC3 and DU145.[44] However, a role for the extrinsic pathway cannot be discounted, as several cytokines and environmental stresses that initiate apoptosis, including tumor necrosis factor (TNF), Fas, ionizing radiation, ultraviolet-C, heat shock, and oxidative stress, also induce rapid ceramide generation.[45]

Studies have shown that phytosterols, in particular beta-sitosterol, inhibit cell proliferation, induce apoptosis, and activate the ceramide cascade in human transformed cell lines cultured *in vitro* (reviewed in Reference 46) (Table 12.3). Significant induction of cellular apoptosis following beta-sitosterol supplementation has been observed in MDA-MB-231 hormone-insensitive human breast adenocarcinoma cells, in metastatic LNCaP hormone-sensitive human prostate adenocarcinoma cells, and in PC-3 hormone-insensitive human prostate adenocarcinoma

## TABLE 12.3
## Phytosterols: Effects on Sphingolipid Metabolism in Human Tissue Culture Cancer Models

| Experimental Human Cell Line | Phytosterol Effect | Ref. |
|---|---|---|
| HT-29 Colon Cancer | | |
|     Cellular sphingomyelin content | Decreased 50% | 50 |
|     ³H-Serine incorporation into ceramide | Increased 45% | 50 |
| LNCaP Prostate Cancer | | |
|     ³H-Serine incorporation into ceramide | Increased 50% | 48 |
|     Ceramide-activated protein phosphatase | Increased 50% | 48 |

*Note:* All experiments utilized 16 μ*M* beta-sitosterol. Experiments are consistent with enhanced *de novo* sphingomyelin production, increased sphingomyelinase activity, and accumulation of ceramide in phytosterol-treated cells. Details can be found in the text and references.

cells.[33,47,48] At least in some systems, this apoptosis-promoting activity of phytosterols appears to be selective for transformed or carcinogenic cells, as beta-sitosterol does not induce apoptosis in normal human mammary epithelial cells, but does promote apoptosis in transformed human mammary carcinoma cells (Awad et al., unpublished).

While the mechanism by which phytosterols induce these effects is not fully understood, some progress has been in this area using *in vitro* and whole animal experiments. The effects of beta-sitosterol on signal transduction enzymes associated with the regulation of cell growth and apoptosis, including protein kinase C, phospholipase C, and sphingomyelinase have been examined. Feeding rats a semisynthetic diet containing a 2% phytosterol mixture in addition to 0.2% cholic acid for 22 days did not affect protein kinase C activity in their colonic mucosa.[29] Similarly, the activity of phospholipase C, a key enzyme that regulates the synthesis of inositol trisphosphate (IP3) and is coupled to the elevation of intracellular $Ca^{2+}$, was unaffected in phytosterol-treated human colonic HT-29 cells. Together these studies suggest a lack of effect of phytosterols on the phospholipase C-protein kinase C pathways, at least in these systems.[49]

However, significant reductions (~50%) in cellular sphingomyelin (SM) content were observed in HT-29 cells supplemented in culture with beta-sitosterol. These observations suggest that activation of sphingomyelinase and the sphingomyelin cycle may be responsible for the reduction in SM and furthermore may play a causative role in beta-sitosterol-mediated apoptosis in transformed cells.[50] Ceramide is a major second messenger generated by the SM cycle.[51] Several direct targets of ceramide are apoptotic mediators including cathepsin D, a lysosomal protease, and the ceramide-activated protein phosphatases comprising serine/threonine protein phosphatases PP1 and PP2A. Ceramide regulation of cathepsin D leads to activation of the pro-apoptotic protein BID, resulting in apoptosis.[38] Activated PP2A mediates the dephosphorylation of BCL-2, culminating in growth arrest, senescence, and apoptosis.[38] In LNCaP cells, beta-sitosterol supplementation resulted both in increased intracellular ceramide as measured by enhanced $^3$H-serine-labeling of the ceramide pool[48] as well as increased activity of ceramide-activated protein phosphatases.[52] These studies suggest that beta-sitosterol, at physiological serum concentration (16 $\mu M$), accelerates sphingomyelin turnover and ceramide accumulation in transformed cells and that these effects may promote enhanced apoptosis in precancerous or transformed cells.

Studies designed to determine the effects of phytosterol supplementation on apoptosis using MDA-MB-231 and MCF7 breast cancer cells in culture demonstrated growth inhibitory effects of beta-sitosterol and effects consistent with activation of both the intrinsic and the extrinsic apoptotic pathways[53] (Awad et al., unpublished). The 3-day supplementation of breast cancer cells with 16 $\mu M$ beta-sitosterol stimulated activities of caspases-3, -8, and -9. Similar observations were made by Choi et al.[54] using HCT 116 human colon cancer cells. In the latter studies, beta-sitosterol supplementation increased the activation and expression of caspases-3 and -9, the proteolytic cleavage of poly(ADP-ribose)-polymerase, the increased expression of the pro-apoptotic BAX and PPAR proteins, the decreased expression of the anti-apoptotic protein BCL-2, and the release of cytochrome c from mitochondria into the cytosol.

## 12.4.2 Effects on Cholesterol Biosynthesis

The effect of phytosterols on *de novo* cholesterol synthesis has been examined in MDA-MB-231 breast cancer cells.[55] The *de novo* cholesterol synthesis pathway serves at least two functions: it produces cholesterol, which is in high demand in proliferating tumor cells, and it provides isoprenyl-derived moieties such as geranyl and farnesyl intermediates for the functioning of specific proteins involved in signal transduction. Supplementation of cells with cholesterol, campesterol, or beta-sitosterol for 3 days inhibited cholesterol synthesis from acetate.[55] Beta-sitosterol was the most potent inhibitor of cholesterol synthesis from mevalonate when compared to cholesterol or campesterol. There was no difference between cholesterol and campesterol in their potency to inhibit cholesterol synthesis from mevalonate. Because this part of the mevalonate pathway is important for downstream isoprenylation of several proteins in the Ras pathway, which, among its varied activities, regulates cell cycle, it was suggested that this could be one of the mechanisms by which beta-sitosterol inhibits cell growth and the progression of cell cycle.[55] Similar results were observed in HT-29 and HCT 116 human colon cancer cells treated with sphinganine, a precursor of ceramide in the *de novo* synthesis pathway. Colonic cancer cell treatment with sphinganine inhibited cell proliferation and induced apoptosis.[56]

## 12.4.3 Effects on Cell Cycle

The balance between proliferation and apoptosis determines the rate of cell growth and the development and maintenance of normal tissues. These processes may be abnormal in tumors: tumor cells often proliferate at higher rates and have low rates of apoptosis. Accordingly, many anticancer drugs have been developed either to inhibit tumor growth or to stimulate apoptosis. Likewise, nutraceuticals and functional foods have been investigated for their effects on tumor cell growth and apoptosis.[57] Our laboratory studies indicate that beta-sitosterol supplementation of MDA-MB-231 human breast carcinoma cells induces cell cycle arrest at the $G_2/M$ phase.[55] Because a crucial event for progression through the $G_2/M$ checkpoint is the activation of the protein phosphatase Cdc25C, which removes cdc2 inhibitory phosphates,[58] it is possible that phytosterol-mediated events in cells may impinge on this phosphatase and account for its effect on cell cycle progression. This is currently under investigation.

### 12.4.4 EFFECTS ON MEMBRANE-BOUND ENZYMES

Phytosterols may affect membrane-dependent enzymatic activities involved in tumor development. Leikin and Brenner[59] fed rats a 5% phytosterol diet for 21 days and examined changes in liver activities. Beta-sitosterol incorporation into hepatic membranes was increased along with the activities of several fatty acid desaturases ($\Delta 9$, $\Delta 6$, and $\Delta 5$ fatty acid desaturases) in the liver. It was postulated that the increase in desaturase activities was triggered by the altered hepatic membrane rigidity in phytosterol-fed animals. Adjusting the fluidity by producing unsaturated fatty acids of the membranes may in turn influence the activities of membrane-bound enzymes.[60] Work from our laboratory indicated that there was an increase in polyunsaturated fatty acids and a decrease in monounsaturated 16:1 fatty acid concentration in membranes from liver, testis, and prostate of rats fed phytosterol supplemented diets for 21 days.[61] Furthermore, in rats fed a diet containing 2% phytosterol for 21 days, there was an observed inhibition of the activities of 5α-reductase and aromatase in the liver and prostate.[62] Hepatic and prostatic 5α-reductase activities were reduced 33 to 44%, and prostatic aromatase activity was reduced 55% in rats fed phytosterol diets. It was postulated that these effects of dietary phytosterols on enzymes involved in the metabolism of testosterone might influence pathways leading to the development of hormone-dependent prostatic cancer. There is also evidence that phytosterols may inhibit Na,K-ATPase activity in the prostate. Hirano et al.[63] demonstrated that *in vitro* incubation with beta-sitosterol at 1 to 1000 $\mu M$ inhibited Na,K-ATPase activity by 23 to 67% in membranes derived from biopsied benign prostatic hyperplastic tissue.

### 12.4.5 EFFECTS ON MODELS OF TUMOR METASTASIS

Often the prognosis of cancer, as well as the effectiveness of therapy, depends largely on whether or not the primary lesion has metastasized to vital organs. Thus, the effect of dietary phytosterol on tumor metastasis has been investigated *in vivo* and *in vitro*. *In vivo* studies have been reviewed in Section 12.3. *In vitro* models of metastasis have used measurements of cell invasion, migration, and adhesion. By using PC-3 human prostatic adenocarcinoma cells and Transwell chambers coated with 8-μm pore size polycarbonate filters coated with Matrigel, invasion of cells supplemented with or without phytosterols was assessed after 20 h using 20% folate binding protein in the underside of the filter as a chemo-attractant.[33] Cholesterol supplementation positively increased cell invasion by 43%, whereas either campesterol or beta-sitosterol supplementation inhibited invasion by 78%. Migration of cells through uncoated membranes was increased by 67% in cells supplemented with cholesterol but reduced by 60 to 93% in cells supplemented with beta-sitosterol or campesterol.

Phytosterols, particularly campesterol more so than beta-sitosterol, also impaired adhesion of PC-3 to extracellular matrix proteins.[33] Beta-sitosterol supplementation of PC-3 reduced the adhesion of cells to laminin by 15 to 38% and to fibronectin by 23%; whereas no effect was observed on the binding of PC-3 cells to either collagen I or collagen IV. The effects of phytosterols in inhibiting cellular invasion, migration, and adhesion using these *in vitro* models are consistent with their effects in inhibiting metastasis observed *in vivo* (see Section 12.3).

### 12.4.6 EFFECTS ON IMMUNE FUNCTION

Observations have suggested that dietary phytosterols function as immune modulators and may play a role in cancer protection by augmenting immune responses involving natural killer (NK) cells.[64] Bouic et al.[65] first reported studies indicating that a mixture of beta-sitosterol and its glucoside derivative stimulated blood lymphocyte proliferation *in vitro*. The proliferation was accompanied by a profile of cytokine secretion indicative of a selective effect on $T_{H1}$ helper cells. Secretion of the $T_{H1}$ helper cell-selective interleukin 2 (IL-2) and interferon γ (IFNγ) was increased, whereas that of the $T_{H2}$ helper cell-selective IL-4 remained unchanged. Additional studies demonstrated greatly enhanced lytic and cytotoxic activities of NK cells against transformed cell lines after NK cell preincubation with the beta-sitosterol–glucoside mixture. The enhanced cytotoxic activity was speculated to be due to the beta-sitosterol-promoted secretion of IL-2 and IFNγ, which are known to promote NK cell activity. Clinical studies showed immunomodulatory effects of phytosterols in pulmonary tuberculosis, feline immunodeficiency virus, human immunodeficiency virus-infected patients, stress-induced immune suppression, rheumatoid arthritis, and allergic rhinitis/sinusitis.[64]

Phytosterols also affect macrophage function. Beta-sitosterol reduced nitric oxide release induced by phorbol ester from RAW 264.7 macrophages, and this was correlated with the impairment of inducible nitric oxide synthase levels and with NF-κB activation.[66] The growth of $P388D_1/MAB$ macrophages in culture and release of the proinflammatory $PGE_2$ were also inhibited by beta-sitosterol.[67]

### 12.4.7 ESTROGENIC ACTIONS

There is conflicting evidence regarding whether phytosterols have estrogenic activity or influence the activity of estrogens at target sites. Besides the structural similarity as sterols, phytosterols could affect endogenous estrogen levels through alterations in enterohepatic recirculation, by effects on bile acid metabolism, by altering estrogen reabsorption, or through competition with cholesterol as a substrate for steroid hormone synthesis.

Limited early studies identified beta-sitosterol as a non-ethanol congener present in bourbon. In these studies, it was determined that beta-sitosterol possessed weak estrogenic activity when tested using ovariectomized rats and estrogen receptor *in vivo* bioassays.[68,69] Subsequent studies that monitored proliferation of human breast adenocarcinoma (MCF7) cells in culture and that included determinations of reporter gene assays and measurements of specific binding to recombinant human estrogen receptors alpha and beta suggested that phytosterols may be functioning as weak estrogen receptor modulators and might function *in vivo* as endocrine disruptors.[70] These studies showed a good correlation among the three estrogenic assays for the potencies of 11 separate putative estrogenic compounds, including 17-beta-estradiol, estrone, estriol, ethinyl estradiol, diethylstilbestrol, beta-sitosterol, octylphenol, and bisphenol A. Other studies confirmed the growth stimulation of estrogen-dependent MCF7 cells in culture by beta-sitosterol; however, dietary phytosterols reduced estradiol-induced MCF7 tumor growth in ovariectomized athymic nude mice.[34]

Other studies failed to show any estrogen potential of phytosterols. Short-term *in vitro* tests of estrogenic potential, as well as standard safety evaluations of phytosterol esters, failed to demonstrate estrogenic activity of phytosterols or phytostanols.[71,72] For estrogenic activities, these studies measured proliferation of MCF7 cells in culture, uterotrophic activity in immature female rats, competitive binding with the immature rat uterine estrogen receptor, and induction of estrogen-inducible genes in yeast. None of these activities was detectable under phytosterol exposure.[71,72] Furthermore, *in vivo* studies monitoring estrogen-dependent embryo implantation in rats failed to demonstrate estrogenic activity of beta-sitosterol at doses of 30 mg/kg.[73] The discrepancies among these studies require further investigation.

### 12.4.8 EFFECTS ON MEMBRANE STRUCTURE

Several studies have indicated that phytosterols such as beta-sitosterol and campesterol can be incorporated into membranes. Incorporation is not accompanied by an increase in total membrane sterols and has no effect on total membrane phospholipids, suggesting that phytosterols may replace some of the membrane cholesterol. The effect of phytosterol on membrane cholesterol may depend on the type of cell and the length of the supplementation. For example, supplementation of HT-29 cells with 16 $\mu M$ beta-sitosterol for 9 days resulted in 32% cholesterol replacement without affecting the total sterols.[50] In P388D1/MAB macrophages supplemented with beta-sitosterol for 5 days, 26% of the membrane cholesterol was replaced by beta-sitosterol without any effect on total sterol or phospholipids.[67] However, similar beta-sitosterol supplementation of HT-29 cells led to a 50% decrease in membrane sphingomyelin and an 8% increase in phosphatidylcholine without an effect on total sterol. The latter effect was associated with an overall increase in polyunsaturated fatty acids and a decrease in 16:1 fatty acid in these membranes. Such structural alterations suggest that phytosterols may affect membrane fluidity, receptor structure and function, and coupling to signal transduction pathways.

## 12.5 CONCLUSIONS

Lifestyle factors play a significant role both in the promotion of most cancers and in the protection from these cancers. Diet and nutrition are perhaps among the most significant of these lifestyle factors. We have reviewed the effects on cancer prevention of one specific dietary component, the phytosterols. Dietary phytosterols, or plant sterols, have been shown by the majority of the experimental data to be protective against specific cancers, including colorectal, breast, prostate, lung, and stomach carcinomas. This protective role of dietary phytosterols appears to be independent on their effects on cholesterol absorption and is supported by the results from large epidemiological studies, as well as from animal studies and laboratory experimentation with *in vitro* tissue culture models. Epidemiological studies have included case-control studies, cohort studies, and randomized placebo-controlled trials. Although one cohort study showed no association between phytosterol intake and cancer incidence, a majority of all epidemiological studies suggest a significant cancer protective effect of phytosterols. Animal experimentation studies have examined the effects of controlled phytosterol-containing diets in models of colon, breast, and prostate cancer. With some exception, these model systems also support a cancer protective effect of dietary phytosterols. The cellular mechanism of action by which dietary phytosterols might protect against specific cancers may be manifold. One of the principal actions of phytosterols is to promote apoptosis, and experimental results suggest that this effect may be selective for precancerous or cancerous cells. Stimulation of sphingomyelin turnover, generation of ceramide, and induction of the intrinsic and extrinsic pathways of apoptosis are biochemical pathways by which phytosterols might check excess abnormal cell proliferation and cancerous transformation. Experimental effects of phytosterols have also been demonstrated on cholesterol biosynthesis, cell cycle regulation, tumor metastasis, immune function, estrogen system signaling, and membrane structure and function. It will be only through continued experimentation in areas of human epidemiology, animal systems, and cellular biochemistry that the cancer preventative actions of dietary phytosterols can be affirmed and understood.

## REFERENCES

1. Davis HR, Zhu L, Hoos LM, Tetzloff G, Maguire M, Liu J, Yao X, Iyer SPN, Lam MH, Lund EG, Detmers PA, Graziano MP, Altmann SW. Niemann-Pick C1 like 1 (NPC1L1) is the intestinal phytosterol and cholesterol transporter and a key modulator of whole-body cholesterol homeostasis. *J Biol Chem* 2004; 279:33586–33592.

2. Salen G, von Bergmann K, Lütjohann D, Kwiterovich P, Kane J, Patel SB, Musliner T, Stein P, Musser B. Multicenter Sitosterolemia Study Group. Ezetimibe effectively reduces plasma plant sterols in patients with sitosterolemia. *Circulation* 2004; 109:966–971.

3. Graf GA, Li WP, Gerard RD, Gelissen I, White A, Cohen JC, Hobbs HH. Coexpression of ATP-binding cassette proteins ABCG5 and ABCG8 permits their rapid transport to the apical cell surface. *J Clin Invest* 2002; 110:659–669.

4. Yu L, Hammer RE, Li-Hawkins J, Von Bergmann K, Lutjohann D, Cohen JC, Hobbs HH. Disruption of Abcg5 and Abcg8 in mice reveals their crucial role in biliary cholesterol secretion. *Proc Natl Acad Sci USA* 2002; 99:16237–16242.

5. Yu L, Li-Hawkins J, Hammer RE, Berge KE, Horton JD, Cohen JC, Hobbs HH. Overexpression of ABCG5 and ABCG8 promotes biliary cholesterol secretion and reduces fractional absorption of dietary cholesterol. *J Clin Invest* 2002; 110:671–680.

6. Plosch T, Bloks VW, Terasawa Y, Berdy S, Siegler K, Van Der Sluijs F, Kema IP, Groen AK, Shan B, Kuipers F, Schwarz M, Schwartz M. Sitosterolemia in ABC-transporter G5-deficient mice is aggravated on activation of the liver-X receptor. *Gastroenterology* 2004; 126:290–300.

7. Sahayek E, Yu HJ, von Bergmann K, Lutjohann D, Stoffel M, Duncan EM, Garcia-Naveda L, Salit J, Blundell ML, Friedman JM, Breslow JL. Phytosterolemia on the island of Kosrae: founder effects for a novel *ABCG8* mutation results in high carrier rate and increased plant sterol levels. *J Lipid Res* 2004; 45:1608–1613.

8. Clifton PM, Noakes M, Ross D, Fassoulakis A, Cehun M, Nestel P. High dietary intake of phytosterol esters decreases carotenoids and increases plasma plant sterol levels with no additional cholesterol lowering. *J Lipid Res* 2004; 45:1493–1499.

9. Muti P, Awad AB, Schünemann H, Fink CS, Hovey K, Freudenheim J, Yow-Wu B, Bellati C, Pala V, Berrino F. A plant food-based diet modifies the serum-sitosterol concentration in hyperandrogenic postmenopausal women. *J Nutr* 2003; 133:4252–4255.

10. Nair PP, Turjman N, Kessie G, Calkins B, Goodman GT, Davidovitz H, Nimmagadda G. Diet, nutrition intake, and metabolism in populations at high and low risk for colon cancer. Dietary cholesterol, $\beta$-sitosterol, and stigmasterol. *Am J Clin Nutr* 1984; 40:927–930.

11. Cohen BI, Raicht RF. Effects of bile acids on colon carcinogenesis in rats treated with carcinogens. *Cancer Res* 1981; 41:3759–3760.

12. Rao AV, Janezic SA. Dose dependent effects of dietary phytosterol on epithelial cell proliferation in the murine colon. *Food Chem Toxicol* 1992; 30:611–616.

13. Berges RR, Windeler J, Trampisch HJ, Senge T. Randomised, placebo-controlled, double-blind clinical trial of beta-sitosterol in patients with benign prostatic hyperplasia. *Lancet* 1995; 345:1529–1532.

14. Klippel KF, Hiltl DM, Schipp B. A multicentric, placebo-controlled, double-blind clinical trial of beta-sitosterol (phytosterol) for the treatment of benign prostatic hyperplasia. *Brit J Urol* 1996; 80:427–432.

15. Jardin A, Bensadoun H, Delauvauche-Cavallier MC, Attali P. Alfuzosin for treatment of benign prostatic hypertrophy. The BPH-ALF group. *Lancet* 1991; 337:1457–1461.

16. Christensen MM, Bendix Holme J, Rasmussen PC, Jacobsen F, Nielsen J, Norgaard JP, Olesen S, Noer I, Wolf H, Husted SE. Doxazosin treatment with patients with obstruction. A double blind placebo-controlled study. *Scand J Urol Nephrol* 1993; 27:39–44.

17. Mendilaharsu M, De Stefani E, Deneo-Pellegrini H, Carzoglio J, Ronco A. Phytosterols and risk of lung cancer: a case-control study in Uruguay. *Lung Cancer* 1998; 21:37–45.

18. Ronco A, De Stefani E, Boffetta P, Deneo-Pellegrini H, Mendilaharsu M, Leborgne F. Vegetables, fruits, and related nutrients and risk of breast cancer: a case-control study in Uruguay. *Nutr Can* 1999; 35:111–119.

19. De Stefani E, Boffetta P, Ronco AL, Brennan P, Deneo-Pellegrini H, Carzoglio JC, Mendilaharsu M. Plant sterols and the risk of stomach cancer: a case-control study in Uruguay. *Nutr Can* 2000; 37:140–144.

20. De Stafani E, Brennan P, Boffeta P, Rono A L, Mendilaharsu M, Deneo-Pellegrini H. Vegetables, fruits, related dietary antioxidants, and the risk of squamous cell carcinoma of the esophagus: a case-control study in Uruguay. *Nutr Cancer* 2000; 38:23–29.

21. Normén AL, Brants HAM, Voorrips LE, Andersson HA, van den Brandt PA, Goldbohm RA. Plant sterol intakes and colorectal cancer risk in the Netherlands Cohort Study on Diet and Cancer. *Am J Clin Nutr* 2001; 74:141–148.

22. Goldbohm RA, van den Brandt PA, Brants HA, van't Veer P, Al M, Sturmans F, Hermus RJ. Validation of a dietary questionnaire used in a large-scale prospective cohort study on diet and cancer. *Eur J Clin Nutr* 1994; 48:253–265.

23. Goldbohm RA, van't Veer P, van den Brandt PA, van't Hof MA, Brants HA, Sturmans F, Hermus RJ. Reproducibility of a food frequency questionnaire and stability of dietary habits determined from five annually repeated measurements. *Eur J Clin Nutr* 1995; 49:420–429.

24. McCann SE, Freudenheim JL, Marshall JR, Graham S. Risk of human ovarian cancer is related to dietary intake of selected nutrients, phytochemicals and food groups. *J Nutr* 2003; 133:1937–1942.

25. Raicht RF, Cohen BI, Fazzini E, Sarwal A, Takehashi M. Protective effect of plant sterols against chemically-induced colon tumors in rats. *Cancer Res* 1980; 40:403–405.

26. Lipkin M. Proliferative changes in the colon. *Am J Digest Dis* 1974; 19:1029–1032.

27. Deschner EE, Cohen BI, Raicht RF. The kinetics of the protective effect of β-sitosterol against MNU-induced colon neoplasia. *J Cancer Res Clin Oncol* 1982; 103:49–54.

28. Janezic SA, Rao AV. Dose-dependent effects of dietary phytosterols on epithelial cell proliferation of the murine colon. *Food Chem Toxicol* 1992; 30:611–616.

29. Awad AB, Tagle-Hernandez AY, Fink CS, Mendel SL. Effect of dietary phytosterols on cell proliferation and protein kinase C activity in rat colonic mucosa. *Nutr Cancer* 1997; 27:210–215.

30. Wargovich MJ, Chen CD, Jimenez A, Steele VE, Velasco M, Stephens LC, Price R, Gray K, Kelloff GJ. Aberrant crypts as a biomarker for colon cancer: evaluation of potential chemoprotective agents in the rat. *Cancer Epidemiol Biomarkers Prev* 1996; 5:355–360.

31. Bird RP. Observation and quantification of aberrant crypts in the murine colon treated with a colon carcinogen: preliminary findings. *Cancer Lett* 1987; 37:147–151.

32. Awad AB, Downie A, Fink CS, Kim U. Dietary phytosterol inhibits the growth and metastasis of MDA-MB-231 human breast cancer cells grown in SCID mice. *Anticancer Res* 2000; 20:821–824.

33. Awad AB, Fink CS, Williams H, Kim U. *In vitro* and *in vivo* (SCID mice) effect of phytosterols on the growth and dissemination of human prostate cancer PC-3 cells. *Eur J Cancer Prev* 2001; 10:507–513.

34. Ju YH, Clausen LM, Allred KF, Almada AL, Helferich WG. Beta-sitosterol, beta-sitosterol glucoside, and a mixture of beta-sitosterol and beta-sitosterol glucoside modulate the growth of estrogen-responsive breast cancer cells *in vitro* and in ovariectomized athymic mice. *J Nutr* 2004; 134:1145–1151.

35. Adams JM. Ways of Dying: multiple pathways to apoptosis. *Genes Devel* 2003; 17:2481–2495.

36. Debatin KM, Krammer PH. Death receptors in chemotherapy and cancer. *Oncogene* 2004; 23; 2950–2966.

37. Adams A. Mitochondria at the crossroads of life and death. *Scientist* 2004; 18:25–29.

38. Ogretmen B, Hannun YA. Biologically active sphingolipids in cancer pathogenesis and treatment. *Nat Rev Cancer* 2004; 4:604–616.

39. Pettus BJ, Chalfant CE, Hannun YA. Ceramide in apoptosis: an overview and current perspectives. *Biochim Biophys Acta* 2002; 1585:114–125.

40. Perry DK, Carlton J, Shah AK, Daniel P, Uhlinger DJ, Hannun YA. Serine palmitoyl transferase regulates *de novo* ceramide synthesis generation during etoposide-induced apoptosis. *J Biol Chem* 2000; 275:9078–9084.

41. Siskind LJ, Kolesnick RN, Colombini M. Ceramide channels increase the permeability of the mitochondrial outer membrane to small proteins. *J Biol Chem* 2002; 277:26798–26803.

42. Zhang J, Alter N, Reed JC, Borner C, Obeid LM, Hannun YA. Bcl-2 interrupts the ceramide-induced pathway of cell death. *Proc Natl Acad Sci USA* 1996; 93:5325–5328.

43. von Haefen C, Wieder T, Gillissen B, Starck L, Graupner V, Dorken V, Daniel PT. Ceramide induces mitochondrial activation and apoptosis via a Bax-dependent pathway in human carcinoma cells. *Oncogene* 2002; 21:4009–4019.

44. Gewies A, Rokhlin OW, Cohen MB. Ceramide induces cell death in the human prostatic carcinoma cell lines PC3 and DU145 but does not seem to be involved in Fas-mediated apoptosis. *Lab Invest* 2000; 80:671–676.

45. Kolesnick RN, Krönke M. Regulation of ceramide production and apoptosis. *Annu Rev Physiol* 1998; 60:643–665.

46. Awad AB, Chinnam M, Fink CS, Bradford PG. Targeting ceramide by dietary means to stimulate apoptosis in tumor cells. *Curr Topics Nutraceutical Res* 2004; 2:93–100.

47. Awad AB, Downie AC, Fink CS. Inhibition of growth and stimulation of apoptosis by β-sitosterol treatment of MDA-MD-231 human breast cancer cells in culture. *Int J Mol Med* 2000; 5:541–545.

48. von Holtz RL, Fink CS, Awad AB. β-Sitosterol activates the sphingomyelin cycle and induces apoptosis in LNCaP human prostate cancer cells. *Nutr Cancer* 1998; 32:8–12.

49. Awad AB, Ntanios FY, Fink CS, Horvath PJ. Effect of membrane lipid alteration on the growth, phospholipase C activity and G-protein of HT-29 tumor cells. *Prostag Leukotr Ess Fatty Acids* 1996; 55:293–302.

50. Awad AB, Chen Y-C, Fink CS, Hennessey T. Beta-sitosterol inhibits HT-29 human colon cancer cell growth and alters membrane lipids. *Anticancer Res* 1996; 16:2797–2804.

51. Hannun YA. The sphingomyelin cycle and the second messenger function of ceramide. *J Biol Chem* 1994; 269:3125–3128.

52. Awad AB, Gan Y, Fink CS. Effects of β-sitosterol, a plant sterol, on growth, protein phophatase 2A and phospholipase D in LNCaP cells. *Nutr Cancer* 1999; 16:74–78.

53. Awad AB, Roy R, Fink CS. Beta-sitosterol, a plant sterol, induces apoptosis and activates key caspases in MDA-MB-231 human breast cancer cells. *Oncology Res* 2003; 10:497–500.

54. Choi YH, Kong KR, Kim YA, Jung KO, Kil JH, Rhee SH, Park KY. Induction of Bax and activation of caspases during beta-sitosterol-mediated apoptosis in human colon cancer cells. *Int J Oncol* 2003; 23:1657–1662.

55. Awad AB, Williams H, Fink CS. Effects of phytosterols on cholesterol metabolism and MAP kinase in MDA-MB-231 human breast cancer cells. *J Nutr Biochem* 2003; 14:111–119.

56. Ahn EH, Schroeder JJ, Sphingoid bases and ceramide induce apoptosis in HT-29 and HCT 116 human colon cancer cells. *Exp Biol Med* 2002; 227:345–353.

57. Gosslau A, Chen KY. Nutraceuticals, apoptosis, and disease prevention. *Nutrition* 2004; 20:95–102.

58. DiPaola RS. To arrest or not to $G_2$-M cell-cycle arrest. *Clin Cancer Res* 2002; 8:3311–3314.

59. Leikin AI, Brenner RR. Fatty acid desaturase activities are modulated by phytosterol incorporation into microsomes. *Biochim Biophys Acta* 1989; 1005:187–191.

60. Spector AA, Yorek MA. Membrane lipid composition and cellular function. *J Lipid Res* 1985; 26:1015–1035.

61. Awad AB, Garcia DM, Fink CS. Effect of dietary phytosterol on rat tissue lipids. *Nutr Cancer* 1997; 29:212–216.

62. Awad AB, Hartati M, Fink CS. Phytosterol feeding induces alteration in testosterone metabolism in rat tissues. *J Nutr Biochem* 1998; 9:712–717.

63. Hirano T, Homma M, Oka K. Effects of stinging nettle root extracts and their steroidal components on the $Na^+$, $K^+$-ATPase of the benign prostatic hyperplasia. *Planta Med* 1994; 60:30–33.

64. Bouic PJD. The role of phytosterols and phytosterolins in immune modulation: a review of the past 10 years. *Curr Opin Clin Nutr Metab Care* 2001; 4:471–475.

65. Bouic PJD, Etsebeth S, Libenberg RW, Albrecht CH, Pegel K, Van Jaarsveld PP. Beta-sitosterol and beta-sitosterol glucoside stimulate human peripheral blood lymphocyte proliferation: implications for their use as an immunomodulatory vitamin combination. *Int J Immunopharmacol* 1996; 18:693–700.

66. Moreno JJ. Effect of olive oil minor components on oxidative stress and arachidonic acid mobilization and metabolism by macrophages RAW 264.7. *Free Radical Biol Med* 2003; 35:1073–1081.

67. Awad AB, Toczek J, Fink CS. Phytosterols decrease prostaglandin release in cultured P388D1/MAB macrophages. *Prostag Leukotr Ess Fatty Acids* 2004; 70:511–520.

68. Gavaler JS, Rosenblum ER, Van Thiel DH, Eagon PK, Pohl CR, Campbell IM, Gavaler J. Biologically active phytoestrogens are present in bourbon. *Alcoholism Clin Exp Res* 1987; 11:399–406.

69. Rosenblum ER, Stauber RE, Van Thiel DH, Campbell IM, Gavaler JS. Assessment of the estrogenic activity of phytoestrogens isolated from bourbon and beer. *Alcoholism Clin Exp Res* 1993; 17:1207–1209.

70. Gutendorf B, Westendorf J. Comparison of an array of in vitro assays for the assessment of the estrogenic potential of natural and synthetic estrogens, phytoestrogens and xenoestrogens. *Toxicology* 2001; 166:79–89.

71. Turnbull D, Frankos VH, Leeman WR, Jonker D. Short-term tests of estrogenic potential of plant stanols and plant stanol esters. *Regul Toxicol Pharmacol* 1999; 29:211–215.

72. Baker VA, Hepburn PA, Kennedy SJ, Jones PA, Lea LJ, Sumpter JP, Ashby J. Safety evaluation of phytosterol esters. Part 1. Assessment of oestrogenicity using a combination of *in vivo* and *in vitro* assays. *Food Chem Toxicol* 1999; 37:13–22.

73. Cummings AM, Laws SC. Assessment of estrogenicity by using the delayed implanting rat models and examples. *Reprod Toxicol* 2000; 14:111–117.

# Part V

*Dietary Components That Protect from Cancer: Polyphenols*

# 13 Classification, Dietary Sources, Absorption, Bioavailability, and Metabolism of Flavonoids

*Jeremy P.E. Spencer*

## CONTENTS

13.1 Introduction .................................................................................273
13.2 Classification and Abundance ...................................................274
13.3 Flavonoids as Classical Antioxidants ......................................275
13.4 Flavonoid Absorption and Metabolism ....................................277
    13.4.1 Upper GI tract ...............................................................278
    13.4.2 Middle GI Tract and Liver ...........................................279
        13.4.2.1 Flavonoid Glycoside Processing ..................279
        13.4.2.2 Flavonoid Metabolism .................................280
    13.4.3 Lower GI Tract ..............................................................281
13.5 Summary .....................................................................................284
References ..............................................................................................287

## 13.1 INTRODUCTION

Flavonoids have been the center of huge research interest over the past decade.[1–6] They have been attributed to a wide range of beneficial properties regarding human health, including effects on cancer,[7–16] cardiovascular diseases,[14,17–19] atherosclerosis,[20,21] inflammation,[14,22] and other diseases in which oxidative stress has been implicated, such as the neurodegenerative disorders.[3,23–26] A large number of *in vitro* studies have characterized flavonoids as powerful antioxidants against both reactive oxygen and reactive nitrogen species.[4,27–32] Until recently, the ability of flavonoids to act as classical H-donating antioxidants was believed to underlie many of their reported health effects.[10,11,18,21,33,34] However, the extent of their antioxidant potential *in vivo* will be dependent on the absorption, metabolism, distribution, and excretion of these compounds within the body after ingestion and the reducing properties of the resulting metabolites. An understanding of the processes involved in the absorption and distribution of polyphenols is essential for determining their bioactivities *in vivo* and their significance. Recently, much data have accumulated on the biotransformation of flavonoids in the small intestine and gastrointestinal tract,[14,35,35–42] as well as the hepatic metabolism.[38,43,44] This chapter attempts to highlight the major sources of flavonoids in the human diet, draw attention to the main sites of biotransformation of flavonoids within the body, and emphasize the major metabolites that may exert biological activity *in vivo*.

## 13.2  CLASSIFICATION AND ABUNDANCE

Flavonoids comprise the most common group of polyphenolic plant secondary metabolites and play an important role in biological processes. Beside their function as pigments in flowers and fruits, to attract pollinators and seed dispersers, flavonoids are involved in protecting the plant against ultraviolet (UV) damage, in fertility and in disease resistance. Flavonoids are synthesized in plants from phenylpropanoid- and acetate-derived precursors and are ubiquitous to green plant cells.[45,46] All flavonoids are derived from chalcone precursors, which in turn are derived from the action of chalcone synthase on phenylpropanoid and three malonyl-CoA units (Figure 13.1). Chalcone synthase is a plant-specific polyketide synthase (named as type III polyketide synthase) and there are many structurally and functionally related enzymes, such as stilbene synthase and coumaroyltriacetic acid synthase. They regulate plant growth by inhibition of the exocytosis of auxin indolyl acetic acid, as well as by induction of gene expression, and they influence other biological cells in numerous ways. They are widely distributed in plant-derived foods including fruits and vegetables and are among the most abundant polyphenols in the human diet. The primary structure of flavonoids consists of two aromatic carbon groups: benzopyran (A and C rings) and benzene (B ring) (Figure 13.2). They can be divided into six main classes based on the degree of oxidation of the C-ring, the hydroxylation pattern of the ring-structure, and the substitution in the 3-position: flavanols (e.g., epicatechin), flavonols (e.g., quercetin), flavones (e.g., luteolin), flavanones (e.g., naringenin), isoflavones (e.g., genistein), and anthocyanidins (e.g., cyanidin)[4] (Figure 13.2).

As discussed, flavonoids have been found in high concentrations in a wide variety of fruits, vegetables, and beverages such as red wine and tea. However, the various classes of flavonoids and specific flavonoids are concentrated in specific foods or beverages. For example, green tea and cocoa are sources of flavanols such as catechin and epicatechin, citrus fruits are excellent sources of flavanones such as naringenin and hesperetin, and berry fruits have high concentrations of anthocyanins such as cyanidin and malvidin. Table 13.1 highlights some of the main dietary sources of the different groups of flavonoids and the polyphenol content of each flavonoid.

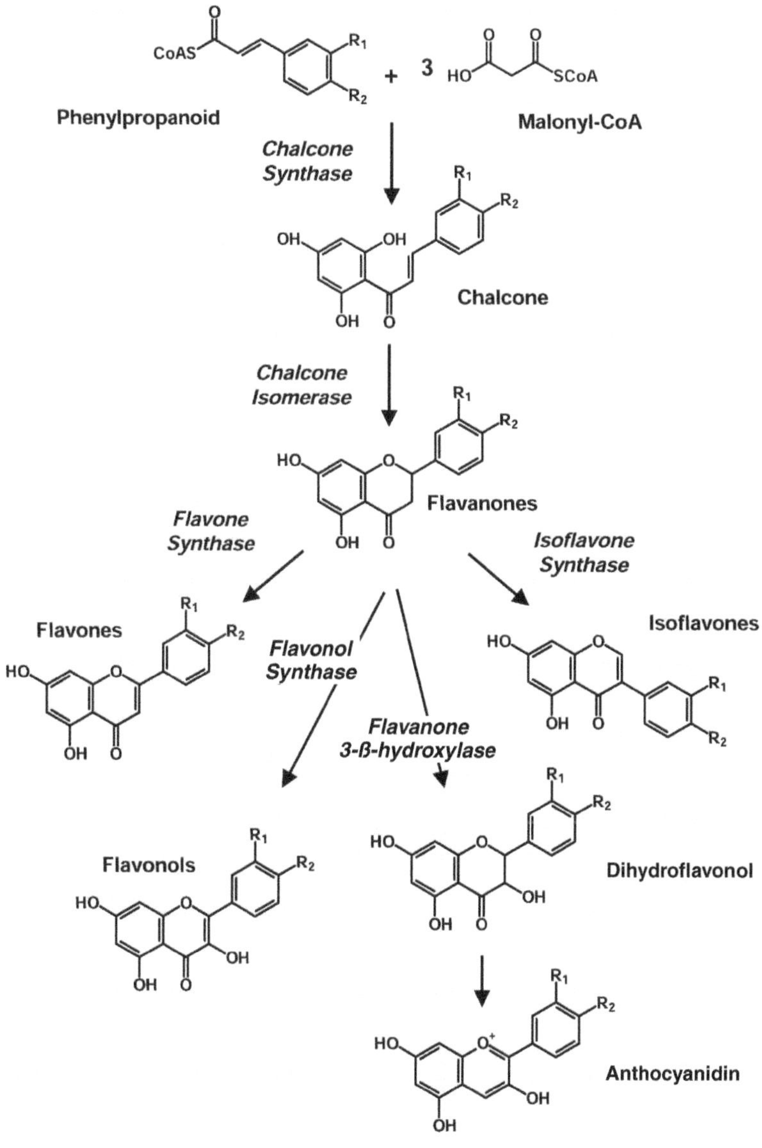

**FIGURE 13.1** The biosynthesis of flavonoids in plants. All flavonoids are derived from chalcone precursors that are derived from phenylpropanoid and three malonyl-CoA and biosynthesized by chalcone synthase (CHS). Various enzymes act to bring about the formation of the various flavonoid classes.

## 13.3 FLAVONOIDS AS CLASSICAL ANTIOXIDANTS

The ability of flavonoids to act as classical electrons (or hydrogen) donating antioxidants *in vitro* has been extensively reported[10,11,18,21,33,34] and used to explain

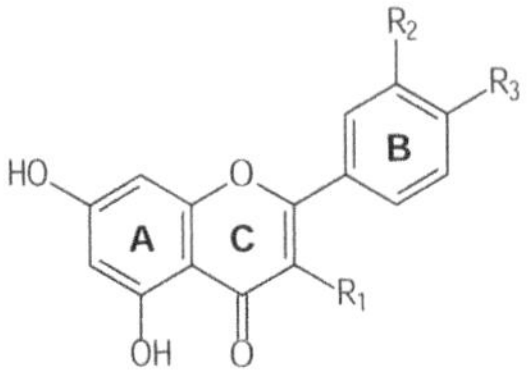

| Flavonols | | | |
|---|---|---|---|
| | R1 | R2 | R3 |
| Quercetin | OH | OH | OH |
| Kaempferol | OH | H | OH |
| **Flavones** | | | |
| Luteolin | H | OH | OH |
| Apigenin | H | H | OH |

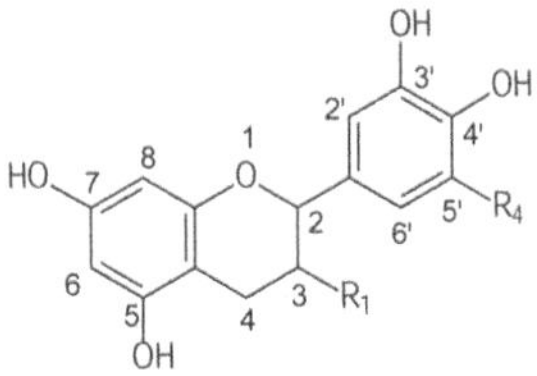

| Flavanols | | |
|---|---|---|
| | R1 | R4 |
| Catechin | OH | H |
| Epicatechin | OH | H |
| EGC | OH | OH |
| ECG | gallate | H |
| EGCG | gallate | OH |

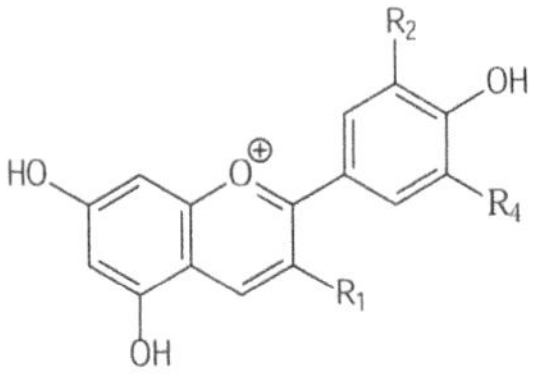

| Anthocyanidins | | | |
|---|---|---|---|
| | R1 | R2 | R4 |
| Cyanidin | OH | OH | H |
| Malvidin | OH | OCH₃ | OCH₃ |
| Delphinidin | OH | OH | OH |

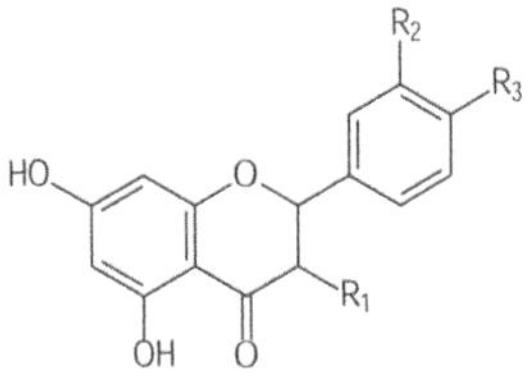

| Flavanones | | | |
|---|---|---|---|
| | R1 | R2 | R3 |
| Taxifolin | OH | OH | OH |
| Naringenin | H | H | OH |
| Hesperetin | H | OCH₃ | H |

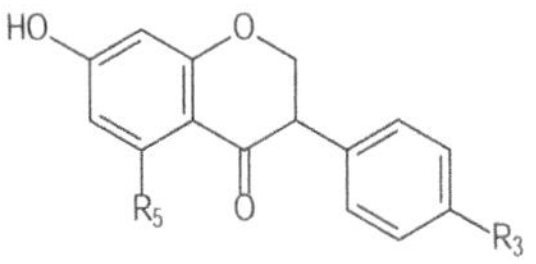

| Isoflavones | | |
|---|---|---|
| | R3 | R5 |
| Genistein | OH | OH |
| Daidzein | OH | H |

**FIGURE 13.2** The structures of the six main classes of flavonoids. The major differences between the individual groups reside in the hydroxylation pattern of the ring-structure, the degree of saturation of the C-ring and the substitution in the 3-position.

**TABLE 13.1**
**Flavonoid-Containing Foods**

| Flavonoid Family | Source | Polyphenol Content (mg/kg or mg/L fresh weight) |
|---|---|---|
| Flavonols | Onion, kale | 300–1200 |
| | Leek, cherry tomato, broccoli, blueberry, black currant, apricot | 50–300 |
| | Apple, green bean, black grape, tomato, black tea, green tea | 0–50 |
| Flavones | Parsley | 200–2000 |
| | Celery | 20–200 |
| | Capsicum pepper | 1–20 |
| Flavanones | Orange, orange juice | 200–1000 |
| | Grapefruit, grapefruit juice | 100–700 |
| | Lemon juice | 50–300 |
| Flavanols | Chocolate, green tea, beans, black tea | 500–1000 |
| | Apricot, cherry, grape, peach, blackberry, apple, red wine, cider | 300–500 10–300 |
| Anthocyanins | Eggplant, blackberry, black currant, blueberry, black grape, cherry | 1000–5000 |
| | Rhubarb | 1000–2000 |
| | Strawberry, red wine, plum, red cabbage | 10–1000 |
| Isoflavones | Soyflour | 1000–2000 |
| | Soybeans, miso, tofu, tempeh, soy milk | 10–1000 |

their protective effects against oxidative stress. Structurally important features that define this antioxidant activity are the hydroxylation pattern, in particular a 3′,4′-dihydroxy catechol structure in the B-ring and the presence of 2,3 unsaturation in conjugation with a 4-oxo-function in the C-ring (Figure 13.3). The antioxidant efficacy of flavonoids has been described for the protection against oxidative damage to a variety of cellular biomolecules. For example, flavonoids inhibit the oxidation of low density lipoprotein[36,47–50] and DNA[51,52] *in vitro*. In addition, flavonoids are effective scavengers of reactive nitrogen species in the form of peroxynitrite[1,53–55] and limit dopamine oxidation mediated by peroxynitrite in a structure-dependent way involving oxidation or nitration of the flavonoid ring system.[56] Furthermore, their antioxidant properties have also been attributed to their abilities to chelate transition metal ions[57–59] and to their potential to quench singlet oxygen.[60,61]

## 13.4 FLAVONOID ABSORPTION AND METABOLISM

Although flavonoids and other polyphenols have been identified as powerful antioxidants *in vitro*, their ability to act as effective antioxidants *in vivo* will be

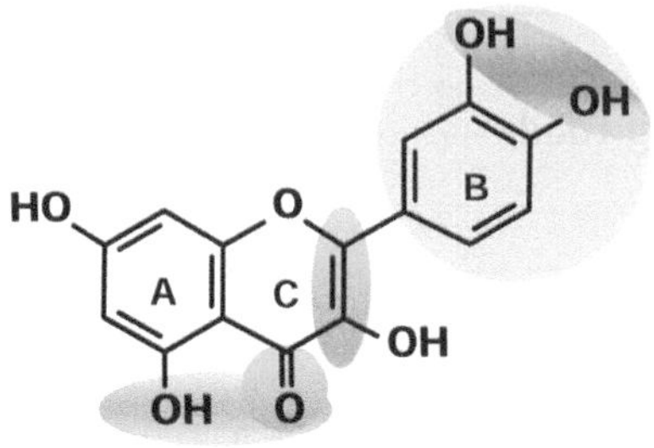

**FIGURE 13.3** Structure of the flavonol quercetin showing features important in defining the classical antioxidant potential of flavonoids. The most important of these is the catechol or dihydroxylated B-ring. Other important features include the presence of unsaturation in the C-ring and the presence of a 4-oxo-function in the C-ring. The catechol group and other functions may also ascribe an ability to chelate transition metal ions such as copper and iron.

dependent on the extent of their biotransformation and conjugation during absorption from the gastrointestinal (GI) tract, in the liver and finally in cells.

### 13.4.1 UPPER GI TRACT

Modifications of flavonoid structure may occur at many points in the GI tract. In the upper GI tract, saliva has been found to cause degalloylation of flavanol gallate esters, such as epigallocatechin gallate[62] but to have little effect on the stability of green tea catechins.[63] The quercetin rutinoside rutin is hydrolyzed by cell-free extracts of human salivary cultures[64,65] and by streptococci isolated from the mouths of normal individuals,[66] but quercetin-3-rhamnoside (quercitrin) is not susceptible to hydrolysis, suggesting that only rutin-glycosidase-elaborating organisms occur in saliva.[65] An interaction of flavanols and procyanidins with salivary proteins has been shown and indicates that (+)-catechin has a higher affinity for proline-rich proteins than (–)-epicatechin and C4–C8-linked procyanidin dimers bind more strongly than their C4–C6 counterparts.[67] This polyphenol–protein binding in the form of adsorption with high-molecular-weight salivary proteins, bacterial cells, and mucous materials may be one explanation for the observed decrease in quercetin mutagenicity after incubation with saliva.[68]

Procyanidin oligomers ranging from a dimer to decamer (isolated from *Theobroma cacao*) have been observed to be unstable under conditions of low pH similar to that present in the gastric juice of the stomach.[69] During incubation of the procyanidins with simulated gastric juice, oligomers rapidly decompose to epicatechin monomeric and dimeric units and also to other oligomeric units primarily, although other oligomeric units, such as trimer and tetramer, were also formed.[69] Thus, absorption of flavanols and procyanidins, for example, after consumption of chocolate or cocoa, are likely to be influenced by preabsorption events in the gastric lumen within the residence time. However, consideration needs to be given to the food matrix, which may influence the pH environment of the procyanidins and their subsequent decomposition. Monomeric flavonoid glycosides have been observed to be stable in the acidic environment of the stomach and are not observed to be undergoing nonenzymatic deglycosylation.[70]

## 13.4.2 MIDDLE GI TRACT AND LIVER

Generally, flavonoids are present in plants conjugated to sugars, and therefore it is these glycosides that are ingested in the diet and enter the GI tract. The exception to this rule is the flavan-3-ols, such as the catechins and procyanidins, which are almost always present in the diet in the nonglycosylated form.[4] There are many factors that influence the extent and rate of absorption of ingested compounds by the small intestine,[53] including physiochemical factors, such as molecular size, lipophilicity, solubility, pKa, and biological factors including gastric and intestinal transit time, lumen pH, membrane permeability, and first-pass metabolism.[71,72]

### 13.4.2.1 Flavonoid Glycoside Processing

Because flavonoid glycosides are relatively polar molecules, their passive diffusion across the membranes of small intestinal brush-border is unlikely. However, many studies have suggested that flavonoid glycosides are subject to the action of β-glucosidases prior to their absorption in the jejunum and ileum,[73–81] and it is generally believed that the removal of the glycosidic moiety is necessary before absorption of the flavonoid can take place. The exceptions to this rule are the anthocyanins that appear to be absorbed intact from the GI tract[82–85] and possibly rutin.[86–88] The cleaved aglycone is thought then to undergo passive diffusion across the intestinal brush-border, although, the exact mechanism of uptake is still unclear. It has been suggested that removal of the sugar and subsequent transport by proteins such as lactate phloridzin hydrolase[77] may occur in the small intestine; however, this process may not occur with all flavonoid glycosides.

Much controversy initially surrounded the absorption of quercetin glucosides in the small intestine[14,74,77] with many initial investigations indicating the absorption of quercetin glucosides in the small intestine.[35,40,41,85,89–92] However, these observations are now questioned. Quercetin glucosides were reported to be absorbed from onions fed to ileotomized volunteers,[90] and recent investigations have postulated that flavonoid glucosides may be absorbed by the small intestine via the sodium-dependent glucose transporter (SGLT-1).[70,93–95] However, a similar study in ileostomy patients, fed a meal containing high concentrations of both quercetin mono- and di-glucosides, resulted in no detection of these compounds in ileostomy fluid.[76] One reason arguing against the uptake of intact quercetin glucosides is that the metabolic capacity of β-glucosidase in the small intestine, and of the liver, is too great for quercetin glucosides to escape deglycosylation.[74] In support of this, the analysis of human plasma using a high-performance liquid chromatography with coularray detection after oral administration of quercetin-3-glucoside or quercetin-4′-glucoside determined that no intact quercetin glucosides were present.[96]

Further investigations into the absorption of quercetin glycosides have been carried out using the caco-2 cell model of the small intestine.[95,97–99] Here observations also suggested the absorption of quercetin glycosides through the human intestinal epithelium via apical MRP2[98] and/or the SGLT-1,[93–95] meaning that the transfer of quercetin glycosides in the small intestine might be possible. However, addition of plasma on the basolateral side significantly reduced the efflux of quercetin by 94%, and therefore the effect of plasma binding can result in an overestimation of basolateral to apical efflux and in misleading net flux calculations in these types of experiments.[99] These studies suggest that quercetin glucosides may be capable of interacting with SGLT-1 in the mucosal epithelium and may therefore be absorbed by the small intestine *in vivo*. Whether they may also escape deglycosylation in the enterocytes and the liver is still to be addressed.

### 13.4.2.2  Flavonoid Metabolism

Many studies have indicated that significant transfer of ingested flavonoids occurs from the lumen of the small intestine to the mesenteric circulation and that extensive metabolism and conjugation of the flavonoid occurs during this transfer.[1,73,100–106] Isolated preparations of rat small intestine[107] have been utilized to study absorption and metabolism in the small intestine and can provide information on events occurring in both the jejunum and ileum.[73,101,106,108–110] Absorption studies, utilizing this model, with a wide range of flavonoids and their glycosides, and hydroxycinnamates show that there was in almost all cases extensive metabolism of the polyphenol in the enterocyte during transfer from the luminal to the serosal side.[73,102,109,111,112] The major products transferred across the small intestinal epithelium were glucuronides of the parent aglycone or of the hydrolyzed glycoside, although *O*-methylated metabolites were also observed[73,101,102,109,111,112] (Figure 13.4). The extent of glucuronidation in these experiments seemed dependent on the flavonoid structure, in that the flavonoids with a substituted hydroxyl group on the B-ring (i.e., hesperetin) were less predisposed to glucuronidation, whereas the flavonoids containing a 3′,4′-ortho-dihydroxy (or catechol) B-ring were transferred predominantly as glucuronides.[73] For example, the jejunal transfer of quercetin resulted in it being almost totally glucuronidated (97.6% of total transferred), whereas the absorption of hesperetin resulted in a much lower level of glucuronidation (17.8%).[73] Monophenolic B-ring flavonoids were also extensively glucuronidated, in particular naringenin, which was only detected in serosal fluid glucuronidated. Similar patterns of metabolism are observed in the ileum;[73] although, in general, glucuronidation occurred to a lesser extent, in line with studies that have recorded lower levels of phase I and II enzymes present in the ileum compared to the jejunum. Glucuronidation of these flavonoids was observed to occur predominantly at the 5- and 7-positions on the A-ring, which would be expected to have little influence on the resulting antioxidant potential of the metabolite. Indeed, recent studies have identified the 5-*O*-β-glucuronide of catechin and epicatechin excreted in the urine of rats post-ingestion and that this does not interfere with their antioxidant properties (as assessed by their ability to scavenge superoxide).[113,114]

While the major metabolites observed on the serosal side after perfusion of the jejunum with catechin or epicatechin were always glucuronidated, there were also high levels of both O-methylated and O-methylated-glucuronide forms.[36,109] 3′-O- and 4′-O-Methylated derivatives of the flavanols were detected at high levels in the serosal fluid (~30% of total transferred) and O-methyl and O-methyl-glucuronidated catechins were the predominant metabolites detected in the serosal fluid (~50%) suggesting these as the most bioavailable forms (Figure 13.4). As with the other flavonoids tested in this model, there was a lower level of metabolism occurring in the ileum, although the total amounts of both catechin and epicatechin absorbed was much higher than in the jejunum. The greater susceptibility to O-methylation of flavanols over other flavonoids in the jejunum presumably resides in the specificity of catechol-O-methyl-transferase (COMT) for these compounds.[115]

Procyanidins have a high affinity for proteins and their absorption through the gut barrier is most likely limited to lower oligomeric forms and to the metabolites formed by the colonic microflora (see Section 13.5). Recently, perfusion of isolated small intestine with the procyanidin dimers B2 and B5 extracted from cocoa indicated that both forms of dimer are transferred to the serosal side of enterocytes, but only to a very small extent (<1% of the total transferred flavanol-like compounds).[116] Perfusion of dimer mainly resulted in large amounts of unmetabolized/unconjugated epicatechin monomer being detected on the serosal side (~95.8%). Low levels of O-methylated dimer were also detected (~3.2%), but no conjugates and metabolites of epicatechin, indicating that metabolism of monomer and dimer is limited during dimer cleavage/translocation. Experiments with normal caco-2 cells and radiolabeled procyanidins suggested that small amounts of dimer and trimer were transferred to the same extent as the epicatechin monomer, whereas oligomers with an average degree of polymerization of 7 were not.[37]

### 13.4.3 Lower GI Tract

Studies have suggested that the extent of absorption of dietary polyphenols in the small intestine is relatively small (10 to 20%).[73,108,109] The implications of this low absorption in the small intestine means that the majority of ingested polyphenols, including those absorbed and conjugated in the enterocytes and/or the liver before transport back out into the lumen either directly or via the bile,[101] will reach the large intestine where they encounter colonic microflora. The colon contains approximately $10^{12}$ microorganisms/cm$^3$, which have enormous catalytic and hydrolytic potential, and the enzymatic degradation of flavonoids by the colonic microflora results in a huge array of new metabolites. For example, bacterial enzymes may catalyze many reactions including hydrolysis, dehydroxylation, demethylation, ring cleavage, and decarboxylation, as well as rapid deconjugation.[44] Unlike human enzymes, the microflora catalyze the breakdown

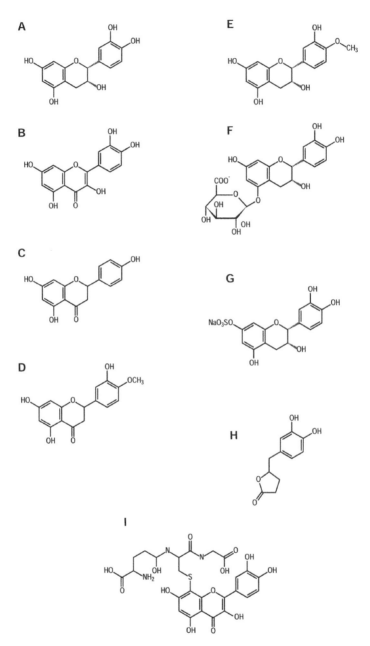

**FIGURE 13.4** Structures of flavonoids and their circulating metabolites: (A) epicatechin, (B) quercetin, (C) naringenin, (D) hesperetin, (E) 3'-O-methyl epicatechin, (F) epicatechin-5-O-β-D-glucuronide, (G) epicatechin-7-sulfate, (H) (−)-5-(3',4'-dihydroxyphenyl)-γ-valerolactone, (I) 8-glutathionyl quercetin. Glucuronide and sulfate conjugates are formed with the majority of flavonoids in the small intestine and liver, whereas O-methylated forms are only formed where the flavonoid has a catechol B-ring.

of the flavonoid backbone itself to simpler molecules such as phenolic acids. Specific metabolites have been observed in urine after consumption of a variety of phenolics. For example, the glycine conjugate of benzoic acid, hippuric acid, is primarily derived from plant phenolics and aromatic amino acids through the action of intestinal bacteria, and consequently, the level of hippuric acid would be expected to increase in the urine of individuals consuming diets rich in flavanols or polyphenols in general. It must be noted, however, that hippuric acid could possibly derive from other sources such as quinic acid or, in quantitative terms, more importantly from the aromatic amino acids tryptophan, tyrosine, and phenylalanine, as well as from the use of benzoic acid as a food preservative. To date, most studies looking at the metabolism of flavonoids in the large intestine have been carried out using either flavanols or flavonols, and there is little data on the metabolism of other commonly consumed flavonoids and other polyphenols.

The 5,7,3′,4′-hydroxylation pattern of flavan-3-ols is believed to enhance ring opening after hydrolysis,[36,44] and metabolism of flavanols by enzymes of the microflora of the large intestine results in many metabolites: 3,4-dihydrophenylacetic acid, 3-hydroxyphenylacetic acid, homovanillic acid, and their conjugates derived from the B-ring[44] and phenolic acids from the C-ring (Figure 13.5). Flavanols because of their structures (no C-4 carbonyl group) can also degrade to the specific metabolites phenylvalerolactones. Phenylpropionic acids (which may undergo further metabolism to benzoic acids) may also be the products of flavanol metabolism in animal studies, which demonstrates fission of the A-ring.[44] The metabolism of flavan-3-ol oligomers may also take place in the colon. Nonlabeled and [14]C-labeled purified proanthocyanidin polymers were almost totally degraded after 48 h of incubation, and meta- or para-monohydroxylated-phenylacetic, phenylpropionic, and phenylvaleric acids were identified as metabolites, providing the first evidence of that dietary procyanidins can be degraded to low-molecular-weight aromatic compounds in the body.[117]

Colonic-derived metabolites of flavanols have been detected in human plasma and urine after a single ingestion of green tea,[118] which suggests that there may be significant metabolism by gut microflora in the colon. The two metabolites, (−)-5-(3′,4′,5′-trihydroxyphenyl)-γ-valerolactone and (−)-5-(3′,4′-dihydroxyphenyl)-γ-valerolactone were identified in urine by both LC-MS/MS and NMR, appearing 7.5 to 13.5 h after ingestion (after a 3-h lag time), whereas epicatechin (EC) and epigallocatechin (EGC) peaked at 2 h. As well as their late excretion profiles, the amounts of metabolite excreted were 8- to 25-fold greater than that of EC and EGC excretion and accounted for 6 to 39% of the EC and EGC ingested. The late excretion and high levels of these metabolites would suggest that they are generated from the precursors EC and EGC by the intestinal microorganisms. A similar observation was made in rats fed labeled catechin where *m*- and *p*-hydroxyphenylproprionic acid, δ-(3-hydroxyphenyl)-γ-valerolactone, and δ-(3,4-dihydroxyphenyl)-γ-valerolactone were identified as metabolites arising due to the action of the colonic microflora.[119]

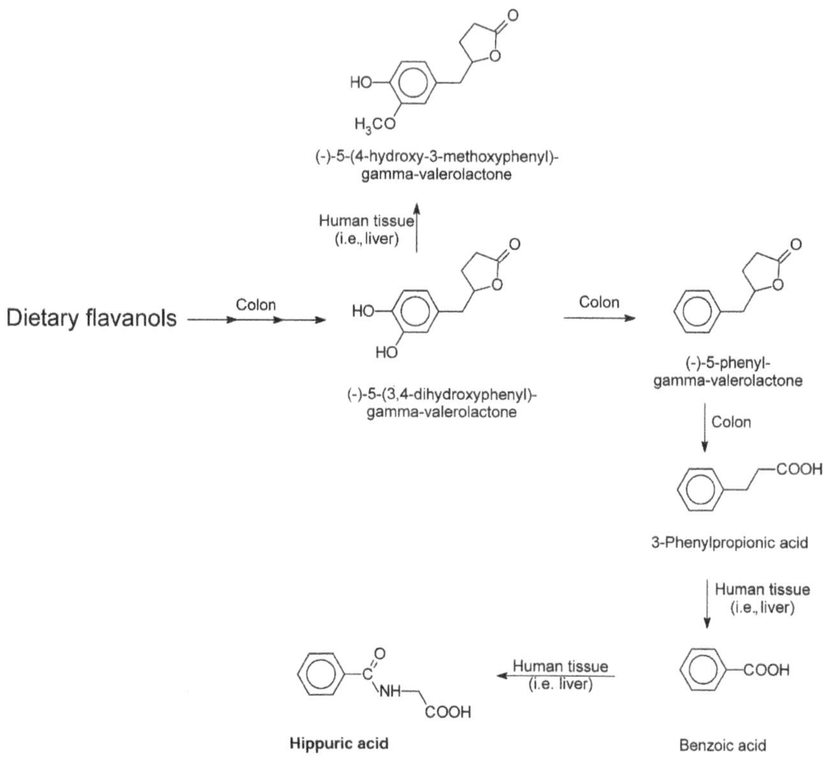

**FIGURE 13.5** Possible pathway of the formation of hippuric acid from flavanols in humans.

Flavonols such as quercetin-3-rhamnoglucoside and quercetin-3-rhamnoside may also undergo metabolism by the colonic flora with *Bacteroides distasonis, B. uniformis,* and *B. ovatus* capable of cleaving the sugar using α-rhamnosidase and β-glucosidase to liberate quercetin aglycone[120] and other phenolic metabolites.[121] Other bacteria, such as *Enterococcus casseliflavus,* have been observed to degrade quercetin-3-glucoside,[122] luteolin-7-glucoside, rutin, quercetin, kaempferol, luteolin, eriodictyol, naringenin, taxifolin, and phloretin[123] to phenolic acids, and *E. ramulus* is capable of degrading the aromatic ring system of quercetin producing the transient intermediate, phloroglucinol.[122] Other flavonoid glycosides, hesperidin, naringin, and poncirin are also metabolized to phenolic acids, via aglycones, by human intestinal microflora that produce α-rhamnosidase, exo-β-glucosidase, endo-β-glucosidase, and/or β-glucuronidase enzymes.[124] In addition, baicalin, puerarin, and daidzin were transformed to their aglycones by the bacteria producing β-glucuronidase, C-glycosidase, and β-glycosidase, respectively.

## 13.5  SUMMARY

It is clear that flavonoids undergo a very significant amount of metabolism and conjugation during absorption from the GI tract and again in the liver

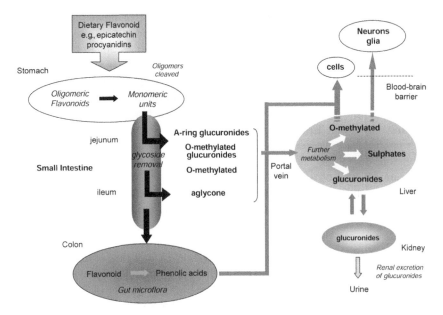

**FIGURE 13.6** Summary of the formation of metabolites and conjugates of flavonoids in humans. Cleavage of procyanidins may occur in the stomach in environments of low pH. All classes of flavonoids undergo extensive metabolism in the jejunum and ileum of the small intestine and resulting metabolites enter the portal vein and undergo further metabolism in the liver. Colonic microflora degrade flavonoids into smaller phenolic acids, which may also be absorbed. The fate of most of these metabolites is renal excretion; however, the extent to which these compounds enter cells and tissues is unknown.

(Figure 13.6). In the jejunum and ileum of the small intestine there is efficient glucuronidation of nearly all flavonoids to differing extents by the action of UDP-glucuronosyltransferase enzymes. In the case of catechol containing B-ring flavonoids there is also extensive *O*-methylation by the action of COMT. Unabsorbed flavonoids, and those taken up, metabolized in the small intestine and liver and transported back into the intestinal lumen, will reach the large intestine where they are further metabolized by the gut microflora to smaller phenolic acids. The extent to which these phenolic acids are absorbed in the colon is unknown; however, they are detected in the plasma and are often further conjugated and metabolized in the liver. Remaining compounds derived from flavonoid intake pass out in the feces.

The action of these flavonoid metabolites, in particular the *O*-methylated and *O*-methylated glucuronide forms, is now of great current interest. For example, the ability of 3′-*O*-methyl epicatechin and epicatechin glucuronides to protect against apoptotic cell death induced by hydrogen peroxide or oxidized LDL has been investigated.[125–127] The emerging view is that flavonoids are likely to exert beneficial and/or toxic actions on cells not through their potential to act as antioxidants but rather through their modulation of protein and lipid kinase signaling cascades. The basis for this conclusion is that flavonoids and their metabolites are unlikely to act as major antioxidants *in vivo* in the presence of small-molecule antioxidants such as ascorbic acid and α-tocopherol are so much higher. However, the concentrations of flavonoids and their metabolites encountered *in vivo* are sufficiently high to have pharmacological activity at receptors, enzymes, and transcription factors. For example, inhibition of Akt/PKB[128] is almost certainly due principally to actions at PI 3-kinase, whereas actions at ERK1/2 may result from flavonoids modulating upstream regulatory kinases, other intermediary molecules within MAP kinase cascades such as GTPases, or by binding directly to receptors. Actions at these cascades may be beneficial in the treatment of proliferative diseases, but could be detrimental to the nervous system where these same pathways control survival and plasticity. Thus, flavonoid interactions with intracellular signaling pathways could have unpredictable outcomes and will be dependent on the cell type, the disease studied, and the stimulus applied.

Recently, the uptake of flavonoids and their *O*-methylated, glucuronidated, and sulfated forms into cells has been addressed as an event that will ultimately determine their biological actions.[127,129] It is clear that uptake of flavonoids into cells is dependent on both the flavonoid and perhaps more importantly the cell type. It seems likely that these differences may reflect the variation in the way different cell populations handle flavonoids. For example, astrocytes metabolize flavonoids intracellularly whereas neurons do not. The generation of such intracellular metabolites, such as 2′-glutathionyl quercetin (Figure 13.4), is of great importance as they may also be capable of mediating potential beneficial or negative actions of flavonoids *in vivo*. Furthermore, intracellularly formed metabolites may represent novel *in vivo* metabolites of flavonoids, and their presence in the circulation and urine may provide important information on the pharmacokinetics of flavonoids following ingestion.

Over the recent years we have gained a greater knowledge of the bioavailable metabolites of dietary flavonoids, and it is now essential to fully evaluate the role of these conjugates and metabolites in disease prevention. It will be important to assess whether the observed metabolism aids entry into cells and/or renders them better or worse at providing protection against different stresses, such as oxidative or nitrative stress. New data in the field are already beginning to suggest that flavonoids may act to protect cells by more complex mechanisms than was once thought.[126,128,130,131] It is evident that flavonoids are potent bioactive molecules and a clear understanding of their mechanisms of action either as antioxidants or modulators of cell signaling is crucial to the evaluation of their potential as anticancer agents and inhibitors of neurodegeneration. Eventually it is hoped that these studies will enable specific dietary recommendations to be made, which will increase general health in the population.

# REFERENCES

1. Rice-Evans C. Flavonoid antioxidants. *Curr Med Chem* 2001; 8(7):797–807.
2. Middleton E. Biological properties of plant flavonoids: an overview. *Int J Pharmacognosy* 1996; 34:344–348.
3. Harborne JB, Williams CA. Advances in flavonoid research since 1992. *Phytochemistry* 2000; 55(6):481–504.
4. Rice-Evans CA, Miller NJ, Paganga G. Structure-antioxidant activity relationships of flavonoids and phenolic acids. *Free Radical Biol Med* 1996; 20(7):933–956.
5. Rice-Evans C. Plant polyphenols: free radical scavengers or chain-breaking antioxidants? *Biochem Soc Symp* 1995; 61:103–116.
6. Croft KD. The chemistry and biological effects of flavonoids and phenolic acids. *Ann NY Acad Sci* 1998; 854:435–442.
7. Abalea V, Cillard J, Dubos MP, Sergent O, Cillard P, Morel I. Repair of iron-induced DNA oxidation by the flavonoid myricetin in primary rat hepatocyte cultures. *Free Radical Biol Med* 1999; 26(11–12):1457–1466.
8. Galati G, O'Brien PJ. Potential toxicity of flavonoids and other dietary phenolics: significance for their chemopreventive and anticancer properties. *Free Radical Biol Med* 2004; 37(3):287–303.
9. Moyers SB, Kumar NB. Green tea polyphenols and cancer chemoprevention: multiple mechanisms and endpoints for phase II trials. *Nutr Rev* 2004; 62(5):204–211.
10. Hollman PC, Feskens EJ, Katan MB. Tea flavonols in cardiovascular disease and cancer epidemiology. *Proc Soc Exp Biol Med* 1999; 220(4):198–202.
11. Arts IC, Hollman PC, Bueno dMH, Feskens EJ, Kromhout D. Dietary catechins and epithelial cancer incidence: the Zutphen elderly study. *Int J Cancer* 2001; 92(2):298–302.
12. Choudhury R, Srai SK, Debnam E, Rice-Evans CA. Urinary excretion of hydroxycinnamates and flavonoids after oral and intravenous administration. *Free Radical Biol Med* 1999; 27:278–286.
13. Spencer JPE, Jenner A, Aruoma OI, Cross CE, Wu R, Halliwell B. Oxidative DNA damage in human respiratory tract epithelial cells. Time course in relation to DNA strand breakage. *Biochem Biophys Res Commun* 1996; 224(1):17–22.
14. Rice-Evans C, Spencer JPE, Schroeter H, Rechner AR. Bioavailability of flavonoids and potential bioactive forms in vivo. *Drug Metab Drug Interact* 2000; 17(1–4):291–310.
15. Basaga H, Poli G, Tekkaya C, Aras I. Free radical scavenging and antioxidative properties of "silibin" complexes on microsomal lipid peroxidation. *Cell Biochem Funct* 1997; 15:27–33.
16. Dragsted LO, Strube M, Leth T. Dietary levels of plant phenols and other non-nutritive components: could they prevent cancer? *Eur J Cancer Prev* 1997; 6(6):522–528.
17. Kris-Etherton PM, Keen CL. Evidence that the antioxidant flavonoids in tea and cocoa are beneficial for cardiovascular health. *Curr Opin Lipidol* 2002; 13(1):41–49.
18. Hertog MG, Feskens EJ, Hollman PC, Katan MB, Kromhout D. Dietary antioxidant flavonoids and risk of coronary heart disease: the Zutphen Elderly Study. *Lancet* 1993; 342(8878):1007–1011.

19. Bolanos-Vasquez MC, Warner D. Effects of *Rhizobium tropici*, *R-etli*, and *R-leguminosarum* bv *phaseoli* on *nod* gene-inducing flavonoids in root exudates of *Phaseolus vulgaris*. *Mol Plant Microbe Interact* 1997; 10:339–346.

20. Wedworth SM, Lynch S. Dietary flavonoids in atherosclerosis prevention. *Ann Pharmacother* 1995; 29(6):627–628.

21. Arts IC, Hollman PC, Feskens EJ, Bueno dMH, Kromhout D. Catechin intake might explain the inverse relation between tea consumption and ischemic heart disease: the Zutphen Elderly Study. *Am J Clin Nutr* 2001; 74(2):227–232.

22. Manthey JA. Biological properties of flavonoids pertaining to inflammation. *Microcirculation* 2000; 7(6 Pt 2):S29–S34.

23. Aruoma OI, Bahorun T, Jen LS. Neuroprotection by bioactive components in medicinal and food plant extracts. *Mutat Res* 2003; 544(2–3):203–215.

24. Pan T, Jankovic J, Le W. Potential therapeutic properties of green tea polyphenols in Parkinson's disease. *Drugs Aging* 2003; 20(10):711–721.

25. Meehan WJ, Spencer JPE, Rannels DE, Welch DR, Knobbe ET, Ostrander GK. Hydrogen peroxide induces oxidative DNA damage in rat type II pulmonary epithelial cells. *Environ Mol Mutagenesis* 1999; 33(4):273–278.

26. Liu L, Castonguay A. Inhibition of the metabolism and genotoxicity of 4-(meth-ylnitrosamino)-1-(3-pyridyl)-1-butanone (Nnk) In rat hepatocytes by (+)-catechin. *Carcinogenesis* 1991; 12:1203–1208.

27. Oldreive C, Zhao K, Paganga G, Halliwell B, Rice-Evans C. Inhibition of nitrous acid-dependent tyrosine nitration and DNA base deamination by flavonoids and other phenolic compounds. *Chem Res Toxicol* 1998; 11(12):1574–1579.

28. Brown JE, Khodr H, Hider RC, Rice-Evans CA. Structural dependence of fla-vonoid interactions with $Cu^{2+}$ ions: implications for their antioxidant properties. *Biochem J* 1998; 330(Pt 3):1173–1178.

29. Rice-Evans CA, Miller NJ, Bolwell PG, Bramley PM, Pridham JB. The relative antioxidant activities of plant-derived polyphenolic flavonoids. *Free Radical Res* 1995; 22(4):375–383.

30. Packer L, Rimbach G, Virgili F. Antioxidant activity and biologic properties of a procyanidin-rich extract from pine (*Pinus maritima*) bark, pycnogenol. *Free Radical Biol Med* 1999; 27:704–724.

31. deOliveira TT, Nagem TJ, daSilva MC, deMiranda LCG, Teixeira MA. Antioxi-dant action of the flavonoids derivatives. *Pesquisa Agropecuaria Bras* 1999; 34:879–883.

32. Bohm H, Boeing H, Hempel J, Raab B, Kroke A. Flavonols, flavones and antho-cyanins as native antioxidants of food and their possible role in the prevention of chronic diseases. *Z Ernahrungswiss* 1998; 37:147–163.

33. Rice-Evans CA, Miller NJ. Antioxidant activities of flavonoids as bioactive com-ponents of food. *Biochem Soc Trans* 1996; 24(3):790–795.

34. Hertog MG, Hollman PC. Potential health effects of the dietary flavonol quercetin. *Eur J Clin Nutr* 1996; 50(2):63–71.

35. Hollman PC, Katan MB. Absorption, metabolism and health effects of dietary flavonoids in man. *Biomed Pharmacother* 1997; 51(8):305–310.

36. Spencer JPE, Schroeter H, Rechner A, Rice-Evans C. Bioavailability of flavan-3-ols and procyanidins: gastrointestinal tract influences and their relevance to bio-active forms *in vivo*. *Antiox Redox Signal* 2001; 3:1023–1040.

37. Scalbert A, Williamson G. Dietary intake and bioavailability of polyphenols. *J Nutr* 2000; 130(8S Suppl):2073S–2085S.

38. Manach C, Donovan JL. Pharmacokinetics and metabolism of dietary flavonoids in humans. *Free Radical Res* 2004; 38(8):771–785.
39. Hollman PCH, Katan MB. Absorption, metabolism and health effects of dietary flavonoids in man. *Biomed Pharmacother* 1997; 51:305–310.
40. Hollman PC, Katan MB. Dietary flavonoids: intake, health effects and bioavailability. *Food Chem Toxicol* 1999; 37(9–10):937–942.
41. Hollman PC, Katan MB. Bioavailability and health effects of dietary flavonols in man. *Arch Toxicol Suppl* 1998; 20:237–248.
42. Hollman PC. Bioavailability of flavonoids. *Eur J Clin Nutr* 1997; 51(Suppl 1):S66–S69.
43. Okushio K, Suzuki M, Matsumoto N, Nanjo F, Hara Y. Methylation of tea catechins by rat liver homogenates. *Biosci Biotech Biochem* 1999; 63:430–432.
44. Scheline RR. Metabolism of oxygen heterocyclic compounds. In: *CRC Handbook of Mammalian Metabolism of Plant Compounds*. Boca Raton, FL: CRC Press; 1999:243–295.
45. Dewick PM. The biosynthesis of shikimate metabolites. *Nat Prod Rep* 1990; 7(3):165–189.
46. Heller W. Flavonoid biosynthesis, an overview. *Prog Clin Biol Res* 1986; 213:25–42.
47. Green ES, Cooper CE, Davies MJ, Rice-Evans C. Antioxidant drugs and the inhibition of low-density lipoprotein oxidation. *Biochem Soc Trans* 1993; 21(2):362–366.
48. Yannai S, Day AJ, Williamson G, Rhodes MJC. Characterization of flavonoids as monofunctional or bifunctional inducers of quinone reductase in murine hepatoma cell lines. *Food Chem Toxicol* 1998; 36:623–630.
49. Yamamoto N, Moon JH, Tsushida T, Nagao A, Terao J. Inhibitory effect of quercetin metabolites and their related derivatives on copper ion-induced lipid peroxidation in human low-density lipoprotein. *Arch Biochem Biophys* 1999; 372:347–354.
50. Hubac C, Ferran J, Tremolieres A, Kondorosi A. Luteolin uptake by rhizobium-meliloti — evidence for several steps including an active extrusion process. *Microbiology-UK* 1994; 140:2769–2774.
51. Duthie SJ, Dobson VL. Dietary flavonoids protect human colonocyte DNA from oxidative attack in vitro. *Eur J Nutr* 1999; 38(1):28–34.
52. Duthie SJ, Collins AR, Duthie GG, Dodson VL. Quercetin and myricetin protect against hydrogen peroxide-induced DNA damage (strand breaks and oxidised pyrimidines) in human lymphocytes. *Mutat Res Gen Toxicol Environ Mutat* 1997; 393:223–231.
53. Lin JH, Chiba M, Baillie TA. Is the role of the small intestine in first-pass metabolism overemphasized? *Pharmacol Rev* 1999; 51(2):135–158.
54. Justesen U. Collision-induced fragmentation of deprotonated methoxylated flavonoids, obtained by electrospray ionization mass spectrometry. *J Mass Spectrom* 2001; 36(2):169–178.
55. Justesen U. Negative atmospheric pressure chemical ionisation low-energy collision activation mass spectrometry for the characterisation of flavonoids in extracts of fresh herbs. *J Chromatogr A* 2000; 902(2):369–379.
56. Weisshaar B, Jenkins GI. Phenylpropanoid biosynthesis and its regulation. *Curr Opin Plant Biol* 1998; 1:251–257.

57. Morel I, Lescoat G, Cillard P, Cillard J. Role of flavonoids and iron chelation in antioxidant action. *Methods Enzymol* 1994; 234:437–443.
58. Bailey DG, Malcolm J, Arnold O, Spence JD. Grapefruit juice-drug interactions. *Br J Clin Pharmacol* 1998; 46:101–110.
59. Vaidyanathan JB, Walle T. Glucuronidation and sulfation of the tea flavonoid (–)-epicatechin by the human and rat enzymes. *Drug Metab Dispos* 2002; 30(8):897–903.
60. Tournaire C, Croux S, Maurette MT et al. Antioxidant activity of flavonoids: efficiency of singlet oxygen (1 delta g) quenching. *J Photochem Photobiol B* 1993; 19(3):205–215.
61. Devasagayam TP, Subramanian M, Singh BB, Ramanathan R, Das NP. Protection of plasmid pBR322 DNA by flavonoids against single-stranded breaks induced by singlet molecular oxygen. *J Photochem Photobiol B* 1995; 30(2–3):97–103.
62. Yang CS, Lee MJ, Chen L. Human salivary tea catechin levels and catechin esterase activities: implication in human cancer prevention studies. *Cancer Epidemiol Biomarkers Prev* 1999; 8(1):83–89.
63. Tsuchiya H, Sato M, Kato H, Okubo T, Juneja LR, Kim M. Simultaneous determination of catechins in human saliva by high-performance liquid chromatography. *J Chromatogr B* 1997; 703:253–258.
64. Laires A, Pacheco P, Rueff J. Mutagenicity of rutin and the glycosidic activity of cultured cell-free microbial preparations of human faeces and saliva. *Food Chem Toxicol* 1989; 27(7):437–443.
65. Macdonald IA, Mader JA, Bussard RG. The role of rutin and quercitrin in stimulating flavonol glycosidase activity by cultured cell-free microbial preparations of human feces and saliva. *Mutat Res* 1983; 122(2):95–102.
66. Parisis DM, Pritchard ET. Activation of rutin by human oral bacterial isolates to the carcinogen-mutagen quercetin. *Arch Oral Biol* 1983; 28(7):583–590.
67. de F, V, Mateus N. Structural features of procyanidin interactions with salivary proteins. *J Agric Food Chem* 2001; 49(2):940–945.
68. Nishioka H, Nishi K, Kyokane K. Human saliva inactivates mutagenicity of carcinogens. *Mutat Res* 1981; 85(5):323–333.
69. Spencer JPE, Chaudry F, Pannala AS, Srai SK, Debnam E, Rice-Evans C. Decomposition of cocoa procyanidins in the gastric milieu. *Biochem Biophys Res Commun* 2000; 272(1):236–241.
70. Gee JM, Dupont MS, Rhodes MJC, Johnson IT. Quercetin glucosides interact with the intestinal glucose transport pathway. *Free Radical Biol Med* 1998; 25:19–25.
71. Higuchi WI, Ho NF, Park JY, Komiya I. Rate-limiting steps and factors in drug absorption. In: Prescott LF, Nimno WS, eds. *Drug Absorption.* New York: ADIS Press; 1981:35–60.
72. Ho NF, Park JY, Ni PF, Higuchi WI. Advancing quantitative and mechanistic approaches in interfacing gastrointestinal drug absorption studies in animals and humans. In: Crouthamel W, Sarapu AC, eds. *Animal Models for Oral Drug Delivery. In Situ and In Vivo Approaches.* Washington, DC: American Pharmaceutics Association; 1983:27–106.
73. Spencer JPE, Chowrimootoo G, Choudhury R, Debnam ES, Srai SK, Rice-Evans C. The small intestine can both absorb and glucuronidate luminal flavonoids. *FEBS Lett* 1999; 458(2):224–230.

74. Day AJ, Williamson G. Biomarkers for exposure to dietary flavonoids: a review of the current evidence for identification of quercetin glycosides in plasma. *Br J Nutr* 2001; 86(Suppl 1):105–110.

75. Hollman PC, Bijsman MN, van Gameren Y, Cnossen EP, de Vries JH, Katan MB. The sugar moiety is a major determinant of the absorption of dietary flavonoid glycosides in man. *Free Radical Res* 1999; 31(6):569–573.

76. Walle T, Otake Y, Walle UK, Wilson FA. Quercetin glucosides are completely hydrolyzed in ileostomy patients before absorption. *J Nutr* 2000; 130(11):2658–2661.

77. Day AJ, Canada FJ, Diaz JC et al. Dietary flavonoid and isoflavone glycosides are hydrolysed by the lactase site of lactase phlorizin hydrolase. *FEBS Lett* 2000; 468(2–3):166–170.

78. Gee JM, Dupont MS, Day AJ, Plumb GW, Williamson G, Johnson IT. Intestinal transport of quercetin glycosides in rats involves both deglycosylation and interaction with the hexose transport pathway. *J Nutr* 2000; 130(11):2765–2771.

79. Morand C, Manach C, Crespy V, Remesy C. Respective bioavailability of quercetin aglycone and its glycosides in a rat model. *BioFactors* 2000; 12(1–4):169–174.

80. Day AJ, Dupont MS, Ridley S et al. Deglycosylation of flavonoid and isoflavonoid glycosides by human small intestine and liver beta-glucosidase activity. *FEBS Lett* 1998; 436(1):71–75.

81. Ioku K, Pongpiriyadacha Y, Konishi Y, Takei Y, Nakatani N, Terao J. beta-Glucosidase activity in the rat small intestine toward quercetin monoglucosides. *Biosci Biotechnol Biochem* 1998; 62(7):1428–1431.

82. Miyazawa T, Nakagawa K, Kudo M, Muraishi K, Someya K. Direct intestinal absorption of red fruit anthocyanins, cyanidin-3-glucoside and cyanidin-3,5-diglucoside, into rats and humans. *J Agric Food Chem* 1999; 47:1083–1091.

83. Tsuda T, Horio F, Osawa T. Absorption and metabolism of cyanidin 3-*O*-beta-D-glucoside in rats. *FEBS Lett* 1999; 449:179–182.

84. Lapidot T, Harel S, Granit R, Kanner J. Bioavailability of red wine anthocyanins as detected in human urine. *J Agric Food Chem* 1998; 46:4297–4302.

85. Paganga G, Rice-Evans CA. The identification of flavonoids as glycosides in human plasma. *FEBS Lett* 1997; 401:78–82.

86. Andlauer W, Stumpf C, Furst P. Intestinal absorption of rutin in free and conjugated forms. *Biochem Pharmacol* 2001; 62(3):369–374.

87. Barzilai A, Rahamimoff H. Inhibition of $Ca^{2+}$-transport ATPase from synaptosomal vesicles by flavonoids. *Biochim Biophys Acta* 1983; 730(2):245–254.

88. Bourne LC, Rice-Evans CA. Detecting and measuring bioavailability of phenolics and flavonoids in humans: pharmacokinetics of urinary excretion of dietary ferulic acid. *Methods Enzymol* 1999; 299:91–106.

89. Hollman PCH, vanderGaag M, Mengelers MJB, vanTrijp JMP, deVries JH, Katan MB. Absorption and disposition kinetics of the dietary antioxidant quercetin in man. *Free Radical Biol Med* 1996; 21:703–707.

90. Hollman PC, de Vries JH, van Leeuwen SD, Mengelers MJ, Katan MB. Absorption of dietary quercetin glycosides and quercetin in healthy ileostomy volunteers. *Am J Clin Nutr* 1995; 62(6):1276–1282.

91. Hollman PC, van Trijp JM, Buysman MN et al. Relative bioavailability of the antioxidant flavonoid quercetin from various foods in man. *FEBS Lett* 1997; 418(1–2):152–156.

92. Hollman PC, Katan MB. Health effects and bioavailability of dietary flavonols. *Free Radical Res* 1999; 31(Suppl):S75–S80.

93. Kobayashi Y, Suzuki M, Satsu H et al. Green tea polyphenols inhibit the sodium-dependent glucose transporter of intestinal epithelial cells by a competitive mechanism. *J Agric Food Chem* 2000; 48(11):5618–5623.

94. Ader P, Block M, Pietzsch S, Wolffram S. Interaction of quercetin glucosides with the intestinal sodium/glucose co-transporter (SGLT-1). *Cancer Lett* 2001; 162(2):175–180.

95. Walgren RA, Lin JT, Kinne RK, Walle T. Cellular uptake of dietary flavonoid quercetin 4'-beta-glucoside by sodium-dependent glucose transporter SGLT1. *J Pharmacol Exp Ther* 2000; 294(3):837–843.

96. Sesink AL, O'Leary KA, Hollman PC. Quercetin glucuronides but not glucosides are present in human plasma after consumption of quercetin-3-glucoside or quercetin-4'-glucoside. *J Nutr* 2001; 131(7):1938–1941.

97. Walgren RA, Walle UK, Walle T. Transport of quercetin and its glucosides across human intestinal epithelial Caco-2 cells. *Biochem Pharmacol* 1998; 55(10):1721–1727.

98. Walgren RA, Karnaky KJJ, Lindenmayer GE, Walle T. Efflux of dietary flavonoid quercetin 4'-beta-glucoside across human intestinal Caco-2 cell monolayers by apical multidrug resistance-associated protein-2. *J Pharmacol Exp Ther* 2000; 294(3):830–836.

99. Walgren RA, Walle T. The influence of plasma binding on absorption/exsorption in the Caco-2 model of human intestinal absorption. *J Pharm Pharmacol* 1999; 51(9):1037–1040.

100. Cheng Z, Radominska-Pandya A, Tephly TR. Studies on the substrate specificity of human intestinal UDP-glucuronosyltransferases 1A8 and 1A10. *Drug Metab Dispos* 1999; 27(10):1165–1170.

101. Crespy V, Morand C, Manach C, Besson C, Demigne C, Remesy C. Part of quercetin absorbed in the small intestine is conjugated and further secreted in the intestinal lumen. *Am J Physiol* 1999; 277(1 Pt 1):G120–G126.

102. Donovan JL, Crespy V, Manach C et al. Catechin is metabolized by both the small intestine and liver of rats. *J Nutr* 2001; 131(6):1753–1757.

103. Windmill KF, McKinnon RA, Zhu X, Gaedigk A, Grant DM, McManus ME. The role of xenobiotic metabolizing enzymes in arylamine toxicity and carcinogenesis: functional and localization studies. *Mutat Res* 1997; 376(1–2):153–160.

104. Franski R, Bednarek P, Siatkowska D, Wojtaszek P, Stobiecki M. Application of mass spectrometry to structural identification of flavonoid monoglycosides isolated from shoot of lupin (*Lupinus luteus* L.). *Acta Biochim Pol* 1999; 46:459–473.

105. Terao J. Dietary flavonoids as antioxidants in vivo: conjugated metabolites of (–)-epicatechin and quercetin participate in antioxidative defense in blood plasma. *J Med Invest* 1999; 46(3–4):159–168.

106. Carbonaro M, Grant G, Pusztai A. Evaluation of polyphenol bioavailability in rat small intestine. *Eur J Nutr* 2001; 40(2):84–90.

107. Fisher RB, Gardner ML. A kinetic approach to the study of absorption of solutes by isolated perfused small intestine. *J Physiol* 1974; 241(1):211–234.

108. Kuhnle G, Spencer JPE, Chowrimootoo G et al. Resveratrol is absorbed in the small intestine as resveratrol glucuronide. *Biochem Biophys Res Commun* 2000; 272(1):212–217.

109. Kuhnle G, Spencer JPE, Schroeter H et al. Epicatechin and catechin are O-methylated and glucuronidated in the small intestine. *Biochem Biophys Res Commun* 2000; 277(2):507–512.

110. Crevoisier C, Buri P, Boucherat J. The transport of three flavonoids across artificial and biological membranes. 5. Transport in situ across the small intestine of the rat. *Pharm Acta Helv* 1975; 50(7–8):231–236.

111. Choudhury R, Chowrimootoo G, Srai K, Debnam E, Rice-Evans CA. Interactions of the flavonoid naringenin in the gastrointestinal tract and the influence of glycosylation. *Biochem Biophys Res Commun* 1999; 265(2):410–415.

112. Shimoi K, Okada H, Furugori M et al. Intestinal absorption of luteolin and luteolin 7-*O*-beta-glucoside in rats and humans. *FEBS Lett* 1998; 438:220–224.

113. Harada M, Kan Y, Naoki H et al. Identification of the major antioxidative metabolites in biological fluids of the rat with ingested (+)-catechin and (–)-epicatechin. *Biosci Biotechnol Biochem* 1999; 63(6):973–977.

114. Okushio K, Suzuki M, Matsumoto N, Nanjo F, Hara Y. Identification of (–)-epicatechin metabolites and their metabolic fate in the rat. *Drug Metab Dispos* 1999; 27(2):309–316.

115. Mannisto PT, Kaakkola S. Catechol-*O*-methyltransferase (COMT): biochemistry, molecular biology, pharmacology, and clinical efficacy of the new selective COMT inhibitors. *Pharmacol Rev* 1999; 51(4):593–628.

116. Spencer JPE, Schroeter H, Shenoy B, Srai SK, Debnam ES, Rice-Evans C. Epicatechin is the primary bioavailable form of the procyanidin dimers B2 and B5 after transfer across the small intestine. *Biochem Biophys Res Commun* 2001; 285(3):588–593.

117. Deprez S, Brezillon C, Rabot S et al. Polymeric proanthocyanidins are catabolized by human colonic microflora into low-molecular-weight phenolic acids. *J Nutr* 2000; 130(11):2733–2738.

118. Li C, Lee MJ, Sheng SQ et al. Structural identification of two metabolites of catechins and their kinetics in human urine and blood after tea ingestion. *Chem Res Toxicol* 2000; 13:177–184.

119. Das NP, Griffiths LA. Studies on flavonoid metabolism. Metabolism of (+)-[14C] catechin in the rat and guinea pig. *Biochem J* 1969; 115(4):831–836.

120. Bokkenheuser VD, Shackleton CH, Winter J. Hydrolysis of dietary flavonoid glycosides by strains of intestinal *Bacteroides* from humans. *Biochem J* 1987; 248(3):953–956.

121. Baba S, Furuta T, Fujioka M, Goromaru T. Studies on drug metabolism by use of isotopes XXVII: urinary metabolites of rutin in rats and the role of intestinal microflora in the metabolism of rutin. *J Pharm Sci* 1983; 72(10):1155–1158.

122. Schneider H, Schwiertz A, Collins MD, Blaut M. Anaerobic transformation of quercetin-3-glucoside by bacteria from the human intestinal tract. *Arch Microbiol* 1999; 171(2):81–91.

123. Schneider H, Blaut M. Anaerobic degradation of flavonoids by *Eubacterium ramulus*. *Arch Microbiol* 2000; 173(1):71–75.

124. Kim DH, Jung EA, Sohng IS, Han JA, Kim TH, Han MJ. Intestinal bacterial metabolism of flavonoids and its relation to some biological activities. *Arch Pharm Res* 1998; 21(1):17–23.

125. Spencer JPE, Schroeter H, Kuhnle G et al. Epicatechin and its in vivo metabolite, 3'-*O*-methyl epicatechin, protect human fibroblasts from oxidative-stress-induced cell death involving caspase-3 activation. *Biochem J* 2001; 354:493–500.

126. Schroeter H, Spencer JPE, Rice-Evans C, Williams RJ. Flavonoids protect neurons from oxidized low-density-lipoprotein-induced apoptosis involving c-Jun N-terminal kinase (JNK), c-Jun and caspase-3. *Biochem J* 2001; 358(Pt 3):547–557.

127. Spencer JPE, Schroeter H, Crossthwaithe AJ, Kuhnle G, Williams RJ, Rice-Evans C. Contrasting influences of glucuronidation and *O*-methylation of epicatechin on hydrogen peroxide-induced cell death in neurons and fibroblasts. *Free Radical Biol Med* 2001; 31(9):1139–1146.

128. Spencer JPE, Rice-Evans C, Williams RJ. Modulation of pro-survival Akt/protein kinase B and ERK1/2 signaling cascades by quercetin and its in vivo metabolites underlie their action on neuronal viability. *J Biol Chem* 2003; 278(37):34783–34793.

129. Spencer JPE, Abd-el-Mohsen MM, Rice-Evans C. Cellular uptake and metabolism of flavonoids and their metabolites: implications for their bioactivity. *Arch Biochem Biophys* 2004; 423(1):148–161.

130. Kong AN, Yu R, Chen C, Mandlekar S, Primiano T. Signal transduction events elicited by natural products: role of MAPK and caspase pathways in homeostatic response and induction of apoptosis. *Arch Pharm Res* 2000; 23(1):1–16.

131. Bastianetto S, Zheng WH, Quirion R. The *Ginkgo biloba* extract (EGb 761) protects and rescues hippocampal cells against nitric oxide-induced toxicity: involvement of its flavonoid constituents and protein kinase C. *J Neurochem* 2000; 74(6):2268–2277.

# 14 Isoflavones, Soybean Phytoestrogens, and Cancer

*Fazlul H. Sarkar and Yiwei Li*

## CONTENTS

14.1　Introduction.................................................................................295
14.2　Source, Absorption, Metabolism, and Bioavailability of Isoflavones ..296
14.3　Isoflavones and Cancers ..............................................................297
　　　14.3.1　Isoflavones and Breast Cancer ...............................................297
　　　14.3.2　Isoflavones and Prostate Cancer.............................................298
　　　14.3.3　Isoflavones and Other Hormone-Related Cancers...................299
　　　14.3.4　Isoflavones and Hormone-Independent Cancers......................299
14.4　Molecular Mechanisms of Action of Isoflavones ..............................300
　　　14.4.1　Regulation of the Expression of Genes Related to Cell Cycle
　　　　　　　and Apoptosis .................................................................300
　　　14.4.2　Regulation of Cell Signaling Pathways ...................................301
　　　　　　　14.4.2.1　NF-κB Pathway...............................................301
　　　　　　　14.4.2.2　Akt Pathway ...................................................302
　　　　　　　14.4.2.3　AR and ER Pathways.........................................302
　　　14.4.3　Regulation of the Expression of Genes Related to
　　　　　　　Angiogenesis and Metastasis ...............................................303
　　　14.4.4　Regulation of Oxidative Stress................................................304
14.5　Conclusion ................................................................................304
Acknowledgment....................................................................................305
References ............................................................................................305

## 14.1　INTRODUCTION

Cancer has become one of the major health problems around the world. In the U.S., about 1,372,910 new cases of cancer will be diagnosed and 570,280 people will die from cancer in 2005.[1] Although cancer occurs in every country around the world, there are wide geographic variations in the incidence of cancer. The incidences of hormone-related cancers including breast, prostate, endometrium, and ovary cancers are much higher in the U.S. and European countries compared to Asian countries such as Japan and China. It has been believed that the difference in the incidences is due to the environmental and lifestyle factors including dietary habits. The Japanese and the Chinese consume a traditional diet high in soy products. Dietary intakes of 39.4 and 47.4 mg soy isoflavone/day in Chinese and Japanese populations, respectively, have been reported, whereas the dietary consumption of soy isoflavones is less than 1 mg/day in the general population in the U.S.[2–4] Epidemiological studies have revealed that high consumption of soybean is inversely associated with the risk of hormone-related cancers.[5–7] Therefore, isoflavones that mainly exist in soybean have received much attention as dietary factors having inhibitory effects on carcinogenesis. In recent years, growing evidence from animal and *in vitro* studies has demonstrated that isoflavones are able to exert their inhibitory effects on the development of cancers, cancer cell growth, and cancer progression, suggesting that isoflavones may be promising agents for cancer prevention and/or treatment.

## 14.2 SOURCE, ABSORPTION, METABOLISM, AND BIOAVAILABILITY OF ISOFLAVONES

Isoflavone is one of the main classes of phytoestrogen. Phytoestrogens possess estrogen-like structure and effect. They are weak estrogens and have been found in a wide variety of plants. However, isoflavones are found primarily in members of the Leguminosae family. Soybean is the food that contains abundant amounts of isoflavones. It has been reported that the levels of isoflavones in soybean vary between 560 and 3810 mg/kg, depending on growing conditions.[8] Some soy products contain more concentrated isoflavones. Soymilk, bean curds, miso, and tofu contain up to 2030 mg isoflavone/kg, depending on the material and the processing.[8] The main isoflavones in soybean are genistein, daidzein, and glycitein. Genistein and daidzein have been found in relatively high concentration in soybeans and most soy-protein products, while much lower amounts of glycitein are present in soybeans. Experimental studies have revealed that isoflavones, particularly genistein, exert significant favorable bioactivity on human health.

The metabolism of isoflavones is an important process creating bioactive molecules for human health. It has been reported that a large amount of isoflavones is present in the inactive form as glycosides in soybeans and soy products. In human intestines, isoflavone glycosides (such as genistin and daidzin) undergo hydrolysis by bacterial beta-glucosidases, releasing corresponding bioactive aglycones (such as genistein and daidzein).[9–11] The aglycones are then absorbed from the intestinal tract to blood and conjugated mainly in liver to glucuronides, which undergo enterohepatic recycling and are excreted in the urine.[12] Genistein and daidzein are the major isoflavones that have been detected in the blood and urine of humans.[13] It has been found that the isoflavone aglycones are absorbed faster and in greater amounts than their glycosides in humans;[14] therefore, isoflavone aglycone-rich products may be more effective than glycoside-rich products in cancer chemoprevention. Among isoflavone aglycones, genistein is the most important isoflavone for human health.

To investigate the effects of isoflavones on reduction of cancer risk, the isoflavone concentration in plasma has been detected in different populations. The physiologic concentration of isoflavones in plasma varies in different populations with different amounts of soy food intake. Plasma concentration of genistein in the nanomolar range has been detected in Americans and Europeans, while $1.4 \pm 0.7$ to $4.09 \pm 0.94$ μmol/L of plasma genistein has been found in various population groups consuming foods rich in isoflavones.[15–19] When investigating the effects of isoflavones on cancers, one major concern is the physiologically achievable concentration of isoflavones in human plasma *in vivo*. An *in vivo* study has shown that up to $27.46 \pm 15.38$ μmol/L of genistein in human plasma can be achieved after receiving genistein supplement at a dose of 16.0 mg/kg,[20] suggesting the bioavailability of genistein from supplement for cancer prevention. The maintenance of high steady-state plasma concentration of isoflavones can be achieved by regular intakes of isoflavone supplement.

## 14.3  ISOFLAVONES AND CANCERS

### 14.3.1  ISOFLAVONES AND BREAST CANCER

The studies on geographical differences in the incidence of breast cancer have shown the preventive effects of soy product on breast cancers. It has been known that the incidence of breast cancer is much higher in Western countries and the U.S. than in China or Japan.[1] A much higher level of isoflavones in plasma has been reported in Asian women with low breast cancer incidence,[5] suggesting a protective role of soy-derived substances against breast cancer. It has been reported that Asian women who emigrated from their native countries to the U.S. and adopted Western lifestyles typically experience increasing breast cancer incidence,[21,22] suggesting that consumption of soy-rich food in their native countries may have a role in reducing the risk of breast cancer. Because of their structural similarity with estrogens, isoflavones bind to estrogen receptors. They initiate only modest response, block the binding of more potent estrogens at same time, and affect estrogen metabolism, thereby exerting a potential role in the prevention of breast cancer.

The data from *in vivo* animal experiments have shown that isoflavones have chemopreventive activity in the rat models of carcinogen-induced breast cancer.[23–26] It has been believed that the timing of the exposure of rats to isoflavones is critical for the prevention of carcinogenesis. Rats treated neonatally or prepubertally with genistein have a longer latency before the occurrence of carcinogen-induced mammary tumors and a marked reduction in tumor number.[23] Isoflavones have also shown the anticarcinogenic effects in mouse breast cancer induced by mouse mammary tumor virus.[27] Moreover, treatment of breast cancer cells with genistein before implantation into nude mice reduces the cells' tumorigenic potential.[28] In addition, isoflavones also inhibit mammary adenocarcinoma growth in syngeneic mouse model,[29] suggesting their inhibitory effects on cancer cell growth *in vivo*.

Isoflavones, in particular genistein, have been shown to inhibit the growth of breast cancer cells *in vitro*.[30] We have found that genistein inhibits the growth of breast cancer cell lines including MDA-MB-231, MDA-MB-435, MCF-7, and MCF10CA1a, regardless of the status of p53 and estrogen receptor (ER).[31-34] Other investigators have also reported similar results in MDA-MB-468, BT20, and T47D breast cancer cells.[35,36] These results suggest that the inhibitory effects of isoflavones on cell growth may be mediated by both ER-dependent and ER-independent pathways. By flow cytometric analysis, we and other investigators have shown that genistein induces a $G_2/M$ cell cycle arrest in MCF-7, MDA-MB-231, MCF10CA1a, and other breast cancer cells,[33,36-38] demonstrating that genistein inhibits the growth of breast cancer cells through induction of $G_2/M$ cell cycle arrest. By using DNA ladder, poly(ADP-ribose) polymerase (PARP), CPP32, and 7AAD assays, we have also found that genistein induces apoptosis in various breast cancer cells,[31-33] suggesting that genistein may inhibit breast cancer cell growth through induction of apoptosis. Other investigations have also observed similar results in genistein-treated breast cancer cells.[39,40]

### 14.3.2  ISOFLAVONES AND PROSTATE CANCER

Epidemiological studies have revealed that soy-rich foods also have a protective role against prostate cancer. Prostate cancer is the most common male cancer in the U.S. and Europe. In contrast, the incidence of prostate cancer in China or Japan is much lower than in the U.S. and Europe. This difference has been believed to be partly due to the dietary factors. A reduced risk of prostate cancer has been associated with consumption of soy foods and isoflavones in China.[41] High consumption of soymilk has also been associated with reduced risk of prostate cancer in the U.S.[42] These finding suggest that isoflavones may be potent agents for prostate cancer chemoprevention.

Soy diets have been shown to inhibit the development of spontaneous and carcinogen-induced prostate cancers in animal models. It has been found that the soy diet significantly prevents spontaneous development of prostate and seminal vesicle cancers in Lobund-Wistar (L-W) rats.[43] In a rat carcinogenesis model induced by 3,2′-dimethyl-4-aminobiphenyl (DMAB), isoflavone supplemented diets prevent the development of adenocarcinomas in the prostate and seminal vesicles.[44] Isoflavones also have been found to suppress other chemical-induced prostate cancer in L-W rats.[45] In addition to the inhibition of carcinogenesis, soy diets also reduce the growth of transplanted prostate adenocarcinomas and inhibit tumor cell proliferation and angiogenesis of transplanted prostate cancer in immunodeficient mice.[46,47] Moreover, animal experiments also showed that isoflavones inhibit orthotopic growth and metastasis of androgen-sensitive human prostate cancers in mice.[48] We also found that dietary genistein significantly inhibited the growth of PC3 bone tumor in SCID-human prostate cancer bone metastasis model.[49] These *in vivo* animal experiments demonstrate that isoflavones can inhibit carcinogenesis and growth of prostate cancer in animal models.

The *in vitro* experiments have also demonstrated that isoflavones inhibit the growth of prostate cancer cells. By MTT cell growth assay, we have found that genistein inhibits the growth of PC3 and LNCaP prostate cancer cells, regardless of the status of p53 and androgen receptor (AR). Flow cytometric analysis showed that genistein induces a $G_2/M$ cell cycle arrest in PC3 and LNCaP cells.[50] Other investigators have also reported similar results in other prostate cancer cell lines,[51–54] showing that genistein inhibits the growth of prostate cancer cells and induces cell cycle arrest. By using DNA ladder, PARP, and 7AAD assays, we have found that genistein induces apoptosis in prostate cancer cells,[50,55] suggesting that genistein may inhibit prostate cancer cell growth through induction of apoptosis. Similar results showing induction of apoptosis in prostate cancer cells by genistein have been also observed by other investigators.[53,56]

### 14.3.3 ISOFLAVONES AND OTHER HORMONE-RELATED CANCERS

In addition to breast and prostate cancer cells, isoflavones also showed inhibitory effects on other hormone-related cancers including endometrial, ovarian, and cervical cancers. It has been found that isoflavone consumptions in the typical American-style diet are inversely related to the risk of endometrial cancer.[57] Animal study has shown that soybean isoflavones have an inhibitory effect on estrogen-related endometrial carcinogenesis, possibly by suppressing estrogen-stimulated gene expression including c-fos, c-jun, interleukin-1α (IL-1α), and tumor necrosis factor-α (TNF-α) in ovariectomized mice uteri.[58] It has been reported that isoflavones exhibit inhibitory effects on the growth of HeLa and ME-180 cervical cancer cells.[59] Treatment of these cell lines with isoflavone genistein also resulted in suppression of invasion through a surrogate membrane in a dose-dependent manner. Several experimental studies also demonstrated that genistein exerts inhibitory effects on ovarian cancer cells. Tanaka et al.[60] have reported that genistein inhibits DMBA-induced ovarian carcinogenesis in rats. Genistein also inhibits the growth of Caov-3, NIH:OVCAR-3, and other ovarian cancer cells.[61,62] These results suggest that soy isoflavones may serve as potent agents for prevention and treatment of estrogen-related cancers.

### 14.3.4 ISOFLAVONES AND HORMONE-INDEPENDENT CANCERS

It has been found that isoflavones not only decrease the risk of hormone-related cancers, but also inhibit hormone-independent cancers including leukemia, lymphoma, melanoma, lung, pancreatic, gastric, intestinal, hepatic, urinary, and head and neck cancer cells.[63–74] Animal experiments have shown that genistein inhibits the growth of human leukemia cells transplanted into mice.[63,75] Dietary soy isoflavones have been known to protect ovariectomized ERαKO and wild-type mice from carcinogen-induced colon cancer.[74] A diet rich in soy has been found to inhibit pulmonary metastasis of melanoma cells in C57Bl/6 mice.[76] In an orthotopic model of pancreatic cancer, genistein increases apoptosis, almost completely inhibits metastasis, and significantly improves survival.[68]

The *in vitro* experimental studies from our laboratory and other investigators have demonstrated that isoflavones inhibit the growth of various hormone-independent cancers.[65–67,70,72,73] Flow cytometric analysis showed that genistein induces a $G_2/M$ cell cycle arrest in nonsmall cell lung cancer,[66] gastric adenocarcinoma,[69] hepatoma,[77] and melanoma cells.[65] By apoptosis assays, we have found that genistein induces apoptosis in lung cancer and head and neck cancer cells,[66,67,73] suggesting that genistein may inhibit cancer cell growth through induction of apoptosis. Other investigators have also reported similar results in isoflavone-treated hepatoma and leukemia cells.[77,78] These results demonstrated that isoflavones have inhibitory effects on both hormone-related and hormone-independent cancers, and may be promising agents against various cancers.

## 14.4 MOLECULAR MECHANISMS OF ACTION OF ISOFLAVONES

### 14.4.1 REGULATION OF THE EXPRESSION OF GENES RELATED TO CELL CYCLE AND APOPTOSIS

To explore the molecular mechanisms by which genistein induces cell cycle arrest, we have examined the expression of cell cycle-related genes including cyclins, CDC2, and cyclin dependent kinase inhibitors (CDKIs). Our results showed that the treatment of cells with different concentrations of genistein caused a dose-dependent decrease in the expression of cyclin $B_1$,[50,66] corresponding with the $G_2/M$ phase cell cycle arrest as observed by flow cytometry. Isoflavone-induced $G_2/M$ arrest has been associated with the inhibition of CDC2 kinase activity.[77,79] We and other investigators have also found significant upregulation of p21[WAF1] expression in genistein-treated cancer cells compared to control cells.[31,32,38,50,51,66,73,79] Moreover, our microarray data showed that genistein inhibited cell growth through downregulation of cell proliferation and cell cycle-related genes (cyclin B, CDC25A, TGF-β, ki67).[80] These results suggest that downregulation of cyclin $B_1$, CDC2, CDC25A, TGF-β, and ki67, and upregulation of p21[WAF1] could be one of the mechanisms by which genistein arrests cancer cells in $G_2/M$ phase and inhibits cancer cell growth.

To explore the molecular mechanisms by which genistein induces apoptosis, our laboratory has examined the expression of genes that are critically involved in the apoptotic pathways after genistein treatment. The results showed that genistein treatment reduced Bcl-2 protein expression and significantly increased expression of Bax in all cancer cells tested.[31,32,50,66,73,81] Other investigators also reported that soy isoflavones could induce apoptosis in human hepatoma cells and breast cancer cells through caspase-3 activation and downregulation of Bcl-2, Bcl-$_{XL}$, and HER-2/neu.[39,77,82] Kazi et al.[83] showed that genistein induced apoptosis by inhibition of proteasome and induction of p27[KIP1], IκB-α, and Bax.[83] These results suggest that caspase activation, inhibition of proteasome, upregulation of

Bax, and downregulation of Bcl-2, Bcl-$_{XL}$, and HER-2/neu may be additional molecular mechanisms by which isoflavones induce apoptosis.

## 14.4.2 REGULATION OF CELL SIGNALING PATHWAYS

### 14.4.2.1 NF-κB Pathway

Nuclear factor-κB (NF-κB) pathway plays important roles in the control of cell growth, differentiation, apoptosis, inflammation, stress response, and many other physiological processes in cellular signaling. Because of its importance in cancer development and progression, NF-κB has been described as a major culprit and a therapeutic target in cancer.[84–88] To investigate whether genistein regulates cell growth and apoptosis through NF-κB pathway, our laboratory examined NF-κB DNA-binding activity in genistein treated PC3 and LNCaP prostate cancer cells by electrophoretic mobility shift assay (EMSA).[89] The results showed that genistein significantly inhibited NF-κB DNA-binding activity in both cell lines and abrogated the induction of NF-κB DNA-binding activity stimulated by either H$_2$O$_2$ or TNF-α. These results demonstrated that genistein inhibits NF-κB DNA-binding activity in both nonstimulated and stimulated conditions.[89] Similar results have been reported by other investigators, showing that NF-κB DNA binding and COX-2 promoter activity were enhanced by TNF-α, and these effects were inhibited by genistein in human lung epithelial cells.[90]

It has been known that NF-κB DNA-binding activity could be activated by IκB phosphorylation, IκB could be phosphorylated by activated IκB kinase (IKK), and IKK could be phosphorylated and activated by an upstream kinase, mitogen-activated kinase kinase 1 (MEKK1).[91–94] The results from our laboratory showed that genistein treatment inhibited MEKK1 kinase activity and reduced the amount of phosphorylated IκB in prostate cancer cells. Cells treated with TNF-α or H$_2$O$_2$ showed increased MEKK1 kinase activity and genistein pretreatment blocked MEKK1 kinase activation stimulated by TNF-α or H$_2$O$_2$. These results suggest that genistein may inhibit MEKK1 kinase activity and subsequent phosphorylation of IκB, thereby resulting in the inactivation of NF-κB.

It has been reported that some chemotherapeutic agents such as cisplatin and docetaxel induce the activation of NF-κB in cancer cells, and this may be responsible for drug resistance in cancer cells. Therefore, inactivation of NF-κB in combination with chemotherapeutic agents may lead to better killing of cancer cells by existing chemotherapeutic agents. Indeed, we have found that the combination treatment of genistein with lower doses of docetaxel or cisplatin elicited significantly greater inhibition of cell growth compared to either agent alone.[95] The combination treatment induced more apoptosis compared to single agents. By EMSA, we found that NF-κB activity was significantly increased by docetaxel or cisplatin treatment, and the NF-κB-inducing activity of these agents was completely abrogated in cells pretreated with genistein. These results clearly suggest that genistein pretreatment, which inactivates NF-κB activity, together with other cellular effects of genistein, may contribute to increased cell growth inhibition and apoptosis with nontoxic doses of docetaxel or cisplatin, which could be a novel strategy for the treatment of cancer.

### 14.4.2.2 Akt Pathway

Akt pathway is an important cell signal transduction pathway. It has been known that Akt is activated by phospholipid binding and phosphorylation at Thr308 by PDK1 or at Ser473 by PDK2.[96] Activated Akt functions to promote cell survival by inhibiting apoptosis through inactivation of pro-apoptotic factors.[97–99] Akt also regulates NF-κB pathway via phosphorylation and activation of molecules in NF-κB pathway. Because of its importance in promoting cell survival, Akt has received much attention and has been believed to be a therapeutic target in cancer.[100,101] We have previously investigated the effects of genistein on Akt pathway in PC3 prostate cancer cells.[55] We found that genistein reduced the level of phosphorylated Akt protein and the Akt kinase activity under nonstimulated condition. Genistein also abrogated Akt activation stimulated by EGF, suggesting the inactivation of Akt kinase under both nonstimulated and stimulated conditions after genistein treatment.

We have further investigated the inhibitory mechanisms of genistein on Akt and NF-κB pathways by transfection experiments.[55] Akt expression construct (pLNCX-Akt) was transiently co-transfected with NF-κB-Luc reporter construct into PC3 prostate cancer cells. Luciferase assay showed an induced luciferase activity in PC3 cells co-transfected with pLNCX-Akt and NF-κB-Luc. However, genistein inhibited the luciferase activity in PC3 cells co-transfected with pLNCX-Akt and NF-κB-Luc. Furthermore, genistein abrogated the activation of Akt in transfected cells stimulated by EGF. EMSA testing for NF-κB DNA-binding activity in transfected cells also showed similar results. These results demonstrate that genistein exerts its inhibitory effects on NF-κB pathway through Akt pathway. Downregulation of NF-κB and Akt signaling pathways by genistein may be one of the molecular mechanisms by which genistein inhibits cancer cell growth and induces apoptosis. Another study by other investigators also demonstrated that genistein could inhibit Akt activation induced by estradiol in MCF-7 cells.[102] These studies provide strong molecular evidence showing the anticancer effects of isoflavone genistein through Akt and NF-κB regulation.

### 14.4.2.3 AR and ER Pathways

It has been known that androgen receptor (AR) signaling pathway is involved in the development and progression of prostate cancer through regulation of transcription of prostate specific antigen (PSA).[103,104] We have investigated the effects of genistein on the expression of PSA through androgen regulation[105] and found that genistein at low concentration (<10 μmol/L) transcriptionally downregulated AR, decreased nuclear protein binding to ARE, and, thereby, inhibited the transcription and protein expression of PSA in androgen-sensitive LNCaP cells. However, higher concentrations (10 to 50 μmol/L) of genistein was needed to significantly inhibit PSA secretion in VeCaP cells, which are androgen-insensitive, and no alternation in the AR expression or ARE binding activity was observed. By transfection experiments, we found that genistein inhibited PSA synthesis in prostate cancer cells through both androgen-dependent and androgen-independent pathways. These results demonstrate the inhibitory effects of genistein on AR and PSA.

Because of its structural similarity to estrogen, isoflavones have been expected to exert their effects through ER signaling pathway. However, an experimental study has found that isoflavones at different concentrations may exhibit different effects. Genistein might either induce breast cancer cell proliferation by estrogenic agonistic properties (at concentrations ≤1 µmol/L) or prevent hormone-dependent growth of breast cancer cells by potential estrogen-antagonistic activity (at concentrations ≥5 µmol/L) dependent on its concentrations.[106] Moreover, experimental studies show that isoflavones also have inhibitory effects on hormone-independent cancers. These results suggest that isoflavones may be potent chemopreventive and/or therapeutic agents for cancers, regardless of hormone responsiveness.

### 14.4.3 REGULATION OF THE EXPRESSION OF GENES RELATED TO ANGIOGENESIS AND METASTASIS

Genistein has been shown to reduce the angiogenic and metastatic potential of cancers.[76,107] We have examined the effect of genistein on the expression of MMPs in MDA-MB-435 breast cancer cells transfected with c-erbB-2,[32] which has been shown to promote secretion of MMPs and subsequent metastasis in experimental models.[108] We found that the expression of c-erbB-2, MMP-2, and MMP-9 in MDA-MB-435 cells stably transfected with c-erbB-2 was much higher than that in parental MDA-MB-435 cells. However, the high expression of c-erbB-2, MMP-2, and MMP-9 in 435 transfectants was significantly downregulated by genistein treatment.[32] These results suggest that genistein may inhibit the expression of c-erbB-2 and subsequently decrease the secretion of MMPs in breast cancer cells.

To further explore the molecular mechanisms by which genistein exerts its anti-angiogenic and anti-metastatic effects on cancer cells, we have utilized microarray to determine the gene expression profile altered by genistein treatment.[109] We found that genistein downregulated the expression of MMP-9, protease M, uPAR, VEGF, neuropilin, TSP, BPGF, LPA, TGF-β, TSP-1, and PAR-2, and upregulated the expression of connective tissue growth factor and connective tissue activation peptide.[109] All of these genes are related to angiogenesis and metastasis. The microarray data were confirmed by RT-PCR, Western blot, and zymographic analysis at the mRNA and protein levels. We have also conducted animal experiment using SCID-human prostate cancer bone metastasis model. We found that dietary genistein significantly inhibited the growth of PC3 bone tumor and the expression of MMPs.[49] Our results demonstrate that genistein regulates the transcription and translation of genes critically involved in the control of angiogenesis, tumor cell invasion and metastasis, and inhibits prostate cancer cell growth in bone metastasis model, suggesting that genistein may be a potent agent against metastatic cancers.

### 14.4.4 REGULATION OF OXIDATIVE STRESS

Isoflavones have been known to function as antioxidants. Since increased oxidative stress is related to carcinogenesis, it has been believed that isoflavones may inhibit carcinogenesis through antioxidative effect of isoflavones. It has been shown that isoflavone reduces hydrogen peroxide-induced DNA damage in sperm[110] and that genistein inhibits tumor promoter, 12-*O*-tetradecanoylphorbol-13-acetate (TPA)-induced hydrogen peroxide production in human polymorpho-nuclear leukocytes and HL-60 cells,[111] suggesting the inhibitory effect of isoflavones on carcinogenesis. Genistein has also shown to stimulate antioxidant gene expression in colon cancer cells,[112] and to inhibit ultraviolet (UV) irradiation-induced oxidative stress in epidermal carcinoma,[113] suggesting its inhibitory effects on cancer cells.

Because oxidative stress activates NF-κB DNA binding activity,[114] we have investigated whether the effect of isoflavone supplementation could inactivate NF-κB and reduce oxidative damage in lymphocytes in human subjects.[115] The lymphocytes from healthy male subjects were harvested from peripheral blood and cultured for 24 h in the absence and presence of genistein. We found that genistein treatment inhibited basal levels of NF-κB DNA binding activity and abrogated TNF-α induced NF-κB activity.[115] When human subjects received 50 mg of isoflavone supplements Novasoy™ twice daily for 3 weeks, TNF-α failed to activate NF-κB activity in lymphocytes harvested from these subjects, while lymphocytes from these subjects collected prior to isoflavone intervention showed activation of NF-κB DNA binding activity upon TNF-α treatment.[115] These results suggest that isoflavone supplementation has a protective effect against TNF-α-induced NF-κB activation in humans both *in vitro* and *in vivo*. We have also investigated the effect of isoflavone supplementation on oxidative DNA damage by measuring the levels of 5-OHmdU, which represents the endogenous status of cellular oxidative stress, in the peripheral blood lymphocytes of normal human subjects before and after isoflavone supplementation. The results showed that 5-OHmdU was significantly decreased after 3 weeks of isoflavone supplementation.[115] These results demonstrate that isoflavones may exert their chemopreventive effects through regulation of oxidative stress.

## 14.5 CONCLUSION

Epidemiological studies and numerous *in vitro* and *in vivo* experiments have clearly indicated that isoflavones exert inhibitory effects on carcinogenesis, cancer cell growth, and cancer progression. These effects of isoflavones have been known to be mediated through the regulation of cell cycle, apoptosis, cell signal transduction pathways, cellular oxidative stress, and cell physiological behaviors. Therefore, isoflavones may be promising agents for prevention and/or treatment of various cancers. Further in-depth experiments and clinical trials will fully evaluate the value of isoflavones as potential chemopreventive or therapeutic agents against cancers.

## ACKNOWLEDGMENT

The authors' work cited in this chapter was partly funded by grants from the National Cancer Institute, NIH (1R01CA101870-01 and 5R01CA083695-03) awarded to F.H.S.

## REFERENCES

1. American Cancer Society. *Cancer Facts & Figures 2005*. Atlanta: American Cancer Society; 2005.
2. Chen Z, Zheng W, Custer LJ, Dai Q, Shu XO, Jin F, Franke AA. Usual dietary consumption of soy foods and its correlation with the excretion rate of isoflavonoids in overnight urine samples among Chinese women in Shanghai. *Nutr Cancer* 1999; 33:82–87.
3. Arai Y, Uehara M, Sato Y, Kimira M, Eboshida A, Adlercreutz H, Watanabe S. Comparison of isoflavones among dietary intake, plasma concentration and urinary excretion for accurate estimation of phytoestrogen intake. *J Epidemiol* 2000; 10:127–135.
4. Setchell KD, Cassidy A. Dietary isoflavones: biological effects and relevance to human health. *J Nutr* 1999; 129:758S–767S.
5. Adlercreutz CH, Goldin BR, Gorbach SL, Hockerstedt KA, Watanabe S, Hamalainen EK, Markkanen MH, Makela TH, Wahala KT, Adlercreutz T. Soybean phytoestrogen intake and cancer risk. *J Nutr* 1995; 125:757S–770S.
6. Jacobsen BK, Knutsen SF, Fraser GE. Does high soy milk intake reduce prostate cancer incidence? The Adventist Health Study (United States). *Cancer Causes Control* 1998; 9:553–557.
7. Lee HP, Gourley L, Duffy SW, Esteve J, Lee J, Day NE. Dietary effects on breast-cancer risk in Singapore. *Lancet* 1991; 337:1197–1200.
8. Fletcher RJ. Food sources of phyto-oestrogens and their precursors in Europe. *Br J Nutr* 2003; 89(Suppl 1):S39–S43.
9. Coldham NG, Darby C, Hows M, King LJ, Zhang AQ, Sauer MJ. Comparative metabolism of genistin by human and rat gut microflora: detection and identification of the end-products of metabolism. *Xenobiotica* 2002; 32:45–62.
10. Coldham NG, Sauer MJ. Identification, quantitation and biological activity of phytoestrogens in a dietary supplement for breast enhancement. *Food Chem Toxicol* 2001; 39:1211–1224.
11. Kulling SE, Lehmann L, Metzler M. Oxidative metabolism and genotoxic potential of major isoflavone phytoestrogens. *J Chromatogr B Anal Technol Biomed Life Sci* 2002; 777:211–218.
12. Kelly GE, Nelson C, Waring MA, Joannou GE, Reeder AY. Metabolites of dietary (soya) isoflavones in human urine. *Clin Chim Acta* 1993; 223:9–22.
13. Lampe JW. Isoflavonoid and lignan phytoestrogens as dietary biomarkers. *J Nutr* 2003; 133(Suppl 3):956S–964S.

14. Izumi T, Piskula MK, Osawa S, Obata A, Tobe K, Saito M, Kataoka S, Kubota Y, Kikuchi M. Soy isoflavone aglycones are absorbed faster and in higher amounts than their glucosides in humans. *J Nutr* 2000; 130:1695–1699.

15. Adlercreutz H, Fotsis T, Watanabe S, Lampe J, Wahala K, Makela T, Hase T. Determination of lignans and isoflavonoids in plasma by isotope dilution gas chromatography-mass spectrometry. *Cancer Detect Prev* 1994; 18:259–271.

16. King RA, Bursill DB. Plasma and urinary kinetics of the isoflavones daidzein and genistein after a single soy meal in humans. *Am J Clin Nutr* 1998; 67:867–872.

17. Morton MS, Wilcox G, Wahlqvist ML, Griffiths K. Determination of lignans and isoflavonoids in human female plasma following dietary supplementation. *J Endocrinol* 1994; 142:251–259.

18. Xu X, Wang HJ, Murphy PA, Hendrich S. Neither background diet nor type of soy food affects short-term isoflavone bioavailability in women. *J Nutr* 2000; 130:798–801.

19. Adlercreutz H, Fotsis T, Lampe J, Wahala K, Makela T, Brunow G, Hase T. Quantitative determination of lignans and isoflavonoids in plasma of omnivorous and vegetarian women by isotope dilution gas chromatography-mass spectrometry. *Scand J Clin Lab Invest Suppl* 1993; 215:5–18.

20. Busby MG, Jeffcoat AR, Bloedon LT, Koch MA, Black T, Dix KJ, Heizer WD, Thomas BF, Hill JM, Crowell JA, Zeisel SH. Clinical characteristics and pharmacokinetics of purified soy isoflavones: single-dose administration to healthy men. *Am J Clin Nutr* 2002; 75:126–136.

21. Deapen D, Liu L, Perkins C, Bernstein L, Ross RK. Rapidly rising breast cancer incidence rates among Asian-American women. *Int J Cancer* 2002; 99:747–750.

22. Ziegler RG, Hoover RN, Pike MC, Hildesheim A, Nomura AM, West DW, Wu-Williams AH, Kolonel LN, Horn-Ross PL, Rosenthal JF. Migration patterns and breast cancer risk in Asian-American women. *J Natl Cancer Inst* 1993; 85:1819–1827.

23. Barnes S. The chemopreventive properties of soy isoflavonoids in animal models of breast cancer. *Breast Cancer Res Treat* 1997; 46:169–179.

24. Hawrylewicz EJ, Zapata JJ, Blair WH. Soy and experimental cancer: animal studies. *J Nutr* 1995; 125:698S–708S.

25. Gotoh T, Yamada K, Yin H, Ito A, Kataoka T, Dohi K. Chemoprevention of *N*-nitroso-*N*-methylurea-induced rat mammary carcinogenesis by soy foods or biochanin A. *Jpn J Cancer Res* 1998; 89:137–142.

26. Constantinou AI, Mehta RG, Vaughan A. Inhibition of N-methyl-N-nitrosourea-induced mammary tumors in rats by the soybean isoflavones. *Anticancer Res* 1996; 16:3293–3298.

27. Mizunuma H, Kanazawa K, Ogura S, Otsuka S, Nagai H. Anticarcinogenic effects of isoflavones may be mediated by genistein in mouse mammary tumor virus-induced breast cancer. *Oncology* 2002; 62:78–84.

28. Constantinou AI, Krygier AE, Mehta RR. Genistein induces maturation of cultured human breast cancer cells and prevents tumor growth in nude mice. *Am J Clin Nutr* 1998; 68:1426S–1430S.

29. Hewitt AL, Singletary KW. Soy extract inhibits mammary adenocarcinoma growth in a syngeneic mouse model. *Cancer Lett* 2003; 192:133–143.

30. Barnes S. Effect of genistein on in vitro and in vivo models of cancer. *J Nutr* 1995; 125:777S–783S.

31. Li Y, Upadhyay S, Bhuiyan M, Sarkar FH. Induction of apoptosis in breast cancer cells MDA-MB-231 by genistein. *Oncogene* 1999; 18:3166–3172.

32. Li Y, Bhuiyan M, Sarkar FH. Induction of apoptosis and inhibition of c-erbB-2 in MDA-MB-435 cells by genistein. *Int J Oncol* 1999; 15:525–533.

33. Upadhyay S, Neburi M, Chinni SR, Alhasan S, Miller F, Sarkar FH. Differential sensitivity of normal and malignant breast epithelial cells to genistein is partly mediated by p21(WAF1). *Clin Cancer Res* 2001; 7:1782–1789.

34. Chinni SR, Alhasan SA, Multani AS, Pathak S, Sarkar FH. Pleotropic effects of genistein on MCF-7 breast cancer cells. *Int J Mol Med* 2003; 12:29–34.

35. Balabhadrapathruni S, Thomas TJ, Yurkow EJ, Amenta PS, Thomas T. Effects of genistein and structurally related phytoestrogens on cell cycle kinetics and apoptosis in MDA-MB-468 human breast cancer cells. *Oncol Rep* 2000; 7:3–12.

36. Cappelletti V, Fioravanti L, Miodini P, Di Fronzo G. Genistein blocks breast cancer cells in the G(2)M phase of the cell cycle. *J Cell Biochem* 2000; 79:594–600.

37. Pagliacci MC, Smacchia M, Migliorati G, Grignani F, Riccardi C, Nicoletti I. Growth-inhibitory effects of the natural phyto-oestrogen genistein in MCF-7 human breast cancer cells. *Eur J Cancer* 1994; 30A:1675–1682.

38. Choi YH, Zhang L, Lee WH, Park KY. Genistein-induced G2/M arrest is associated with the inhibition of cyclin B1 and the induction of p21 in human breast carcinoma cells. *Int J Oncol* 1998; 13:391–396.

39. Katdare M, Osborne M, Telang NT. Soy isoflavone genistein modulates cell cycle progression and induces apoptosis in HER-2/neu oncogene expressing human breast epithelial cells. *Int J Oncol* 2002; 21:809–815.

40. Shao ZM, Alpaugh ML, Fontana JA, Barsky SH. Genistein inhibits proliferation similarly in estrogen receptor-positive and negative human breast carcinoma cell lines characterized by P21WAF1/CIP1 induction, G2/M arrest, and apoptosis. *J Cell Biochem* 1998; 69:44–54.

41. Lee MM, Gomez SL, Chang JS, Wey M, Wang RT, Hsing AW. Soy and isoflavone consumption in relation to prostate cancer risk in China. *Cancer Epidemiol Biomarkers Prev* 2003; 12:665–668.

42. Jacobsen BK, Knutsen SF, Fraser GE. Does high soy milk intake reduce prostate cancer incidence? The Adventist Health Study (United States). *Cancer Causes Control* 1998; 9:553–557.

43. Pollard M, Wolter W. Prevention of spontaneous prostate-related cancer in Lobund-Wistar rats by a soy protein isolate/isoflavone diet. *Prostate* 2000; 45:101–105.

44. Onozawa M, Kawamori T, Baba M, Fukuda K, Toda T, Sato H, Ohtani M, Akaza H, Sugimura T, Wakabayashi K. Effects of a soybean isoflavone mixture on carcinogenesis in prostate and seminal vesicles of F344 rats. *Jpn J Cancer Res* 1999; 90:393–398.

45. Wang J, Eltoum IE, Lamartiniere CA. Dietary genistein suppresses chemically induced prostate cancer in Lobund-Wistar rats. *Cancer Lett* 2002; 186:11–18.

46. Landstrom M, Zhang JX, Hallmans G, Aman P, Bergh A, Damber JE, Mazur W, Wahala K, Adlercreutz H. Inhibitory effects of soy and rye diets on the development of Dunning R3327 prostate adenocarcinoma in rats. *Prostate* 1998; 36:151–161.

47. Zhou JR, Gugger ET, Tanaka T, Guo Y, Blackburn GL, Clinton SK. Soybean phytochemicals inhibit the growth of transplantable human prostate carcinoma and tumor angiogenesis in mice. *J Nutr* 1999; 129:1628–1635.

48. Zhou JR, Yu L, Zhong Y, Nassr RL, Franke AA, Gaston SM, Blackburn GL. Inhibition of orthotopic growth and metastasis of androgen-sensitive human prostate tumors in mice by bioactive soybean components. *Prostate* 2002; 53:143–153.

49. Li Y, Che M, Bhagat S, Ellis K, Kucuk O, Doerge DR, Abrams J, Cher ML, Sarkar FH. Regulation of gene expression and inhibition of experimental prostate cancer bone metastasis by dietary genistein. *Neoplasia* 2004; 6:354–363.

50. Davis JN, Singh B, Bhuiyan M, Sarkar FH. Genistein-induced upregulation of p21WAF1, downregulation of cyclin B, and induction of apoptosis in prostate cancer cells. *Nutr Cancer* 1998; 32:123–131.

51. Choi YH, Lee WH, Park KY, Zhang L. p53-independent induction of p21 (WAF1/CIP1), reduction of cyclin B1 and G2/M arrest by the isoflavone genistein in human prostate carcinoma cells. *Jpn J Cancer Res* 2000; 91:164–173.

52. Ejima Y, Yan S, Sasaki R, Nishimura H, Demizu Y, Okamoto Y, Matsumoto A, Soejima T, Sugimura K. Combination of genistein with ionizing radiation on surviving fraction, apoptosis and cell-cycle alterations on Du-145 prostate cancer cells. *Int J Radiat Oncol Biol Phys* 2003; 57:S353.

53. Kyle E, Neckers L, Takimoto C, Curt G, Bergan R. Genistein-induced apoptosis of prostate cancer cells is preceded by a specific decrease in focal adhesion kinase activity. *Mol Pharmacol* 1997; 51:193–200.

54. Peterson G, Barnes S. Genistein and biochanin A inhibit the growth of human prostate cancer cells but not epidermal growth factor receptor tyrosine autophosphorylation. *Prostate* 1993; 22:335–345.

55. Li Y, Sarkar FH. Inhibition of nuclear factor κB activation in PC3 cells by genistein is mediated via Akt signaling pathway. *Clin Cancer Res* 2002; 8:2369–2377.

56. Kumi-Diaka J, Sanderson NA, Hall A. The mediating role of caspase-3 protease in the intracellular mechanism of genistein-induced apoptosis in human prostatic carcinoma cell lines, DU145 and LNCaP. *Biol Cell* 2000; 92:595–604.

57. Horn-Ross PL, John EM, Canchola AJ, Stewart SL, Lee MM. Phytoestrogen intake and endometrial cancer risk. *J Natl Cancer Inst* 2003; 95:1158–1164.

58. Lian Z, Niwa K, Tagami K, Hashimoto M, Gao J, Yokoyama Y, Mori H, Tamaya T. Preventive effects of isoflavones, genistein and daidzein, on estradiol-17beta-related endometrial carcinogenesis in mice. *Jpn J Cancer Res* 2001; 92:726–734.

59. Wang SY, Yang KW, Hsu YT, Chang CL, Yang YC. The differential inhibitory effects of genistein on the growth of cervical cancer cells *in vitro*. *Neoplasma* 2001; 48:227–233.

60. Tanaka T, Kohno H, Tanino M, Yanaida Y. Inhibitory effects of estrogenic compounds, 4-nonylphenol and genistein, on 7,12-dimethylbenz[a]anthracene-induced ovarian carcinogenesis in rats. *Ecotoxicol Environ Saf* 2002; 52:38–45.

61. Chen X, Anderson JJ. Isoflavones inhibit proliferation of ovarian cancer cells *in vitro* via an estrogen receptor-dependent pathway. *Nutr Cancer* 2001; 41:165–171.

62. Gercel-Taylor C, Feitelson AK, Taylor DD. Inhibitory effect of genistein and daidzein on ovarian cancer cell growth. *Anticancer Res* 2004; 24:795–800.

63. Uckun FM, Evans WE, Forsyth CJ, Waddick KG, Ahlgren LT, Chelstrom LM, Burkhardt A, Bolen J, Myers DE. Biotherapy of B-cell precursor leukemia by targeting genistein to CD19-associated tyrosine kinases. *Science* 1995; 267:886–891.

64. Buckley AR, Buckley DJ, Gout PW, Liang H, Rao YP, Blake MJ. Inhibition by genistein of prolactin-induced Nb2 lymphoma cell mitogenesis. *Mol Cell Endocrinol* 1993; 98:17–25.

65. Casagrande F, Darbon JM. p21CIP1 is dispensable for the G2 arrest caused by genistein in human melanoma cells. *Exp Cell Res* 2000; 258:101–108.

66. Lian F, Bhuiyan M, Li YW, Wall N, Kraut M, Sarkar FH. Genistein-induced G2-M arrest, p21WAF1 upregulation, and apoptosis in a non-small-cell lung cancer cell line. *Nutr Cancer* 1998; 31:184–191.

67. Lian F, Li Y, Bhuiyan M, Sarkar FH. p53-independent apoptosis induced by genistein in lung cancer cells. *Nutr Cancer* 1999; 33:125–131.

68. Buchler P, Gukovskaya AS, Mouria M, Buchler MC, Buchler MW, Friess H, Pandol SJ, Reber HA, Hines OJ. Prevention of metastatic pancreatic cancer growth in vivo by induction of apoptosis with genistein, a naturally occurring isoflavonoid. *Pancreas* 2003; 26:264–273.

69. Matsukawa Y, Marui N, Sakai T, Satomi Y, Yoshida M, Matsumoto K, Nishino H, Aoike A. Genistein arrests cell cycle progression at G2-M. *Cancer Res* 1993; 53:1328–1331.

70. Yanagihara K, Ito A, Toge T, Numoto M. Antiproliferative effects of isoflavones on human cancer cell lines established from the gastrointestinal tract. *Cancer Res* 1993; 53:5815–5821.

71. Lei B, Roncaglia V, Vigano R, Cremonini C, De Maria N, Del Buono MG, Manenti F, Villa E. Phytoestrogens and liver disease. *Mol Cell Endocrinol* 2002; 193:81–84.

72. Su SJ, Yeh TM, Lei HY, Chow NH. The potential of soybean foods as a chemo-prevention approach for human urinary tract cancer. *Clin Cancer Res* 2000; 6:230–236.

73. Alhasan SA, Pietrasczkiwicz H, Alonso MD, Ensley J, Sarkar FH. Genistein-induced cell cycle arrest and apoptosis in a head and neck squamous cell carcinoma cell line. *Nutr Cancer* 1999; 34:12–19.

74. Guo JY, Li X, Browning JD Jr, Rottinghaus GE, Lubahn DB, Constantinou A, Bennink M, MacDonald RS. Dietary soy isoflavones and estrone protect ovariectomized ERαKO and wild-type mice from carcinogen-induced colon cancer. *J Nutr* 2004; 134:179–182.

75. Lamartiniere CA, Moore JB, Brown NM, Thompson R, Hardin MJ, Barnes S. Genistein suppresses mammary cancer in rats. *Carcinogenesis* 1995; 16:2833–2840.

76. Li D, Yee JA, McGuire MH, Murphy PA, Yan L. Soybean isoflavones reduce experimental metastasis in mice. *J Nutr* 1999; 129:1075–1078.

77. Su SJ, Chow NH, Kung ML, Hung TC, Chang KL. Effects of soy isoflavones on apoptosis induction and G2-M arrest in human hepatoma cells involvement of caspase-3 activation, Bcl-2 and Bcl-XL downregulation, and Cdc2 kinase activity. *Nutr Cancer* 2003; 45:113–123.

78. Spinozzi F, Pagliacci MC, Migliorati G, Moraca R, Grignani F, Riccardi C, Nicoletti I. The natural tyrosine kinase inhibitor genistein produces cell cycle arrest and apoptosis in Jurkat T-leukemia cells. *Leukemia Res* 1994; 18:431–439.

79. Frey RS, Li J, Singletary KW. Effects of genistein on cell proliferation and cell cycle arrest in nonneoplastic human mammary epithelial cells: involvement of Cdc2, p21(waf/cip1), p27(kip1), and Cdc25C expression. *Biochem Pharmacol* 2001; 61:979–989.

80. Li Y, Sarkar FH. Gene expression profiles of genistein-treated PC3 prostate cancer cells. *J Nutr* 2002; 132:3623–3631.

81. Upadhyay S, Li G, Liu H, Chen YQ, Sarkar FH, Kim HR. bcl-2 suppresses expression of p21WAF1/CIP1 in breast epithelial cells. *Cancer Res* 1995; 55:4520–4524.

82. Po LS, Wang TT, Chen ZY, Leung LK. Genistein-induced apoptosis in MCF-7 cells involves changes in Bak and Bcl-x without evidence of anti-oestrogenic effects. *Br J Nutr* 2002; 88:463–469.

83. Kazi A, Daniel KG, Smith DM, Kumar NB, Dou QP. Inhibition of the proteasome activity, a novel mechanism associated with the tumor cell apoptosis-inducing ability of genistein. *Biochem Pharmacol* 2003; 66:965–976.

84. Bharti AC, Aggarwal BB. Nuclear factor-κB and cancer: its role in prevention and therapy. *Biochem Pharmacol* 2002; 64:883–888.

85. Biswas DK, Dai SC, Cruz A, Weiser B, Graner E, Pardee AB. The nuclear factor κB (NF-κB): a potential therapeutic target for estrogen receptor negative breast cancers. *Proc Natl Acad Sci USA* 2001; 98:10386–10391.

86. Haefner B. NF-κB: arresting a major culprit in cancer. *Drug Discovery Today* 2002; 7:653–663.

87. Hideshima T, Chauhan D, Richardson P, Mitsiades C, Mitsiades N, Hayashi T, Munshi N, Dang L, Castro A, Palombella V, Adams J, Anderson KC. NF-κB as a therapeutic target in multiple myeloma. *J Biol Chem* 2002; 277:16639–16647.

88. Orlowski RZ, Baldwin AS. NF-κB as a therapeutic target in cancer. *Trends Mol Med* 2002; 8:385–389.

89. Davis JN, Kucuk O, Sarkar FH. Genistein inhibits NF-κB activation in prostate cancer cells. *Nutr Cancer* 1999; 35:167–174.

90. Chen CC, Sun YT, Chen JJ, Chiu KT. TNF-α-induced cyclooxygenase-2 expression in human lung epithelial cells: involvement of the phospholipase C-γ 2, protein kinase C-α, tyrosine kinase, NF-κB-inducing kinase, and I-κB kinase 1/2 pathway. *J Immunol* 2000; 165:2719–2728.

91. Zandi E, Chen Y, Karin M. Direct phosphorylation of IκB by IKKα and IKKbeta: discrimination between free and NF-κB-bound substrate. *Science* 1998; 281:1360–1363.

92. Karin M, Delhase M. The I κB kinase (IKK) and NF-κB: key elements of proinflammatory signalling. *Semin Immunol* 2000; 12:85–98.

93. Lee FS, Peters RT, Dang LC, Maniatis T. MEKK1 activates both IκB kinase α and IκB kinase beta. *Proc Natl Acad Sci USA* 1998; 95:9319–9324.

94. Nakano H, Shindo M, Sakon S, Nishinaka S, Mihara M, Yagita H, Okumura K. Differential regulation of IκB kinase α and β by two upstream kinases, NF-κB-inducing kinase and mitogen-activated protein kinase/ERK kinase kinase-1. *Proc Natl Acad Sci USA* 1998; 95:3537–3542.

95. Li Y, Ellis KL, Ali S, El Rayes BF, Nedeljkovic-Kurepa A, Kucuk O, Philip PA, Sarkar FH. Apoptosis-inducing effect of chemotherapeutic agents is potentiated by soy isoflavone genistein, a natural inhibitor of NF-κB in BxPC-3 pancreatic cancer cell line. *Pancreas* 2004; 28:e90–e95.

96. Alessi DR, Andjelkovic M, Caudwell B, Cron P, Morrice N, Cohen P, Hemmings BA. Mechanism of activation of protein kinase B by insulin and IGF-1. *EMBO J* 1996; 15:6541–6551.

97. Cardone MH, Roy N, Stennicke HR, Salvesen GS, Franke TF, Stanbridge E, Frisch S, Reed JC. Regulation of cell death protease caspase-9 by phosphorylation. *Science* 1998; 282:1318–1321.

98. Brunet A, Bonni A, Zigmond MJ, Lin MZ, Juo P, Hu LS, Anderson MJ, Arden KC, Blenis J, Greenberg ME. Akt promotes cell survival by phosphorylating and inhibiting a Forkhead transcription factor. *Cell* 1999; 96:857–868.

99. Rommel C, Clarke BA, Zimmermann S, Nunez L, Rossman R, Reid K, Moelling K, Yancopoulos GD, Glass DJ. Differentiation stage-specific inhibition of the Raf-MEK-ERK pathway by Akt. *Science* 1999; 286:1738–1741.

100. Romashkova JA, Makarov SS. NF-κB is a target of AKT in anti-apoptotic PDGF signalling. *Nature* 1999; 401:86–90.

101. Ozes ON, Mayo LD, Gustin JA, Pfeffer SR, Pfeffer LM, Donner DB. NF-κB activation by tumour necrosis factor requires the Akt serine-threonine kinase. *Nature* 1999; 401:82–85.

102. Stoica GE, Franke TF, Wellstein A, Czubayko F, List HJ, Reiter R, Morgan E, Martin MB, Stoica A. Estradiol rapidly activates Akt via the ErbB2 signaling pathway. *Mol Endocrinol* 2003; 17:818–830.

103. Kupelian P, Katcher J, Levin H, Zippe C, Klein E. Correlation of clinical and pathologic factors with rising prostate-specific antigen profiles after radical prostatectomy alone for clinically localized prostate cancer. *Urology* 1996; 48:249–260.

104. Sato N, Gleave ME, Bruchovsky N, Rennie PS, Goldenberg SL, Lange PH, Sullivan LD. Intermittent androgen suppression delays progression to androgen-independent regulation of prostate-specific antigen gene in the LNCaP prostate tumour model. *J Steroid Biochem Mol Biol* 1996; 58:139–146.

105. Davis JN, Kucuk O, Sarkar FH. Expression of prostate-specific antigen is transcriptionally regulated by genistein in prostate cancer cells. *Mol Carcinogen* 2002; 34:91–101.

106. Martin PM, Horwitz KB, Ryan DS, McGuire WL. Phytoestrogen interaction with estrogen receptors in human breast cancer cells. *Endocrinology* 1978; 103:1860–1867.

107. Fotsis T, Pepper M, Adlercreutz H, Hase T, Montesano R, Schweigerer L. Genistein, a dietary ingested isoflavonoid, inhibits cell proliferation and in vitro angiogenesis. *J Nutr* 1995; 125:790S–797S.

108. Tan M, Yao J, Yu D. Overexpression of the c-erbB-2 gene enhanced intrinsic metastasis potential in human breast cancer cells without increasing their transformation abilities. *Cancer Res* 1997; 57:1199–1205.

109. Li Y, Sarkar FH. Down-regulation of invasion and angiogenesis-related genes identified by cDNA microarray analysis of PC3 prostate cancer cells treated with genistein. *Cancer Lett* 2002; 186:157–164.

110. Sierens J, Hartley JA, Campbell MJ, Leathem AJ, Woodside JV. *In vitro* isoflavone supplementation reduces hydrogen peroxide-induced DNA damage in sperm. *Teratog Carcinogen Mutagen* 2002; 22:227–234.

111. Wei H, Wei L, Frenkel K, Bowen R, Barnes S. Inhibition of tumor promoter-induced hydrogen peroxide formation in vitro and in vivo by genistein. *Nutr Cancer* 1993; 20:1–12.

112. Kameoka S, Leavitt P, Chang C, Kuo SM. Expression of antioxidant proteins in human intestinal Caco-2 cells treated with dietary flavonoids. *Cancer Lett* 1999; 146:161–167.

113. Chan WH, Yu JS. Inhibition of UV irradiation-induced oxidative stress and apoptotic biochemical changes in human epidermal carcinoma A431 cells by genistein. *J Cell Biochem* 2000; 78:73–84.

114. Dudek EJ, Shang F, Taylor A. $H_2O_2$-mediated oxidative stress activates NF-κB in lens epithelial cells. *Free Radical Biol Med* 2001; 31:651–658.

115. Davis JN, Kucuk O, Djuric Z, Sarkar FH. Soy isoflavone supplementation in healthy men prevents NF-κB activation by TNF-α in blood lymphocytes. *Free Radical Biol Med* 2001; 30:1293–1302.

# 15 Implications of Flavonoids as a Sex Hormone Source

## David Jenkins and Roxanne LaBelle

## CONTENTS

15.1 Introduction ............................................................................................313
15.2 Isoflavones, Natural Selective Estrogen Receptor Modulators
(SERMs)..............................................................................................314
15.3 Cancer and Phytoestrogens.................................................................315
    15.3.1 Breast Cancer............................................................................315
    15.3.2 Prostate Cancer .........................................................................317
    15.3.3 Other Cancers ...........................................................................317
15.4 Rat Models............................................................................................318
15.5 Trends in Cancer Incidence.................................................................320
15.6 Conclusion ...........................................................................................320
References ......................................................................................................322

## 15.1 INTRODUCTION

In recent years there has been much interest in the potential health effects of phytoestrogens. Much of the interest has centered on the structural similarity between estrogens and plant phenolics such as the isoflavones (Figure 15.1). The topic of phytoestrogens and health has recently been reviewed in detail by Setchell.[1] Although there are many different classes of plant phenolics, most of the clinical and nutritional interest has focused on the lignans that are found in high concentration in flaxseed[2] and the isoflavones that are abundant in soy protein-containing foods.[3] Similarly, the effects of flaxseed phytoestrogens have been reviewed recently by Thompson.[4] Flaxseed has 75 to 800 times the phytoestrogens content that of other common plant foods.[5–7] Both isoflavones and lignans have been suggested to have anticancer effects.[4,8,9] The levels in serum of these biologically active phytoestrogens may exceed by many orders of magnitude the levels of endogenous estrogens. Typical concentrations of soy isoflavones can exceed endogenous estradiol concentrations by 10,000- to 20,000-fold in

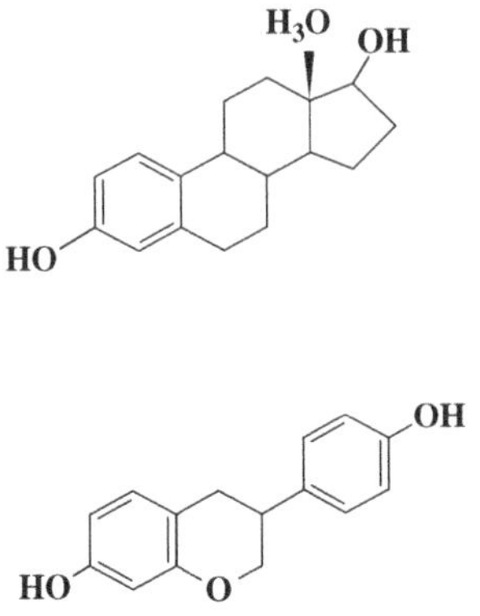

**17 β-Estradiol**

**Equol**

**FIGURE 15.1** Structure of estrogen and equol.

adults[5,10–12] and infants[13] and, as such, might be expected to exert biological effects at the molecular, cellular, or physiological level. However, their biological activity is low and this, combined with their affinity for estrogen receptors, makes them inhibitors by blocking the binding of mammalian (endogenous) estrogens. In this discussion the focus is the lignans of flaxseed and the isoflavones of soy that are the most concentrated sources of phytoestrogens, and their implications for different dietary patterns and incidence of cancers.

## 15.2 ISOFLAVONES, NATURAL SELECTIVE ESTROGEN RECEPTOR MODULATORS (SERMs)

The classification of flaxseed lignans and soy isoflavones as "estrogens" is technically incorrect. Isoflavones are nonsteroidal in chemical structure. However, due to the presence of the phenolic rings, particularly the 4´-hydroxyl group, they have the ability to bind to estrogen receptors (ERs), as do many substances, including antiestrogens such as tamoxifen, used successfully to treat breast cancer. Isoflavones also show a higher relative affinity for binding to the receptor than estrogens although with less biological activity than endogenous mammalian estrogens.[14] X-ray crystallographic studies have compared the conformational binding of estrogens,[15] the SERM raloxifene, and the isoflavone genistein.[16] These studies demonstrated differences in the position of the isoflavone within the dimerized ER-complex. It has been demonstrated that genistein is similar to raloxifene in the way it binds to the ER-complex.[16] Thus, soy isoflavones should be classified as natural SERMs, as originally proposed.[17] Because of this it has been suggested that soy isoflavones are likely to have the beneficial effects of estrogen without the disadvantages, especially in tissues such as the endometrium and breast.[18]

## 15.3 CANCER AND PHYTOESTROGENS

Phytoestrogens have been considered to have a preventive effect against various cancers. The consumption of phytoestrogen-rich foods such as soy, a source of isoflavones, and whole grain products, which contain lignans, is thought to play a role in the prevention of breast, prostate, and colon cancer. Other cancers also may be influenced by the presence of dietary phytoestrogens, but the studies in humans are comparatively few.

### 15.3.1 BREAST CANCER

Early studies by Axelson and Setchell[19] suggested that vegetarian women had a higher urinary secretion of lignans than omnivores. Later studies demonstrated lower urinary outputs of lignans in women diagnosed with breast cancer.[19] The question arose whether these compounds exerted a tamoxifen-like action on breast cancer tissue related to low dose stimulation of the ER and higher dose blocking or whether other direct or indirect actions were responsible, such as increasing the concentration of serum hormone binding proteins.

Soy isoflavones may also reduce breast cancer risk by affecting endogenous sex hormone concentrations and prolonging the menstrual cycle. There is evidence from early studies *in vitro* and *in vivo* that suggests that phytoestrogens stimulate the production of sex hormone-binding globulin (SHBG) in liver cells.[20] An increase in SHBG would lead to lower free-sex hormone concentrations. Longer menstrual cycles, which would lower breast cancer risk, have been seen in young women placed on soy experimentally. [21]

The increased production of equol in the gut has been associated with a lower risk of breast cancer.[20] Equol, known to be estrogenic, is a metabolite produced *in vivo* from the soy phytoestrogen, daidzein, by the action of gut microflora.[22] Equol concentrations are high in people consuming diets rich in plant proteins, carbohydrates, and fiber, but low in those on a high-fat diet. High equol producers also have a slightly higher concentration of SHBG than low equol producers.

In a study to examine whether soy in the diet is related to mammographic parenchymal patterns, which have been shown to predict breast cancer, 406 women ages 45 to 74 were randomly selected from among 3421 women.[23] These women were classified as displaying either high-risk (cases) or low-risk (controls) parenchymal patterns. Women with lower soy intake had higher percentage mammographic densities. The mammographically dense patterns, which are known to be associated with increased risk of breast cancer, are Tabar patterns IV and V.[23,24] The Tabar IV pattern represents fibrous proliferation and the Tabar V pattern represents dense fibrosis. There was a reduction of these patterns with high intake of soy, which would be considered to be protective against breast cancer development.[23] Ironically, a reduction in the risk of the Tabar IV and V patterns was also associated with high fat intakes. However, mammographic density can be reduced by an increase of fatty tissue in the breast as a result of a high-fat diet. In postmenopausal women, breast cancer risk increased linearly with increasing weight. Therefore the association of high body mass index (BMI) with increased risk may not be through increasingly dense mammographic patterns in postmenopausal women due to the increase of fatty tissue in the breast.[23] High-risk patterns and high BMI, although both risk factors, are negatively confounding.[24] Thus, the reduced occurrence of dense patterns with increasing age is consistent with the mammographically dense tissue being replaced by fatty tissue after menopause.[23]

In the Shanghai breast cancer study soyfood intake was associated with a decreased risk of breast cancer.[25] The study included 1459 cases and 1556 age-matched controls. Women in Shanghai had levels of soy intake considered high; i.e., soy consumption was at least once a week. The women with the highest consumption had a 30% reduced risk of breast cancer with stronger reduction for ER-positive subjects compared to subjects who were ER negative. In this situation there was even greater reduction among women with a higher BMI. But perhaps the most protective effect of soy was found in the offspring of women who had significant soy intake during pregnancy.[25] No association was found for women who increased their usual soy intake. It has been reasoned that women were required to eat soy at least once a week to maintain a constant level of isoflavonoids in their body, as most isoflavonoids are excreted in the urine within 96 hours. There was no additional benefit seen with increasing soy intake among women who already took soy weekly.[25]

A further human study in Hiroshima and Nagasaki showed no significant association between reported consumption of soy and breast cancer risk.[26] The 34,759 women in the Life Span Study cohort in Hiroshima and Nagasaki, who were alive at the time the atomic bombs were dropped and therefore exposed to radiation, completed dietary questionnaires in 1969–1970 or 1979–1981 and were followed until 1993. Among the 19 foods examined, the only statistically significant associations between breast cancer risk and diet were an increase in risk with increasing consumption of pickled vegetables and a decrease in risk with an increasing consumption of dried fish. These associations may be due to chance because of the large number of comparisons and because no plausible explanation can be given for pickled vegetables. There was no significant association between tofu or miso soup and reduction of breast cancer risk. The radiation exposure from the 1945 atomic bombs was a potential confounder of any association of soy consumption with breast cancer risk. However, it could be argued that this cohort would be more susceptible to breast cancer and thus act as a sensitive dietary indicator. All the analyses were adjusted for radiation exposure, and similar results were found in the subgroup of women exposed to very little radiation. It seems that even in potentially sensitive subjects soy consumption does not increase the risk of cancer.[26]

Finally, studies in the early 1990s noted a reduction in risk of breast cancer among premenopausal women with high soy intake in Singapore, with no relationship among postmenopausal women.[27,28] Similar investigations in Japan and China found a significant association of a reduced risk with high tofu consumption in premenopausal women.[29,30] These human studies therefore suggest that soy consumption at least once a week prior to menopause had no adverse effect and possibly a protective effect on breast cancer.

## 15.3.2 Prostate Cancer

Two studies have been carried out to examine the effect of soy consumption with and without high levels of isoflavones to determine whether over a period of months prostate specific antigen (PSA) levels could be reduced. [31,32] No effect was observed in serum PSA levels either in the men with high starting levels of PSA or in those with low levels.[33] More hopeful data were obtained by Kumar et al.[33] They assessed the effect of a soy beverage containing 60 mg genistein vs. the control in 12-week studies in 76 men with prostate cancer and Gleeson score of 6 or below. PSA was reduced or unchanged in 69% of the test subjects compared to 55% in the placebo group. In this group mean starting PSA levels were in the 7.4 µg/L range (total) with a free PSA of 0.99 to 1.03 µg/L.[33] These data therefore support a possibly protective effect for soy in prostate cancer.

Reanalyses of the Seventh-day Adventist men provide some suggestion for this conclusion. The relationship between soy milk consumption and the risk of prostate cancer within this population was evaluated. This study involved 12,395 men and 225 incident cases of prostate cancer over a total of 15 years of observation. There was a 70% reduction in risk of prostate cancer in the men who drank soy milk several times a day. Total intake needed for a protective effect cannot be calculated due to the lack of information about exact portion sizes. Assuming a daily intake of 400 g of soy milk, then men who drank soy milk several times a day would have had a total isoflavone intake of approximately 7 mg daidzein and 10 mg genistein for a protective effect.[34] An earlier cohort study including 7999 men with Japanese ancestry in Hawaii found that men who consumed tofu five or more times per week had a 65% reduction in cancer risk.[35] However, no association was found with the other popular soy item, miso soup, and prostate cancer risk.[35] It has also reported that a weekly intake of 160 mg of isoflavonoids in men prior to prostatectomy resulted in apoptosis of an adenocarcinoma of the prostate, which is a similar effect to estrogen therapy.[36] This further suggests a protective effect of isoflavones on prostate cancer and justifies additional study.

## 15.3.3 Other Cancers

The isoflavonoids have been found to have antiproliferative activity in two human intestinal tumor cell lines, Caco-2 and HT-29. Baicalein, genistein, bavachinin, and myricetin all increase apoptotic activity in the intestinal cell lines reaching significance for all four flavonoids in HT-29 but only for baicalein and myricetin in Caco-2 cells.[37] This has led to the suggestion that flavonoids may reduce colon cancer risk by blocking hyperproliferation of the epithelium and by promoting apoptosis.[38]

At least one study has also indicated a protective effect of soy intake on gastric cancer.[39] The study was a prospective study of a cohort of 30,304 men and women over 35 years old in Takayama, Japan. They were followed for 7 years during which time 121 deaths from stomach cancer occurred. A significant inverse relation was found between soy intake and stomach cancer in men with a relative risk for the highest vs. the lowest intake of soy of 0.50 (CI: 0.26 to 0.93) (P for trend = 0.030). Assessed separately, the women showed a similar effect but this did not reach significance.[39] This study is of particular interest since it shows a protective effect of a traditional food, soy, despite a historically high level of gastric cancer in the region.

The consumption of soy foods has also been associated with a lower risk of endometrial cancer. An observational study including 832 women diagnosed with endometrial cancer aged 30 to 69 and 846 age-matched controls suggested a significantly lower risk of cancer with higher intakes of soy protein and fiber, but not significantly with higher intakes of soy isoflavones. The association of soy protein intake and endometrial cancer was also found to be similar for both pre- and postmenopausal women.[40] More support for a protective effect came from a study of non-Asian women from California. It was found that higher intakes of phytoestrogens reduced the incidence of endometrial cancer.[41] Two subject groups were assessed, the first consisted of 500 women aged 35 to 79 of African American, Latino, and Caucasian descent and the second consisted of 470 women age- and ethnicity-matched with 75% of all subjects postmenopausal. The endometrial cancer risk was significantly lower in the women with highest soy intake.[41]

It has been suggested that infant leukemia may be induced by exposure to DNA topoisomerase II inhibitors, which include flavonoids.[42] Approximately 80% of infant leukemias have chromosome translocations involving the MLL gene. Patients with cancer treated with chemotherapeutic agents such as etoposide (VP16) or doxorubicin (Dox) can develop therapy-related leukemia. A proposed cause of infant leukemia includes maternal exposure to flavonoids. Maternal ingestion of flavonoids may induce damage at the MLL break point cluster region (BCR) of the DNA strand by inhibiting topoisomerase II and possibly leading to chromosomal translocations, which result in leukemia.[42,43] Schroder-van der Elst et al.[44] demonstrated that flavonoids do cross the placental barrier in a study where pregnant rats were injected with a radioactive flavonoid, which was found present in all fetal tissues.[44] However, the exact significance of these findings remains uncertain and whether this also applies to other phenolics and lignans from fruit and vegetable consumption cannot be determined.

## 15.4 RAT MODELS

Much of the work in animal models has involved breast cancer, and because of the number of studies, the present discussion of animal models is limited to this condition as an example of the animal work. In a review of the literature, Barnes[45] concluded that in two thirds of studies on the effect of genistein-containing soy materials in animal models of cancer, the risk of cancer (incidence, latency, or tumor number) was significantly reduced.[45] Thus, in a study in which the growth and metastasis of the ER-negative human breast cancer cells MDA MB 435 were investigated using the athymic immunodeficient mouse model,[46] flaxseed feeding resulted in significant reductions in established tumor growth rate of these ER-negative cells and a 45% reduction in total incidence of metastasis. Reductions in cell proliferation and expression of insulin-like growth factor-1 and epidermal growth factor receptor were observed on flaxseed feeding, suggesting that the effect of flaxseed was to some extent the result of downregulation of these growth factors. The concentration of vascular endothelial growth factor (VEGF) in the extracellular fluid was lower in the tumors. VEGF is a known stimulator of angiogenesis.[47] Hence, the study suggested that the slower tumor growth rate and lower metastasis caused by flaxseed may be attributed to its effect on tumor growth and the inhibition of growth of the tumor blood supply.[4,45]

On the other hand when ER-positive human breast cells were implanted in ovariectomized athymic mice, the tumors were larger in the genistein-treated group than in the negatively treated group. The results showed that genistein can act as an estrogen agonist in the total absence of estrogen. The relevance of this in the human situation when detectable estrogen levels are present is uncertain. However, with detectable levels of circulating estrogen, it remains likely that there would be inhibition of cell growth due to blocking by flavonoids of the action of endogenous (mammalian) estrogen.[48]

In rats, studies by Thompson have indicated that feeding 5% flaxseed during the preinitiation stage, using the chemical carcinogen DMBA (i.e., 4 weeks before DMBA injection) or in the early promotion stage of carcinogenesis (20 weeks after DMBA injection), resulted in a 21 to 32% reduction in tumor incidence. When the lignans were tested separately from flaxseed, the lignans, secoisolariciresinol diglycoside (SDG), resulted in a 46% reduction in the number of tumors per rat.[4]

The effects on tumor inhibition may be related to the action of phytoestrogens in breast development. A reduction in the number of highly proliferative terminal end bud (TEB) structures in the developing mammary gland through differentiation to the less proliferative alveolar buds and lobules has been suggested to be protective against mammary cancer. Exposure to 5 to 10% flaxseed during gestation and suckling or throughout life significantly reduced TEB density in the mammary gland, whereas exposure after weaning had no effect. When the experiment was repeated with rats exposed to flaxseed only during gestation or gestation to postnatal day 50, the data indicated that the critical period for enhancing the mammary gland differentiation was during suckling. The flaxseed and SDG diets reduced the tumor incidence by 31.3 and 42%, respectively, total tumor load by 50.8 and 62.5%, respectively, and mean tumor size by 43.9 and 67.7%, respectively. These findings supported the hypothesis that exposure to flaxseed during an early stage of mammary gland development (i.e., suckling) can enhance mammary gland differentiation. In turn, this development of the glandular tissue may reduce the risk of breast cancer in adulthood, an effect that may be mediated by lignans.[4]

## 15.5  TRENDS IN CANCER INCIDENCE

The IARC data for cancer incidence in 1990 and 2002 are of interest in relation to the links among diet, isoflavones and lignans, and cancer.[49,50] Data are presented from U.S. and U.K. to contrast to traditionally high-soy-eating parts of the world, Japan and China. Recognizing that traditional habits are changing in Asia, especially Japan, a further contrast is the comparison of findings from Japan and China. These data are presented on the understanding that the China data are likely to be less robust than those of the other three nations. The most significant finding was the rise in colon cancer in Japan, which now leads the world in both gastric and colon cancer incidence (Figure 15.2). This is of particular concern since epidemiologically the incidence of colon cancer has usually been related inversely with that of stomach cancer. Furthermore, the relative lack of increase in all cancers in China contrasts to the sharp rise of cancers in Japan, which in most instances shows a similar percentage increase to that seen in the U.S. and U.K. For Japan, it might be argued that these changes are due to the increased caloric consumption associated with rising height and increasing bodyweight, but it may also be related to the increased consumption of a more Westernized diet with reduced soy consumption and therefore lower isoflavone intake.

## 15.6  CONCLUSION

Adlercreutz[20] in a review of the literature concluded that there was no convincing evidence to suggest that soy or isoflavone consumption during adult life was protective against breast cancer for women living in Western countries. However, moderate lifelong intake of soy products or isoflavone supplements may have beneficial effects on the cardiovascular system and bone metabolism, but negative effects on the breast could not be completely excluded, although equally positive findings are also present in the literature.[20] The epidemiological data indicate that in the context of a healthy lifestyle soy consumption does not preclude low levels of breast cancer incidence. Furthermore, affluence and Westernization, in the absence of increased soy consumption seem to be the major drivers for increases in breast cancer. For other cancers such as prostate, and possibly colon and stomach, soy may well turn out to have beneficial effects. The alarming rise in colon cancer in Japan at a time of increasing Westernization perhaps hints that traditional Japanese habits, which include soy consumption, may be protective. However, there are no long-term, randomized, controlled trials of isoflavone or lignan consumption on cancer incidence or surrogate markers, such as aberrant crypt foci or polyps in the case of colon cancer. Future recommendations must be based on trial experience. In the absence of these there seems no reason to cease recommending to the public to eat more whole grains, seeds, and legumes, foods high in lignans and isoflavones.

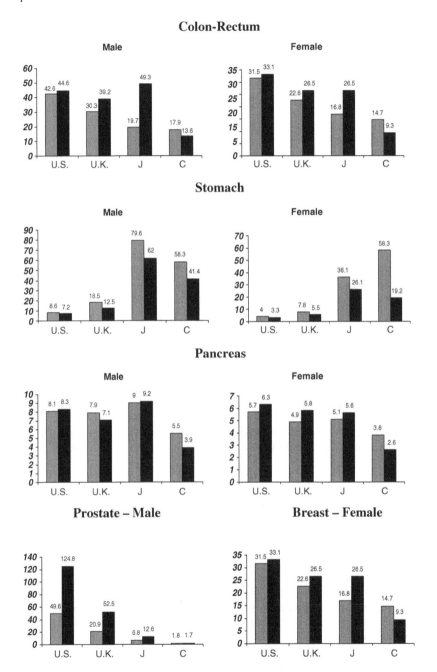

**FIGURE 15.2** Age-adjusted incidence of cancer (per 100,000) according to the 1990 (striped bars) and 2002 (solid bars) IARC reports.[47,48]

## REFERENCES

1. Setchell KDR. Soy isoflavones — benefits and risks from nature's selective estrogen receptor modulators (SERMs). *J Am Coll Nutr* 2001; 20(5 Suppl):354S–362S.
2. Setchell KDR, Lawson AM, Mitchell FL, Adlercreutz H, Kirk DN, Axelson M. Lignans in man and in animal species. *Nature* 1980; 287:740–742.
3. Setchell KDR, Borriello SP, Hulme P, Kirk DN, Axelson M. Nonsteroidal estrogens of dietary origin: possible roles in hormone-dependent disease. *Am J Clin Nutr* 1984; 40:569–578.
4. Thompson L. Flaxseed, lignans, and cancer. In *Flaxseed in Human Nutrition*, 2nd ed. SC Cunnane, LU Thompson, eds. Champaign, IL: AOCS Press; 2003:194–222.
5. Bhatty RS. Nutrient composition of whole flaxseed and flaxseed meal. In *Flaxseed in Human Nutrition*. SC Cunnane, LU Thompson, eds. Champaign, IL: AOCS Press; 1995:22–42.
6. Thompson LU, Robb P, Serriano M, and Cheung F. Mammalian lignan production for various foods. *Nutr Cancer* 1991; 16:43–52.
7. Mazur W. Phytoestrogen content in foods. *Bailliere's Clin Endocrin Metab* 1998; 12:729–742.
8. Adlercreutz H, Fotsis T, Heikkinen B, Dwyer JR, Wood M, Goldin BR, Gorbach SL. Excretion of the lignans enterolactone and enterdiol and of equol in omnivorous and vegetarian women and in women with breast cancer. *Lancet* 1982; 2:1295–1299.
9. Johnston PV. Flaxseed oil and cancer: α-linolenic acid and carcinogenesis. In *Flaxseed in Human Nutrition*. SC Cunnane, LU Thompson, eds. Champaign, IL: AOCS Press; 1995:207–218.
10. Setchell KDR. Discovery and potential clinical importance of mammalian lignans. In *Flaxseed in Human Nutrition*. SC Cunnane, LU Thompson, eds. Champaign, IL: AOCS Press; 1995:82–98.
11. Meagher LP, Beecher GR, Flanagan VP, Li BW. Isolation and characterization of the lignans, isolariciresinol and pinoresinol, in flaxseed meal. *J Agric Food Chem* 1999; 47:3173–3180.
12. Thompson LU. Analysis and bioavailability of lignans. In *Flaxseed in Human Nutrition*, 2nd ed. SC Cunnane, LU Thompson, eds. Champaign, IL: AOCS Press; 2003:92–116.
13. Rickard SE, Orcheson LJ, Seidl MM, Luyengi L, Fong HH, Thompson LU. Dose-dependent production of mammalian lignans in rats and in-vitro from the purified precursor secoisolariciresinol diglycoside from flaxseed. *J Nutr* 1996; 126:2012–2019.
14. Jordan VC, Morrow M. Tamoxifen, raloxifene, and the prevention of breast cancer. *Endocr Rev* 1989; 20:253–278.
15. Brzozowski AM, Pike AC, Dauter Z, Hubbard RE, Bonn T, Engstorm O, Ohman L, Greene GL, Gustafsson JA, Carlquist M. Molecular basis of agonism and antagonism in the oestrogen receptor. *Nature* 1997; 389:753–758.
16. Pike AC, Brzozowski AM, Hubbard RE, Bonn T, Thorsell AG, Engstorm O, Ljunngren J, Gustafsson JA, Carlquist M. Structure of the ligand-binding domain of oestrogen receptor beta in the presence of a partial agonist and a full antagonist. *EMBO J* 1999; 18:4608–4618.
17. Brzezinski A, Debi A. Phytoestrogens: the "natural" selective estrogen receptor modulators? *Eur J Obstet Gynecol Reprod Biol* 1999; 85:47–51.

18. Cummings SR, Eckert S, Krueger KA, Grady D, Powles TJ, Cauley JA, Norton L, Nickelsen T, Bjarnason NH, Morrow M, Lippman ME, Black D, Glusman JE, Costa A, Jordan VC. The effect of raloxifene on risk of breast cancer in post-menopausal women: results from the MORE randomized trial. Multiple outcomes of raloxifene evaluations. *J Am Med Assoc* 1999; 281:2189–2197.

19. Axelson M, Setchell KD. Conjugation of lignans in human urine. *FEBS Lett* 1980; 122:49–53.

20. Adlercreutz H. Phyto-oestrogens and cancer. *Lancet Oncol* 2002; 3:364–373.

21. Cassidy A, Bingham S, Setchell KD. Biological effects of a diet of soy protein rich in isoflavones on the menstrual cycle of premenopausal women. *Am J Clin Nutr* 1994; 60:333–340.

22. Muthyala RS, Ju YH, Sheng S, Williams LD, Doerge DR, Katzenellenbogen BS, Helferich WG, Katzenellenbogen JA. Equol, a natural estrogenic metabolite from soy isoflavones: convenient preparation and resolution of R- and S-equols and their differing binding and biological activity through estrogen receptors alpha and beta. *Bioorg Med Chem* 2004; 12:1559–1567.

23. Jakes RW, Duffy SW, Ng FC, Gao F, Ng EH, Seow A, Lee HP, Yu MC. Mammographic parenchymal patterns and self-reported soy intake in Singapore Chinese women. *Cancer Epidemiol Biomarkers Prev* 2002; 11:608–613.

24. Boyd NF, Stone J, Vogt KN, Connelly BS, Martin LJ, Minkin S. Dietary fat and breast cancer risk revisited: a meta-analysis of the published literature. *Br J Cancer* 2003; 89:1672–1685.

25. Dai Q, Shu XO, Jin F, Potter JD, Kushi LH, Teas J, Gao YT, Zheng W. Population-based case-control study of soyfood intake and breast cancer risk in Shanghai. *Br J Cancer* 2001; 85:372–378.

26. Key TJ, Sharp GB, Appleby PN, Beral V, Goodman MT, Soda M, Mabuchi K. Soya foods and breast cancer risk: a prospective study in Hiroshima and Nagasaki, Japan. *Br J Cancer* 1999; 81:1248–1256.

27. Lee HP, Gourley L, Duffy SW, Esteve J, Lee J, Day NE. Dietary effects on breast-cancer risk in Singapore. *Lancet* 1991; 337:1197–1200.

28. Lee HP, Gourley L, Duffy SW, Esteve J, Lee J, Day NE. Risk factors for breast cancer by age and menopausal status: a case-control study in Singapore. *Cancer Causes Control* 1992; 3:313–322.

29. Hirose K, Tajima K, Hamajima N, Inoue M, Takezaki T, Kuroishi T, Yoshida M, Tokudome S. A large-scale, hospital-based case-control study of risk factors of breast cancer according to menopausal status. *Jpn J Cancer Res* 1995; 86:146–154.

30. Yuan J-M, Wang Q-S, Ross RK, Henderson BE, Yu MC. Diet and breast cancer in Shanghai and Tiajin. China. *Br J Cancer* 1995; 71:1353–1358.

31. Jenkins DJ, Kendall CW, D'Costa MA, Jackson CJ, Vidgen E, Singer W, Silverman JA, Koumbridis G, Honey J, Rao AV, Fleshner N, Klotz L. Soy consumption and phytoestrogens: effect on serum prostate specific antigen when blood lipids and oxidized low-density lipoprotein are reduced in hyperlipidemic men. *J Urol* 2003; 169:507–511.

32. Urban D, Irwin W, Kirk M, Markiewicz MA, Myers R, Smith M, Weiss H, Grizzle WE, Barnes S. The effect of isolated soy protein on plasma biomarkers in elderly men with elevated serum prostate specific antigen. *J Urol* 2001; 165:294–300.

33. Kumar NB, Cantor A, Allen K, Riccardi D, Besterman-Dahan K, Seigne J, Helal M, Salup R, Pow-Sang J. The specific role of isoflavones in reducing prostate cancer risk. *Prostate* 2004; 59(2):141–147.

34. Reinli K, Block G. Phytoestrogen content of foods — a compendium of literature values. *Nutr Cancer* 1996; 26:123–148.

35. Severson RK, Nomura AMY, Grove JS, Stemmermann GN. A prospective study of demographics, diet, and prostate cancer among men of Japanese ancestry in Hawaii. *Cancer Res* 1989; 9:545–552.

36. Jacobsen BK, Knutsen SF, Fraser GE. Does high soy milk intake reduce prostate cancer incidence? The Adventist Health Study (United States). *Cancer Causes Control* 1998; 9:553–557.

37. Matsuzaki Y, Kurokawa N, Terai S, Matsumura Y, Kobayashi N, Okita K. Cell death induced by baicalein in human hepatocellular carcinoma cell lines. *Jpn J Cancer Res* 1996; 87:170–177.

38. Kuntz S, Wenzel U, Daniel H. Comparative analysis of the effects of flavonoids on proliferation, cytotoxicity, and apoptosis in human colon cancer cell lines. *Eur J Nutr* 1999; 38:133–142.

39. Nagata C, Takatsuka N, Kawakami N, Shimizu H. A prospective cohort study of soy product intake and stomach cancer death. *Br J Cancer* 2002; 87:31–36.

40. Xu WH, Zheng W, Xiang YB, Ruan ZX, Cheng JR, Dai Q, Gao YT, Shu XO. Soya food intake and risk of endometrial cancer among Chinese women in Shanghai: population based case-control study. *Br Med J* 2004 May 29; 328(7541):1285.

41. Horn-Ross PL, John EM, Canchola AJ, Stewart SL, Lee MM. Phytoestrogen intake and endometrial cancer risk. *J Natl Cancer Inst* 2003; 95:1158–1164.

42. Ross JA. Dietary flavonoids and the MLL gene: A pathway to infant leukemia? *Proc Natl Acad Sci USA* 2000; 97:4411–4413.

43. Strick R, Strissel PL, Borgers S, Smith SL, Rowley JD. Dietary bioflavonoids induce cleavage in the MLL gene and may contribute to infant leukemia. *Proc Natl Acad Sci USA* 2000; 97:4790–4795.

44. Schroder-van der Elst JP, van der Heide D, Rokos H, Morreale de Escobar G, Kohrle J. Synthetic flavonoids cross the placenta in the rat and are found in fetal brain. *Am J Physiol* 1998; 274:E253–E256.

45. Barnes S. Effect of genistein on in vitro and in vivo models of cancer. *J Nutr* 1995; 125(3 Suppl):777S–783S.

46. Chen JM, Stavro M, Thompson LU. Dietary flaxseed inhibits breast cancer growth and metastasis and downregulates expression of epidermal growth factor receptor and insulin-like growth factor. *Nutr Cancer* 2002; 43;187–192.

47. Yoshji H, Gomez DE, Shibuya M, Thorgeirsson UP. Expression of vascular endothelial growth factor, its receptor, and other angiogenic factors in human breast cancer. *Cancer Res* 1996; 56:2013–2016.

48. Hsieh CY, Santell RC, Haslam SZ, Helferich WG. Estrogenic effects of genistein on the growth of estrogen receptor-positive human breast cancer (MCF-7) cells *in vitro* and in vivo. *Cancer Res* 1998; 58:3833–3838. Erratum, *Cancer Res* 1999; 59:1388.

49. Whelan SL, Parkin DM, Masoyer E. *Patterns of Cancer in Five Continents.* WHO-IRAC. Lyon: IARC; 1990.

50. IRAC. Globocan 2002. [Online]. Available from http://www-depdb.iarc.fr/globocan/GLOBOframe.htm 2004, Oct. 27.

# 16 Flavonoids as Inhibitors of Tumor Metastasis

*Jin-Rong Zhou*

## CONTENTS

16.1 Introduction ...................................................................................326
16.2 Critical Review of the Roles of Flavonoids in Tumor Metastasis:
Evidence from *in Vitro* and *in Vivo* Studies .......................................328
   16.2.1 Tea Polyphenols and Antimetastasis ........................................328
      16.2.1.1 Effects of Tea Polyphenols on Invasion and
               Metastasis of Melanoma ...............................................332
      16.2.1.2 Effects of Tea Polyphenols on Invasion and
               Metastasis of Prostate Cancer .......................................332
      16.2.1.3 Effects of Tea Polyphenols on Invasion and
               Metastasis of Other Types of Cancer .........................333
   16.2.2 Soy Isoflavones and Antimetastasis .........................................334
      16.2.2.1 Effects of Soy Isoflavones on Invasion and
               Metastasis of Breast Cancer .........................................334
      16.2.2.2 Effects of Soy Isoflavones on Invasion and
               Metastasis of Prostate Cancer .......................................334
      16.2.2.3 Effects of Soy Isoflavones on Invasion and
               Metastasis of Melanoma ...............................................335
      16.2.2.4 Effects of Soy Isoflavones on Invasion and
               Metastasis of Other Types of Cancer .........................335
   16.2.3 Apigenin and Quercetin and Antimetastasis ............................336
      16.2.3.1 Effects of Apigenin on Invasion and Metastasis of
               Cancer.............................................................................336
      16.2.3.2 Effects of Quercetin on Invasion and Metastasis
               of Cancer ........................................................................336
16.3 Mechanisms by Which Flavonoids Inhibit Tumor Metastasis.............337
   16.3.1 Flavonoids and Angiogenesis...................................................337
      16.3.1.1 Effects of Tea Polyphenols on Angiogenesis ..............338
      16.3.1.2 Effects of Soy Isoflavones on Angiogenesis ..............338
   16.3.2 Flavonoids and Proteolytic Enzymes .......................................339
      16.3.2.1 Effects of Tea Polyphenols on MMP Activities..........340
      16.3.2.2 Effects of Soy Isoflavones on MMP Activities..........340

        16.3.3  Flavonoids and Cancer Cell Adhesion ....................................341
                16.3.3.1  Effects of Tea Polyphenols on Cancer Cell
                          Adhesion ....................................................................341
                16.3.3.2  Effects of Soy Isoflavones on Cancer Cell Adhesion ...341
16.4    Critical Issues and Future Directions in Research on Flavonoids and
        Tumor Metastasis ..............................................................................342
        16.4.1  Identification of Flavonoids for Inhibition of Cancer-Specific
                Metastasis ...............................................................................342
        16.4.2  Verification of Antimetastasis Activities of Flavonoids ...........343
        16.4.3  Further Elucidation of Mechanisms .........................................343
        16.4.4  Interactive Effects of Flavonoids with Other Dietary
                Bioactives ...............................................................................344
16.5    Conclusions .....................................................................................344
References ...................................................................................................344

## 16.1  INTRODUCTION

Flavonoids, a family of phytochemical compounds, are widely distributed in foods of plant origin such as vegetables, fruits, soy, nuts, tea, onions, and red wine, and are consumed regularly as a part of the human diet. More than 4000 different flavonoids have been characterized, and the major flavonoid classes include flavones, flavanones, catechins, anthocyanidins, isoflavones, and chalcones.[1] Flavonoid structure is typically composed of two benzene rings (a and b rings in Figure 16.1A) linked through a heterocyclic pyran or pyrone ring (c).

Flavonoids display a variety of biological activities with antioxidative and antiproliferative activities the most extensively studied.[2] Recently, more research has been focused on the role of flavonoids in cancer prevention because epidemiological investigations suggest that increased intake of fruits and vegetables is associated with the reduced risks of certain cancers. *In vitro* and animal studies in general suggest that some dietary flavonoids have potent cancer chemoprevention activities.[2]

Cancer metastasis, which involves multiple processes and various cytophysiological changes, is a primary cause of cancer death. Currently available therapeutic drugs have limited effects on metastatic tumors. Therefore, there is an urgent need for novel therapeutic approaches to treat tumor metastasis. Search for effective agents from plant resources, such as flavonoids and other phytochemicals, for treatment of cancer metastasis has become one of the top priorities in cancer research. Accumulating evidence from *in vitro* and animal studies suggests that some plant flavonoids possess anti-invasion activities *in vitro* and antimetastasis activities in animal models. Tea catechins and soy isoflavones are among the most extensively studied flavonoids that show anti-invasive and antimetastatic activities. Other flavonoids such as apigenin and quercetin have also demonstrated anti-invasion and antimetastasis activities. Figure 16.1 shows the structures of commonly studied flavonoids. The objectives of this chapter are to provide an

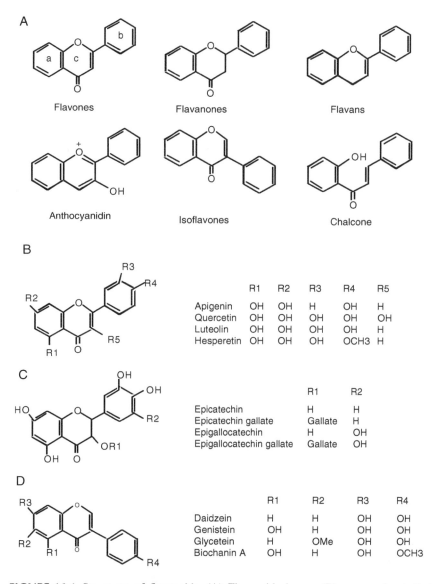

**FIGURE 16.1** Structures of flavonoids. (A) Flavonoid classes; (B) commonly studied flavonoids; (C) tea polyphenols; (D) soy isoflavones.

up-to-date review of available *in vitro* and *in vivo* evidence on anti-invasion and antimetastasis activities of these flavonoids, to elucidate the underlying mechanisms by which these flavonoids inhibit cancer cell invasion/metastasis, and to identify several critical issues in this research field so that future research directions can be highlighted.

## 16.2 CRITICAL REVIEW OF THE ROLES OF FLAVONOIDS IN TUMOR METASTASIS: EVIDENCE FROM *IN VITRO* AND *IN VIVO* STUDIES

A series of *in vitro* and animal studies has been conducted to evaluate the anti-invasion and antimetastasis activities of flavonoids in recent years. Most of the experimental evidence is derived from the *in vitro* studies that evaluate the effects of flavonoids on invasive potentials of cancer cells by determining the ability of cancer cells to invade through a reconstituted basement membrane (Matrigel). The antimetastasis activities of some flavonoids are further confirmed in appropriate animal models. Tea polyphenols and soy isoflavones are two groups of most extensively investigated flavonoids for their anti-invasion and antimetastasis activities in various types of cancer cells. In addition, the flavonoids apigenin and quercetin have shown potent anti-invasion and antimetastasis activities. In this section, the evidence from both *in vitro* and animal studies is reviewed with particular emphasis on the *in vivo* evidence. The animal studies on flavonoids and tumor metastasis are summarized in Table 16.1.

### 16.2.1 TEA POLYPHENOLS AND ANTIMETASTASIS

Tea consumption as a beverage in the world is very high and ranks second only to water consumption.[3] Tea contains a variety of components with flavonoids the major constituents. Green tea is the rich source of flavonoids, namely, catechins and flavonols. Black tea is subjected to a more extensive fermentation process than green tea. During the fermentation process, tea catechins are converted to complex condensation products, namely, theaflavins, theaflavic acids, and thearubigen polymers. The major green tea catechins are epigallocatechin gallate (EGCG), epicatechin gallate (ECG), epigallocatechin (EGC), and epicatechin (EC), which, altogether, may constitute up to 30% of the dry leaf weight.[4] Typically, green tea flavonoids is composed of 90% of catechins and 10% flavonols; and black tea flavonoids is composed of 30% catechins, 47% of thearubigins, 13% theaflavins, and 10% of flavonols.[5]

Previous studies have primarily focused on the cancer-prevention effect of green tea in part due to its high content of EGCG, a putative chemopreventive agent and a major component of green tea. Most epidemiological studies have looked at the associations of tea, especially green tea, with certain types of cancers such as skin cancer and colorectal cancer.[6,7] Experimental studies suggest that tea contains bioactive components that inhibit the development, growth, and progression/metastasis of prostate cancer. Among tea components, EGCG has been the most frequently used pure tea compound for the *in vitro* and *in vivo* studies. Although thearubigins represent the highest proportion of black tea polyphenols, they are very difficult to purify; therefore their role in cancer prevention has not been well studied. Another black tea component, theaflavins, has been isolated and used for some *in vitro* studies. Most anti-invasion and antimetastasis

**TABLE 16.1**

**Effects of Flavonoids on Antimetastasis of Several Types of Tumors in Animal Studies**

| Study | Animal Models | Flavonoids | Diet | Results |
|---|---|---|---|---|
| **Tea Polyphenols and Tumor Metastasis** | | | | |
| Caltagirone et al.[10] | B16-BL6 melanoma, iv inoculation | EGCG (50 mg/kg), ip administration | 0 | EGCG and lung metastasis |
| Gupta et al.[13] | TRAMP | GTP (0.1% in drinking water) | — | GTP and lung metastases |
| Liu et al.[8] | B16-F3m melanoma, ip implantation | EGCG (ip. 2 mg/d, three times/wk for 11 wk) | — | EGCG and lung metastases |
| Menon et al.[9] | B16-F10 melanoma, iv implantation | Catechin or curcumin (ip. 200 μmol/kg BW) | — | Catechin and lung metastasis |
| | | | — | Curcumin and lung metastasis |
| Sartor et al.[14] | TRAMP | Decaffeinated green tea extract (59% EGCG, 86% total catechins, 0.5% caffeine) | 0 | Green tea extract and growth or metastasis |
| Sazuka et al.[16] | Lewis lung carcinoma | Green tea infusion (2%) | — | Green tea and lung metastasis |
| Sazuka et al.[15] | Lewis lung carcinoma LL2-Lu3 cells | Theaflavins | — | Theaflavins and lung metastasis |
| Taniguchi et al.[11] | B16-F10 in experimental metastasis (iv injection); B16-BL6 cells in spontaneous metastasis (after removal of primary tumor) | EGCG (0.05% or 0.1% in drinking water) | — | EGCG and experimental lung metastasis |
| | | | — | EGCG and spontaneous lung metastasis |
| Zhou et al.[12] | Orthotopic LNCaP tumor | Green tea (1.5%) and soy phytochemical concentrate (SPC, 0.5%), black tea (1.5%) and SPC (0.5%) | 0 | Black tea or green tea and lymph node metastasis |
| | | | — | Tea and soy combinations and lymph node metastasis |

(continued)

**TABLE 16.1 (CONTINUED)**
**Effects of Flavonoids on Antimetastasis of Several Types of Tumors in Animal Studies**

| Study | Animal Models | Flavonoids | Diet | Results |
|---|---|---|---|---|
| **Soy Isoflavones and Tumor Metastasis** | | | | |
| Buchler et al.[44] | Orthotopic pancreatic tumors | Genistein (1.3 mg/mouse/d, ip) | — | Genistein and growth and liver metastasis |
| Charland et al.[29] | MAC-33 mammary tumor, sc implantation | Soybean extract and heat-stable soybean extract | + | Soy extracts and lung metastasis |
| Iishi et al.[45] | AOM-induced intestinal adenocarcinoma | Genistein (5. and 10 mg/kg BW) | — | Genistein and incidence of metastasis |
| | | | 0 | Genistein and growth of intestinal tumors |
| Li et al.[34] | B16-BL6 melanoma, iv | Genistein (450 and 900 µg/kg diet) | — | Genistein and lung metastasis |
| Menon et al.[36] | B16-F10 melanoma, iv | Genistein (200 µmol/kg BW) | — | Genistein and lung metastasis |
| Myoung et al.[42] | Oral squamous cell carcinoma | Genistein (0.5 mg/kg BW) | 0 | Genistein and growth or metastasis |
| Schleicher et al.[31] | Sex gland carcinoma | Genistein (ip, 50 mg/kg BW) | — | Genistein and tumor growth, and metastasis to LN, lung |
| Wietrzyk et al.[35] | B16-BL6 melanoma, iv; LL2 lung carcinoma, iv or sc | Genistein | — | Genistein and lung metastasis of melanoma cells |
| | | | — | Genistein and lung metastasis of lung carcinoma cells |
| Yan et al.[32] | B16-BL6 melanoma, iv | Genistein (ip, 20 and 30 µM/d) | — | Genistein and lung metastasis |
| | | | — | SPC and lymph node and lung metastasis |
| Zhou et al.[30] | Orthotopic LNCaP tumors | Genistin (0.14%), soy phytochemical concentrate (SPC, 0.5%) | 0 | Genistin and lymph node or lung metastasis |

### Apigenin and Quercetin and Tumor Metastasis

| Reference | Model | Treatment | Result | Comments |
|---|---|---|---|---|
| Caltagirone et al.[10] | B16-BL6, iv implantation | Apigenin (25, 50 mg/kg), quercetin (25, 50 mg/kg) | — | Quercetin and lung metastasis |
| | | | — | Apigenin and lung metastasis |
| Tatsuta et al.[53] | AOM-induced and bombesin-enhanced intestinal adenocarcinoma | Apigenin (0.75, 1.5 mg/kg BW) | — | Apigenin and incidence of metastasis |
| | | | 0 | Apigenin and growth of intestinal tumors |
| Menon et al.[58] | B16-F10 melanoma, iv implantation | Rutin, quercetin, catechin, curcumin (all at 200 nmol/kg BW) | — | Catechin, rutin, and curcumin and lung metastasis |
| | | | 0 | Quercetin and lung metastasis |

*Abbreviations*: AOM, azoxymethane; BW, body weight; EGCG, epigallocatechin gallate; GTP, green tea polyphenols; ip, intraperitoneal; iv, intravenous; sc, subcutaneous; SPC, soy phytochemical concentrate.

studies have also used EGCG as a major tea bioactive compound. In addition, EGCG-rich green tea polyphenol extract and whole tea have been used in some animal studies.

### 16.2.1.1 Effects of Tea Polyphenols on Invasion and Metastasis of Melanoma

A series of studies has been conducted to determine the anti-invasion activities *in vitro* and antimetastasis activities *in vivo* of tea polyphenols, especially EGCG, in several cancer types. Because of the highly metastatic potential of melanoma cells, the effects of tea polyphenols on melanoma cell invasion and metastasis are among the most extensively studied cancer types. Murine B16 melanoma cell line and its highly metastatic sublines, such as B16-F3m, B16-F10, and B16-BL6 cells, have been used for evaluation. EGCG significantly inhibited B16-F3m cell migration and invasion *in vitro;*[8] tea catechin significantly inhibited the invasion of B16-F10 melanoma cells *in vitro.*[9] On the other hand, EGCG did not inhibit invasion of highly metastatic B16-BL6 cells *in vitro.*[10]

Besides the *in vitro* anti-invasion studies, tea polyphenols have been evaluated for their antimetastasis activities in several animal models. In one animal study,[8] the B16-F3m cells were implanted intraperitoneally into the mice to develop metastases, and the mice were treated with EGCG at 2 mg/day, three times/week for 11 weeks. EGCG significantly reduced lung metastases in mice bearing B16-F3m melanomas.[8] In another animal study,[9] B16-F10 melanoma cells were intravenously inoculated into the mice to develop lung metastases, and tea catechin was administered orally at 200 μmol/kg body weight for 10 alternate days. The lung metastases were significantly inhibited by catechin treatment.[9] Taniguchi and co-workers applied two animal models of metastasis to evaluate the antimetastasis effects of EGCG.[11] In the experimental metastasis model, B16-F10 melanoma cells were inoculated intravenously to develop lung metastases, and in the spontaneous metastasis model, the more metastatic B16-BL6 melanoma cells were inoculated subcutaneously into the mouse footpad to develop primary tumors, followed by removal of the primary tumors to develop lung metastases.[11] Per oral administration of EGCG (0.05 and 0.1%) significantly inhibited lung metastasis of both B16-F10 and B16-BL6 melanoma tumors in both lung metastasis animal models.[11] However, EGCG did not show inhibitory effect on lung metastasis of B16-BL6 cells in one animal study in which lung metastases were developed by intravenous inoculation of cancer cells.[10]

### 16.2.1.2 Effects of Tea Polyphenols on Invasion and Metastasis of Prostate Cancer

Several animal studies have been conducted to determine the effects of tea on prostate tumor metastasis. We studied the effects of green tea and black tea, alone or in combination with soy isoflavone-enriched phytochemical extract, soy phytochemical concentrate (SPC), which contains 50% total isoflavones by weight, on the growth and metastasis of androgen-sensitive LNCaP human prostate tumors in an orthotopic tumor model. We found that the combination of tea (1.5% tea infusion) with SPC (0.5% of the diet) significantly inhibited lymph node metastases of LNCaP tumors.[12] The transgenic mouse model for prostate tumors, the transgenic adenocarcinoma of the mouse prostate (TRAMP) model, was also used to determine the effect of green tea polyphenols (GTPs) on the growth and metastasis of prostate tumors. Oral infusion of a polyphenolic fraction isolated from green tea at a human achievable dose (0.1% in drinking water, equivalent to 6 cups of green tea per day) significantly inhibited prostate tumor development and increased survival in these mice. GTP infusion resulted in almost complete inhibition of distant site metastases.[13] On the other hand, the decaffeinated green tea extract (59% EGCG, 86% total catechins, and 0.5% caffeine) did not inhibit the growth or metastasis of xenografts of TRAMP-C1 cells in mice,[14] although EGCG inhibited invasion of TRAMP-C1 cells *in vitro*.[14]

### 16.2.1.3 Effects of Tea Polyphenols on Invasion and Metastasis of Other Types of Cancer

Lewis lung carcinoma is another type of highly metastatic tumor that is used for invasion/metastasis studies. Green tea infusion, EGCG, and black tea polyphenols, theaflavin and theaflavin digallate, significantly inhibited invasion of highly metastatic mouse Lewis lung carcinoma LL2-Lu3 cells *in vitro*.[15,16] The per oral administration of green tea infusion (2%) significantly reduced the number of lung colonies of mouse Lewis lung carcinoma cells *in vivo*.[16]

Tea polyphenols (EGCG, theaflavins, or green tea polyphenol extracts) also inhibited invasion of other types of cancer cells *in vitro*, such as biliary carcinoma cells,[17] fibrosarcoma cells,[18] gastric cancer cells,[19] hepatoma cells,[20] medulloblastoma cells,[21] oral carcinoma cells,[22] and pancreatic carcinoma cells.[23]

It is surprising that few studies have investigated the effects of tea polyphenols on invasion and metastasis of breast cancer. On the other hand, in an epidemiological study, increased consumption of green tea was closely associated with decreased numbers of axillary lymph node metastases among premenopausal patients with stage I and II breast cancer.[24] Further follow-up study showed that increased consumption of green tea was significantly correlated with decreased recurrence of stage I and II breast cancer.[24]

In summary, available *in vitro* and animal studies provide promising evidence that tea polyphenols may have potent anticancer metastasis activities. On the other hand, because many *in vitro* studies used high levels of tea polyphenols, their antimetastasis activities need to be further verified in animal models at appropriate levels of supplementation. In particular, because of the prevalence of breast cancer, more effort should be made to determine the effects of tea polyphenols on breast cancer invasion and metastasis.

## 16.2.2 SOY ISOFLAVONES AND ANTIMETASTASIS

Soy isoflavones comprise of genistein, daidzein, and in less content, glycitein. They exist mainly in the glycoside forms in the soybean called genistin, daidzin, and glycitin, respectively. Upon intestinal bacterial action, the glycosides are converted to their biologically active aglycone forms. Genistein is one of the predominant soy isoflavones, and is shown to have variety types of biological functions that are related to its anticarcinogenesis activity.[25] Moreover, genistein is also found to be a potent inhibitor of cancer cell metastasis. In this part of the review, the anti-invasion and antimetastasis activities of genistein and other soy isoflavones will be summarized.

### 16.2.2.1 Effects of Soy Isoflavones on Invasion and Metastasis of Breast Cancer

A series of *in vitro* studies has been conducted to determine the effects of soy isoflavones, especially genistein, on invasion of breast cancer cells. Genistein inhibited invasion of a highly metastatic subline of BALB/c mammary carcinoma 410.4 cells with an $EC_{50}$ of approximately 1 µ$M$, at which genistein showed little effect on cell growth.[26] On the other hand, daidzein was much less potent than genistein on inhibiting 410.4 cell invasion, and most of the effect on invasion was apparently due to its effect on growth inhibition.[26] Magee and co-workers[27] determined the effects of soy isoflavones (genistein, daidzein, glycitein, equol, *O*-desmethylangolensin) on invasion of a breast cancer cell-line MDA-MB-231 *in vitro*, and found that soy isoflavones exerted a potent inhibitory effect on cell invasion without affecting cell growth. Genistein inhibited both constitutive as well as epidermal growth factor (EGF)-stimulated invasion of estrogen receptor (ER)-negative human breast carcinoma lines MDA-MB-231 and MDA-MB-468 *in vitro*.[28]

Despite the *in vitro* effects of soy isoflavones on breast cancer cell invasion, their antimetastasis activities on breast cancer cells *in vivo* have not been reported. On the other hand, one animal study reported possible metastasis-promoting effects of soy isoflavones.[29] In the study, a soybean extract enriched in isoflavones was further heated to denature protease inhibitors, and both heated and unheated extracts were determined for their effects on the growth and metastasis of a mammary tumor MAC-33 in mice. Soy isoflavones did not inhibit the tumor growth, and heated soybean extract significantly increased the number of lung metastases.[29] Clearly, more *in vitro* and *in vivo* studies are urgently required to determine the role of soy isoflavones in metastasis of breast cancer.

### 16.2.2.2 Effects of Soy Isoflavones on Invasion and Metastasis of Prostate Cancer

Although the effects of soy isoflavones on prostate cancer cell invasion have not been adequately studied, the effects of soy isoflavones on prostate cancer metastasis were determined in two animal studies. We have studied the effects of genistin and an isoflavone-enriched SPC on orthotopic growth and metastasis of LNCaP human prostate tumors.[30] SPC at 0.5% of the diet significantly inhibited both lymph node and lung metastases, whereas genistin at the same level as that in the SPC diet did not significantly inhibit lymph node or lung metastases.[30] These data suggest that soybean contains bioactive components other than genistein that have significant antimetastasis activity. In another study, a cell line, K1 that was derived from a carcinogen-induced accessory sex gland carcinoma, was used to examine the effects of genistein on tumor growth and metastasis. Genistein (50 mg/kg body weight) significantly inhibited tumor growth, lymph node metastases, and lung metastases, suggesting that genistein may be a useful chemotherapeutic agent to inhibit the growth and metastasis of accessory sex gland cancers, such as those derived from the prostate.[31]

### 16.2.2.3  Effects of Soy Isoflavones on Invasion and Metastasis of Melanoma

Several *in vitro* and *in vivo* studies have evaluated the effects of genistein on invasion and metastasis of melanoma cells. Genistein significantly inhibited invasion of B16-BL6 mouse melanoma cells *in vitro*.[32,33] In the animal model in which the lung metastasis was developed by intravenous inoculation of B16-BL6 melanoma cells, genistein significantly inhibited the lung metastases.[32,34] Similarly, B16-F10 melanoma cells were inoculated intravenously to develop lung metastases, and genistein significantly inhibited lung metastases of B16-F10 cells in mice.[35,36] On the other hand, the isoflavone daidzein had no significant effect on the reduction of lung metastasis induced by melanoma cells.[36]

### 16.2.2.4  Effects of Soy Isoflavones on Invasion and Metastasis of Other Types of Cancer

The effects of genistein on invasion and metastasis of other types of cancer cells were also evaluated. Genistein significantly inhibited invasion of fibrosarcoma cell line HT1080 *in vitro*,[37] highly invasive lung carcinoma LL2 cells *in vitro*,[35] cervical cancer cells *in vitro*,[38] glioblastoma cells *in vitro*,[39] head and neck cancer cells *in vitro*,[40] transformed keratinocytes *in vitro*,[41] and oral squamous cell carcinoma *in vitro*.[42] Both genistein and glycitein also inhibited Jurkat cell invasion at a similar extent *in vitro*.[43]

Two animal studies showed that genistein inhibited metastasis of pancreatic cancer and intestinal tumors *in vivo*. Pancreatic tumors were orthotopically implanted in mice, and intraperitoneal administration of genistein (1.3 mg/mouse/day) significantly inhibited tumor metastasis to liver.[44] In an animal study of azoxymethane (AOM)-induced intestinal adenocarcinoma, genistein (5 or 10 mg/kg body weight) significantly inhibited the incidence of metastasis of tumors to peritoneum and significantly reduced lymphatic vessel invasion of adenocarcinomas, without significant inhibition on the growth of intestinal cancer.[45] On the other hand, genistein did not inhibit metastasis of oral squamous cell carcinoma *in vivo*.[42]

In summary, available evidence from *in vitro* and animal studies in general supports the antimetastasis role of soy isoflavones. Although genistein is the major bioactive component in soy, soy may contain other antimetastasis components, and the combination of soy bioactive components may have more potent antimetastasis activities than any single component. More *in vivo* studies should be conducted to evaluate the effects of soy bioactives combinations on the metastasis of various types of cancer.

### 16.2.3 APIGENIN AND QUERCETIN AND ANTIMETASTASIS

#### 16.2.3.1 Effects of Apigenin on Invasion and Metastasis of Cancer

Apigenin is a natural plant flavonoid present in the leaves and stems of vascular plants, including fruits and vegetables. Previous studies have suggested that apigenin has cancer chemopreventive activities, which include antimutagenesis,[46] inhibition of ornithine decarboxylase,[47] COX-2,[48] and aromatase,[49] increase of gap junction communication,[50] and inhibition of cell cycle progression by arresting cancer cells at G2/M phases.[51] Its anti-invasion and antimetastasis activities have been investigated in recent years.

Apigenin was shown to significantly inhibit the protease-mediated invasiveness of estrogen-insensitive MDA-MB-231 human breast cancer cells *in vitro*[52] and invasion of B16-BL6 melanoma cells *in vitro*.[10] Two animal studies evaluated the effects of apigenin on tumor metastasis. In one animal study using intravenous inoculation of B16-BL6 melanoma cells to develop lung metastases, apigenin administration at 25 and 50 mg/kg body weight significantly inhibited lung metastasis of B16-BL6 melanoma tumors.[10] Another animal study using an AOM-induced and bombesin-enhanced intestinal adenocarcinoma and metastasis rat model, subcutaneous injection of apigenin at 0.75 or 1.5 mg/kg body weight significantly inhibited the incidence of peritoneal metastasis and the incidence of lymphatic vessel invasion of adenocarcinomas in rats.[53]

#### 16.2.3.2 Effects of Quercetin on Invasion and Metastasis of Cancer

Quercetin is a plant flavonoid found in most edible fruits and vegetables. Daily human consumption has been estimated to be ~25 mg including its glycoside, rutin.[54] Quercetin has demonstrated chemopreventive activity in a variety of laboratory animal models, including tumorigenesis induced by AOM in the colon of mice[55] and human breast tumor xenografts.[56] The possible anti-invasion and antimetastasis of quercetin have been studied recently. Quercetin inhibited the invasion of murine melanoma B16-BL6 cells *in vitro*.[57] Quercetin also significantly inhibited lung metastasis of B16-BL6 melanoma tumors in mice.[10] When administered at 200 nmol/kg body weight, quercetin did not inhibit lung metastasis of B16-F10 melanoma cells, but its glycoside rutin at the same dose significantly inhibited lung metastasis by 72%.[58]

In summary, despite promising *in vitro* and especially *in vivo* evidence to suggest that apigenin and quercetin may be potent antimetastasis agents, the evidence is still insufficient and more *in vitro* and animal studies are required to further evaluate the antimetastasis activities of apigenin and quercetin.

## 16.3  MECHANISMS BY WHICH FLAVONOIDS INHIBIT TUMOR METASTASIS

Cancer mortality is primarily due to metastasis. In order for cancer cells to metastasize they must be able to degrade the basement membrane (BM), traverse the extracellular matrix (ECM), enter the lymphatic or vascular system, adhere to a distant site, and then invade the local tissue. BM and ECM are composed of several proteins with type IV collagen the major structural component. Penetration of BM and ECM by cancer cells through proteolytic degradation has been suggested to be the first step in invasion and metastasis. One of the important groups of proteolytic enzymes involving tumor invasion/metastasis is matrix metalloproteinases (MMPs). Another proteolytic enzyme is urokinase-type plasminogen activator (uPA). Besides proteolytic enzymes, tumor angiogenesis and cancer cell adhesion to ECM also play critical roles in cancer metastasis. Understanding the basic principles by which flavonoids inhibit tumor invasion and metastasis may lead to the development of new therapeutic strategies, in addition to supporting the role of flavonoids as cancer chemopreventive agents. Available evidence suggests that flavonoids may exert their anti-invasion and antimetastasis activities by modulating some of these critical events. In this section, the evidence of flavonoids on modulating the activities of proteolytic enzymes, angiogenesis, and adhesion is discussed.

### 16.3.1  FLAVONOIDS AND ANGIOGENESIS

Angiogenesis, the formation of new blood vessels by sprouting from preexisting endothelium, is a critical event for tumor growth and metastasis. Angiogenesis is a complex process involving a series of cellular events other than proliferation. Formation of new capillaries begins with a localized breakdown of the basement membrane of the parent vessel via the finely tuned elaboration of proteolytic enzymes and their inhibitors, followed by migration of endothelial cells and invasion to the surrounding ECM. The proteolytic degradation of ECM components by capillary endothelial cells is one of the key prerequisites of the angiogenic process. In tumors angiogenesis is persistently upregulated. Although the mechanisms leading to persistent pathological angiogenesis are still unclear, resulting evidence indicates that it is due to an imbalance between angiogenic factors and inhibitors.[59]

Available evidence has demonstrated that one of the mechanisms by which flavonoids inhibit cancer cell invasion and metastasis is via inhibition of angiogenesis. Among flavonoids, EGCG and genistein have been shown to be potent anti-angiogenic compounds, and may be responsible, at least in part, to the antigrowth and antimetastasis effects of tea and soy products, respectively. On the other hand, there is no sufficient evidence to demonstrate whether apigenin or quercetin has anti-angiogenesis activity. Therefore in this section, we focus on the experimental evidence on anti-angiogenesis activities of tea polyphenols and soy isoflavones.

### 16.3.1.1 Effects of Tea Polyphenols on Angiogenesis

Because the angiogenesis process involves a series of cellular events, a series of *in vitro* and *in vivo* methods is commonly used to identify potential anti-angiogenic agents. These assays include *in vitro* proliferation, migration, invasion, and tube formation of endothelial cells, *in vivo* angiogenesis assays, and *in vivo* tumor growth inhibition associated with modulation of markers for angiogenesis. The anti-angiogenesis activity of tea polyphenols, especially EGCG, has been evaluated by using these *in vitro* and *in vivo* angiogenesis assays. EGCG significantly inhibited the endothelial cell proliferation,[60] migration,[61] and invasion[62] *in vitro*, suppressed endothelial cell tube formation[61,62] *in vitro*, and inhibited angiogenesis *in vivo*.[62] Further tumor growth inhibition studies showed that EGCG inhibited the growth of both colon 26 NL17 carcinoma and Meth A sarcoma, in part through the inhibition of angiogenesis.[62] In addition, drinking green tea also significantly inhibited angiogenesis *in vivo*.[60]

Several *in vitro* studies also determined whether the inhibitory effect of EGCG on invasion of endothelial cells is via downregulation of MMP, and found that EGCG inhibited MMP activities in endothelial cells *in vitro*.[61,63,64] It suggests the possibility that tea polyphenols suppress angiogenesis and metastasis in part via inhibition of MMP activities in endothelial cells.

### 16.3.1.2 Effects of Soy Isoflavones on Angiogenesis

Among soy isoflavones, genistein has been shown to be a potent anti-angiogenic isoflavone. The anti-angiogenic ability of soy isoflavones was first identified by Fotsis and co-workers.[65] They fractionated the urine samples of human subjects consuming a diet rich in plant products and found that fractions containing soy isoflavones and metabolites (genistein, daidzein, *O*-desmethylangolensin, or equol) inhibited basic fibroblast growth factor-stimulated proliferation of bovine brain-derived capillary endothelial cells (BBCE).[65] Further studies indicated that pure genistein had a potent and dose-dependent inhibitory effect on proliferation of BBCE at $IC_{50}$ of 5 $\mu M$.[66] Genistein also inhibited the proliferation of other vascular endothelial cells such as that derived from bovine adrenal cortex, and aorta.[66]

The effects of genistein on angiogenic factors were determined to elucidate the mechanisms by which genistein might inhibit angiogenesis. Tumor cells produce angiogenic factors that include platelet-derived growth factor, vascular endothelial growth factor (VEGF), basic fibroblast growth factor, and platelet-derived endothelial cell growth factor, to stimulate neovascularization. Among angiogenic factors, VEGF, an endothelial cell-specific mitogen and a vascular permeability, plays an important role in tumor angiogenesis. Genistein inhibited angiogenesis by reducing VEGF levels via post-transcriptional regulation of VEGF expression[67] *in vitro*. Genistein also inhibited VEGF-promoted endothelial cell proliferation[68,68a] and basic fibroblast growth factor–mediated vascular endothelial cell proliferation[69] *in vitro*.

Besides its anti-angiogenic activity *in vitro*, genistein has shown anti-angiogenesis activity *in vivo*. Wietrzyk and co-workers[70] measured the volume of blood present in tumor tissue as a marker of angiogenesis, and found that genistein treatment reduced tumor blood supply by 35%. We studied the anti-angiogenic activities of both genistein and genistein-enriched SPC in a series of animal tumor models, and found that their antigrowth and anti-angiogenesis effects on bladder tumors and prostate tumors were associated with significant inhibition of tumor microvessel density, a marker of angiogenesis *in vivo*.[12,30,71,72] Although genistein and SPC did not significantly reduce angiogenesis in MCF-7 tumors, the combination of SPC with tea significantly reduced angiogenesis,[73] which suggests that one possible mechanism by which soy and tea synergistically suppress estrogen-dependent breast tumors may be via interactions that impede tumor angiogenesis. We also determined the molecular targets that may be responsible for anti-angiogenesis activity of soy components and found that the expression of basic fibroblast growth factor, not VEGF, was slightly but significantly down-regulated by genistein *in vivo*.[30]

## 16.3.2 FLAVONOIDS AND PROTEOLYTIC ENZYMES

MMPs are naturally occurring, $Zn^{2+}$-dependent, endopeptidases, involved in normal turnover of connective tissue matrix, as well as in certain disease processes such as cancer cell invasion and metastasis. MMPs are secreted in proenzyme forms and activated extracellularly. The activated forms of MMPs can be inhibited by tissue inhibitors of metalloproteinases (TIMPs). uPA is a serine proteinase that functions in conversion of the circulating zymogen plasminogen to the active serine proteinase plasmin. The biological activity of uPA is regulated by a functional interplay between the proteinase, its receptor, uPA receptor (uPAR), and the uPA inhibitor 1 (PAI-1).

One of the most important aspects for tumor metastasis is via its invasion through the ECM. MMPs produced by tumor and stromal cells are believed to play a key role in the degradation of ECM instrumental to invasion. Both *in vitro* and *in vivo* studies have suggested that one of the mechanisms by which flavonoids inhibit tumor metastasis may be via inhibition of MMP activity. Among these flavonoids, tea polyphenol EGCG and soy isoflavone genistein have been shown to be potent inhibitors of MMPs. Although flavonoids apigenin and quercetin have anti-invasion and antimetastasis activities, their effects on MMPs have not been adequately studied. On the other hand, the effects of flavonoids on uPA activity have not been adequately studied and experimental results have been insufficient for discussion. This part of the chapter will primarily focus on modulation of MMP activities by tea polyphenols and soy isoflavones.

### 16.3.2.1   Effects of Tea Polyphenols on MMP Activities

A series of *in vitro* studies has been conducted to determine the effects of tea polyphenols, especially EGCG on the expression and activity of MMP. The MMP expression is usually determined by RNA and/or protein levels, whereas its activity is measured by zymography. Tea catechin significantly inhibited B16-F10 melanoma cell invasion *in vitro* by inhibition of the activities of MMP-2 and MMP-9.[9] EGCG significantly inhibited the invasion of B16-F3m melanoma cells and MMP-9 activity,[8] inhibited invasion of TRAMP-C1 prostate cancer cells *in vitro* and downregulation of MMP-2 activity,[14] and inhibited the gastric cancer cell invasiveness and MMP-9 expression.[19] EGCG, theaflavin, and theaflavin digallate significantly inhibited invasion of mouse Lewis lung carcinoma LL2-Lu3 cells *in vitro* in part by inhibition of MMP activities.[15] ECG, EGCG, and theaflavin significantly suppressed the invasion of fibrosarcoma HT1080 cells and the expression and activity of MMP-2 and MMP-9.[18]

More *in vitro* studies have further determined how tea polyphenols modulate the activities of MMP-2 and MMP-9. The membrane type 1 matrix metalloproteinase (MT1-MMP) is the receptor and the major activator of MMP-2. EGCG inhibited MMP-2 activity in part by significant inhibition of MT1-MMP activity.[74,75] Other studies showed that EGCG inhibited MMP-9 expression through the suppression of MAP kinase via inhibition of the phosphorylation of extracellular signal-regulated kinases 1 and 2 (ERK1/2)[75] and/or activator protein (AP)-1 activation.[19]

Despite promising data from the *in vitro* studies, few animal studies have determined the correlation between the antimetastasis effect of tea polyphenols and the inhibition of MMP activities. In one animal study, oral feeding of green tea polyphenols as the sole source of drinking fluid to TRAMP mice resulted in significant inhibition of the tumor metastasis and MMP-2 and MMP-9 expression.[76]

### 16.3.2.2   Effects of Soy Isoflavones on MMP Activities

Some *in vitro* studies have been conducted to determine the effects of soy isoflavones, especially genistein, on the expression and/or activity of MMPs. Genistein inhibited both constitutive and EGF-stimulated invasion in ER-negative human breast carcinoma lines and the downregulation of MMP-9 and upregulation of TIMP-1 *in vitro*,[28] inhibited invasion of HT1080 fibrosarcoma cells *in vitro* by suppression of conversion of latent forms of MMP-2 and MMP-9 into active forms and by increase of TIMP-1 expression,[37] and inhibited invasion of head and neck cancer cells by downregulation of MMP-2 and MMP-9 secretion.[40] Genistein and glycitein inhibited Jurkat cell invasion, in part through the down-regulation of MMP-13 activity and MMP-8 expression.[43,77] Genistein inhibited transforming growth factor-beta-1 (TGF-$\beta$1)-stimulated cell migration and invasiveness of mouse transformed keratinocytes *in vitro* and increased uPA expression/secretion.[41]

In contrast to *in vitro* studies, few animal studies have determined the correlation between antimetastasis activities of soy isoflavones to their inhibition of MMPs. Although genistein inhibited invasion of oral squamous cell carcinoma cells *in vitro*,[42] the animal study failed to show the significant effects of genistein supplementation on inhibition of tumor growth and metastasis, or the expression of MMP-2 and basic fibroblast growth factor.[42]

## 16.3.3 FLAVONOIDS AND CANCER CELL ADHESION

Altered cell adhesion ability is suggested to play a critical role in cancer cell migration, proliferation, invasion, and metastasis. The invasiveness of cancer cells strongly depends on their ability to migrate and to adhere to the ECM. Cell adhesion is primarily mediated by a class of proteins called integrins. Integrins are cell surface $\alpha\beta$-heterodimeric glycoproteins. To date, 24 $\alpha\beta$-heterodimers formed by 8 $\beta$ and 18 $\alpha$ subunits are identified.[78] Integrins bind to various ECM proteins such as collagen, fibronectin, laminin, and vitronectin, and their binding activates important intracellular signaling pathways that regulate cell proliferation, migration, invasion, and metastasis. Experimental evidence suggests that one of the mechanisms by which flavonoids such as tea polyphenols and soy isoflavones inhibit cancer cell invasion and metastasis may be via modulation of the expression of integrins.

### 16.3.3.1 Effects of Tea Polyphenols on Cancer Cell Adhesion

The effects of EGCG on modulation of integrins have been studied in several cancer cell types *in vitro*. EGCG inhibited invasion of the pediatric brain tumor-derived medulloblastoma cells *in vitro*, in part via modulation of specific cell surface integrins, notably upregulation of $\beta$1 integrin.[21] Laminin is a major glycoprotein of basement membrane and plays significant roles during cancer cell invasion and metastases. Tea catechin inhibited laminin-promoted MO4 brain cancer cell attachment *in vitro*.[79] EGCG also inhibited the adhesion of mouse melanoma B16 cells to laminin *in vitro*.[80]

### 16.3.3.2 Effects of Soy Isoflavones on Cancer Cell Adhesion

The effects of genistein on modulation of cancer cell adhesion are basically dependent on its protein tyrosine kinase activity. Protein tyrosine phosphorylation occurs as one of the earlier events in cancer-ECM interaction.[59] Genistein, as a protein tyrosine kinase inhibitor,[81] significantly inhibited invasion of B16-BL6 melanoma cells *in vitro* associated with suppression of the tyrosine phosphory-lation of proteins located at the cell periphery when cells attached to and interacted with ECM.[32,33] Focal adhesion kinase (FAK) is a protein tyrosine kinase located at the focal adhesion sites of spreading cells. It is a pivotal element in the signaling cascade associated with cell–ECM interaction. It is suggested that suppression of adhesion-induced tyrosine phosphorylation of FAK may interrupt cancer cell–ECM interaction and subsequent invasion and metastasis potential of cancer cells. Genistein inhibited FAK activity *in vitro*.[82]

## 16.4  CRITICAL ISSUES AND FUTURE DIRECTIONS IN RESEARCH ON FLAVONOIDS AND TUMOR METASTASIS

Previous research has indicated that flavonoids such as tea polyphenols, soy isoflavones, apigenin, and quercetin have significant anti-invasion activities *in vitro* associated with inhibition of angiogenesis, proteolytic enzymes activities, and enhancement of cell–ECM interactions. Some *in vitro* anti-invasion activities of flavonoids are confirmed in animal models. These studies suggest that some flavonoids may play a significant role in prevention of cancer metastasis, in addition to prevention of cancer development. On the other hand, research in this exciting field is still preliminary and large gaps in data exist among *in vitro*, animal, and human studies that are barriers to advancing the flavonoids and prevention of tumor metastasis hypothesis. Identification of these critical issues will provide the directions of future research priorities in this field.

### 16.4.1  IDENTIFICATION OF FLAVONOIDS FOR INHIBITION OF CANCER-SPECIFIC METASTASIS

Previous *in vitro* studies have provided promising evidence to support that fla-vonoids have anti-invasion activities. Although it would be ideal to identify flavonoids that have anti-invasion activities for all types of cancer, it is more likely that some flavonoids are potent anti-invasive agents for certain types of cancer, or certain cancer phenotypes. In addition, some flavonoids have anti-invasion activities only at high concentrations, either at superphysiological or pharmacological levels. It is possible that the combination of certain flavonoids may reach significant activities at physiologically achievable doses. Therefore, one of the future research priorities should be identification of specific flavonoids and/or the combinations of flavonoids that have the most potent anti-invasive activities for each type of cancer or each phenotype. A series of *in vitro* assays, such as those for proliferation, migration, and invasion of both cancer cells and endothelial cells, should be used to identify the candidate flavonoids or the combinations in a systematic approach. The identified candidates will be subject to *in vivo* verification of activities.

## 16.4.2 Verification of Antimetastasis Activities of Flavonoids

Successful identification of potent antimetastasis flavonoids requires application of appropriate testing systems, both *in vitro* and animal models. Although *in vitro* cell culture systems provide a fast and inexpensive screening system and are essential for identification of candidate regimens, it should be recognized that cell culture is an artificial system with different metabolic and biological processes from the *in vivo* system. Simple extrapolation of *in vitro* results to *in vivo* effects may be misleading. Appropriate animal models are thus required to confirm the efficacy of identified flavonoids or their combinations from the cell culture studies, to elucidate the *in vivo* mechanisms of action, and to monitor possible adverse effects or toxicities.

A series of animal models should be applied to represent growth and metastasis of different types of cancer. It is true that each animal model has its strengths and weaknesses. Therefore, it is important to use as clinically relevant tumor models as possible. For example, an orthotopic (intra-organ) tumor implantation model for growth and metastasis may be more clinically relevant than a subcutaneous tumor model because the orthotopic tumor model may mimic the tumor microenvironment and epithelial/stromal cell interactions in humans. Besides xenografts and orthotopic implantation tumor models, a series of transgenic animal models for different types of cancer and different phenotypes with specific degrees of metastasis have been established.

## 16.4.3 Further Elucidation of Mechanisms

Despite progression in the mechanistic research *in vitro*, the *in vivo* mechanisms by which bioactive flavonoids, such as tea polyphenols, soy isoflavones, apigenin, and quercetin, prevent tumor metastasis are largely unknown. Efficacy confirmation of identified potent flavonoids regimens also requires appropriate understanding of their mechanisms of action *in vivo*. Traditional methods of analysis of gene expression patterns have imposed a practical limit on the number of candidate genes. Highly parallel technologies exploiting sample hybridization to oligonucleotide or cDNA arrays permit the expression levels of tens of thousands of genes to be monitored simultaneously and rapidly. With the advent of DNA microarray technology, quantitative comparisons of thousands of genes can be made at one time. The application of this technology and/or other advanced technologies such as proteomics will greatly facilitate our mechanistic research and identification of biomarkers that could be used as intermediate end points.

Future research should involve application of advanced technologies in genomics and proteomics to identify the molecular markers that are responsive to the effective flavonoid treatments, and functional assays such as RNA interference to further identify the functional markers that are responsible for the effective treatment.

### 16.4.4 INTERACTIVE EFFECTS OF FLAVONOIDS WITH OTHER DIETARY BIOACTIVES

Besides flavonoids, fruits and vegetables, like other foods, contain a diverse array of other components. It is possible that the interactions between dietary bioactive components are largely responsible for the effective anticancer and antimetastasis activities of diets. Therefore, in addition to studying the combined effects of flavonoids on tumor metastasis, the interactive effects between flavonoids and other dietary bioactives should be encouraged. Similar to flavonoid combinations studies, a series of *in vitro* assays should be first applied to identify possible synergistic combinations between flavonoids and other bioactives for specific cancer types or phenotypes, and to further verify the efficacy of these combinations in clinically relevant animal models. Advanced technologies in genomics and proteomics should be applied to elucidate the mechanisms of action.

## 16.5 CONCLUSIONS

Previous research has provided important scientific evidence to support the role of flavonoids in antimetastasis. On the other hand, more systematic approaches are required to further identify more potent dietary bioactive components and their combinations for effective inhibition of tumor growth and metastasis. The availability of a diverse array of dietary bioactive components such as flavonoids and other phytochemicals ensures the success of identification of effective regimens. Although intake of various types of fruits and vegetables provides effective prevention of cancer development and metastasis, bioactivity-guided isolation of bioactives-enriched fractions should be encouraged and will be expected to provide potent activities. However, whether a specific bioactives-containing extract is safe and efficacious requires comprehensive evaluation.

## REFERENCES

1. Cook NC, Samman S. Flavonoids — chemistry, metabolism, cardioprotective effects, and dietary sources. *J Nutr Biochem* 1996; 7:66–76.
2. Middleton E, Kandaswami C, Theoharides TC. The effects of plant flavonoids on mammalian cells: implications for inflammation, heart disease, and cancer. *Pharmacol Rev* 2000; 52:673–751.
3. Mitscher LA, Jung M, Shankel D, Dou JH, Steele L, Pillai SP. Chemoprotection: a review of the potential therapeutic antioxidant properties of green tea (*Camellia sinensis*) and certain of its constituents. *Med Res Rev* 1997; 17(4):327–365.
4. Graham HN. Green tea composition, consumption, and polyphenol chemistry. *Prev Med* 1992; 21:334–350.
5. Tijburg LB, Mattern T, Folts JD, Weisgerber UM, Katan MB. Tea flavonoids and cardiovascular disease: a review. *Crit Rev Food Sci Nutr* 1997; 37(8):771–785.
6. Yang CS, Wang ZY. Tea and cancer. *J Natl Cancer Inst* 1993; 85(13):1038–1049.

7. Blot WJ, McLaughlin JK, Chow WH. Cancer rates among drinkers of black tea. *Crit Rev Food Sci Nutr* 1997; 37(8):739–760.

8. Liu JD, Chen SH, Lin CL, Tsai SH, Liang YC. Inhibition of melanoma growth and metastasis by combination with (–)-epigallocatechin-3-gallate and dacarbazine in mice. *J Cell Biochem* 2001; 83(4):631–642.

9. Menon LG, Kuttan R, Kuttan G. Anti-metastatic activity of curcumin and catechin. *Cancer Lett* 1999; 141(1–2):159–165.

10. Caltagirone S, Rossi C, Poggi A et al. Flavonoids apigenin and quercetin inhibit melanoma growth and metastatic potential. *Int J Cancer* 2000; 87(4):595–600.

11. Taniguchi S, Fujiki H, Kobayashi H, et al. Effect of (–)-epigallocatechin gallate, the main constituent of green tea, on lung metastasis with mouse B16 melanoma cell lines. *Cancer Lett* 1992; 65(1):51–54.

12. Zhou J-R, Yu L, Zhong Y, Blackburn GL. Soy phytochemicals and tea bioactive components synergistically inhibit androgen-sensitive human prostate tumors in mice. *J Nutr* 2003; 133:516–521.

13. Gupta S, Hastak K, Ahmad N, Lewin JS, Mukhtar H. Inhibition of prostate carcinogenesis in TRAMP mice by oral infusion of green tea polyphenols. *Proc Natl Acad Sci USA* 2001; 98(18):10350–10355.

14. Sartor L, Pezzato E, Dona M et al. Prostate carcinoma and green tea: (–)epigallocatechin-3-gallate inhibits inflammation-triggered MMP-2 activation and invasion in murine TRAMP model. *Int J Cancer* 2004; 112(5):823–829.

15. Sazuka M, Imazawa H, Shoji Y, Mita T, Hara Y, Isemura M. Inhibition of collagenases from mouse lung carcinoma cells by green tea catechins and black tea theaflavins. *Biosci Biotechnol Biochem* 1997; 61(9):1504–1506.

16. Sazuka M, Murakami S, Isemura M, Satoh K, Nukiwa T. Inhibitory effects of green tea infusion on *in vitro* invasion and *in vivo* metastasis of mouse lung carcinoma cells. *Cancer Lett* 1995; 98(1):27–31.

17. Takada M, Ku Y, Habara K, Ajiki T, Suzuki Y, Kuroda Y. Inhibitory effect of epigallocatechin-3-gallate on growth and invasion in human biliary tract carcinoma cells. *World J Surg* 2002; 26(6):683–686.

18. Maeda-Yamamoto M, Kawahara H, Tahara N, Tsuji K, Hara Y, Isemura M. Effects of tea polyphenols on the invasion and matrix metalloproteinases activities of human fibrosarcoma HT1080 cells. *J Agric Food Chem* 1999; 47(6):2350–2354.

19. Kim HS, Kim MH, Jeong M et al. EGCG blocks tumor promoter-induced MMP-9 expression via suppression of MAPK and AP-1 activation in human gastric AGS cells. *Anticancer Res* 2004; 24(2B):747–753.

20. Zhang G, Miura Y, Yagasaki K. Suppression of adhesion and invasion of hepatoma cells in culture by tea compounds through antioxidative activity. *Cancer Lett* 2000; 159(2):169–173.

21. Pilorget A, Berthet V, Luis J, Moghrabi A, Annabi B, Beliveau R. Medulloblastoma cell invasion is inhibited by green tea (–)epigallocatechin-3-gallate. *J Cell Biochem* 2003; 90(4):745–755.

22. Hsu SD, Singh BB, Lewis JB et al. Chemoprevention of oral cancer by green tea. *Gen Dent* 2002; 50(2):140–146.

23. Takada M, Nakamura Y, Koizumi T et al. Suppression of human pancreatic carcinoma cell growth and invasion by epigallocatechin-3-gallate. *Pancreas* 2002; 25(1):45–48.

24. Nakachi K, Suemasu K, Suga K, Takeo T, Imai K, Higashi Y. Influence of drinking green tea on breast cancer malignancy among Japanese patients. *Jpn J Cancer Res* 1998; 89(3):254–261.

25. Messina MJ, Persky V, Setchell KD, Barnes S. Soy intake and cancer risk: a review of the *in vitro* and *in vivo* data. *Nutr Cancer* 1994; 21(2):113–131.

26. Scholar EM, Toews ML. Inhibition of invasion of murine mammary carcinoma cells by the tyrosine kinase inhibitor genistein. *Cancer Lett* 1994; 87(2):159–162.

27. Magee PJ, McGlynn H, Rowland IR. Differential effects of isoflavones and lignans on invasiveness of MDA-MB-231 breast cancer cells *in vitro*. *Cancer Lett* 2004; 208(1):35–41.

28. Shao ZM, Wu J, Shen ZZ, Barsky SH. Genistein inhibits both constitutive and EGF-stimulated invasion in ER-negative human breast carcinoma cell lines. *Anticancer Res* 1998; 18(3A):1435–1439.

29. Charland SL, Hui JW, Torosian MH. The effects of a soybean extract on tumor growth and metastasis. *Int J Mol Med* 1998; 2(2):225–228.

30. Zhou J-R, Yu L, Zhong Y et al. Inhibition of orthotopic growth and metastasis of androgen-sensitive human prostate tumors in mice by bioactive soybean components. *Prostate* 2002; 53:143–153.

31. Schleicher RL, Lamartiniere CA, Zheng M, Zhang M. The inhibitory effect of genistein on the growth and metastasis of a transplantable rat accessory sex gland carcinoma. *Cancer Lett* 1999; 136(2):195–201.

32. Yan C, Han R. Suppression of adhesion-induced protein tyrosine phosphorylation decreases invasive and metastatic potentials of B16-BL6 melanoma cells by protein tyrosine kinase inhibitor genistein. *Invasion Metastasis* 1997; 17(4):189–198.

33. Yan C, Han R. Genistein suppresses adhesion-induced protein tyrosine phosphorylation and invasion of B16-BL6 melanoma cells. *Cancer Lett* 1998; 129(1):117–124.

34. Li D, Yee JA, McGuire MH, Murphy PA, Yan L. Soybean isoflavones reduce experimental metastasis in mice. *J Nutr* 1999; 129(5):1075–1078.

35. Wietrzyk J, Opolski A, Madej J, Radzikowski C. Antitumour and antimetastatic effect of genistein alone or combined with cyclophosphamide in mice transplanted with various tumours depends on the route of tumour transplantation. *In Vivo* 2000; 14(2):357–362.

36. Menon LG, Kuttan R, Nair MG, Chang YC, Kuttan G. Effect of isoflavones genistein and daidzein in the inhibition of lung metastasis in mice induced by B16F-10 melanoma cells. *Nutr Cancer* 1998; 30(1):74–77.

37. Yan C, Han R. Effects of genistein on invasion and matrix metalloproteinase activities of HT1080 human fibrosarcoma cells. *Chin Med Sci J* 1999; 14(3):129–133.

38. Wang SY, Yang KW, Hsu YT, Chang CL, Yang YC. The differential inhibitory effects of genistein on the growth of cervical cancer cells *in vitro*. *Neoplasma* 2001; 48(3):227–233.

39. Penar PL, Khoshyomn S, Bhushan A, Tritton TR. Inhibition of epidermal growth factor receptor-associated tyrosine kinase blocks glioblastoma invasion of the brain. *Neurosurgery* 1997; 40(1):141–151.

40. Alhasan SA, Aranha O, Sarkar FH. Genistein elicits pleiotropic molecular effects on head and neck cancer cells. *Clin Cancer Res* 2001; 7(12):4174–4181.

41. Santibanez JF, Quintanilla M, Martinez J. Genistein and curcumin block TGF-beta 1-induced u-PA expression and migratory and invasive phenotype in mouse epidermal keratinocytes. *Nutr Cancer* 2000; 37(1):49–54.

42. Myoung H, Hong SP, Yun PY, Lee JH, Kim MJ. Anti-cancer effect of genistein in oral squamous cell carcinoma with respect to angiogenesis and *in vitro* invasion. *Cancer Sci* 2003; 94(2):215–220.

43. Kim MH, Gutierrez AM, Goldfarb RH. Different mechanisms of soy isoflavones in cell cycle regulation and inhibition of invasion. *Anticancer Res* 2002; 22(6C):3811–3817.

44. Buchler P, Gukovskaya AS, Mouria M et al. Prevention of metastatic pancreatic cancer growth *in vivo* by induction of apoptosis with genistein, a naturally occurring isoflavonoid. *Pancreas* 2003; 26(3):264–273.

45. Iishi H, Tatsuta M, Baba M, Yano H, Sakai N, Akedo H. Genistein attenuates peritoneal metastasis of azoxymethane-induced intestinal adenocarcinomas in Wistar rats. *Int J Cancer* 2000; 86(3):416–420.

46. Kuo ML, Lee KC, Lin JK. Genotoxicities of nitropyrenes and their modulation by apigenin, tannic acid, ellagic acid and indole-3-carbinol in the *Salmonella* and CHO systems. *Mutat Res* 1992; 270(2):87–95.

47. Wei H, Tye L, Bresnick E, Birt DF. Inhibitory effect of apigenin, a plant flavonoid, on epidermal ornithine decarboxylase and skin tumor promotion in mice. *Cancer Res* 1990; 50(3):499–502.

48. Liang YC, Huang YT, Tsai SH, Lin-Shiau SY, Chen CF, Lin JK. Suppression of inducible cyclooxygenase and inducible nitric oxide synthase by apigenin and related flavonoids in mouse macrophages. *Carcinogenesis* 1999; 20(10):1945–1952.

49. Pelissero C, Lenczowski M, Chinzi D, Davailcuisset B, Sumpter JP, Fostier A. Effects of flavonoids on aromatase activity, an *in vitro* study. *J Steroid Biochem Mol Biol* 1996; 57(3–4):215–223.

50. Chaumontet C, Bex V, Gaillard SI, Seillan HC, Suschetet M, Martel P. Apigenin and tangeretin enhance gap junctional intercellular communication in rat liver epithelial cells. *Carcinogenesis* 1994; 15(10):2325–2330.

51. Lepley DM, Li B, Birt DF, Pelling JC. The chemopreventive flavonoid apigenin induces G2/M arrest in keratinocytes. *Carcinogenesis* 1996; 17(11):2367–2375.

52. Lindenmeyer F, Li H, Menashi S, Soria C, Lu H. Apigenin acts on the tumor cell invasion process and regulates protease production. *Nutr Cancer* 2001; 39(1):139–147.

53. Tatsuta A, Iishi H, Baba M et al. Suppression by apigenin of peritoneal metastasis of intestinal adenocarcinomas induced by azoxymethane in Wistar rats. *Clin Exp Metastasis* 2000; 18(8):657–662.

54. Kuhnau J. The flavonoids. A class of semi-essential food components: their role in human nutrition. *World Rev Nutr Diet* 1976; 24:711–791.

55. Matsukawa Y, Nishino H, Okuyama Y et al. Effects of quercetin and/or restraint stress on formation of aberrant crypt foci induced by azoxymethane in rat colons. *Oncology* 1997; 54(2):118–121.

56. Zhong X, Wu K, He S, Ma S, Kong L. Effects of quercetin on the proliferation and apoptosis in transplantation tumor of breast cancer in nude mice. *Sichuan Da Xue Xue Bao Yi Xue Ban* 2003; 34(3):439–442.

57. Zhang X, Xu Q, Saiki I. Quercetin inhibits the invasion and mobility of murine melanoma B16-BL6 cells through inducing apoptosis via decreasing Bcl-2 expression. *Clin Exp Metastasis* 2000; 18(5):415–421.

58. Menon LG, Kuttan R, Kuttan G. Inhibition of lung metastasis in mice induced by B16F10 melanoma cells by polyphenolic compounds. *Cancer Lett* 1995; 95(1–2):221–225.

59. Liotta LA, Steeg PS, Stetler-Stevenson WG. Cancer metastasis and angiogenesis: an imbalance of positive and negative regulation. *Cell* 1991; 64:327–336.

60. Cao Y, Cao R. Angiogenesis inhibited by drinking tea. *Nature* 1999; 398:381.

61. Singh AK, Seth P, Anthony P et al. Green tea constituent epigallocatechin-3-gallate inhibits angiogenic differentiation of human endothelial cells. *Arch Biochem Biophys* 2002; 401(1):29–37.

62. Yamakawa S, Asai T, Uchida T, Matsukawa M, Akizawa T, Oku N. (–)-Epigallocatechin gallate inhibits membrane-type 1 matrix metalloproteinase, MT1-MMP, and tumor angiogenesis. *Cancer Lett* 2004; 210(1):47–55.

63. Oku N, Matsukawa M, Yamakawa S et al. Inhibitory effect of green tea polyphenols on membrane-type 1 matrix metalloproteinase, MT1-MMP. *Biol Pharm Bull* 2003; 26(9):1235–1238.

64. Tosetti F, Ferrari N, De Flora S, Albini A. Angioprevention: angiogenesis is a common and key target for cancer chemopreventive agents. *FASEB J* 2002; 16(1):2–14.

65. Fotsis T, Pepper M, Adlercreutz H et al. Genistein, a dietary-derived inhibitor of *in vitro* angiogenesis. *Proc Natl Acad Sci USA* 1993; 90(7):2690–2694.

66. Fotsis T, Pepper M, Adlercreutz H, Hase T, Montesano R, Schweigerer L. Genistein, a dietary ingested isoflavonoid, inhibits cell proliferation and *in vitro* angiogenesis. *J Nutr* 1995; 125(3 Suppl):790S–797S.

67. Levy AP, Levy NS, Goldberg MA. Post-transcriptional regulation of vascular endothelial growth factor by hypoxia. *J Biol Chem* 1996; 271(5):2746–2753.

68. Guo D, Jia Q, Song HY, Warren RS, Donner DB. Vascular endothelial cell growth factor promotes tyrosine phosphorylation of mediators of signal transduction that contain SH2 domains. Association with endothelial cell proliferation. *J Biol Chem* 1995; 270(12):6729–6733.

68a. Xia P, Aiello LP, Ishii H et al. Characterization of vascular endothelial growth factor's effect on the activation of protein kinase C, its isoforms, and endothelial cell growth. *J Clin Invest* 1996; 98:2018–2026.

69. Koroma BM de, Juan E Jr. Phosphotyrosine inhibition and control of vascular endothelial cell proliferation by genistein. *Biochem Pharmacol* 1994; 48(4):809–818.

70. Wietrzyk J, Boratynski J, Grynkiewicz G, Ryczynski A, Radzikowski C, Opolski A. Antiangiogenic and antitumour effects *in vivo* of genistein applied alone or combined with cyclophosphamide. *Anticancer Res* 2001; 21(6A):3893–3896.

71. Zhou J-R, Mukherjee P, Gugger ET, Tanaka T, Blackburn GL, Clinton SK. The inhibition of murine bladder tumorigenesis by soy isoflavones via alterations in the cell cycle, apoptosis, and angiogenesis. *Cancer Res* 1998; 58:5231–5238.

72. Zhou J-R, Gugger ET, Tanaka T, Guo Y, Blackburn GL, Clinton SK. Soybean phytochemicals inhibit the growth of transplantable human prostate carcinoma and tumor angiogenesis in mice. *J Nutr* 1999; 129:1628–1635.

73. Zhou J-R, Yu L, Mai Z, Blackburn GL. Combined inhibition of estrogen-dependent human breast carcinoma by soy and tea bioactive components in mice. *Int J Cancer* 2004; 108(1):8–14.

74. Dell'Aica I, Dona M, Sartor L, Pezzato E, Garbisa S. (–)Epigallocatechin-3-gallate directly inhibits MT1-MMP activity, leading to accumulation of nonactivated MMP-2 at the cell surface. *Lab Invest* 2002; 82(12):1685–1693.

75. Maeda-Yamamoto M, Suzuki N, Sawai Y et al. Association of suppression of extracellular signal-regulated kinase phosphorylation by epigallocatechin gallate with the reduction of matrix metalloproteinase activities in human fibrosarcoma HT1080 cells. *J Agric Food Chem* 2003; 51(7):1858–1863.

76. Adhami VM, Ahmad N, Mukhtar H. Molecular targets for green tea in prostate cancer prevention. *J Nutr* 2003; 133(7 Suppl):2417S–2424S.

77. Kim MH, Albertsson P, Xue Y, Nannmark U, Kitson RP, Goldfarb RH. Expression of neutrophil collagenase (MMP-8) in Jurkat T leukemia cells and its role in invasion. *Anticancer Res* 2001; 21(1A):45–50.

78. Brakebusch C, Bouvard D, Stanchi F, Sakai T, Fassler R. Integrins in invasive growth. *J Clin Invest* 2002; 109:999–1006.

79. Castronovo V, Bracke ME, Mareel MM, Reznik M, Foidart JM. Absence of laminin deposition in breast cancer and metastases except to the brain. *Pathol Res Pract* 1991; 187(2–3):201–208.

80. Suzuki Y, Isemura M. Inhibitory effect of epigallocatechin gallate on adhesion of murine melanoma cells to laminin. *Cancer Lett* 2001; 173(1):15–20.

81. Akiyama T, Ishida J, Nakagawa S et al. Genistein, a specific inhibitor of tyrosine-specific protein kinases. *J Biol Chem* 1987; 262(12):5592–5595.

82. Kyle E, Neckers L, Takimoto C, Curt G, Bergan R. Genistein-induced apoptosis of prostate cancer cells is preceded by a specific decrease in focal adhesion kinase activity. *Mol Pharmacol* 1997; 51(2):193–200.

# 17 Catechins and Inhibitory Activity against Carcinogenesis

*Jen-Kun Lin*

## CONTENTS

Abstract ...................................................................................................................351
17.1 Introduction..................................................................................................352
17.2 Occurrence of Catechins...............................................................................354
17.3 Chemical Structures of Catechins and Their Biological Activities......354
17.4 Inhibition of Carcinogenesis by Catechins in Animal Models............355
17.5 Chemoprevention of Human Cancer by Tea Drinking.........................355
17.6 Biochemical and Molecular Mechanisms of Cancer
     Chemoprevention by Catechins................................................................356
     17.6.1 Antioxidant Effects of Catechins .................................................356
     17.6.2 Pro-Oxidant Effects of Catechins................................................357
     17.6.3 Induction of Apoptosis and Cell Cycle Arrest..........................358
     17.6.4 Inhibition of Cellular Proliferation and Tumor Progression
            through Suppressing EGFR Signaling .......................................358
     17.6.5 Inhibition of iNOS through Downregulating NFκB
            Activation....................................................................................359
     17.6.6 Inhibition of Tumor Promotion and Cell Transformation
            through Suppressing AP-1 Activation .......................................359
     17.6.7 Suppression of Fatty Acid Synthase Expression by
            Catechins and Theaflavins.........................................................360
     17.6.8 Inhibition of Ubiquitin–Proteasome Pathway by Catechins.....361
17.7 Discussion of the Action Mechanisms of Catechins ...........................361
Acknowledgments .................................................................................................362
References ..............................................................................................................362

## ABSTRACT

Catechins are a group of compounds that naturally occur in the plant kingdom. These compounds are called tea polyphenols and are rich in tea beverages that are consumed daily by most people. The health effects of teas are attributed to their tea polyphenols, namely, catechins from green tea and theaflavins from black tea. Recently, catechins have been intensively investigated and showed many profound biochemical and pharmacological activities including antioxidant and pro-oxidant effects, induction of apoptosis and arrest of cell cycle in cancer cells, inhibition of cellular proliferation and tumor progression through suppression of the epidermal growth factor receptor signaling pathway, suppression of inducible nitric oxide synthase expression through downregulation of nuclear factor κB (NFκB) activation, inhibition of tumor promotion through suppression of activator protein-1 (AP-1) activation and fatty acid synthase expression, and inhibition of tumor promotion and cellular proliferation through suppression of the function of the ubiquitin–proteasome pathway. The mechanisms of action involved in these biochemical and pharmacological activities of catechins have been described and discussed. Tea is a heavily consumed beverage worldwide because of its unique aroma, low cost, and broad availability. Tea and tea polyphenols have been considered potential cancer chemopreventive and anti-obesity agents in the general population. Furthermore, the mechanisms of cancer chemoprevention by tea and tea polyphenols might be via blocking cellular signal transduction pathways.

## 17.1  INTRODUCTION

Several epidemiologic and laboratory data suggest that long-term tea drinking may reduce the incidence of several types of cancer.[1] Case-control and cohort studies report benefits for those consuming green tea regarding cancers of the breast,[2] colon and rectum, pancreas, stomach, ovary, and lung.[1] The health effects of green tea are attributed to tea polyphenols, which comprise 30% of dried leaf extract.[3] These compounds include flavanoids, flavanols, flavonoids, and phenolic acids; however, most tea polyphenols isolated from green tea are monomeric flavan-3-ols, commonly known as catechins (Figure 17.1) including (+)-catechin (C), (–)-epicatechin (EC), (+)-gallocatechin (GC), (–)-epigallocatechin (EGC), (–)-epicatechin-3-gallate (ECG), and (–)-epigallocatechin-3-gallate (EGCG). Among the catechins in green tea, EGCG is most abundant and is the representative compound for biomedical research.[3] In an analysis of EGCG biotransformation products in rats, five biliary methylated metabolites (Figure 17.1) were identified as 3′-$O$-methyl-EGCG, 4′-$O$-methyl-EGCG, 3″-$O$-methyl-EGCG, 4″-$O$-methyl-EGCG, and 4′,4″$O$,$O$-dimethyl-EGCG.[4]

Development in molecular oncology has provided profound basis for understanding the mechanisms of multistep carcinogenesis including tumor initiation, tumor promotion, and tumor progression.[3] Chemoprevention of carcinogenesis is one of the major strategies for cancer control. Many studies have shown that tea and tea polyphenols have inhibitory effects on carcinogenesis in rodent models,[5] and an antipromoting effect of EGCG has been demonstrated.[6] The molecular mechanism of its antipromoting effect on tumor growth and proliferation might be through blocking the signal transduction pathways,[7] leading to the activation of important transcription factors such as activator protein-1 (AP-1) and nuclear factor κB (NFκB).[6,8,9] On the other hand, black tea is reported to significantly

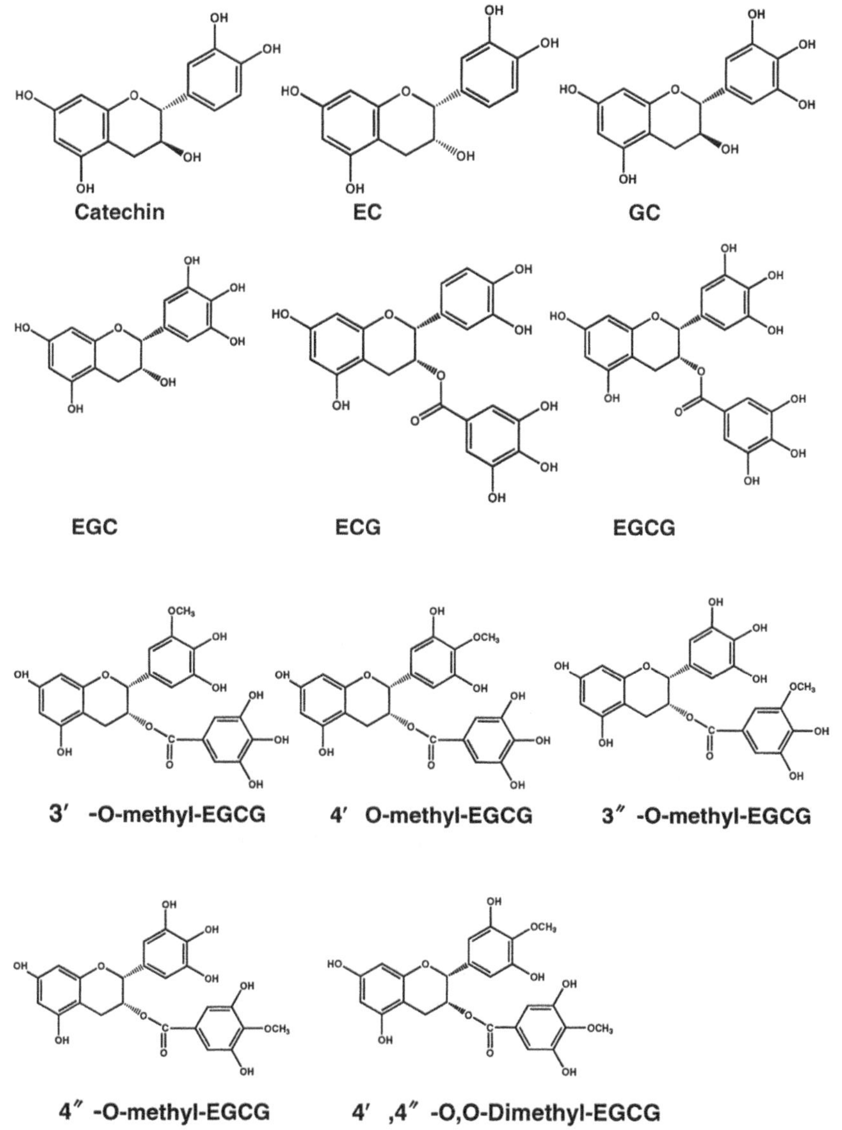

**FIGURE 17.1** Structures of catechins from tea.

inhibit proliferation and enhance apoptosis of skin tumors in mice.[10] Among the black tea polyphenols, theaflavins including theaflavin (TF-1), theaflavin-3-gallate (TF-2a), theaflavin-3'-gallate (TF-2b), and theaflavin-3,3'-digallate (TF-3) are generally considered to be the active principles for the inhibition of carcinogenesis.[11] Because of space limitations, only the green tea polyphenols catechins are discussed in this chapter.

## 17.2  OCCURRENCE OF CATECHINS

Phytopolyphenolic compounds are widespread in the plant kingdom. The major groups of this category are the flavanoids and flavonoids, which are important in contributing the flavor and color of many fruits and vegetables.[12] Some of them are important for the normal growth, development, and defense of plants.[13] They are found in several medicinal plants and herbal remedies that are used in folk medicine throughout the world.[14] It has been reported that diets rich in fruits and vegetables appear to protect against cardiovascular disease and some forms of cancer.[15,16]

The important group of phytopolyphenolics in food are flavonoids and flavanoids, which consist mainly of flavones, flavanones, flavanonols, isoflavones, flavanols, and anthrocyanidins.[12] Although flavanols, also called catechins, seem to be widely distributed in plants, they are rich only in tea leaves, where they may constitute up to 30% of the dry leaf weight. It has been demonstrated that levels of catechins in the tea tree varies with species, season, weather, and horticultural conditions.

## 17.3  CHEMICAL STRUCTURES OF CATECHINS AND THEIR BIOLOGICAL ACTIVITIES

Studies on the structure–activity relationship with catechins such as EGCG indicate that a linear increase of the rate constants with OH radical correlates with the number of reactive hydroxyl groups (such as the number of catechol or pyrogallol moieties), suggesting the importance of the structure of flavan-3-ol linked to gallic acid for the antioxidant activity of EGCG[17] (Figure 17.1). Methylation at the 4″ position of EGCG resulted in loss of the antioxidant activity,[18] whereas methylation at 3″ position did not.[19] Whether anticancer activities of EGCG are different by methyl substitutions remains to be systematically elucidated.

Highest antiproliferative activity was found with the presence of three adjacent hydroxyl groups. However, O-methyl EGCG had a stronger anti-allergic activity than EGCG against Type I allergy in mice[20] and in the activation and degranulation of basophilic KU812 cells.[21,22] Suppression of cancer via inhibition of AP-1 activity by EGCG and related tea catechins has been attributed to inhibition of phosphorylation of c-jun by the galloyl structure on the B ring or the gallate moiety.[23] It has been suggested that the minimal motif to mediate cell apoptosis is a pyrogallol-type B ring structure, and activity is enhanced with a 3-O-gallate group in cis configuration to the B ring. Catechins without a pyrogallol-type structure showed no enhancement or suppression of apoptosis.[24]

Tea polyphenols inhibited AP-1 activity and the mitogen-activated protein (MAP) kinase pathway, which contributed to the growth inhibition; however, different mechanisms may be involved in the inhibition by catechins and theaflavins. Theaflavins may be considered the oxidized derivatives of catechins, but they are different in chemical structural nucleus, and this variation may cause their different action mechanisms at target cells. Further investigations are needed to resolve this issue.

## 17.4 INHIBITION OF CARCINOGENESIS BY CATECHINS IN ANIMAL MODELS

The anticarcinogenic effects of catechins on various organs including skin, glandular stomach, duodenum, colon, liver, pancreas, and lung in rats and mice have been reported in several laboratories.[24–27] Recent studies provide evidence that tea catechins including EGCG, EGC, and ECG may have the potential to lower the risk of prostate cancer in the human population. It has been shown that green tea polyphenols when given to a transgenic mouse model that mimics progressive forms of human prostate cancer exert remarkable preventive effects against prostate cancer development.[28] There are multiple targets for prostate cancer chemoprevention by green tea, and its catechins, highlighting the need for further studies to identify novel pathways that may be modulated by green tea catechins.[29]

Sugimura's group[30] was first to use a two-stage skin carcinogenesis mouse model to demonstrate that topical application of EGCG inhibited tumor promotion induced by teleocidin in DMBA-initiated mouse skin. EGCG inhibited the growth of established skin tumors induced chemically or by ultraviolet (UV) light.[31] Oral, subcutaneous, or intraperitoneal administration of EGCG or other green tea catechins in mice also resulted in significant suppression of the growth of implanted tumor cells.[32] Peroral administration of green tea infusion or EGCG inhibited lung metastasis in mouse melanoma and Lewis lung carcinoma cells.[33,34]

## 17.5 CHEMOPREVENTION OF HUMAN CANCER BY TEA DRINKING

This is the most important issue in the cancer chemoprevention of tea.

For years, the preventive effects of tea drinking on cancer development in humans have not been conclusive. Many epidemiologic studies in certain countries reported no significant association; in others, a positive association, and in still others, a negative association between tea consumption and cancer incidence were observed.[27,35] The discrepancy among these different epidemiologic studies on the association of tea drinking with cancer incidence may arise from their different study subjects and different questionnaire designs. It is worth noting that the frequency and quantity of tea drinking daily in a population might affect the outcome of cancer chemoprevention. There are many lifetime tea-drinkers in Asian countries such as China, Japan, Korea, and Taiwan. They drink tea every day, even every hour during the daytime! This may be one of the reasons that previous published studies from Asian populations gave definitively positive prevention effects of tea on cancer incidence.[36,37] It is necessary to point out that the tea polyphenols contents in bottled tea (on sale in most supermarkets) and freshly prepared hot tea (homemade) may be quite different in quality and quantity. It is well known that a part of tea polyphenols may be precipitated out and filtered away during the manufacturing of bottled tea.

A recent cohort study has shown that the slowdown in increase of cancer incidence with age observed among females who consumed more than 10 cups a day is consistent with the finding that increased consumption of green tea is associated with later onset of cancer.[38]

## 17.6 BIOCHEMICAL AND MOLECULAR MECHANISMS OF CANCER CHEMOPREVENTION BY CATECHINS

The development of genetic oncology has demonstrated that damage to numerous regulatory genes may result in induction of invasive and metastatic cancer. It has been established that the pathological processes of multistep carcinogenesis comprises initiation, promotion, and progression.[7] The natural history of carcinogenesis and cancer development provides a strong rationale for a preventive approach to the control of this disease and leads one to consider the possibility of active pharmacological intervention to arrest or reverse the processes of carcinogenesis before invasion and metastasis occur. The inhibitory effects of tea against carcinogenesis have been attributed to the biologic activities of the polyphenolic catechins in the tea. However, the biochemical and molecular mechanisms of cancer chemoprevention by tea catechins are not fully elucidated. Some of the recent developments in our laboratory and others are discussed in the following.

### 17.6.1 ANTIOXIDANT EFFECTS OF CATECHINS

Tea is particularly rich in polyphenols, including catechins, theaflavins, and thearubigins, which are thought to contribute to the health benefits of tea. Tea polyphenols act as antioxidants *in vitro* by scavenging reactive oxygen and nitrogen species and chelating redox-active transition metal ions. They may also function indirectly as antioxidants through inhibition of the redox sensitive transcription factors, NFκB, and AP-1; inhibition of pro-oxidant enzymes such as inducible nitric oxide synthase (iNOS), lipoxygenase, cyclooxygenase, and xanthine oxidase; and induction of phase II and antioxidant enzymes, such as glutathione *S*-transferases and superoxide dismutases. The fact that catechins are rapidly and extensively metabolized emphasizes the importance of demonstrating their antioxidant activity *in vivo*.[39]

Tea catechins show remarkable antioxidative effects in various systems. Tea catechins are strong scavengers against superoxide, hydrogen peroxide, hydroxyl radicals, nitric oxide, and peroxynitrite produced by various chemicals and biological systems. Chen and Ho[40] showed that the 1,1-diphenyl-2-picrylhydrazyl (DPPH) radical-scavenging ability of various tea polyphenols was proportional to the number of –OH groups in the catechins or theaflavins. Recent studies show that catechins in green tea are highly active in reducing the amount of oxidative damage sustained by DNA through hydroxyl radical (OH) attack. Catechins when compared with other classes of flavonoids are found to be very active in reducing the amount of strand breakage and residual base damage by a mechanism other than direct scavenging of hydroxyl radicals before they react with DNA.[41] Pulse radiolysis data support the mechanism of electron transfer (or H-transfer) from catechins to radical sites on DNA.[42] These results support an antioxidant role of catechins in their direct interaction with DNA radicals.

The inhibitory effects of tea polyphenols on xanthine oxidase (XO) were investigated.[43] Catechins and theaflavins inhibit XO to produce uric acid and also act as scavengers of superoxide. The antioxidative activity of tea catechins is due not only to their ability to scavenge superoxides, but also to their ability to block XO and related oxidative signal transducers.[43] It has been demonstrated that tea or tea catechins inhibit $Cu^{2+}$-mediated LDL oxidation *in vitro*[44] and induction of atherogenesis in mice.[39] To determine whether tea catechins act as effective antioxidants *in vivo*, future studies in animals and humans should employ sensitive and specific biomarkers of oxidative damage to DNA, proteins, and lipids.

## 17.6.2 PRO-OXIDANT EFFECTS OF CATECHINS

Biologically important ROS that can damage DNA and, thereby, alter gene expression in cell growth and differentiation include the hydroxyl radical, superoxide, peroxyradical, singlet oxygen, peroxynitrite, and hydrogen peroxide.[42] As oxidative DNA damage is considered to be a pathogenic event in the induction of many cancers,[45] a reduction in the rate of such damage by catechins acting as antioxidants may lead to a reduced risk of cancer.

On the contrary, recent studies have demonstrated the pro-oxidant effects of green tea catechins.[46,47] Green tea catechins enhanced colon carcinogenesis in rats.[48] Experiments using [32]P-labeled DNA fragments obtained from human cancer-related genes showed that catechins induced DNA damage in the presence of metals such as Cu(II) and Fe(III) complexes.[46] It is concluded that EGCG can induce hydrogen peroxide generation and subsequent damage to isolated and cellular DNA, and that oxidative DNA damage may mediate the potential carcinogenicity of EGCG.[46] EGCG (12.5 to 50 $\mu M$) decreased the viability of Jurkat cells and caused concomitant increase in cellular caspase 3 activity. Catalase and Fe(II) chelating reagent $O$-phenanthroline suppressed the EGCG effects, indicating involvements of both hydrogen peroxide and Fe(II) in the mechanism. Unexpectedly, ECG, which has Fe(III)-reducing potency comparable to EGCG, failed to decrease viability of Jurkat cells, while EGC, which has low capacity to reduce Fe(III), showed a cytotoxic effect similar to EGCG. These results suggest that a mechanism other than Fe(III) reduction plays a role in catechin-mediated Jurkat cell death. EGCG causes an elevation of hydrogen peroxide levels (a pro-oxidant effect) in Jurkat cell culture, in cell-free culture medium, and sodium phosphate buffer. Catechins with higher ability to produce hydrogen peroxide were more cytotoxic to Jurkat cells. Hydrogen peroxide itself exerted Fe(II)-dependent cytotoxicity. Among human and normal cell lines tested, cells exhibiting lower hydrogen peroxide-eliminating activity were more sensitive to EGCG. It is proposed that cytotoxicity of catechins in certain tumor cells is due to their ability to produce hydrogen peroxide and that the resulting increase in hydrogen peroxide levels triggers Fe(II)-dependent formation of highly toxic hydroxyl radicals, which in turn induces apoptosis in the target cells.[47]

### 17.6.3 INDUCTION OF APOPTOSIS AND CELL CYCLE ARREST

We have examined the apoptotic inducing effects of EGCG, theaflavins, and theasinensin A (from oolong tea) in the human cancer cell lines histolytic lymphoma U937 and acute T-cell leukemia Jurkat cells.[49] The action mechanisms of tea polyphenols induced apoptosis as determined by annexin V apoptosis assay; DNA fragmentation and caspase activation were further investigated. Loss of membrane potential and ROS generation were also detected by flow cytometry. Treatment with tea polyphenols caused rapid induction of caspase-3, but not caspase-1, activity and stimulated proteolytic cleavage of poly(ADP-ribose)-polymerase (PARP).[49]

Recent studies on apoptosis and cell cycle arrest in cancer cells by *in vivo* metabolites of teas have been described.[50] The tea extracts from green, oolong, and black teas were prepared. The rat sera obtained after oral intubation of the prepared tea extracts, and tea polyphenolic compounds EGCG, EGC, ECG, and theaflavins were used in the related tests. All these tea samples significantly inhibited the proliferation of a rat hepatoma cell line (AH 109A) and murine B16 melanoma cells, but not normal rat mesothelial (M) cells.

EGCG was found to inhibit the growth of the transformed W138VA cells, but not of their normal counterparts. A similar growth inhibitory effect of EGCG between human colorectal cancer (Caco-2) cells, breast cancer (Hs578T) cells, and their respective normal counterparts were observed.[51] EGCG treatment also induced apoptosis, and enhanced serum-induced expression of c-fos and c-myc genes in transformed W138VA cells, but not in the normal W138 cells. EGCG and other catechins inhibit growth of human lung cancer (PC-9) cells with a $G_2/M$ phase arrest of the cell cycle.[52]

### 17.6.4 INHIBITION OF CELLULAR PROLIFERATION AND TUMOR PROGRESSION THROUGH SUPPRESSING EGFR SIGNALING

Multiple data have demonstrated the pivotal role of mitogenic signal transduction in controlling the tumor proliferation.[3,35] The induction of ornithine decarboxylase (ODC), PKC, protein kinase activities, and oxidative stress by TPA is believed to be closely related to the tumor promotion activity of this compound.[7,53] Topical application of green tea catechins to mouse skin was found to inhibit TPA-caused induction of ODC activity in a dose-dependent manner.[54] Our studies have demonstrated that EGCG and theaflavins inhibited TPA-induced transformation, PKC activation, and AP-1 binding activities in mouse fibroblast cells.[55,56] We have investigated the effects of EGCG on the proliferation of human epidermoid cancer cell line A431.[9] EGCG strongly inhibited the DNA synthesis and protein tyrosine kinase activities of epidermal growth factor (EGF)-receptor, platelet derived growth factor (PDGF)-receptor, and fibroblast growth factor (FGF)-receptor. In an *in vivo* assay, EGCG could reduce the auto-phosphorylation level of EGF-receptor by EGF. EGCG inhibited the EGF-stimulated increase in phosphotyrosine level in A431 cells. EGCG also blocked EGF-binding to its receptor. These results suggested that the inhibition of proliferation and suppression of the EGF signaling by EGCG might mainly mediate dose-dependent blocking of ligand binding to its receptor, and subsequently through inhibition of EGF-receptor kinase activity and its signaling.[9]

### 17.6.5 INHIBITION OF iNOS THROUGH DOWNREGULATING NFκB ACTIVATION

Nitric oxide (NO) is a small bioactive molecule that plays an important role in inflammation and multistep carcinogenesis. We have investigated the effects of tea polyphenols on the induction of iNOS in thioglycolate-elicited and lipopolysaccharide (LPS)-activated peritoneal macrophage.[8,57] Gallic acid, EGC, EGCG, and theaflavins have found to inhibit nitrite production, iNOS protein, and mRNA in activated macrophages. Western blot, reverse transcriptase-polymerase chain reaction (RT-PCR), and Northern blot analyses demonstrated that significantly reduced 130-kDa protein and 4.5-kb mRNA levels of iNOS were expressed in LPS-activated macrophages with EGCG or theaflavins compared with those without tea polyphenols. Electrophoretic mobility shift assay (EMSA) indicated that EGCG blocked the activation of NFκB, a transcription factor necessary for iNOS induction.[8] EGCG and theaflavins also blocked the disappearance of inhibitor IκB from the cytosolic fraction.[57] These results suggest that EGCG and theaflavins decrease the activity and protein levels of iNOS by reducing the expression of iNOS mRNA and the reduction could occur through prevention of the binding of NFκB to the iNOS promoter, thereby inhibiting the induction of iNOS expression.[8]

### 17.6.6 INHIBITION OF TUMOR PROMOTION AND CELL TRANSFORMATION THROUGH SUPPRESSING AP-1 ACTIVATION

A number of studies have suggested that the activation of AP-1 plays an important role in tumor promotion; the downregulation of this transcription factor is now thought to be a general therapeutic strategy against cancer.[58,59] Dong et al.[60] investigated the anticancer-promoting effects of EGCG and theaflavins. Both were found to inhibit EGF- or TPA-induced cell transformation as well as AP-1-dependent transcriptional activity and DNA-binding activity. This study further showed that the inhibition of AP-1 activation occurs via the inhibition of a c-Jun NH$_2$-terminal kinase (JNK)-dependent pathway.[60] EGCG and theaflavins inhibited TPA-induced NFκB activity in a concentration-dependent manner. These tea polyphenols blocked TPA-induced phosphorylation of IκBα at Ser-32 in the same concentration range. These results suggest that inhibition of NFκB activation is also important in accounting for the antitumor promotion effects of EGCG and theaflavins.[56,57,61]

### 17.6.7 SUPPRESSION OF FATTY ACID SYNTHASE EXPRESSION BY CATECHINS AND THEAFLAVINS

Fatty acid synthase (FAS) is a key enzyme in lipogenesis. FAS is highly expressed in the proliferative normal tissues and malignant tumors, is overexpressed in the malignant human breast carcinoma MCF-7 cells, and its expression is further enhanced by EGF. The EGF-induced expression of FAS was inhibited by green and black tea extracts. The expression of FAS was also suppressed by the catechins and theaflavins at both protein and mRNA levels that may lead to the inhibition of cell lipogenesis and proliferation.[62] Both EGCG and theaflavin-3,3′-digallate inhibit the activation of AKt and block the binding of SP-1 to its target site at transcription promoter region. Furthermore, the EGF-induced biosynthesis of lipids and cell proliferation were significantly suppressed by EGCG and theaflavins.[9,60] These findings suggest that tea polyphenols suppress FAS expression by downregulating the EGF-receptor/PI3K/AKt/Sp-1 signal transduction pathway; and tea and tea polyphenols might induce hypolipidemic and antiproliferative effects by suppressing FAS.[62]

Several reports have demonstrated that EGCG is a natural inhibitor of FAS *in vitro*. EGCG is an inhibitor of FAS from chicken liver.[63] The marked inhibition of ketoacyl reduction shows that the inhibition is related to β-ketoacyl reductase of FAS. The observable protection of NADPH and competitive inhibition of NADPH for ketoacyl reduction indicate that EGCG may compete with NADPH for the same binding site.[63] The analogs of galloyl moiety without the catechin skeleton such as propyl gallate also showed obvious slow-binding inhibition, whereas the green tea ungallated catechin did not.

Atomic orbital energy analyses suggest that the positive charge is more distinctly distributed on the carbon atom of ester bond of galloyl moiety of gallate catechins, and that gallated forms are more susceptible for a nucleophilic attack than other catechins.[64] Thus, gallated catechins provide a nucleophilic target for the ketoacyl reductase of FAS that lead to the inhibition of the enzyme. EGCG also showed profound inhibition on the bacterial type II fatty acid synthase.[65] EGCG and the related tea catechins potently inhibit both the FabG and FabI reductase steps in the fatty acid elongation cycle with $IC_{50}$ values between 5 and 15 μM. The presence of the galloyl moiety was essential for activity.

Chemical inhibitors of FAS inhibit growth and induce apoptosis in several cancer cell lines *in vitro*[66] and in tumor xenografts *in vivo*.[67] EGCG inhibits FAS activity as efficiently as currently known synthetic inhibitors and selectively causes apoptosis in LNPaP cells but not in nontumoral fibroblasts. These findings establish EGCG as a potent natural inhibitor of FAS in intact cells and strengthen the molecular basis for the use of EGCG as a chemopreventive agent.[68]

### 17.6.8 Inhibition of Ubiquitin–Proteasome Pathway by Catechins

Many cell-cycle and cell-death regulators are identified as targets of the ubiquitin–proteasome-mediated degradation pathway. Proteasome inhibitors are able to induce tumor growth arrest, and tea consumption is correlated with cancer prevention.[1,29] It has been demonstrated that ester bond-containing tea polyphenols such as EGCG potently and specifically inhibit the chymotrypsin-like activity of the proteasome *in vitro* at concentrations that are found in the serum of green tea drinkers.[69] Atomic orbital energy analyses and high-performance liquid chromatography suggest that the carbon of the polyphenol ester bond is essential for targeting and thereby inhibiting the proteasome in cancer cells. This inhibition of the proteasome results in accumulation of two proteasome substrates p27/kip1 and IκBα, an inhibitor of NFκB, and this inhibition is followed by growth arrest in the $G_1$ phase of the cell cycle. Tea polyphenols without an ester bond were inactive in this capacity. It is estimated that 20S proteasome inhibition is achieved via acylation of the catalytic N-terminal threonine on the proteasome's β5 subunit, wherein the A ring of (–)-EGCG acts as a tyrosine mimic to bind the hydrophobic S1 pocket of β5, which is the location of the chymotrypsin active site.[69] Eight potential hydrogen bonds support docking of the complex. Synthetic (+)-EGCG was more potent to purified 20S proteasome than normal *cis*(–)-EGCG. Furthermore, compared with their simian virus-transformed counterparts, the parental normal human fibroblasts are much more resistant to EGCG-induced p27/kip1 protein accumulation and $G_1$ arrest.[69] This study suggests that proteasome is a cancer-related molecular target of tea polyphenols and that inhibition of proteasome activity by ester bond-containing polyphenols may contribute to the cancer chemopreventive effects of tea. It is interesting to note that the naturally occurring ester bond containing polyphenol pentagalloylglucose has been shown to be a strong inhibitor of 26S proteasome in our laboratory.[70]

## 17.7 DISCUSSION OF THE ACTION MECHANISMS OF CATECHINS

As described above, the action mechanisms of catechins are multiple pathways through multiple targets.[1,3,35] The new developments on the inhibition of catechins on the function of ubiquitin–proteasome pathways are critically interesting and deserve further discussion. The proteasome is an essential component of the ATP-dependent proteolytic pathway in the nucleus and cytoplasm of eukaryotic cells and is responsible for the degradation of most cellular proteins.[71] The 20S (700-kDa) proteasome contains multiple peptidase activities that function through a new type of proteolytic mechanism involving a threonine active site. The 26S (2000-kDa) complex, which degrades ubiquitinated proteins, contains in addition to the 20S proteasome, a 19S regulatory complex composed of multiple ATPases and components necessary for binding protein substrates.

Proteasomal degradation of proteins is critical for the regulation of cellular proteins and homeostasis such as progression of the cell cycle,[72] apoptosis,[73] oncogenesis, transcription, cell adhesion, migration, angiogenesis, and antigen presentation. Proteasome plays a central role in the regulation of proteins that control cell cycle progression and apoptosis and has therefore become an important target for anticancer therapy.[72] The central role of the proteasome in controlling the expression of regulators of cell proliferation and survival has led to interest in developing proteasome inhibitors as novel anticancer agents. *In vitro* and *in vivo* studies have shown that proteasome inhibitors have activity against a variety of tumor types.[74] It is encouraging to demonstrate that tea catechins have a profound inhibitory effect on the proteasome chymotryptic activity.[69] These findings have provided another molecular basis for the cancer chemopreventive effects of tea and tea polyphenols.

In summary, the cancer chemopreventive agents such as tea catechins can inhibit tumor growth and tumor promotion through arresting cell cycle and inducing cell apoptosis. During the past few years, experimental results from our laboratory and others have demonstrated that cancer chemoprevention by tea polyphenols can be achieved by signal transduction blockade.[3,35] Discovering novel therapeutics and chemopreventive agents with clinical utility continues to be the focus of biochemical and pharmacological scientists working in the signal transduction therapy. Recent developments in FAS inhibitors and inhibitors in ubiquitin–proteasome pathways have provided additional potential fields for further exploration.[66,67,75]

## ACKNOWLEDGMENTS

This study was supported by the National Science Council: NSC 93-2311-B-002-001, NSC 93-2320-B-002-111, and NSC 93-2320-B-002-127. The author takes this opportunity to express his sincere appreciation to his research associates Prof. S. Y. Lin-Shiau, Prof. Y. S. Ho, Prof. Y. C. Liang, Dr. Y. L. Lin, Dr. S. F. Lee, and others for their excellent collaboration, which made the completion of this chapter possible.

## REFERENCES

1. Moyers SB, Kumar N. Green tea polyphenols and cancer chemoprevention: multiple mechanisms and endpoints for phase II trials. *Nutr Rev* 2004; 62(5):204–211.
2. Wu AH, Yu MC, Tseng CC, Hankin J, Pike MC. Green tea and risk of breast cancer in Asian Americans. *Int J Cancer* 2003; 106: 574–579.
3. Lin JK, Liang YC, Lin-Shiau SY. Cancer chemoprevention by tea polyphenols through mitotic signal transduction blockade. *Biochem Pharmacol* 1999; 59: 911–915.
4. Kida K, Suzuki M, Matsumoto N, Nanjo F, Hara Y. Identification of biliary metabolites of (–)-epigallocatechin gallate in rats. *J Agric Food Chem* 200; 48: 4151–4155.

5. Yang CS, Wang ZY. Tea and cancer. *J Natl Cancer Inst* 1993: 85:1038–1049.
6. Dong Z, Ma WY, Huang C, Yang CS. Inhibition of tumor promoter-induced activator protein-1 activities and cell transformation by tea polyphenols EGCG and theaflavins. *Cancer Res* 1997; 57: 4444–4449.
7. Lin JK, Lee SF. Inhibition of tumor promotion through blocking signal transduction. *Zool Stud* 1995; 34: 67–81.
8. Lin YL, Lin JK. (–)-epigallocatechin 3-gallate blocks the induction of nitric oxide synthase by down-regulating lipopolysaccharide-induced activity of transcription factor nuclear factor-κB. *Mol Pharmacol* 1997; 52: 465–472.
9. Liang YC, Lin-Shiau SY, Chen CF, Lin JK. Suppression of extracellular signals and cell proliferation through EGF-receptor binding by (–)-epigallocatechin 3-gallate in human A431 epidermoid carcinoma cells. *J Cell Biochem* 1997; 67: 55–65.
10. Lu YP, Lou YR, Xie JG, Yen P, Huang MT, Conney AH. Inhibitory effect of black tea on the growth of established skin tumors in mice: effects on tumor size, apoptosis, mitosis and bromodeoxyuridine incorporation into DNA. *Carcinogenesis* 1997; 18: 2163–2169.
11. Morse MA, Kresty LA, Steele VE, Kelloff GJ, Boone CW, Balentine DA, Harbowy ME, Stoner GD. Effects of theaflavins on *N*-nitroso-methylbenzylamine- induced esophageal tumorigenesis. *Nutr Cancer* 1997; 29: 7–12.
12. Ho CT, Chang YL, Huang MT, (eds.). Phenolic compounds in food and their effects on health, I. *Analysis, Occurrence and Chemistry.* ACS Symposium Series 506. Washington, DC: American Chemical Society; 1992.
13. Lin JK, Tsai SH, Lin-Shiau SY. Anti-inflammatory and anti-tumor effects of flavonoids and flavanoids. *Drug Future* 2001; 26: 145–152.
14. Huang MT, Ho CT, Lee YL (eds.). Phenolic compounds in food and their effects on health, II. *Antioxidants & Cancer Chemoprevention.* ACS Symposium Series 507. Washington, DC: American Chemical Society; 1992.
15. Block GA. A role of anti-oxidants in reducing cancer risk. *Nutr Rev* 1992; 50: 207–213.
16. Hertog MGL, Feskens EJM, Holman PCH, Kalan MB, Kromhout D. Dietary antioxidants flavonoids and risk of coronary heart disease. The Eulphen Elderly Study. *Lancet* 1993; 342: 1007–1011.
17. Plumb GW, De Pascual-Teresa S. Santos-Buelga C, Cheynier V, Williamson G. Anti-oxidant properties of catechins and pro-anthocyanidins. *Free Radical Res* 1998; 29: 351–358.
18. Nanjo F, Goto K, Seto R. Scavenging effects of tea catechins and their derivatives on 1,1-diphenyl-2-picrylhydrazyl radical. *Free Radical Biol Med* 1996; 21: 895–902.
19. Kawase M, Wang R, Shiomi T, Saizo R, Yagi K. Anti-oxidative activity of (–)-epigallocatechin-3-(3″-O-methyl)-gallate isolated from fresh tea leaf and preliminary results on its biological activity. *Biosci Biotechnol Biochem* 2000; 64: 2218–2220.
20. Sano M, Suzuki M, Miyase T, Yoshino K, Maeda-Yamamoto M. Novel anti-allergic catechin derivatives isolated from oolong tea. *J Agric Food Chem* 2000; 47: 1906–1910.

21. Fujimura Y, Tachibana H, Maeda-Yamamoto M. Miyase T, Sano M, Yamada K. Anti-allergic tea catechin (–)-epigallocatechin-3-$O$-(3″-$O$-methyl)-gallate, suppresses FcεRI expression in human basophilic KU812 cells. *J Agric Food Chem* 2002; 50: 5729–5734.

22. Tachibana H, Sunada Y, Miyase T, Sano M, Maeda-Yamamoto M, Yamada K. Identification of a methylated tea catechin as an inhibitor of degranulation in human basophilic KU812 cells. *Biosci Biotechnol Biochem* 2000; 64: 452–454.

23. Chung JY, Hwang C, Meng X, Dong Z, Yang CS. Inhibition of activator protein 1 activity and cell growth by purified green tea and black tea polyphenols in H-ras transformed cells: structure–activity relationship and mechanisms involved. *Cancer Res* 1999; 59: 4610–4617.

24. Xu Y, Ho CT, Amin SG, Han C, Chung FL. Inhibition of tobacco-specific nitrosamine-induced lung tumorigenesis in A/J mice by green tea and its major polyphenol as anti-oxidant. *Cancer Res* 1992; 52: 3875–3879.

25. Yamane T, Hagiwara N, Taleishi M, Akuchi S, Rim M, Okuzumi J, Kitao Y, Inugake M, Kuwata K, Takahashi T. Inhibition of azomethane-induced colon carcinogenesis in rat by green tea polyphenol fraction. *Jpn J Cancer Res* 1991; 82: 1336–1339.

26. Lin JK. Mechanisms of cancer chemoprevention by phytochemicals and phytopolyphenols. *Food Sci Agric Chem* 2000; 2(4): 189–201.

27. Lin JK, Liang YC. Cancer chemoprevention by tea polyphenols. *Proc Natl Sci Council ROC (B)* 2000; 24: 1–13.

28. Saleem M, Adhami VM, Siddiqui IA, Mukhtar H. Tea beverage in chemoprevention of prostate cancer: a minireview. *Nutr Cancer* 2003; 47(1): 13–23.

29. Adhmi VM, Ahmad N, Mukhtar H. Molecular targets for green tea in prostate cancer prevention. *J Nutr* 2003; 133: 2417s–2424s.

30. Yoshizawa S, Horiuchi T, Sugimura T. Antitumor promoting activity of (–)-epigallocatechin-3-gallate the main constituted of "tannin" in green tea. *Phytother Res* 1987; 1: 44–47.

31. Wang ZY, Huang MT, Ferraro T, Wong Q, Lou TR, Reubl R, Yang CS, Conney AH. Inhibitory effect of green tea in the drinking water on tumorigenesis by ultraviolet light and 12-$O$-tetradecanoylphorbol-13-acetate in the skin of SKH-1 mice. *Cancer Res* 1992; 52: 1162–1170.

32. Oguni I, Naus K, Yamamoto S, Nomura T. On the antitumor activity of fresh green tea leaf. *Agric Biol Chem* 1988; 52: 1879–1880.

33. Taniguchi S, Fujiki H, Kobayshi H, Go H, Miyado K, Sadano H, Shimokawa R. Effect of (–)-epigallocatechin gallate, the main constituent of green tea, on lung metastasis with mouse B16 melanoma cell lines. *Cancer Lett* 1992; 65: 51–54.

34. Sazuka M, Murakami S, Iseumura M, Satoh K, Nukiwa T. Inhibitory effects of green tea infusion on *in vitro* invasion and *in vivo* metastasis of mouse lung carcinoma cells. *Cancer Lett* 1995; 98: 27–31.

35. Lin JK. Cancer chemoprevention by tea polyphenols through modulating signal transduction pathways. *Arch Pharm Res* 2002; 25(5): 561–571.

36. Gao YT, McLaughlin JK, Blot WJ, Ji BT, Dai Q, Fraumeni JF Jr. Reduced risk of esophageal cancer associated with green tea consumption. *J Natl Cancer Inst* 1994; 86: 855–858.

37. Nakachi K, Matsuyama S, Miyake S, Suganuma M, Imai K. Protective effects of drinking green tea on cancer and cardiovascular disease: epidemiological evidence for multiple targeting prevention. *BioFactors* 2000; 13: 49–54.

38. Imai K, Suga K, Nakachi K. Cancer preventive effects of drinking green tea among Japanese population. *Prev Med* 1997; 26: 769–775.
39. Frei B, Higdon JV. Anti-oxidant activity of tea polyphenols *in vivo*: evidence from animal studies. *J Nutr* 2003; 133: 3275s–3284s.
40. Chen CW, Ho CT. Anti-oxidant properties of polyphenols extracted from green and black teas. *J Food Lipid* 1994; 2: 35–46.
41. Anderson RF, Amarasinghe C, Fisher LJ, Mak WB, Packer JE. Reduction in free-radicals induced DNA strand breaks and base damage through fast chemical repair by flavonoids. *Free Radical Res* 2000; 33: 91–103.
42. Anderson RF, Fisher LJ, Hara Y, Harris T, Mak WB, Melton LD, Packer JE. Green tea catechins partially protect DNA from hydroxyl radical-induced strand breaks and base damage through fast chemical repair of DNA radicals. *Carcinogenesis* 2001; 22(8): 1189–1193.
43. Lin JK, Chen PC, Ho CT, Lin-Shiau SY. Inhibition of xanthine oxidase and suppression of intracellular reactive oxygen species in HL-60 cells by theaflavin-3,3′-digallate, (–)-epigallocatechin-3-gallate and propyl gallate. *J Agric Food Chem* 2000; 48: 2736–2743.
44. Leung LK, Su Y, Chen R, Zhang Z, Huang Y, Chen ZY. Theaflavins in black tea and catechins in green tea are equally effective anti-oxidants. *J Nutr* 2001; 131: 2248–2251.
45. Ames B, Gold LS. Endogenous mutagens and the causes of aging and cancer. *Mutat Res* 1991; 250: 3–16.
46. Furukawa A, Okawa S, Murata M, Hiraka Y, Kawanishi S. (–)-Epigallocatechin gallate causes oxidative damage to isolated and cellular DNA. *Biochem Pharmacol* 2003; 66: 1769–1778.
47. Nakagawa H, Hasumi K, Woo JT, Nagai K, Wachi M. Generation of hydrogen peroxide primarily contributes to the induction of Fe(II)-dependent apoptosis in Jurkat cells by (–)-epigallocatechin gallate. *Carcinogenesis* 2004; 25(9): 1567–1574.
48. Hirose M, Hoshiya T, Mizoguchi Y, Nakamura A, Akagi K, Shirai T. Green tea catechins-enhance tumor development in the colon without effect in the lung or thyroid after pretreatment with 1,2-dimethylhydrazine or 2,2-dihydroxy-di-*n*-propylnitrosamine in male F344 rats. *Cancer Lett* 2001; 168: 23–29.
49. Pan MH, Liang YC. Lin-Shiau SY, Zhu NQ, Ho CT, Lin JK. Induction of apoptosis by the oolong tea polyphenol theasinensin A through cytochrome c release and activation of caspase-9 and caspase-3 in human U-937 cells. *J Agric Food Chem* 2000; 48: 6337–6346.
50. Zhang G, Miura Y, Yagasaki K. Induction of apoptosis and cell cycle arrest in cancer cells *in vivo* metabolites of teas. *Nutr Cancer* 2000; 38(2): 265–273.
51. Chen ZP, Schell JB, Ho CT, Chen KY. Green tea epigallocatechin gallate shows a pronounced growth inhibitory effect on cancerous cells but not on their normal counterparts. *Cancer Lett* 1978; 129: 173–179.
52. Fujiki H, Suganuma M, Okabe M, Sueoka N, Komori A. Cancer inhibition by green tea. *Mutat Res* 1998; 402: 307–310.
53. Balmain A, Brown K. Oncogene activation and chemical carcinogenesis. *Adv Cancer Res* 1988; 51: 147–182.

54. Agarwal R, Katiyar SK, Zaidi S, Mukhtar H. Induction of tumor promoter-caused induction of ornithine decarboxylase activity in Sencar mice by phenolic fraction isolated from green tea and its individual epicatechin derivatives. *Cancer Res* 1992; 52: 3582–3588.

55. Lee SF, Lin JK. Inhibitory effects of phytopolyphenols on TPA-induced transformation, PKC activation and c-jun expression in mouse fibroblast cells. *Nutr Cancer* 1997; 28: 177–183.

56. Chen YC, Liang YC, Lin-Shiau SY, Ho CT, Lin JK. Inhibition of TPA-induced PKC and AP-1 binding activities by the theaflavin-3,3′-digallate from black tea in NIH3T3 cells. *J Agric Food Chem* 1999; 47: 1416–1421.

57. Lin YL, Tsai SH, Lin-Shiau SY, Ho CT, Lin JK. Theaflavin-3,3′-digallate from black tea blocks the nitric oxide synthase by down-regulating the activation of NFκB in macrophages. *Eur J Pharmacol* 1999; 367: 379–388.

58. Huang TS, Lee SC, Lin JK. Suppression of c-jun/AP-1 activation by an inhibitor of tumor promotion in mouse fibroblast cells. *Proc Natl Acad Sci USA* 1991; 88: 5292–5296.

59. McCarty MF. Polyphenol-mediated inhibition of AP-1 transactivating activity may slow cancer growth by impeding angiogenesis and tumor invasiveness. *Med Hypothesis* 1998; 50: 511–514.

60. Dong Z, Ma WY, Huang C, Yang CS. Inhibition of tumor promoter-induced activator protein 1 activation and cell transformation by tea polyphenols EGCG and theaflavins. *Cancer Res* 1997; 57: 4414–4419.

61. Nomura M, Ma WY, Chen N, Bode AM, Dong Z. Inhibition of 12-*O*-tetradecanoyl- phorbol-13-acetate-induced NFκB activation by tea polyphenols EGCG and theaflavins. *Carcinogenesis* 2000; 21(10): 1855–1890.

62. Yeh CW, Chen WJ, Chiang CT, Lin-Shiau SY, Lin JK. Suppression of fatty acid synthase in MCF-7 breast cancer cells by tea and tea polyphenols: a possible mechanism for their hypolipidemic effects. *Pharmocogenomics J* 2003; 3: 267–276.

63. Wang X, Tian WX. Green tea epigallocatechin gallate: a natural inhibitor of fatty acid synthase. *Biochem Biophys Res Commun* 2001; 288: 1200–1206.

64. Wang X, Song KS, Guo QX, Tian WX. The galloyl moiety of green tea catechins is the critical structural feature to inhibit fatty acid synthase. *Biochem Pharmacol* 2003; 66: 2039–2047.

65. Zhang YM, Rock CO. Evaluation of epigallocatechin gallate and related plant polyphenols as inhibitors of the FabG and FabI reductases of bacterial type II fatty acid synthase. *J Biol Chem* 2004; 279(30): 30994–31001.

66. Kuhajda FP, Pizer ES, Li JN, Man NS, Frehywot GL, Townsend CA. Synthesis and anti-tumor activity of an inhibitor of fatty acid synthase. *Proc Natl Acad Sci USA* 2000; 97: 3450–3454.

67. Pizer ES, Thupari J, Han WF, Pinn ML, Chrest FJ, Frehywort GL, Townsend CA, Kuhajda FP. Malonyl-coenzyme A is a potential mediator of cytotoxicity induced by fatty acid synthase inhibition in human breast cancer cells and xenografts. *Cancer Res* 2000; 60: 213–218.

68. Brusselmans K, De Schriver E, Heyns W, Verhoeven G, Swinnen JV. Epigallocatechin-3-gallate is a potent natural inhibitor of fatty acid synthase in intact cells and effectively induces apoptosis in prostate cancer cells. *Int J Cancer* 2003; 106: 856–862.

69. Nam S, Smith DM, Dou QP. Ester bond-containing tea polyphenols potently inhibit proteasome activity *in vitro* and *in vivo*. *J Biol Chem* 2001; 276: 13322–13330.

70. Chen WJ, Lin JK. Induction of G1 arrest and apoptosis in human Jurkat T cells by pentagalloylglucose through inhibiting proteasome activity and elevating p27/kipl, p21/Cip1/WAF1 and Bax proteins. *J Biol Chem* 2004; 279(14): 13496–13505.

71. Coux O, Tanaka K, Goldberg AL. Structure and functions of the 20S and 26S proteasomes. *Annu Rev Biochem* 1996; 65: 801–847.

72. Adams J. The proteasome: structure, function and role in the cell. *Cancer Treatment Rev* 2003; 27(Suppl. 1): 3–9.

73. Naujokat C, Hoffmann S. Role and function of the 26S proteasome in proliferation and apoptosis. *Lab Invest* 2002; 82(8): 965–980.

74. Adams J. Proteasome inhibition: a novel approach to cancer therapy. *Trends Mol Med* 2002; 8(4 Suppl 1): S49–S54.

75. Kisselev AF, Goldberg AL. Proteasome inhibitors: from research tools to drug candidates. *Chem Biol* 2001; 8:739–758.

# 18 Cancer Chemoprotective Activity of Stilbenes: Resveratrol

*Catherine A. O'Brian, Jubilee R. Stewart, and Feng Chu*

## CONTENTS

Abstract ..................................................................................................................369
18.1 Nutritional Sources of Resveratrol.....................................................370
18.2 The Resveratrol–Cancer Prevention Connection: Where It Began ......370
18.3 Intrinsic Antioxidant Activity of Resveratrol.....................................371
18.4 Effects of Resveratrol on the Cell Cycle Machinery..........................372
18.5 Resveratrol-Induced Cancer Cell Apoptosis .......................................373
18.6 NF-κB Survival Pathway Suppression by Resveratrol........................374
18.7 Effects of Resveratrol on Cyclooxygenase Activity and Expression ...375
18.8 Modulation of Estrogen-Dependent Gene Regulation by Resveratrol...376
18.9 Inhibition of Protein Kinase C (PKC) Isozymes by Resveratrol ........376
18.10 Cancer Prevention by Resveratrol *in Vivo*............................................377
Acknowledgments .................................................................................................379
References ..............................................................................................................379

### ABSTRACT

*trans*-3,5,4′-Trihydroxystilbene, commonly referred to as resveratrol, has attracted great attention as a cancer preventive nutritional substance. Grapes, red wine, and peanuts are rich in resveratrol and resveratrol glucosides. Resveratrol potently activates sirtuins, $NAD^+$-dependent deacetylases implicated in the lifespan-extending effects of caloric restriction. Resveratrol has been shown to induce $G_1$- or S-phase arrest of more than a dozen unrelated cancer cell lines. WAF1/p21 induction accompanied both $G_1$ arrest in cultured cells and resveratrol amelioration of ultraviolet B-induced damage to mouse skin, and was p53-independent in some instances. Resveratrol-induced $G_1$ arrest sensitizes cancer cells but not normal cells to apoptosis by TRAIL, in association with survivin down-regulation. Resveratrol also downregulated survivin in ultraviolet B-damaged mouse skin. Resveratrol induces apoptosis of diverse leukemia and epithelial cancer cell lines by (1) p53-dependent, JNK-dependent and (2) Fas/Fas-ligand-independent, FADD-dependent mechanisms, and it suppresses the NF-κB sur-vival pathway. Studies in human breast and endometrial cancer cell lines have shown that resveratrol is a phytoestrogen with mixed estrogen-receptor ago-nist/antagonist activity, suggesting some potential for increased cancer risk. Enthusiasm for translation to chemopreventive intervention in humans is also tempered by the concern that resveratrol bioavailability in humans may be insuf-ficient to effect chemoprotection achieved in several rodent models of carcino-genesis. A study in human volunteers established that a 25-mg oral dose of [$^{14}$C] resveratrol was absorbed >70%, but rapidly metabolized to sulfates and glucu-ronic conjugates. Efforts are under way by a team led by G.R. Pettit to develop new resveratrol analogs for use as antineoplastic drugs in humans.

## 18.1   NUTRITIONAL SOURCES OF RESVERATROL

*trans*-Resveratrol (3,5,4'-trihydroxystilbene), commonly referred to as resvera-trol, has attracted great attention in recent years as a cancer preventive and cardioprotective nutritional substance. Resveratrol is a phytoalexin produced in some plants, such as grapevines, in response to fungal infection, ultraviolet light, and other types of stress, e.g., mechanical. Commercial food sources rich in resveratrol and closely related, bioactive forms of the stilbene, e.g., the *cis* isomer of resveratrol and the glucoside of resveratrol known as piceid, include grapes, red wine, and peanuts.[1,2] Because the stilbene content of grapes is primarily in the grape skin, white wines have low amounts of resveratrol compared to red.[1] Surveys of the resveratrol content of these food sources have indicated ranges of 0.02 to 1.79 μg resveratrol/g in peanuts, 0.6 to 6.8 μg/ ml in French red wines, and 0 to 2.1 μg/ml in various white wines.[1,2] Glucosides of resveratrol are on average several-fold more abundant than resveratrol in red wine, indicating the importance of also measuring glucosides when evaluating the resveratrol content of food products.[1]

## 18.2   THE RESVERATROL–CANCER PREVENTION CONNECTION: WHERE IT BEGAN

Neoplastic disease development is characterized by three distinct stages: tumor initiation, promotion, and progression. In 1997, Pezzuto's group[3] reported in *Science* that resveratrol antagonizes each stage of carcinogenesis, based on an analysis of the stilbene in an array of *in vitro* and *in vivo* bioassays, including the mouse-skin model of chemical carcinogenesis. At the time this chapter was written, a PubMed search of "resveratrol and cancer" yielded 337 reports, with the Pezzuto report[3] the first chronologically, indicating the excitement generated in the field by the seminal report. Cancer is often a disease related to aging, and recent reports identify resveratrol as potentially protective against aging-related pathological conditions through its capacity to activate Sir2-like proteins (sirtuins). Sirtuins are $NAD^+$-dependent deacetylases implicated in the lifespan-extending effects of caloric restriction in yeast, nematodes, flies, and mammals.[4–6] Resveratrol potently stimulates sirtuins expressed across the spectrum of these organisms. Resveratrol extends the lifespan of yeast up to 70% by mimicry of calorie restriction through sirtuin activation.[4] Resveratrol also extends nematode (*Caenorhabditis elegans*) and fly (*Drosophila*) lifespans without reducing fecundity in a sirtuin-dependent manner.[5] In mice, sirtuin activation by either resveratrol or caloric restriction induces a fat mobilization response that has the effect of reducing body fat. Because reduced body fat is implicated in the lifespan-extending effects of caloric restriction in mammals, this suggests that resveratrol may protect against aging-related pathological changes such as neoplastic development in humans.[6]

## 18.3 INTRINSIC ANTIOXIDANT ACTIVITY OF RESVERATROL

Potent antioxidant activity of resveratrol observed in eukaryotic cells and *in vivo* models involves effects of resveratrol on particular redox-regulatory targets, such as the cyclooxygenases COX-1 and COX-2 (discussed in Section 18.7) and the intrinsic antioxidant activity of the polyphenol. Illustrative of the antioxidant action of resveratrol in cells, the stilbene potently suppresses the production of superoxide anion, hypochlorous acid, and nitric oxide in isolated human neutrophils.[7] The contribution of the intrinsic antioxidant activity of resveratrol to its suppression of reactive oxygen species (ROS) in cells has been inferred from the ability of the polyphenol to scavenge superoxide anion produced by the xanthine/xanthine oxidase system and hydroxyl radical, whether produced by the Fenton reaction ($Fe^{2+} + H_2O_2 \rightarrow Fe^{3+} + \cdot OH + OH^-$) or by the transition metal Cr(VI) in the presence of NADPH and glutathione reductase.[8] Resveratrol is a potent ROS scavenger in each of these systems. Reaction rate measurements establish resveratrol as comparable in potency to the antioxidants ascorbate and glutathione in scavenging hydroxyl radical.[8] Like other polyphenols, resveratrol can exhibit either pro-oxidant or antioxidant activity under artificial conditions. A concern that resveratrol could have pro-oxidant effects detrimental to health was raised by the observation that resveratrol actually promoted hydroxyl radical formation in the presence of Cu(II) and plasmid DNA, suggestive of potential mutagenic activity. This concern was put to rest by establishing that resveratrol switches from pro-oxidant to antioxidant activity when either ascorbate or glutathione is introduced in this system at physiologically relevant concentrations.[9] Still, the caveat remains that resveratrol could exert detrimental, pro-oxidant effects under aberrant pathophysiological conditions.

## 18.4 EFFECTS OF RESVERATROL ON THE CELL CYCLE MACHINERY

Resveratrol has been reported to induce growth arrest of more than a dozen diverse cancer cell lines, with arrest primarily in the $G_1$[10–12] or S phase of the cell cycle.[13,14] Growth arrest may involve direct inhibitory effects of resveratrol against ribonucleotide reductase ($IC_{50} = 100$ $\mu M$),[15] which is vital to DNA synthesis owing to its catalysis of the reduction of ribonucleotides to deoxyribonucleotides, and resveratrol suppression of ornithine decarboxylase (ODC) induction, evidently through attenuation of myc expression.[16] Resveratrol has profound effects on the cell cycle machinery. Resveratrol induction of the cyclin kinase inhibitor (CKI) WAF1/p21 accompanied the $G_1$ arrest response to the polyphenol in cultured cells[10–12] and was also associated with resveratrol amelioration of ultraviolet B-induced damage to mouse skin.[17] Studies with p53-null cells indicate that, in at least some cases, resveratrol induces $G_1$ arrest and WAF1/p21 expression in a p53-independent manner,[12] while retinoblastoma (pRb) hypophosphorylation was implicated in resveratrol-induced WAF/p21 upregulation in studies with human A431 epidermoid carcinoma cells.[11] Complete loss of the $G_1$ arrest response to resveratrol in p21-deficient colon carcinoma cells established WAF1/p21 as crucial to the response.[12] Resveratrol arrest of A431 cell growth and suppression of ultraviolet B-induced mouse skin damage were associated with loss of cyclin-dependent kinases (CDKs) and cyclins that operate in the $G_1$ phase of the cell cycle.[10,17] Highly significant from the perspective of cancer prevention, resveratrol-induced $G_1$ arrest sensitized cancer cells but not normal cells to apoptosis by tumor necrosis factor-related apoptosis-inducing ligand (TRAIL), an inducer of cancer cell apoptosis that leaves normal tissues unharmed; apoptosis potentiation by resveratrol required WAF1/p21, was p53-independent, and was accompanied by downregulation of the inhibitor of apoptosis protein (IAP), survivin.[12] The significance of resveratrol-mediated survivin downregulation to cancer prevention is also suggested by observations that survivin upregulation in preneoplastic, ultraviolet B-damaged mouse skin is abrogated by resveratrol, while the apoptotic response of the damaged tissue to ultraviolet B radiation is increased by the polyphenol, suggesting surveillance against cancer through clearance of damaged cells.[18]

Resveratrol-induced arrest of cell growth in S phase was associated with decreased expression of the $G_1$-phase protein cyclin D1 and the $G_2$-phase protein cyclin B1 in several diverse cancer cell lines, suggesting loss of these proteins as possible surrogate markers of resveratrol sensitivity.[14] Furthermore, resveratrol-induced S phase arrest was accompanied by apoptosis induction and survivin downregulation.[13,14] In summary, the efficacy of resveratrol in arresting cancer cell growth by interference with the cell cycle machinery and ancillary pathways, together with the association of this response with survivin downregulation and apoptosis induction, suggests the potential for implementation of resveratrol or related stilbenes in cancer preventive surveillance and destruction of cancer cells without harm to normal tissues.

## 18.5 RESVERATROL-INDUCED CANCER CELL APOPTOSIS

Resveratrol induces apoptosis of diverse leukemia and epithelial cancer cell lines. Leukemia cells subject to resveratrol-induced apoptosis include early myeloid (K562, KCL22, HL60), monocytic (U937, THP1), B-lymphoid (WSU-CLL), and T-lymphoid (Jurkat).[14,19,20] Human carcinoma cell lines that apoptose in response to resveratrol span human breast cancer (MCF-7), prostate cancer (LNCaP, DU145), colorectal cancer (SW480), pancreatic cancer (PANC-1, AsPC-1), and esophageal cancer (Bic-1, Seg-1, HCE7).[14,21–25]

Resveratrol induces apoptosis of MCF-7 cells by a p53-dependent mechanism. Induction of MCF-7 cell apoptosis by resveratrol was accompanied by induction of p53 phosphorylation and acetylation, post-translational modifications implicated in stabilization of p53 and consequent increased p53 abundance. Pifithrin-$\alpha$, a selective p53 inhibitor, blocked resveratrol-induced p53 post-translational modification and apoptosis of the MCF-7 cells.[24] MCF-7 cells express wild-type p53.[26] Resveratrol also induces p53-dependent apoptosis of DU145 cells, which harbor a mutated form of p53. Resveratrol-induced DU145 cell apoptosis was blocked by pifithrin-$\alpha$, as were resveratrol-induced p53 phosphorylation at serine-15, p53 accumulation, and p53 transcriptional activity in the prostate cancer cells.[22] Activation of the Jun-NH2 kinase (JNK) pathway, which is triggered by various forms of stress, has been shown to stabilize p53, enhance p53 transcriptional activity, and potentiate p53-dependent apoptosis.[27] Resveratrol potently induced JNK activation in mouse epidermal JB6 cells, and resveratrol-induced p53-dependent apoptosis was attenuated in JB6 cells transfected with dominant-negative JNK1 and in JNK1–/– and JNK2–/– mouse embryo fibroblasts.[28]

An analysis of resveratrol-induced apoptosis of seven human leukemia cell lines (K562, KCL22, HL60, U937, THP1, WSU-CLL, and Jurkat) determined that Fas/Fas-ligand (FasL) did not contribute to the apoptotic responses of the cells, and that resveratrol induced caspase activity in each case. Interestingly, Z-VAD-FMK, a nondiscriminating inhibitor of caspases, did not increase the survival of resveratrol-treated K562 cells unless administered with the promiscuous protease-inhibitor leupeptin, which was also ineffective alone.[20] A study focused on resveratrol-induced apoptosis of U937 cells found that apoptosis was associated with caspase-3 activation and was blocked by Z-VAD-FMK as well as by enforced Bcl-2 expression. Resveratrol-induced apoptosis was associated with loss of the IAPs cIAP1 and cIAP2, but XIAP and survivin levels were unchanged.[19] A safety concern noted in Ferry-Dumazet et al.[20] is that, although resveratrol did not affect resting normal human peripheral blood lymphocytes (PBL), PHA-activated normal PBL were more sensitive to resveratrol-induced growth suppression/apoptosis than several leukemia cell lines.

A detailed analysis of resveratrol-induced apoptosis in human colon cancer SW480 cells revealed that resveratrol activates the death-receptor apoptosis pathway Fas/FasL by recruiting the death-receptor Fas to cluster and enter the death-inducing signaling complex (DISC) with the adaptor molecule FADD (Fas-associating protein with death domain) and caspase-8; interestingly, resveratrol-induced SW480 apoptosis was unaffected by an antagonistic Fas Ab and by ligand sequestration by FasL Ab, but was abrogated by dominant-negative FADD.[23] While the focus of this chapter is cancer prevention, there is growing interest in the use of resveratrol and other cancer-preventive phytochemicals in cancer therapy. Remarkably, the action of resveratrol in SW480 cells bears some resemblance to apoptosis induction by the highly effective cancer therapeutic taxol, which triggers leukemia cell apoptosis primarily through caspase-10 activation by a death receptor-independent, FADD-dependent mechanism.[29]

## 18.6  NF-κB SURVIVAL PATHWAY SUPPRESSION BY RESVERATROL

The transcription-factor NF-κB (nuclear factor-κB) induces the expression of key survival genes, e.g., Bcl-XL, XIAP, and cFLIP, pro-inflammatory cytokines, e.g., interleukin-1 (IL-1) and tumor necrosis factor (TNF), and other genes involved in cell proliferation, e.g., cyclin D1.[30] Based on its pro-inflammatory, anti-apoptotic, and oncogenic activity, NF-κB is viewed as an important target in cancer prevention and therapy.[30] NF-κB is sequestered in the cytoplasm in an inactive state as a complex with the inhibitory protein IκBα. NF-κB activation entails IκBα phosphorylation by the kinase complex IKK. This triggers ubiquitination and proteasomal degradation of IκBα, thus liberating NF-κB to translocate to the nucleus and activate expression of target genes. A study in human monocyte THP-1 cells revealed that resveratrol potently suppresses NF-κB-dependent gene expression, whether induced by TNF or LPS (lipopolysaccharide) by targeting the NF-κB pathway at a point upstream of IKK. This was demonstrated by showing that resveratrol inhibition of TNF-induced NF-κB activation was associated with suppression of IKK activation, IκBα phosphorylation, and IκBα degradation. IKK was ruled out as the direct target by showing that resveratrol had no effect on the activity of the isolated kinase complex, with the implication that the resveratrol target was upstream of IKK in the NF-κB pathway.[31]

A number of NF-κB-inducible genes correspond to gene products that induce NF-κB activation, forming a positive feedback loop, e.g., TNF and IL-1β. IL-1β is a critical cytokine in the proliferation of acute myeloid leukemia (AML) cells. Estrov et al.[32] have established that resveratrol suppresses IL-1β-induced NF-κB activation in the AML cell line OCIM2 and concomitantly attenuates production of the IL-1β protein by the cells. The significance of these findings to cancer prevention is strongly suggested by the analysis of clinical AML specimens in the report. Resveratrol inhibited the colony-forming growth of freshly isolated AML blast colony-forming cells in a concentration-dependent manner, and colony formation was partially rescued by exogenous IL-1β.[32]

## 18.7 EFFECTS OF RESVERATROL ON CYCLOOXYGENASE ACTIVITY AND EXPRESSION

Cyclooxygenases catalyze the formation of prostaglandins from arachidonic acid. COX-1 is expressed constitutively as a housekeeping gene in most normal tissues, while COX-2 expression is induced by pro-inflammatory and other mitogenic signals. Aberrant COX-2 upregulation is a common feature of cancer cells and potentially preneoplastic conditions such as tissue inflammation. COX-2 has been causally linked to epithelial tumorigenesis and is under investigation as a target for cancer prevention and therapy (reviewed in Reference 33). COX-catalyzed conversion of arachidonic acid to prostaglandin involves two sequential reactions at spatially distinct active sites, i.e., a cyclooxygenase reaction followed by a hydroperoxidase reaction. In assessing resveratrol as a cancer preventive agent, the Pezzuto team reported that resveratrol inhibited the cyclooxygenase and hydroperoxidase activities of COX-1 but exhibited much weaker effects against COX-2 activity.[3] More recently, a detailed mechanistic analysis established that resveratrol is a mechanism-based inactivator of COX-1 peroxidase catalysis. Resveratrol was oxidized at the peroxidase active site in a manner dependent on the presence of the substrate hydrogen peroxide, with concomitant inactivation of COX-1 peroxidase and cyclooxygenase activities. The authors hypothesized that inactivation entailed generation of resveratrol and protein radical species. COX-2 was more efficient than COX-1 in catalyzing peroxide-dependent resveratrol oxidation but was not inactivated by the polyphenol.[34] Interestingly, COX-1 inactivation by resveratrol is distinct from classical nonsteroidal anti-inflammatory drug (NSAID) action, in that classical NSAIDs target the cyclooxygenase active site of COX isoforms.

While resveratrol potently inhibits COX-1 but not COX-2, it suppresses the expression of COX-2 but not COX-1. This is illustrated by the results of a study employing an experimental model of ulcerative colitis, which is a nonspecific inflammatory disorder of the colonic mucosa and submucosa. The model involves intracolonic administration of trinitrobenzenesulfonic acid (TNBS) in rats, thus effecting colonic inflammation and injury. Resveratrol attenuated TNBS-induced colonic inflammation and injury, and this was associated with suppression of TNBS-induced COX-2 expression and no change in COX-1 expression in the colonic epithelial cells.[35] Similarly, the chemoprotective effects of resveratrol on ultraviolet B-damaged mouse skin were associated with attenuated COX-2 expression.[18] Consistent with these *in vivo* models, resveratrol has been shown to inhibit TGFα-stimulated and basal human COX-2 promoter activity in a reporter gene assay in human colon cancer DLD-1 cells.[36] In summary, studies of resveratrol effects on COX-1 and COX-2 indicate that COX-1 inhibition may reinforce the anti-inflammatory effects of COX-2 suppression by resveratrol, suggesting COX isoforms as important targets in the cancer preventive action of stilbenes.

## 18.8  MODULATION OF ESTROGEN-DEPENDENT GENE REGULATION BY RESVERATROL

The structural similarity between resveratrol and the synthetic estrogen diethyl-stilbestrol provided the first clue that resveratrol may function as a phytoestrogen. Estrogen-receptor (ER) agonists bind to the receptor and induce ER binding to estrogen response elements (EREs) in the promoters of target genes with the effect of promoter activation. Phytoestrogens are dietary nonsteroidal agents with ER agonist or mixed ER agonist/antagonist activity. In the first definitive analysis of resveratrol effects on the transcriptional activity of the ER, Jameson's group[37] established that resveratrol competitively bound ER expressed by MCF7 cells, and activated an ERE-containing promoter-reporter gene construct in MCF7 cells but not a derived construct with the ERE deleted. Furthermore, resveratrol-induced activation of the ERE-containing promoter was abrogated by the pure antiestrogen ICI 182780, indicating that transcriptional activation entailed resveratrol binding to the ER and thus identifying resveratrol as a phytoestrogen.[37] Studies in a human endometrial cancer cell line, Ishikawa cells, established that resveratrol can also function as an ER antagonist. Resveratrol antagonized estrogen-induced expression of the endogenous genes alkaline phosphatase and progesterone receptor, and the polyphenol also antagonized estrogen-induced activation of an ERE-containing promoter-reporter construct. Furthermore, resveratrol showed no ER agonist activity in these experiments when tested in the absence of estrogen.[38] Collectively, the studies in MCF7 and Ishikawa cells established resveratrol as a mixed ER agonist/antagonist. Recently, an analysis of ER-negative human breast cancer MDA-MB-231 cells stably transfected with human ER$\alpha$ established that resveratrol acts as an ER$\alpha$ agonist in the cells to induce expression of an endogenous ER target gene, transforming growth factor-$\alpha$ (TGF$\alpha$). Resveratrol induction of the TGF$\alpha$ gene was blocked by the pure antiestrogen ICI 182780, and resveratrol did not antagonize TGF$\alpha$ induction by estrogen.[39] While phytoestrogens are widely viewed as healthful and cardioprotective, the mixed ER agonist/antagonist activity of resveratrol suggests potential for increased cancer risk, a possibility that warrants caution in the implementation of dietary stilbenes as cancer preventive agents or health-promoting dietary supplements in women.

## 18.9  INHIBITION OF PROTEIN KINASE C (PKC) ISOZYMES BY RESVERATROL

Protein kinase C (PKC) is a family of ten isozymes that play critical roles in the regulation of cell growth and survival. Most PKC isozymes are activated by phosphatidylserine-dependent mechanisms that involve binding of the stimulatory cofactors $sn$-1,2-diacylglycerol (DAG) and Ca$^{2+}$ to the regulatory domain; PKC$\alpha$, PKC$\beta$1, PKC$\beta$2, and PKC$\gamma$ are activated by Ca$^{2+}$ and DAG, and PKC$\delta$, PKC$\epsilon$, PKC$\theta$, and PKC$\eta$ are activated by DAG alone.[40] The discovery that phorbol-ester tumor promoters, such as 12-$O$-tetradecanoyl phorbol-13-acetate (TPA), could substitute for DAG and activate PKC isozymes at nanomolar concentrations[41] led to the consideration of PKC as a target for cancer prevention or therapy. Subsequent studies established that the PKC family includes oncogenic isozymes, e.g., PKCε,[42,43] and tumor-suppressive isozymes, e.g., PKCδ,[44] indicating the need for isozyme-selective PKC targeting in designing strategies of cancer prevention and therapy. A study of resveratrol effects on purified PKC isozymes established that resveratrol is PKC inhibitory, but the inhibitory potency of the polyphenol was similar against the seven isozymes surveyed, which were the $Ca^{2+}$, DAG-activated isozymes PKCα, PKCβ1, PKCβ2, and PKCγ, the DAG-activated isozymes PKCδ and PKCε, and the DAG-independent isozyme PKCζ. PKC inhibition by resveratrol entailed competition with ATP substrate.[45]

Protein kinase D (PKD) is a family of three isozymes, PKD1–3, that have in common with PKC a conserved DAG/TPA binding-site. However, PKD is not activated by DAG/TPA, and is instead activated downstream of PKC by phosphorylation at activation-loop residues serine 744/748. PKD is involved in the transmission of PKC-dependent cell proliferative and survival signals.[46] Interestingly, cell survival signaling by PKD may involve suppression of the JNK signaling pathway through PKD–JNK complex formation.[47] A comparison of the inhibitory effects of resveratrol against purified PKD-1 (formerly called PKCμ) vs. the PKC isozymes analyzed in Reference 45 determined that the polyphenol is somewhat more potent against PKD-1, and markedly so with respect to the kinase autophosphorylation reaction.[48] This suggested that resveratrol inhibition of PKC might be reinforced in cells by coordinate inhibition of the PKC effector PKD. A recent analysis of growth-suppressive effects of resveratrol in the androgen-independent human prostate cancer cell line PC-3 established that resveratrol blocked TPA-induced PKCα activation without any effect on the other phorbol ester-activated protein kinases in the cells (PKD, PKCε).[49] These findings are consistent with a recent report identifying PKCε as the endogenous activator of PKD.[50] Furthermore, they reveal that, although an indiscriminate inhibitor of purified PKC/PKD species, resveratrol selectively inhibits a subset of these targets in cells. The strong suppression of DMBA (7,12-dimethyl-benz(a)anthracene)/TPA-induced papilloma formation achieved by resveratrol, when co-administered with TPA in the promotion phase of the two-stage mouse skin carcinogenesis model, offers evidence that, in at least some tissues, the sum total of resveratrol inhibitory effects against TPA-responsive PKC isozymes and PKD may be cancer preventive.[3]

## 18.10  CANCER PREVENTION BY RESVERATROL IN VIVO

The first demonstration that resveratrol has cancer preventive activity *in vivo* was the aforementioned finding by Pezzuto and co-workers[3] that co-administration of resveratrol and TPA in the tumor-promotion phase of the two-stage mouse skin model potently suppressed tumor formation; two subsequent reports confirmed that resveratrol has cancer preventive activity in the DMBA/TPA mouse skin model.[51,52] In the mouse skin model, resveratrol is directly applied to the DMBA/TPA-treated skin, so that the issues of resveratrol metabolism and bio-availability in the circulation are minimized. Thus, the finding that orally administered resveratrol has cancer preventive activity in the azoxymethane (AOM)-induced colon carcinogenesis model in F344 rats was a significant advance. In that study, Tessitore et al.[53] established that intake of resveratrol in the drinking water, while having no effect on body weight, suppressed AOM induction of aberrant crypt foci, which are preneoplastic lesions in the colonic epithelium.[53] The cancer preventive activity of resveratrol against intestinal tumor development was also demonstrated in an analysis of *Min* (multiple intestinal neoplasia) mice, which harbor a mutated *Apc* (adenomatous polyposis coli) gene and, as a result, spontaneously develop tumors in the small intestine and, to a lesser extent, in the colon. Oral intake of resveratrol in the drinking water did not significantly affect body weight but sharply reduced the incidence of tumors in the small intestine as well as the colon of *Min* mice, in a 7-week timeframe.[54] Resveratrol has also been shown to have cancer preventive activity in the upper digestive tract. Intra-peritoneal delivery of resveratrol significantly reduced the incidence and size of *N*-nitrosomethylbenzamine (NMBA)-induced esophageal tumors in F344 rats.[55]

As mentioned in Section 18.8, the mixed estrogen agonist/antagonist activity of resveratrol has raised the concern that some dietary stilbenes may increase breast cancer risk. Therefore, the demonstration that oral intake of resveratrol dramatically suppresses DMBA-induced mammary tumor incidence in female Sprague-Dawley rats without affecting body weight[56] is an important advance that should encourage further research in this area.

Despite the efficacy of resveratrol as a cancer preventive agent in rodent models of carcinogenesis, enthusiasm for translation to cancer preventive intervention in humans has been tempered by the valid concern that resveratrol bioavailability in humans may be too limited to effect cancer prevention.[57] Still, from the perspective that the glass is half-full rather than half-empty, target organs with relatively limited dependence on systemic delivery, e.g., the upper digestive tract, are likely to benefit from chemoprotection by dietary resveratrol.[58,59] Recently, a study of the absorption, bioavailability, and metabolism of [$^{14}$C] resveratrol in human volunteers established that a 25-mg oral dose was absorbed >70%, generating peak plasma levels of total radioactivity of 2 $\mu M$ at 1 h and 1.3 $\mu M$ at 6 h, followed by an exponential decline in the plasma concentration; most of the radioactivity was recovered in the urine within 12 h of ingestion.[59] However, the bioavailability of *trans*-resveratrol was very low, with only trace amounts in the plasma within 30 min of intravenous delivery, despite high retention of resveratrol metabolites. While not specifically identified, major metabolites were established as resveratrol sulfates and glucuronic conjugates.[59] Identification and analysis of the bioactivity of these metabolites and analysis of bioactive metabolite accumulation in target tissues will be important in the assessment of resveratrol as a cancer preventive agent in humans.

Some resveratrol analogs may be more effective than resveratrol itself for cancer prevention in humans. For example, piceid and other glucosides of resveratrol are more hydrophilic than the aglycone and may have superior oral bioavailability.[60] With respect to the issue of stilbene solubility, a survey of red grape juices determined that *trans*-piceid is present on average at 3.4 µg/ml, despite the absence of the ethanol solvent that contributes to the stilbene content of wine.[61] Piceatannol is a tetrahydroxy resveratrol metabolite (trans-3,4,3′,5′-tetrahydroxystilbene) produced by CYP1B1-catalyzed hydroxylation of resveratrol[62] that has been shown to be more potent than resveratrol in inducing apoptosis of primary leukemic lymphoblasts isolated from patients with acute lymphoblastic leukemia (ALL).[63] Attempts to develop resveratrol analogs for use as antineoplastic drugs in humans by chemical synthesis and preclinical screening are under way by a team led by G.R. Pettit.[64] Through a similar approach, they isolated a bioactive cis-stilbene from a Zulu medicinal plant and then developed a water-soluble antineoplastic prodrug form of the agent, combretastatin A-4 phosphate [*cis*-1-(3,4,5,-trimethoxyphenyl)-2-(4′-methoxyphenyl) ethene-3′-*O*-phosphate],[65] which is under evaluation in clinical trials.[64]

## ACKNOWLEDGMENTS

Supported by the Robert A. Welch Foundation and the Elsa U. Pardee Foundation.

## REFERENCES

1. Ribeiro de Lima MT, Waffo-Teguo P, Teissedre PL, Pujolas A, Vercauteren J, Cabanis JC, Merillon JM. Determination of stilbenes (trans-astringin, cis- and trans-piceid, and cis- and trans-resveratrol) in Portuguese wines. *J Agric Food Chem* 1999; 47:2666–2670.
2. Sanders TH, McMichael RW Jr, Hendrix KW. Occurrence of resveratrol in edible peanuts. *J Agric Food Chem* 2000; 48:1243–1246.
3. Jang M, Cai L, Udeani GO, Slowing KV, Thomas CF, Beecher CW, Fong HH, Farnsworth NR, Kinghorn AD, Mehta RG, Moon RC, Pezzuto JM. Cancer chemo-preventive activity of resveratrol, a natural product derived from grapes. *Science* 1997; 275:218–220.
4. Howitz KT, Bitterman KJ, Cohen HY, Lamming DW, Lavu S, Wood JG, Zipkin RE, Chung P, Kisielewski A, Zhang LL, Scherer B, Sinclair DA. Small molecule activators of sirtuins extend *Saccharomyces cerevisiae* lifespan. *Nature* 2003; 425:191–196.
5. Wood JG, Rogina B, Lavu S, Howitz K, Helfand SL, Tatar M, Sinclair D. Sirtuin activators mimic caloric restriction and delay ageing in metazoans. *Nature* 2004; 430:686–689.
6. Picard F, Kurtev M, Chung N, Topark-Ngarm A, Senawong T, Machado De Oliveira R, Leid M, McBurney MW, Guarente L. Sirt1 promotes fat mobilization in white adipocytes by repressing PPAR-gamma. *Nature* 2004; 429:771–776.
7. Cavallaro A, Ainis T, Bottari C, Fimiani V. Effect of resveratrol on some activities of isolated and in whole blood human neutrophils. *Physiol Res* 2003; 52:555–562.

8.  Leonard SS, Xia C, Jiang BH, Stinefelt B, Klandorf H, Harris GK, Shi X. Resveratrol scavenges reactive oxygen species and effects radical-induced cellular responses. *Biochem Biophys Res Commun* 2003; 309:1017–1026.

9.  Burkitt MJ, Duncan J. Effects of trans-resveratrol on copper-dependent hydroxyl-radical formation and DNA damage: evidence for hydroxyl-radical scavenging and a novel, glutathione-sparing mechanism of action. *Arch Biochem Biophys* 2000; 381:253–263.

10. Ahmad N, Adhami VM, Afaq F, Feyes DK, Mukhtar H. Resveratrol causes WAF-1/p21-mediated G(1)-phase arrest of cell cycle and induction of apoptosis in human epidermoid carcinoma A431 cells. *Clin Cancer Res* 2001; 7:1466–1473.

11. Adhami VM, Afaq F, Ahmad N. Involvement of the retinoblastoma (pRb)-E2F/DP pathway during antiproliferative effects of resveratrol in human epidermoid carcinoma (A431) cells. *Biochem Biophys Res Commun* 2001; 288:579–585.

12. Fulda S, Debatin KM. Sensitization for tumor necrosis factor-related apoptosis-inducing ligand-induced apoptosis by the chemopreventive agent resveratrol. *Cancer Res* 2004; 64:337–346.

13. Fulda S, Debatin KM. Sensitization for anticancer drug-induced apoptosis by the chemopreventive agent resveratrol. *Oncogene* 2004; 23:6702–6711.

14. Joe AK, Liu H, Suzui M, Vural ME, Xiao D, Weinstein IB. Resveratrol induces growth inhibition, S-phase arrest, apoptosis, and changes in biomarker expression in several human cancer cell lines. *Clin Cancer Res* 2002; 8:893–903.

15. Fontecave M, Lepoivre M, Elleingand E, Gerez C, Guittet O. Resveratrol, a remarkable inhibitor of ribonucleotide reductase. *FEBS Lett* 1998; 421:277–279.

16. Wolter F, Turchanowa L, Stein J. Resveratrol-induced modification of polyamine metabolism is accompanied by induction of c-Fos. *Carcinogenesis* 2003; 24:469–474.

17. Reagan-Shaw S, Afaq F, Aziz MH, Ahmad N. Modulations of critical cell cycle regulatory events during chemoprevention of ultraviolet B-mediated responses by resveratrol in SKH-1 hairless mouse skin. *Oncogene* 2004; 23:5151–5160.

18. Aziz MH, Afaq F, Ahmad N. Prevention of ultraviolet-B radiation — damage by resveratrol in mouse skin is mediated via modulation in survivin. *Photochem Photobiol* 2005; 81:25–31.

19. Park JW, Choi YJ, Suh SI, Baek WK, Suh MH, Jin IN, Min DS, Woo JH, Chang JS, Passaniti A, Lee YH, Kwon TK. Bcl-2 overexpression attenuates resveratrol-induced apoptosis in U937 cells by inhibition of caspase-3 activity. *Carcinogenesis* 2001; 22:1633–1639.

20. Ferry-Dumazet H, Garnier O, Mamani-Matsuda M, Vercauteren J, Belloc F, Billiard C, Dupouy M, Thiolat D, Kolb JP, Marit G, Reiffers J, Mossalayi MD. Resveratrol inhibits the growth and induces the apoptosis of both normal and leukemic hematopoietic cells. *Carcinogenesis* 2002; 23:1327–1333.

21. Morris GZ, Williams RL, Elliott MS, Beebe SJ. Resveratrol induces apoptosis in LNCaP cells and requires hydroxyl groups to decrease viability in LNCaP and DU 145 cells. *Prostate* 2002; 52:319–329.

22. Lin HY, Shih A, Davis FB, Tang HY, Martino LJ, Bennett JA, Davis PJ. Resveratrol induced serine phosphorylation of p53 causes apoptosis in a mutant p53 prostate cancer cell line. *J Urol* 2002; 168:748–755.

23. Delmas D, Rebe C, Lacour S, Filomenko R, Athis A, Gambert P, Cherkaoui-Malki M, Jannin B, Dubrez-Daloz L, Latruffe N, Solary E. Resveratrol-induced apoptosis is associated with Fas redistribution in the rafts and the formation of a death-inducing signaling complex in colon cancer cells. *J Biol Chem* 2003; 278:41482–41490.

24. Zhang S, Cao HJ, Davis FB, Tang HY, Davis PJ, Lin HY. Oestrogen inhibits resveratrol-induced post-translational modification of p53 and apoptosis in breast cancer cells. *Br J Cancer* 2004; 91:178–185.

25. Ding XZ, Adrian TE. Resveratrol inhibits proliferation and induces apoptosis in human pancreatic cancer cells. *Pancreas* 2002; 25:71–76.

26. Pati D, Haddad BR, Haegele A, Thompson H, Kittrell FS, Shepard A, Montagna C, Zhang N, Ge G, Otta SK, McCarthy M, Ullrich RL, Medina D. Hormone-induced chromosomal instability in p53-null mammary epithelium. *Cancer Res* 2004; 64:5608–5616.

27. Fuchs SY, Adler V, Pincus MR, Ronai Z. MEKK1/JNK signaling stabilizes and activates p53. *Proc Natl Acad Sci USA* 1998; 95:10541–10546.

28. She QB, Huang C, Zhang Y, Dong Z. Involvement of c-jun NH(2)-terminal kinases in resveratrol-induced activation of p53 and apoptosis. *Mol Carcinogen* 2002; 33:244–250.

29. Park SJ, Wu CH, Gordon JD, Zhong X, Emami A, Safa AR. Taxol induces caspase-10-dependent apoptosis. *J Biol Chem* 2004; 279:51057–51067.

30. Aggarwal BB. Nuclear factor-κB: the enemy within. *Cancer Cell* 2004; 6:203–208.

31. Holmes-McNary M, Baldwin AS. Chemopreventive properties of trans-resveratrol are associated with inhibition of activation of the IκB kinase. *Cancer Res* 2000; 60:3477–3483.

32. Estrov Z, Shishodia S, Faderl S, Harris D, Van Q, Kantarjian HM, Talpaz M, Aggarwal BB. Resveratrol blocks interleukin-1β-induced activation of the nuclear transcription factor NF-κB, inhibits proliferation, causes S-phase arrest, and induces apoptosis of acute myeloid leukemia cells. *Blood* 2003; 102:987–995.

33. Sinicrope FA, Gill S. Role of cyclooxygenase-2 in colorectal cancer. *Cancer Metastasis Rev* 2004; 23:63–75.

34. Szewczuk LM, Forti L, Stivala LA, Penning TM. Resveratrol is a peroxidase-mediated inactivator of COX-1 but not COX-2: a mechanistic approach to the design of COX-1 selective agents. *J Biol Chem* 2004; 279:22727–22737.

35. Martin AR, Villegas I, La Casa C, de la Lastra CA. Resveratrol, a polyphenol found in grapes, suppresses oxidative damage and stimulates apoptosis during early colonic inflammation in rats. *Biochem Pharmacol* 2004; 67:1399–1410.

36. Mutoh M, Takahashi M, Fukuda K, Matsushima-Hibiya Y, Mutoh H, Sugimura T, Wakabayashi K. Suppression of cyclooxygenase-2 promoter-dependent transcriptional activity in colon cancer cells by chemopreventive agents with a resorcin-type structure. *Carcinogenesis* 2000; 21:959–963.

37. Gehm BD, McAndrews JM, Chien PY, Jameson JL. Resveratrol, a polyphenolic compound found in grapes and wine, is an agonist for the estrogen receptor. *Proc Natl Acad Sci USA* 1997; 94:14138–14143.

38. Bhat KP, Pezzuto JM. Resveratrol exhibits cytostatic and antiestrogenic properties with human endometrial adenocarcinoma (Ishikawa) cells. *Cancer Res* 2001; 61:6137–6144.

39. Levenson AS, Gehm BD, Pearce ST, Horiguchi J, Simons LA, Ward JE, Jameson JL, Jordan VC. Resveratrol acts as an estrogen receptor (ER) agonist in breast cancer cells stably transfected with ERα. *Intl J Cancer* 2003; 104:587–596.

40. Ron D, Kazanietz MG. New insights into the regulation of protein kinase C and novel phorbol ester receptors. *FASEB J* 1999; 13:1658–1676.

41. Castagna M, Takai Y, Kaibuchi K, Sano K, Kikkawa U, Nishizuka Y. Direct activation of calcium-activated, phospholipid-dependent protein kinase by tumor-promoting phorbol esters. *J Biol Chem* 1982; 257:7847–7851.

42. Cacace AM, Ueffing M, Philipp A, Han EK, Kolch W, Weinstein IB. PKC epsilon functions as an oncogene by enhancing activation of the Raf kinase. *Oncogene* 1996; 13:2517–2526.

43. Reddig PJ, Dreckschmidt NE, Zou J, Bourguignon SE, Oberley TD, Verma AK. Transgenic mice overexpressing protein kinase Cε in their epidermis exhibit reduced papilloma burden but enhanced carcinoma formation after tumor promotion. *Cancer Res* 2000; 60:595–602.

44. Reddig PJ, Dreckschimdt NE, Ahrens H, Simsiman R, Tseng C-P, Zou J, Oberley TD, Verma AK. Transgenic mice overexpressing protein kinase Cδ in the epidermis are resistant to skin tumor promotion by 12-*O*-tetradecanoylphorbol-13-acetate. *Cancer Res* 1999; 59:5710–5718.

45. Stewart JR, Ward NE, Ioannides CG, O'Brian CA. Resveratrol preferentially inhibits protein kinase C-catalyzed phosphorylation of a cofactor-independent, arginine-rich protein substrate by a novel mechanism. *Biochemistry* 1999, 38:13244–13251.

46. Rykx A, De Kimpe L, Mikhalap S, Vantus T, Seufferlein T, Vandenheede JR, Van Lint J. Protein kinase D: a family affair. *FEBS Lett* 2003; 546:81–86.

47. Hurd C, Waldron RT, Rozengurt E. Protein kinase D complexes with c-Jun N-terminal kinase via activation loop phosphorylation and phosphorylates the c-Jun N-terminus. *Oncogene* 2002; 21:2154–2160.

48. Stewart JR, Christman KL, O'Brian CA. Effects of resveratrol on the autophosphorylation of phorbol ester-responsive protein kinases: inhibition of protein kinase D but not protein kinase C isozyme autophosphorylation. *Biochem Pharmacol* 2000; 60:1355–1359.

49. Stewart JR, O'Brian CA. Resveratrol antagonizes EGFR-dependent Erk1/2 activation in human androgen-independent prostate cancer cells with associated isozyme-selective PKC alpha inhibition. *Invest New Drugs* 2004; 22:107–117.

50. Rey O, Reeve JR, Zhukova E, Sinnett-Smith J, Rozengurt E. G protein-coupled receptor-mediated phosphorylation of the activation loop of protein kinase D: dependence on plasma membrane translocation and protein kinase Cε. *J Biol Chem* 2004; 279:34361–34372.

51. Kapadia GJ, Azuine MA, Tokuda H, Takasaki M, Mukainaka T, Konoshima T, Nishino H. Chemopreventive effect of resveratrol, sesamol, sesame oil and sunflower oil in the Epstein-Barr virus early antigen activation assay and the mouse skin two-stage carcinogenesis. *Pharmacological Res* 2002; 45:499–505.

52. Soleas GJ, Grass L, Josephy PD, Goldberg DM, Diamandis EP. A comparison of the anticarcinogenic properties of four red wine polyphenols. *Clin Biochem* 2002; 35:119–124.

53. Tessitore L, Davit A, Sarotto I, Caderni G. Resveratrol depresses the growth of colorectal aberrant crypt foci by affecting bax and p21(CIP) expression. *Carcinogenesis* 2000; 21:1619–1622.

54. Schneider Y, Duranton B, Gosse F, Schleiffer R, Seiler N, Raul F. Resveratrol inhibits intestinal tumorigenesis and modulates host-defense-related gene expression in an animal model of human familial adenomatous polyposis. *Nutr Cancer* 2001; 39:102–107.

55. Li ZG, Hong T, Shimada Y, Komoto I, Kawabe A, Ding Y, Kaganoi J, Hashimoto Y, Imamura M. Suppression of N-nitrosomethylbenzylamine (NMBA)-induced esophageal tumorigenesis in F344 rats by resveratrol. *Carcinogenesis* 2002; 23(9):1531–1536.

56. Banerjee S, Bueso-Ramos C, Aggarwal BB. Suppression of 7,12-dimethyl-benz(a)anthracene-induced mammary carcinogenesis in rats by resveratrol: role of nuclear factor-κB, cyclooxygenase 2, and matrix metalloprotease 9. *Cancer Research* 2002; 62:4945–4954.

57. Gescher AJ, Steward WP. Relationship between mechanisms, bioavailability, and preclinical chemopreventive efficacy of resveratrol: a conundrum. *Cancer Epidemiol Biomarkers Prev* 2003; 12:953–957.

58. Red wine may reduce oral cancer risks. *J Am Dent Assoc* 2000; 131:729.

59. Walle T, Hsieh F, DeLegge MH, Oatis JE, Jr, Walle UK. High absorption but very low bioavailability of oral resveratrol in humans. *Drug Metab Dispos* 2004; 32:1377–1382.

60. Krasnow MN, Murphy TM. Polyphenol glucosylating activity in cell suspensions of grape (*Vitis vinifera*). *J Agric Food Chem* 2004; 52:3467–3472.

61. Romero-Perez AI, Ibern-Gomez M, Lamuela-Raventos RM, de La Torre-Boronat MC. Piceid, the major resveratrol derivative in grape juices. *J Agric Food Chem* 1999; 47:1533–1536.

62. Potter GA, Patterson LH, Wanogho E, Perry PJ, Butler PC, Ijaz T, Ruparelia KC, Lamb JH, Farmer PB, Stanley LA, Burke MD. The cancer preventative agent resveratrol is converted to the anticancer agent piceatannol by the cytochrome P450 enzyme CYP1B1. *Br J Cancer* 2002; 86:774–778.

63. Wieder T, Prokop A, Bagci B, Essmann F, Bernicke D, Schulze-Osthoff K, Dorken B, Schmalz HG, Daniel PT, Henze G. Piceatannol, a hydroxylated analog of the chemopreventive agent resveratrol, is a potent inducer of apoptosis in the lymphoma cell line BJAB and in primary, leukemic lymphoblasts. *Leukemia* 2001; 15:1735–1742.

64. Pettit GR, Grealish MP, Jung MK, Hamel E, Pettit RK, Chapuis JC, Schmidt JM. Antineoplastic agents 465. Structural modification of resveratrol: sodium resverastatin phosphate. *J Med Chem* 2002; 45:2534–2542.

65. Pettit GR, Rhodes MR. Antineoplastic agents 389. New syntheses of the combretastatin A-4 prodrug. *Anti-Cancer Drug Design* 1998; 13:183–191.

# 19 Flaxseed and Lignans: Effects on Breast Cancer

*Krista A. Power and Lilian U. Thompson*

## CONTENTS

19.1 Introduction .................................................................................................385
19.2 Epidemiological Studies ............................................................................387
    19.2.1 Lignan Intake ...................................................................................392
    19.2.2 Serum Lignans .................................................................................393
19.3 Experimental Studies .................................................................................394
    19.3.1 FS and Lignans and Breast Cancer Prevention .....................394
        19.3.1.1 FS and Lignans and Mammary Gland
                 Development................................................................394
        19.3.1.2 FS and Lignans and Tumor Initiation and
                 Promotion ...................................................................396
    19.3.2 FS and Lignans and Breast Cancer Treatment .....................397
        19.3.2.1 FS and Lignans in Carcinogen-Treated
                 Rat Model......................................................................397
        19.3.2.2 Lignans and Athymic Nude Mice Model..................397
        19.3.2.3 Clinical Study................................................................400
19.4 Mechanisms ................................................................................................400
    19.4.1 Altering Estrogen Bioavailability................................................400
    19.4.2 Altering Estrogen Synthesis and Metabolism..........................401
        19.4.2.1 Estrogen Synthesis .....................................................401
        19.4.2.2 Estrogen Metabolism .................................................402
    19.4.3 Altering Estrogen Action................................................................402
    19.4.4 Non-ER-Mediated Mechanisms .................................................403
        19.4.4.1 Effects on Metastasis .................................................403
        19.4.4.2 Effects on Growth Factors .........................................404
19.5 Conclusion .................................................................................................405
References ............................................................................................................405

## 19.1 INTRODUCTION

Flaxseed (FS) (*Linum usitatissimum*) has recently gained recognition as a food with disease risk-reducing capabilities.[1] FS contains about 30% dietary fiber, 20%

protein, and 40% oil of which 50% is α-linolenic acid (ALA). In addition, it contains plant lignans such as secoisolariciresinol diglycoside (SDG), matairesinol (MAT), isolariciresinol, and pinoresinol, with SDG in the highest concentration. Although lignans are found in the highest concentration in FS, they are ubiquitously present in most food, including fruits and vegetables, nuts and seeds, berries, whole grains, and cereals.[2]

The absorption and metabolism of lignans involve multiple steps and the complete mechanism has yet to be elucidated. A major requirement for lignan metabolism and absorption is the presence of colonic bacteria, as it was shown that germ-free rodents[3] and humans who have taken antimicrobials[4] have lower excretion of mammalian lignans compared to their normal controls. Bacterial activity is needed for the removal of glucose residues (to form aglycones), demethylation, and dehydroxylation of the plant lignans to the diphenolic mammalian lignans enterolactone (ENL) and enterodiol (END) (Figure 19.1). SDG is metabolized to the aglycone secoisolariciresinol (SECO), then to END and to ENL. MAT can be directly converted to ENL. END and ENL are absorbed from the colon, transported to the liver, where they are conjugated, enter the circulation, and then are partly excreted in the urine, or secreted in bile to undergo enterohepatic circulation.[5] The degree of conversion of mammalian lignans from plant lignans depends on the type of plant lignan precursor ingested.[6]

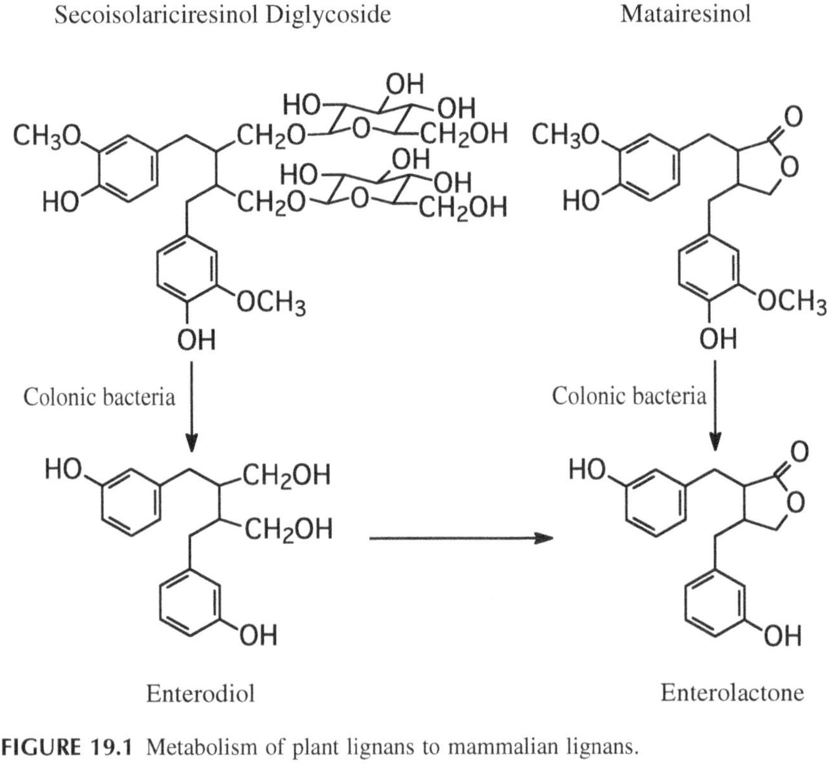

Secoisolariciresinol Diglycoside                Matairesinol

FIGURE 19.1 Metabolism of plant lignans to mammalian lignans.

Like the isoflavones found primarily in soy and coumestans found in high concentrations in clover, the lignans are classified as phytoestrogens due to their structural similarity to the steroid hormone estrogen. Ingestion of foods containing phytoestrogens has been associated with a lower incidence of many types of cancer, especially hormone-related cancers such as the breast[7] and prostate.[8] Their incidence is lower in Asia, where the phytoestrogen intake is high, compared to where the phytoestrogen intake is low, such as in North America and Europe.[9] Because estrogen is known to influence the growth and development of these cancers, phytoestrogens are also thought to influence cancer development. However, the mechanism of phytoestrogen action can also be both hormone and nonhormone related.[10] This chapter discusses epidemiological and experimental studies on the effects of FS and, more specifically the lignans, on the growth and development of breast cancer. Potential mechanisms of lignan action are also discussed.

## 19.2  EPIDEMIOLOGICAL STUDIES

Adlercreutz et al.[7] first showed in 1982, in a small number of subjects, that postmenopausal Finnish women with breast cancer ($n = 7$) had a lower urinary mammalian lignan excretion compared to healthy controls ($n = 20$), suggesting that the lignans are associated with a reduced risk of breast cancer. More studies, detailed in Table 19.1, have since been conducted, utilizing larger sample sizes and either urinary or serum lignans levels, or lignan intake as biomarkers, to determine if the lignans are associated with breast cancer risk. From 1997–2002, three case-control studies[11–13] showed negative association between urinary lignans or lignan intake and breast cancer risk, while a case-control study[14] showed no association between lignan intake and breast cancer risk in pre- and postmenopausal women. In another case-control study, when both pre- and postmenopausal women were combined, there was a significant negative association between serum lignans and breast cancer risk.[15] A prospective study[16] showed no association between urinary lignans and breast cancer risk in a group of postmenopausal women, while in another prospective study[17] utilizing three separate cohorts in Sweden, two of the cohorts showed a weak positive association between serum lignans and breast cancer risk, while the other showed a negative association between serum lignans and breast cancer risk. However, the authors[17] stated that their results should be viewed with caution due to the small sample sizes in each cohort.

The above six studies gave contradictory results regarding the association between lignans and breast cancer risk. Therefore, more epidemiological studies, further described in greater detail below, were conducted in recent years using newer methods of estimating lignan exposure (i.e., intake and serum levels), in hopes to clarify the lignan and breast cancer association.

**TABLE 19.1**
**Epidemiological Studies Relating Lignans and Breast Cancer**

| Study Design Location | Subjects | Source of Lignan | Lignan Levels | Outcome | Ref. |
|---|---|---|---|---|---|
| Case control Australia | Pre- and postmenopausal breast cancer (BC) cases ($n = 144$) and controls ($n = 144$) | Urinary ENL, END, MAT | Median: BC cases = 282 nmol END/24 h; 1973 nmol ENL/24h; 28.9 nmol MAT/24 h; controls= 316.5 nmol END/24 h; 3097.7 nmol ENL/24 h; 29.3 nmol MAT/24 h | Negative association between BC risk and ENL excretion (OR 0.36, 95% CI: 0.15–0.86, $p_{trend}$ = 0.013); no significant association between END (OR 0.73, 95% CI: 0.33–1.64, $p_{trend}$ = 0.288) or MAT (OR 2.18, 95% CI: 0.83–5.76, $p_{trend}$ = 0.308) excretion and BC risk | Ingram et al., 1997[11] |
| Case control Shanghai | Pre- and postmenopausal BC cases ($n = 250$) and controls ($n = 250$) | Urinary ENL and END | Mean: BC cases = 0.86 nmol END/mg creatinine; 3.59 nmol ENL/mg creatinine; controls = 0.9 nmol END/mg creatinine; 6.28 nmol ENL/mg creatinine | Negative association between premenopausal BC risk and ENL + END excretion (OR 0.62, 95% CI: 0.12–0.50, $p_{trend}$ < 0.01); no significant association between ENL + END excretion and postmenopausal BC risk (OR 0.62, 95% CI: 0.31–1.26, $p_{trend}$ = 0.16) | Dai et al., 2002[12] |
| Prospective Netherlands | Postmenopausal BC cases ($n = 88$) and controls ($n = 268$) | Urinary ENL | Range of ENL excretion 7.16–2334.9 μmol/mol creatinine | No significant association between lignan excretion and BC risk (OR 1.43, 95% CI: 0.79–2.59, $p_{trend}$ = 0.25) | den Tonkelaar et al., 2001[16] |
| Case control USA | Pre- and postmenopausal BC cases ($n = 1272$) and controls ($n = 1610$) | FFQ | Range of total lignan intake for pre- and postmenopausal BC cases and controls: <1.05 to ≥2.78 mg/day | No significant association between plant lignan intake and pre- or postmenopausal BC risk (OR 1.3, 95% CI: 1.0–1.6) | Horn-Ross et al., 2001[14] |

| Study / Country | Subjects | Method | Values | Results | Reference |
|---|---|---|---|---|---|
| Case control USA | Pre- and postmenopausal BC cases ($n = 740$) and controls ($n = 810$) | FFQ | Range of total lignan intake for pre- and postmenopausal BC cases and controls: 0.06–2.48 mg/day | Negative association between lignan intake and premenopausal BC risk (OR 0.49, 95% CI: 0.32–0.75, $p < 0.05$); no significant association between plant lignan intake and postmenopausal BC risk (OR 0.72; 95% CI: 0.51–1.02) | McCann et al., 2002[13] |
| Prospective (EPIC) Netherlands | Pre- and postmenopausal BC cases ($n = 280$) and controls ($n = 15,275$) | FFQ | Median: estimated ENL + END = 0.67 mg/day | Nonsignificant negative association between estimated ENL + END and BC risk (OR 0.7, 95% CI: 0.46–1.09, $p_{trend} = 0.06$) | Keinan-Boker et al., 2004[22] |
| Case control Germany | Premenopausal BC cases ($n = 278$) and controls ($n = 666$) | FFQ | Median: SECO + MAT: premenopausal BC cases = 570.3 µg/day, controls = 563.1 µg/day; estimated ENL + END: premenopausal BC cases = 726.1 µg/day, controls = 752.1 µg/day | Negative association between BC risk and MAT intake (OR 0.58, 95% CI: 0.37–0.94, $p_{trend} = 0.025$) Negative association between BC risk and estimated ENL (OR 0.57, 95% CI: 0.35–0.92, $p_{trend} = 0.008$) and END (OR 0.61, 95% CI: 0.39–0.98, $p_{trend} = 0.034$) | Linseisen et al., 2004[21] |
| Case control USA | pre- ($n = 315$) and postmenopausal ($n = 807$) breast cancer patients and matched controls ($n = 593$ and $n = 1443$, respectively) | FFQ | Mean: SECO + MAT: premenopausal BC cases = 509.6 µg/day, controls 537.2 µg/day; postmenopausal BC cases = 575.8 µg/day, controls = 570.5 µg/day | Premenopausal: negative association between BC risk and SECO + MAT intake (OR 0.66, 95% CI: 0.44–0.98). Postmenopausal: no significant association (OR = 0.93; 95% CI: 0.71–1.22) | McCann et al., 2004[20] |
| Case control Finland | Pre- and postmenopausal BC cases ($n = 194$) and controls ($n = 208$) | Serum ENL | Mean ENL: All cases = 19.6 nM, controls = 25.9 nM ($p = 0.003$) | Negative association between combined pre- and postmenopausal BC risk and ENL levels (OR 0.38, 95% CI: 0.18–0.77, $p_{trend} = 0.03$) | Pietinen et al., 2001[15] |

*(continued)*

**TABLE 19.1 (CONTINUED)**
**Epidemiological Studies Relating Lignans and Breast Cancer**

| Study Design Location | Subjects | Source of Lignan | Lignan Levels | Outcome | Ref. |
|---|---|---|---|---|---|
| Prospective Sweden 3 cohorts: 1. Västerbotten intervention project (VIP) 2. Monitoring of trends and cardiovascular disease study (MONICA) 3. Mammary screening project (MSP) | Pre- and postmenopausal BC cases VIP and MONICA: BC cases (n = 155) and controls (n = 308) MSP: BC cases (n = 93) and controls (n = 185) | Serum ENL | VIP and MONICA: Mean: BC cases = 26.8 nmol/L, controls = 22.9 nmol/L MSP: Mean: BC cases = 19.3 nmol/L, controls = 20.4 nmol/L | Positive association between BC risk and ENL levels for combined cohorts (OR 1.8, 95% CI: 1.4–4.3) VIP and MONICA: positive association between BC risk and ENL levels (OR 2.4, 95% CI: 1.4–4.3) MSP: negative association between ENL levels and BC risk (OR 0.9, 95% CI: 0.4–2.3) | Hulten et al., 2002[17] |
| Prospective USA | 417 BC cases from 14,275 participants; premenopausal BC (n = 189) and postmenopausal BC (n = 228) | Serum ENL | Mean: Premenopausal BC cases = 18.3 nmol/L, control = 15.1 nmol/L (p = 0.01); Postmenopausal BC cases = 18.6 nmol/L, controls = 18.9 nmol/L | Premenopausal: Weak positive association between ENL levels and BC risk (OR 1.6, 95% CI: 0.7–3.4, $p_{trend}$ = 0.13) Postmenopausal: No significant difference | Zeleniuch-Jacquotte et al., 2004[27] |

| Prospective Italy | 383 women with palpable cyst, 18 of which developed BC | Serum ENL | Median: BC cases = 8.5 nmol/L, controls = 16.0 nmol/L | Negative association between serum ENL and BC risk (OR 0.36, 95% CI: 0.14–0.925, p = 0.03) | Boccardo et al., 2004[29] |
|---|---|---|---|---|---|
| Case control Finland | Pre- and postmenopausal BC cases (n = 206) and control (n = 215) | Serum ENL | Mean ENL: BC cases = 25.2 nmol/L, controls = 24 nmol/L | Nonsignificant negative association between serum ENL and premenopausal BC cases (OR 0.73, 95% CI: 0.34–1.59, p = 0.42) Nonsignificant positive association between serum ENL and postmenopausal breast cancer cases (OR 1.22, 95% CI: 0.69–2.16, p = 0.50) | Kilkkinen et al., 2004[28] |

*Abbreviations:* BC = breast cancer, FFQ = food frequency questionnaire, ENL = enterolactone, END = enterodiol, SECO = secoisolariciresinol, MAT = matairesinol, OR = odds ratio, CI = confidence interval.

## 19.2.1 LIGNAN INTAKE

Because FS has only recently been recognized as a food source with the highest concentration of lignans,[2] it has not been consumed in large quantities for very long. Thus, many epidemiological studies have focused on other food sources of lignans to determine associations with breast cancer risk. With the availability of several databases that include values for the plant lignans SDG, its aglycone SECO and MAT,[18,19] or actual mammalian lignans produced from different plant foods,[2] several recent studies have used food frequency questionnaires (FFQs) and these published databases to estimate lignan intake and relate it to breast cancer risk.

In a case-control study, McCann et al.[20] analyzed lignan intake from FFQ completed by both pre- and postmenopausal patients with breast cancer and matched controls (Table 19.1). The mean total plant lignan intakes (SECO + MAT) in the cases were not significantly different from their matched controls. However, when the data were divided into quartiles, lignan intake was negatively associated with premenopausal breast cancer risk, but not with postmenopausal breast cancer risk. The authors suggest that the menopausal status-dependent effects of the lignans indicate that the lignan may be protective only when circulating estradiol is high.

In another case-control study, German premenopausal women with breast cancer and matched controls completed an FFQ, no more than 2 years after diagnosis, to determine intake of phytoestrogens during the year prior to breast cancer diagnosis[21] (Table 19.1). The median intakes of each lignan (estimated from plant lignans or mammalian lignans) did not differ significantly between cases or controls. However, when quartiles were assessed using intake data calculated from plant lignan content of foods, MAT intake, but not SECO, was negatively associated with breast cancer risk. The lignan intake calculated from the amount of mammalian lignans, ENL and END, produced from the foods was also associated with a decreased risk of premenopausal breast cancer risk.

A prospective study in the Netherlands asked women participating in the European Prospective Investigation into Cancer and Nutrition (EPIC) study to fill out an FFQ, and once breast cancer developed, cancer risk was determined[22] (Table 19.1). A total of 15,555 women participated in the study and a total of 280 (1.8%) women developed their first incident of breast cancer during the follow-up period, which was a median of 5.2 years. There was no significant association between plant lignan (SECO + MAT) intake and breast cancer risk in these women. A tendency for breast cancer protective effect of high lignan intake estimated from the mammalian lignan database (ENL + END) was observed when quartiles were assessed, but the results did not reach significance.

The use of FFQ with lignan databases is beneficial in that it estimates long-term lignan intake. However, although current databases are useful, they are still incomplete, as many foods have yet to be analyzed for their lignan contents. In addition, the amount of other mammalian lignan precursors, such as pinoresinol and lariciresinol, has yet to be determined in foods. Current databases contain primarily values for the plant lignans SECO and MAT. These may have contributed to the inconsistent results obtained in the above studies and may be considered a limitation in the McCann et al. study,[20] which estimated lignan intake primarily from plant lignan database. Linseisen et al.[21] and Keinan-Boker et al.,[22] who reported different conclusions, determined the lignan intake using both the plant lignan database[19,23,24] and the database developed by Thompson et al.,[2] which estimates the amount of mammalian lignans produced from foods after incubation with human fecal inoculum. The data take into account all the mammalian lignan precursors in foods. However, the conversion of plant lignans to mammalian lignans is dependent on the individuals' colonic microflora, which varies from person to person. Thus, this database also has some limitations.

## 19.2.2 SERUM LIGNANS

Since the development of the time-resolved fluoroimmunoassay (TR-FIA) method for ENL analysis,[25,26] several studies have recently been conducted to determine the relationship between serum ENL concentrations and breast cancer risk. This assay is advantageous over traditional GC-MS and HPLC methods used in earlier studies[11] because of the small volume of serum and a shorter time needed to run the assay, and its potential for analyzing multiple samples simultaneously from large population studies.

In a prospective study conducted in both pre- and postmenopausal patients with breast cancer from the New York University Women's Health Cohort Study, a single blood sample was taken prior to breast cancer diagnosis and plasma ENL was measured and correlated with breast cancer risk[27] (Table 19.1). Circulating ENL levels were higher in cases than in the matched controls. When the women were separated by menopausal status, only the premenopausal cases had serum ENL levels that differed from their controls. Although the effect of lignans was stronger in premenopausal women, after the data were divided into quintiles, the positive association with breast cancer risk between low and high serum lignan levels no longer was significant.

In Finland, a prospective study was conducted on women participating in an independent cross-sectional population survey[28] (Table 19.1). Serum samples were collected in four different cohorts and analyzed for ENL levels by the TR-FIA method. After the exclusion process, a total of 206 breast cancer cases and 215 matched controls were included in the study, with two thirds of the women classified as postmenopausal. Mean serum ENL levels did not differ significantly between cases and control. When the women were separated by menopausal status, serum ENL levels were nonsignificantly negatively associated with premenopausal breast cancer risk and were nonsignificantly positively associated with postmenopausal breast cancer risk in the cases.

Another prospective study analyzed serum ENL in women with a high risk of breast cancer development, i.e., women with palpable cysts[29] (Table 19.1). After a follow-up period of approximately 6.5 years, 18 women had developed breast cancer. The serum ENL of those women that subsequently developed cancer was significantly lower than those that did not develop cancer, suggesting that ENL may be protective against breast cancer development in high-risk women.

Although the prospective design of the above experiments allows for an unbiased look at cases vs. control, a single blood measurement of ENL levels may not have been adequate to draw conclusion concerning risk of cancer development. A study was recently conducted to determine the reliability of single time point serum ENL measurements in healthy postmenopausal women.[30] The subjects ingested a standardized low lignan diet and blood was taken, after a 12-hour fast, at time points 0, 4, 8, 12, and 24 hours on three separate days. Large intraindividual variations in serum ENL concentrations were observed. In addition, a 31% variation in within-day serum levels and 56% variation in day-to-day serum ENL levels were observed. The authors concluded that a single time point measurement of serum ENL was inadequate to determine an individual's circulating ENL concentrations. Therefore the results of the prospective studies described above[28,29] may have made conclusions on associations between breast cancer risk and serum levels of ENL, that do not accurately reflect normal ENL levels.

In summary, the results of epidemiological studies are inconsistent. Although both the early and later studies have limitations, more than half of the studies (7 of 12) suggest a negative association between lignan exposure and breast cancer risk. However, epidemiological studies do not provide direct evidence of cause and effect. Hence, experimental studies still need to be conducted to establish a conclusive relationship between lignan exposure and breast cancer risk. The next section reviews the experimental studies on the effects of FS and its lignans in the prevention and treatment of breast cancer. Because FS contains the highest concentration of lignans, it has been used as a food model system to study the effects of lignans in the experimental studies.

## 19.3  EXPERIMENTAL STUDIES

### 19.3.1  FS AND LIGNANS AND BREAST CANCER PREVENTION

FS and lignans affect breast cancer prevention at several levels, including altering the development of the mammary gland and inducing effects on the early stages of carcinogenesis (initiation and promotion). The following are animal studies conducted to determine their effects.

#### 19.3.1.1  FS and Lignans and Mammary Gland Development

One suggested hypothesis regarding why Asian women have a lower incidence of breast cancer compared to European and American women is that exposure to phytoestrogens at an early age enhances the development of the mammary gland thereby making it less susceptible to carcinogens.[31] The rat mammary gland has been utilized for decades as a model of the human breast. Mammary gland development begins with the branching of the mammary ducts. The branch endings are termed terminal end buds (TEBs), which are highly proliferative and vulnerable to carcinogens. With stimulation by estrogens, the TEBs later differentiate to less proliferative structures called alveolar buds (ABs) and lobules. Because the latter are less susceptible to carcinogens, it has been hypothesized that compounds that can enhance the differentiation of the TEBs can reduce the risk of breast cancer.

Lignans are estrogen-like in structure and thus early exposure to FS or its lignans may enhance the development of the mammary gland. It has been shown that lignans can be transferred from rat dams to offspring through the breast milk;[32] thus, they are available to alter the mammary gland development in the offspring.

Several comprehensive studies have been performed to determine at which stage of the rodent life FS and its lignan SDG could modulate mammary gland development and subsequent breast cancer development. In one study, a 5 or 10% FS diet, or the equivalent amount of SDG, was fed (1) to pregnant rat dams during pregnancy and lactation, (2) to the female offspring after weaning from postnatal day (PND) 21 to 50, or (3) from gestation to PND 50.[33] The results show that FS and SDG can reduce the number of TEB and increase the number of the less proliferative ABs in the mammary glands of the adult offspring that were exposed to the compounds during gestation and lactation but not when exposed to the FS or SDG after weaning.

In another study, Ward et al.[34] differentiated the effect of exposure to lignans during gestation or during suckling on the mammary gland of the offspring. Pregnant rat dams were fed a basal diet (BD) for the entire duration of pregnancy. Following delivery, the rat dams were randomized and fed the BD, or a 10% FS diet, or BD supplemented with SDG, at the level found in a 10% FS diet, until offspring were weaned at PND 21. Offspring either continued on their mothers' diets or switched to BD until PND 50. This study design allows for some offspring to be exposed to FS or SDG during suckling only or during suckling and continuing until PND 50. The results showed that rats exposed to FS or SDG during suckling only or continuously until PND 50 had mammary glands with less TEB and an increased AB density. The same results were obtained when the study was repeated;[35] i.e., the mammary glands of offspring exposed to FS or SDG during suckling had a lower number of TEB at PND 50 compared to the BD group. These results as well as those from the study conducted by Tou et al.[36] stressed the significance of exposure timing in inducing an effect on mammary gland development by FS and SDG. Lactation appears to be a crucial time for the diet to alter mammary gland structures of the offspring and potentially reduce the risk of breast cancer.

To determine whether lignan exposure during suckling could indeed prevent breast tumorigenesis,[37] rat dams were fed the BD during pregnancy and then, following birth of the pups, divided into groups and fed a 10% FS diet, or the BD supplemented with SDG (equivalent to the amount in 10% FS diet), or remained on the BD. All female pups were fed the BD upon weaning and thus were only exposed to FS or SDG during suckling. At PND 50, the female offspring were given a breast carcinogen 9,10-dimethyl-1,2-benzanthracene (DMBA) and were sacrificed 21 weeks later. The results showed that both FS- and SDG-treated groups had lower tumor incidence (31.3 and 42.0%, respectively), total tumor load (50.8 and 62.5%, respectively), tumor number (46.9 and 44.8%, respectively), and mean tumor size (43.9 and 67.7%, respectively) compared to the rats exposed to BD only during lactation. Thus the study showed that lignan exposure during the lactation period enhances the mammary gland development in the offspring, which ultimately protects them against breast cancer at adulthood.

### 19.3.1.2   FS and Lignans and Tumor Initiation and Promotion

Breast carcinogenesis involves multiple steps including initiation, promotion, progression, and metastasis. However, in discussing breast cancer prevention, only the initiation and promotion stages of carcinogenesis are discussed here. Rats given DMBA for 24 hours after feeding them either 5 or 10% FS or defatted FS meal diet for 4 weeks had significant reduction in nuclear aberration and cell proliferation in the epithelial cells of the mammary gland TEB in the rats fed the 5% FS diet.[38] Furthermore, in rats fed a 5% FS diet 4 weeks before DMBA injection (preinitiation), which was then switched to a BD at the promotion stage (20 weeks following DMBA administration), a lower tumor incidence and multiplicity were observed compared to the control group.[39] In addition, when the treatment period was reversed, i.e., BD was fed at the preinitiation period and 5% FS at the promotion period, significant reduction in tumor size was observed.[39] In a further study, 1.5 mg/day SDG (equivalent to the amount of SDG found in 5% FS diet) was given to rats starting 1 week after DMBA administration.[40] After 20 weeks, the SDG group had significantly lower tumor multiplicity and number of tumors per group. The above studies suggest that the effect of FS and its lignan on cancer prevention depends on the dose and timing of treatment.

Utilizing the $N$-methyl-$N$-nitrosourea (MNU)-induced breast cancer rat model, 50-day-old rats were given MNU carcinogen and 2 days later (representing early promotion period of carcinogenesis) rats were fed a BD, 2.5 or 5% FS diet, or given a daily gavage of SDG equivalent to the amount in the 2.5% (LSDG) or 5% (HSDG) FS diet for 22 weeks.[41] The results showed that all treatment groups had less-invasive tumors, but only the HSDG group had lower tumor multiplicity compared to the BD group. Although the 5% FS-fed rats had tumors that were smaller than the BD group throughout the study, final tumor volume, weight, and incidence were not significantly affected by the FS or lignan treatment. However, all treatments reduced the invasiveness and grade of the MNU tumors, suggesting that tumor progression was reduced. The authors conclude that the study design and the dose of the carcinogen may be the reason for the lack of significance. It may also be plausible that FS and the lignans are less effective during the promotion period of MNU-induced tumors compared to DMBA-induced tumors.

## 19.3.2 FS AND LIGNANS AND BREAST CANCER TREATMENT

Two experimental animal models have been used to determine if FS or its lignans can modulate breast cancer treatment: (1) the DMBA- or MNU-carcinogen-induced tumor models, which involve administration of the carcinogen, allowing the tumors to become established, and then feeding or administering the FS or lignans to determine if they affect tumor growth; and (2) a model utilizing athymic nude mice in which human breast cancer cells are implanted and allowed to develop into tumors, at which time the animals are fed or administered FS or the lignans.

### 19.3.2.1 FS and Lignans in Carcinogen-Treated Rat Model

In one study, rats were fed a 2.5 or 5% FS diet or SDG (at the level found in the 5% FS diet) 9 weeks after DMBA administration so that mammary tumors are already established.[42] After 7 weeks, all treatment groups had tumors that were >50% smaller than the control group that was fed the BD. In addition, the SDG group had the lowest number of tumors, suggesting that the lignan component of FS was in part responsible for the tumor reducing effects of FS. In another study,[43] using a similar model as above, rats with established tumors were given a daily gavage of ENL (10 mg/kg body weight, BW) for 9 weeks following DMBA administration. After 7 weeks treatment, the ENL group had smaller established tumors and had less new tumor growth. These studies suggest that treatment with FS and the lignans can reduce the development of breast cancer in the carcinogen-treated rat model.

### 19.3.2.2 Lignans and Athymic Nude Mice Model

#### 19.3.2.2.1 Estrogen Receptor-Negative Human Breast Tumors

The athymic nude mice model is a useful model to determine the effect of compounds on human tumors *in vivo*. Depending on the type of breast cancer cells implanted into the mice, different mechanisms of action can be elucidated for FS and the lignans. For example, the MDA-MB-435 human breast cancer cell line is not responsive to estrogen, does not contain estrogen receptors (ERs), and is highly metastatic; thus it can be used to determine the effect of FS lignans on metastasis and other non-ER mediated mechanisms.

Athymic nude mice with established MDA-MB-435 tumors were then divided into two groups: a BD group and a 10% FS group.[44] The mice remained on the diets for 7 weeks and palpable tumors were measured weekly. The mice fed the FS diet not only had smaller tumors but also had a 45% less incidence of total metastasis (including lung and lymph node) compared to the BD-fed mice. Similar results were obtained when the study was repeated, showing that FS reduced MDA-MB-435 breast tumor metastasis incidence by 60% compared to the BD control.[45]

Using the same study design as above, two more studies were conducted in which mice with established MDA-MB-435 tumors were divided into five groups and treated with BD, 10% FS, SDG, FS oil (FO), or SDG + FO.[46] The levels of SDG and FO were equivalent to that found in the 10% FS diet. After 6 weeks, the 10% FS and SDG + FO groups had significant reductions in metastasis incidence, suggesting that both the lignan and the ALA-rich oil components contribute to the antimetastatic effect of FS.

In the second study, tumors were excised prior to randomization into the same five treatment groups as above to determine if FS and its components could reduce the tumor recurrence and metastasis.[47] After 6 weeks treatment, no significant effect of FS or its components on recurrent tumor incidence was observed compared to the BD control. However, when the treatment groups were subdivided according to the size of the primary tumors that were excised i.e., ≤9 or >9 g, FS and SDG diets significantly lowered the recurrent tumor incidence in mice with ≤9 g tumors compared to those with >9 g tumors. No such difference was observed in the BD control, FO, and SDG + FO groups. In addition, all treatment groups reduced the incidence of total metastasis (lymph node, lung, and other organs). This study suggests that FS and its components may affect tumor metastasis to a greater extent than tumor recurrence. However, the results on tumor recurrence incidence indicate that smaller tumors may be more susceptible to the effects of FS and its lignan.

### 19.3.2.2.2 ER-Positive Human Breast Tumors

Another human breast cancer cell line commonly utilized in the athymic nude mouse model is MCF-7. This cell line requires estrogen to stimulate growth, contains both ERα and ERβ, but does not metastasize and is therefore used to establish the estrogenic or antiestrogenic potential of compounds. There are two general study designs used when MCF-7 cells are implanted into athymic nude mice. In both cases the mice are ovariectomized and implanted with an estradiol (E2) pellet, which is used to stimulate growth of MCF-7 tumors. Once the tumors are established, the E2 pellet is either removed, to establish a low circulating estrogen level, which simulates a postmenopausal condition, or a new pellet is implanted, which simulates a premenopausal condition.

TAM has been used for decades as an adjuvant therapy for ER+ breast cancers. In patients with breast cancer, tumor regression initially results; however, some exhibit resistance to TAM treatment after a period of 5 years of use, in addition to an increased risk of uterine cancer.[48] TAM also induces menopausal-like symptoms, as it is an antiestrogen.[49] Therefore, some patients use complementary alternative treatments, such as phytoestrogen-rich soy and FS, to alleviate the symptoms.

Recent studies in our laboratory demonstrate the effect of a 10% FS diet alone or in combination with TAM, on the growth of MCF-7 tumors implanted into ovariectomized athymic nude mice.[50] In one study, ovariectomized athymic nude mice were implanted with MCF-7 breast cancer cells and an estradiol (E2) pellet. When the tumors reached an area of ~40 mm$^2$, all E2 pellets were removed (simulating postmenopausal conditions) and the mice were divided into five treatment groups: negative control group fed the BD (E2$^-$); group fed BD supplemented with 10% FS (FS); group given a TAM pellet (5 mg; 60 day release) implant (TAM); and a group given TAM and fed the FS diet (TAM + FS). One group was given a fresh E2 pellet (E2$^+$) and fed the BD to serve as positive control. During the 7 weeks treatment period all tumors initially regressed in size, with the exception of the E2$^+$ group, which increased throughout the duration of the study. The tumors in the FS group regressed continuously to the level of the negative control group. However, the tumors of the TAM group started to grow at week 4, demonstrating TAM resistance. When FS was combined with TAM (TAM + FS), the growth stimulatory effect of TAM was negated. Hence, the final tumor volume and weight in the TAM group were significantly larger than those in the TAM + FS, FS, and negative control groups.

In another study,[50] the design was the same as above with the following exception: after tumors were established, all mice received a fresh E2 pellet (simulating a premenopausal condition) except for the E2 group. The treatment period continued for 6 weeks at which time the animals were sacrificed and tumor volume and weight were recorded. The final tumor volume and weight were the smallest in the FS + TAM group, followed by the TAM, and then the FS group compared to the positive control group. Although the tumor volume and weight of the TAM + FS group were not significantly different from the TAM alone group, further analysis of the tumor proliferation index (measured by Ki67) showed that the TAM + FS tumors had a significantly lower index than the TAM or FS groups alone. This suggests that FS in combination with TAM is more effective in reducing tumor growth, than either one alone, when E2 was high. Although under both the pre- and postmenopausal conditions FS appears to induce more favorable effects on tumor growth when combined with TAM, clinical studies still need to be conducted to confirm these effects seen in animal studies.

FS and the lignans have also been shown to interact with soy and its isoflavone GEN.[51,52] Although many studies have shown a protective effect of soy and GEN on breast cancer growth,[53] some recent studies have shown that they induce growth of MCF-7 tumors in mice[54,55] and MNU-induced tumors in rats.[56] Utilizing the same athymic nude mouse model described above, ovariectomized mice with established MCF-7 tumors had the E2 pellet removed (i.e., simulating postmenopausal conditions) and were fed a 20% soy protein isolate (SPI) diet (containing isoflavones), a 10% FS diet, or 10% FS + SPI diet for 25 weeks.[51] While tumors initially regressed in all treatment groups, by week 12, the tumors of the mice fed the SPI diet started to increase in size and finally had significantly greater weight and volume at the end of the treatment period compared with the negative control group. The 10% FS regressed the tumors when given alone and also prevented the regrowth of the SPI-induced tumor growth (10% FS + SPI).

The same growth pattern was observed when the mice were given daily injections of ENL, END, GEN, or ENL + END + GEN (10 mg/kg BW) for 22 weeks.[52] While all tumors regressed in size at the start of the treatment period, the GEN treated animals had significantly larger tumors than all other treatment groups. The mice that were given a combination of lignans and isoflavones (ENL + END + GEN) had tumors that did not differ in size compared to the BD-fed animals, showing a more beneficial effect on breast tumor growth when these phytoestrogens are consumed in combination as opposed to genistein alone.

### 19.3.2.3 Clinical Study

In a randomized, double-blind, placebo-controlled clinical trial,[57] women with newly diagnosed breast cancer were assigned to eat either a muffin containing 25 g FS or placebo for a mean duration of 32 and 39 days, respectively, to determine if FS could alter tumor biomarkers on tumor biopsies taken at diagnosis and at time of surgery (end of treatment period). While the placebo did not cause significant changes in the tumors, FS treatment significantly reduced tumor cell proliferation (34%) (Ki67 labeling index), increased apoptosis (30.7%), and decreased the expression of c-erbB2 (71%). In addition, urinary lignans increased by 1300% in the FS-treated patients and the intake of FS was significantly correlated with changes in c-erbB2 score and apoptotic index. These results suggest that the lignans, perhaps in combination with other components such as the oil in FS, may in part be responsible for the changes in tumor biomarkers.

In summary, several experimental studies, described above, showed that FS and its lignans have both preventative and treatment roles in breast cancer. However, the mechanisms of action still remain unclear. Several studies, discussed below, have been conducted, primarily using *in vitro* models, to help elucidate the potential mechanisms of lignan action.

## 19.4  MECHANISMS

Several mechanisms have been suggested regarding how lignans may achieve their protective effects on breast cancer. Due to the structural similarities between lignans and estrogens, it has been hypothesized that the lignans may interfere and/or interact with endogenous estrogen by altering estrogen bioavailability, modulating estrogen synthesis, and altering estrogen action. However, other non-hormone-related mechanisms have also been suggested including antimetastatic and anti-angiogenic.

### 19.4.1  ALTERING ESTROGEN BIOAVAILABILITY

Estrogen is a major stimulus of breast cancer proliferation and thus reducing its availability may reduce its action on breast tumors.[58] This may be accomplished by altering the production or availability of sex hormone-binding globulin (SHBG). Of the circulating estrogens only 2 to 3% is free or biologically active, as most of the hormone is bound to albumin or SHBG. SHBG is a plasma glycoprotein that binds with high affinity to steroid hormones, such as estrogen and testosterone, thus regulating their free concentration in plasma. *In vitro* studies have shown that ENL stimulates the production of SHBG.[59] An increase in SHBG would potentially increase the amount of bound estrogen therefore decreasing the amount of free biologically active estrogen. This would reduce the ability of estrogen to reach target tissues and thus reduce estrogenic effects.

Human studies conducted to evaluate this mechanism have been inconsistent. Phipps et al.[60] showed that although urinary lignan excretion increased following FS ingestion by premenopausal women, plasma levels of SHBG did not change. However, Adlercreutz et al.[61] observed a positive correlation between plasma SHBG and urinary excretion of lignans, suggesting that the lignans may be able to alter biologically active estrogen levels by modulating SHBG production. Hutchins et al.[62] conducted a cross-over study design where 28 postmenopausal women were fed either a control (usual diet), 5 g ground FS, or 10 g ground FS per day for 7 weeks, with 7 to 14 week washout periods between each treatment. Although there was no difference in SHBG levels, serum E2 was decreased in the women who consumed either the 5 or 10 g ground FS per day compared to the controls. The difference between the results of these studies may be related to the difference between the subjects' hormonal status, the dose of FS used, and the length of FS exposure.

### 19.4.2 Altering Estrogen Synthesis and Metabolism

#### 19.4.2.1 Estrogen Synthesis

There are two main enzymes involved in the synthesis and regulation of estrogen synthesis: aromatase and 17-hydroxysteroid dehydrogenase (HSD). Aromatase is a cytochrome P450 enzyme responsible for the conversion of androstenedione and testosterone, to estrone (E1) and E2, respectively, while HSD controls the balance between E2 and the less biologically active E1. Present-day interest in aromatase is due to the findings that human breast cancers have increased aromatase expression[63] and that postmenopausal patients with breast cancer have higher levels of estradiol in the breast tissue compared to plasma,[64] suggesting local estradiol production. Therefore, aromatase inhibitors may benefit some patients with breast cancer by inhibiting aromatase conversion of androgens to estrogens, the main proliferative stimulator of some breast cancers.[58] Because ENL and END have been shown to be inhibitors of human placental aromatase,[65] and HSD in genital skin fibroblast,[66] ingestion of FS or lignans may induce these effects in breast cancer cells, and thus inhibit estrogen stimulated growth.

An *in vitro* study was conducted to determine the effect of ENL and END on aromatase and HSD activity, and subsequent proliferation of MCF-7.[67] ENL and END (10 $\mu M$) were shown to reduce the production of E1 from androstenedione, by 37 and 81%, respectively, indicating decreased aromatase activity in MCF-7 cells. ENL (50 $\mu M$) also reduced the conversion of E2 from E1 by 84%, thereby indicating an inhibition of HSD. When changes in enzyme activity were related to changes in cell proliferation, significant positive correlations were observed for ENL inhibition of aromatase activity, ENL inhibition of HSD activity, and the reduction in MCF-7 cell proliferation, indicating that the mammalian lignans reduce the proliferation of MCF-7 cells in part by inhibiting enzymes involved in estrogen synthesis and thus may be a mechanism for their role in decreasing breast cancer growth.

## 19.4.2.2  Estrogen Metabolism

The metabolism of estrogen results in the production of the two major estrogen metabolites, 2-hydroxyestrone (2OHE1) and 16-hydroxyestrone (16OHE1), with low biological activity associated with 2OHE1 and estrogenic activity associated with 16OHE1 as indicated by induction of breast cancer cell growth.[68] It was therefore hypothesized that the ratio of these two metabolites may be a useful biomarker of breast cancer risk; with a low 2OHE1:16OHE1 corresponding to an increased breast cancer risk.[69] The daily intake of 25 g FS for 16 weeks by postmenopausal women has been shown to increase urinary 2OHE1:16OHE1 ratio, by increasing the excretion of the less biological active estrogen metabolite 2OHE1.[70] The increased ratio was positively correlated with urinary lignan levels, suggesting that the lignans may be partially responsible for the changes in estrogen metabolism. Haggans et al.[71] observed similar effects in premenopausal women who consumed 10 g FS/day lasting over two menstrual cycles, i.e., significant increase in the 2OHE1:16OHE1 ratio, with an increase of the 2OHE1 metabolite during the luteal phase of the menstrual cycle.

## 19.4.3  Altering Estrogen Action

The lignans have been shown in several studies[72,73] to either induce estrogenic effects or interfere with estrogen action in breast cancer cells and thus have been characterized as having both weak estrogenic and antiestrogenic activities. The effect of ENL and END on DNA synthesis in MCF-7 cells was analyzed and it was found that ~10 $\mu M$ ENL stimulated DNA synthesis to a level that was ~60% of that stimulated by estradiol. However, when TAM, a known inhibitor of estrogen action, was combined with 10 $\mu M$ ENL, DNA synthesis was inhibited, suggesting that ENL was acting through an estrogenic pathway.[72] Wang and Kurzer[73] also analyzed the effect of the lignan ENL on DNA synthesis in both MCF-7 cells and in an estrogen-independent cell line MDA-MB-231. While 10 $\mu M$ ENL induced DNA synthesis in the MCF-7 cells, it did not in the MDA-MB-231 cells, further suggesting that the lignan acts through an estrogenic pathway. However, at higher concentrations ENL reduced the growth of both cell lines, suggesting that at high concentrations the mechanism of action is through non-ER-mediated pathways.

Estrogen action can be altered by compounds that are estrogen-like in structure (i.e., phytoestrogens) that compete with or inhibit estrogen from binding to the ER (ERα or ERβ), thus decreasing its proliferative stimulus. The ER is a member of the steroid nuclear receptor superfamily of ligand inducible transcription factors.[74] Estrogen binds to the ligand-binding domain of the ER inducing a conformational change that enables binding of certain coactivators or corepressors. The

ER can also dimerize as either ERα or ERβ homodimers or ERα/ERβ heterodimers.[75] ER dimers bind to DNA response elements located upstream of estrogen-sensitive genes, causing either activation or repression of gene transcription, which modulates the growth and development of cells. Genes that are regulated by the ER include genes involved in signaling cell proliferation and cell cycle regulation (TGFβ, IGF, EGF, cyclin D1, c-fos, c-jun, and c-myc).[76]

Competition with estrogen for binding to the ER, at target tissues, can modulate estrogen activity and inhibit estrogen action or potentially activate the ER in a way similar to estrogen. It has been shown previously that other phytoestrogens, such as the isoflavones GEN and equol, bind to ERβ with a higher affinity than to ERα.[77] This finding suggests that the phytoestrogens may elicit their estrogenic or antiestrogenic effects through this ER subtype. Mueller et al.[78] recently determined the binding affinity of the lignan ENL and its hydroxylated metabolite 6OH-ENL, for ERα and ERβ. Both ENL and 6OH-ENL appear to have a higher affinity to ERα compared to ERβ. These results do not agree with the general understanding that the phytoestrogens have preferential binding affinity for ERβ, which suggests that the lignans may act through the ER differently compared to other phytoestrogens.

The transcriptional activation potential of ENL and END were studied in an ERα or ERβ transfected cell line.[79] The authors concluded that there was no transcriptional activation through either ER subtype at lignan concentrations <1 μM; however, at ENL concentrations >1 μM activation through both ERα and ERβ was observed, while END only induced transcriptional activation through ERα at concentrations >1 μM. This suggests that the lignans may be weak agonists of ER-mediated activities. In addition, ENL and END were unable to inhibit E2 transcriptional activation through the ERs, suggesting that the lignans may not act as antiestrogens.

## 19.4.4 Non-ER-Mediated Mechanisms

### 19.4.4.1 Effects on Metastasis

Although proliferation is a major outcome of breast cancer development, studying other aspects of breast cancer biology is also important in determining the effects of lignans. As described above (see Section 19.3.2.2.1), FS and its components can reduce the incidence of metastasis of ER-human tumors in mice. However, the cellular mechanisms behind this effect are unclear. Magee et al.[80] analyzed the effect of lignans on breast cancer cell invasion. Invasion, along with adhesion and motility or migration, is one of the primary steps leading to the metastasis of cancer cells to other tissues. The cell line MDA-MB-231 has been shown to be highly metastatic in comparison to the MCF-7 cell line and is therefore used as a model system to determine the effects of compounds on the steps in metastasis. In this study the lignans SECO, MAT, ENL, and END were analyzed for their ability to inhibit the cells from invading through the basement membrane and thus inhibit the initiation of the metastasis process. It was found that only high concentrations of SECO and END (50 μ$M$) could inhibit invasion of MDA-MB-231 cells, suggesting that the main role of lignans as anticancer agents is not through the modulation of the invasion process of metastasis.

A similar study was conducted by Chen and Thompson,[81] in which two ER-human breast cancer cells lines (MDA-MB-435 and MDA-MB-231) were treated with ENL, END, and TAM, alone and in combination, to determine their effects on the metastasis process. Three experiments were carried out to help elucidate which steps (cell adhesion, invasion, and migration) in the metastasis process were affected by these compounds. ENL, END, and TAM significantly reduced cell adhesion at concentrations of 1 or 5 μ$M$; however, this effect differed between the two cell lines, with END and TAM being more effective in the MDA-MB-435 cells. When the cells were treated with END, ENL, and TAM in combination (1 μ$M$), there was a greater reduction in cell adhesion than with any of the three compounds alone. Cell invasion was also reduced by the compounds with the greatest effect seen at 5 μ$M$. When the compounds were given in combination, invasion was further decreased compared to ENL or TAM alone but not compared to END. Cell migration was decreased by ENL and END (0.1 to 10 μ$M$) but was unaffected by TAM at concentrations (0.1 to 1 μ$M$); however, at 10 μ$M$, TAM significantly increased cell migration. The authors concluded that the lignans affect the metastasis process at multiple levels and that the effect may be enhanced when combined with the breast cancer drug TAM.

Although the studies above[80,81] have contrasting conclusions on the effect of lignans on cell invasion, several differences in study design can be noted, particularly in the concentrations of ENL and END and cell lines used (Chen and Thompson: 0.1, 1, 5, 10 μ$M$; Magee et al.: 2.5, 10, 50 μ$M$). Chen and Thompson[81] observed reductions in MDA-MB-435 cell invasion at low concentrations (5 μ$M$) but not in the MDA-MD-231 cell line at 10 μ$M$, which agrees with the finding by Magee et al.,[80] who observed in MDA-MB-231 reductions only at 50 μ$M$. Therefore, the effects of the lignans on cell invasion may be concentration and cell line dependent.

### 19.4.4.2   Effects on Growth Factors

Several growth factors have been correlated with breast cancer risk. In particular, insulin-like growth factor 1 (IGF-1), epidermal growth factor (EGF), and vascular endothelial growth factor (VEGF) are positively associated with breast cancer risk.[82,83] Thus, if FS or the lignans can alter the level of certain growth factors, it may be one of the mechanisms of their anticancer effects. In one study, rats fed a 5% FS diet or its equivalent amount of SDG for 4 weeks had reduced serum IGF-1 compared to the control group.[84] However, when the rats received a MNU carcinogen, only the 5% FS diet reduced serum IGF-1 levels. As described previously, a 5% FS diet reduced the MNU tumor invasiveness and grade;[41] therefore, a reduction in IGF-1 may be a potential mechanism for reducing tumor progression.

Tumor cell proliferation, IGF-1, and EGF receptor (EGFR), but not VEGF, were also reduced in nude mice with established MDA-MB-435 tumors fed a 10% FS diet compared to control.[44] In this study, tumor growth and metastasis incidence was reduced by FS and thus may be, in part, related to the FS-induced reduction in EGF and IGF signaling pathways. When this study was repeated and VEGF was measured in the tumor extracellular fluid[45] as opposed to within tumor sections,[44] VEGF was significantly lower in the FS compared to BD group. VEGF is a promoter of angiogenesis, the formation of new blood vessels necessary for metastasis to occur, indicating that FS may decrease the incidence of metastasis by decreasing angiogenesis.

Growth factors were also reduced in the mammary gland of rats that were exposed to FS and SDG during suckling.[35] While 10% FS decreased EGF in TEB and lobules at PND 49-51, SDG increased EGFR in rat mammary gland (TEB and TD) at PND 21 but reduced EGFR in TEB and LOB at PND 49-51. Since early exposure to FS or SDG is protective against breast carcinogenesis,[37] altering the mammary gland EGF pathway may be a potential mechanism.

## 19.5 CONCLUSION

Epidemiological studies did not show a consistent relationship between risk of breast cancer and lignan exposure based on lignan intake, urinary lignan excretion, or plasma lignan levels. However, a majority of the studies show a negative relationship. On the other hand, experimental studies using either FS or the lignans have shown that both can prevent tumor development and decrease tumor growth, although a clear mechanism of action is yet to be established. Because the lignans are phytoestrogens, they are thought to act through the ER pathway; however, other nonhormone-mediated effects have also been observed. Gene array analysis of tumors treated with FS may be useful in identifying pathways that are affected by FS. With encouraging results from animal studies, clinical studies on the effect of FS and lignans on breast cancer should be conducted in the future. In particular, the interesting finding that FS in combination with TAM is more beneficial than TAM alone in reducing tumor growth and TAM resistance suggests a potentially good treatment regimen for patients with breast cancer. More research on FS or lignan interactions with other cancer drugs needs to be explored in the future.

## REFERENCES

1. Thompson L, Cunanne S, eds. *Flaxseed in Human Nutrition*; 2nd ed. Champaign, Illinois: AOCS Press; 2004.
2. Thompson L, Robb P, Serraino M, Cheung F. Mammalian lignan production from various foods. *Nutr Cancer* 1991; 16:43–52.
3. Bowey E, Adlercreutz H, Rowland I. Metabolism of isoflavones and lignans by the gut microflora: a study in germ-free and human flora associated rats. *Food Chem Toxicol* 2003; 41:631–636.

4. Kilkkinen A, Pietinen P, Klaukka T, Virtamo J, Korhonen P, Adlercreutz H. Use of oral antimicrobials decreases serum enterolactone concentration. *Am J Epidemiol* 2002; 155:472–477.

5. Adlercreutz H, van der Wildt J, Kinzel J, Attalla H, Wahala K, Makela T, Hase T, Fotsis T. Lignan and isoflavonoid conjugates in human urine. *J Steroid Biochem Mol Biol* 1995; 52:97–103.

6. Saarinen N, Smeds A, Makela S, Ammala J, Hakala K, Pihlava J, Ryhanen E, Sjoholm R, Santti R. Structural determinants of plant lignans for the formation of enterolactone *in vivo*. *J Chromatogr B Anal Technol Biomed Life Sci* 2002; 777:311–319.

7. Adlercreutz H, Fotsis T, Heikkinen R, Dwyer J, Woods M, Goldin B, Gorbach S. Excretion of the lignans enterolactone and enterodiol and of equol in omnivorous and vegetarian postmenopausal women and in women with breast cancer. *Lancet* 1982; 2:1295–1299.

8. Morton M, Chan P, Cheng C, Blacklock N, Matos-Ferreira A, Abranches-Montero L, Correia R, Lloyd S, Griffiths K. Lignans and isoflavonoids in plasma and prostatic fluid in men: samples from Portugal, Hong Kong, and the United Kingdom. *Prostate* 1997; 32:122–128.

9. Adlercreutz H. Review: phyto-oestrogens and cancer. *Lancet Oncol* 2002; 3:364–373.

10. Magee P, Rowland I. Phyto-oestrogens, their mechanism of action: current evidence for a role in breast and prostate cancer. *Br J Nutr* 2004; 9:513–531.

11. Ingram D, Sanders K, Kolybaba M, Lopez D. Case-control study of phyto-oestrogens and breast cancer. *Lancet* 1997; 350:990–994.

12. Dai Q, Franke A, Jin F, Shu X, Hebert J, Custer L, Cheng J, Gao Y, Zheng W. Urinary excretion of phytoestrogens and risk of breast cancer among Chinese women in Shanghai. *Cancer Epidemiol Biomarkers Prev* 2002; 11:815–821.

13. McCann S, Moysich K, Freudenheim J, Ambrosone C, Shields P. The risk of breast cancer associated with dietary lignans differs by CYP17 genotype in women. *J Nutr* 2002; 132:3036–3041.

14. Horn-Ross P, John E, Lee M, Steward S, Koo J, Sakoda L, Shiau A, Goldstein J, Davis P, Perez-Stable E. Phytoestrogen consumption and breast cancer risk in a multiethnic population. *Am J Epidemiol* 2001; 154:434–441.

15. Pietinen P, Stumpf K, Mannisto S, Kataja V, Uusitupa M, Adlercreutz H. Serum enterolactone and the risk of breast cancer. A case control study in eastern Finland. *Cancer Epidemiol Biomarkers Prev* 2001; 10:339–344.

16. Tonkelaar den I, Keinan-Boker L, Veer van't P, Arts C, Adlercreutz H, Thijssen J, Peeters P. Urinary phyto-oestrogens and postmenopausal breast cancer risk. *Cancer Epidemiol Biomarkers Prev* 2001; 10:223–228.

17. Hulten K, Winkvist A, Lenner P, Johansson R, Adlercreutz H, Hallmans G. An incident case-referent study on plasma enterolactone and breast cancer risk. *Eur J Nutr* 2002; 41:168–176.

18. Horn-Ross P, Barnes S, Lee M, Coward L, Mandel J, Koo J, John E, Smith M. Assessing phytoestrogen exposure in epidemiological studies: development of a database (United States). *Cancer Causes Control* 2000; 11:289–298.

19. Mazur W., Fotsis T., Wahala K., Ojala S., Salakka A., Adlercreutz H. Isotope dilution gas chromatographic-mass spectrometric method for the determination of isoflavonoids, coumestrol, and lignans in food samples. *Anal Biochem* 1996; 233:169–180.

20. McCann S, Muti P, Vitp D, Edge S, Trevisan M, Freudenheim J. Dietary lignan intakes and risk of pre- and postmenopausal breast cancer. *Int J Cancer* 2004; 111:440–443.

21. Linseisen J, Piller R, Hermann S, Chang-Claude J. Dietary phytoestrogen intake and premenopausal breast cancer risk in a German case-control study. *Int J Cancer* 2004; 110:284–290.

22. Keinan-Boker L, van der Schouw Y, Grobbee D, Peeters P. Dietary phytoestrogens and breast cancer risk. *Am J Clin Nutr* 2004; 79:282–288.

23. De Kleijn M, van Der Schouw Y, Wilson P, Adlercreutz H, Mazur W, Grobbee D, Jacques P. Intake of dietary phytoestrogens is low in postmenopausal women in the United States: the Framingham study. *J Nutr* 2001; 131:1826–1832.

24. Mazur W, Fotsis T, Wahala K, Ojala S, Salakka A, Adlercreutz H. Isotope dilution gas chromatographic-mass spectrometric method for the determination of isoflavonoids, coumestrol, and lignans in food samples. *Anal Biochem* 1996; 233:169–180.

25. Adlercreutz H, Wang G, Lapcik O, Hampl R, Wahala K, Makela T, Lusa K, Talme M, Mikola H. Time-resolved fluoroimmunoassay for plasma enterolactone. *Anal Biochem* 1998; 265:208–213.

26. Stumpf K, Uehara M, Nurmi T, Adlercreutz H. Changes in the time-resolved fluoroimmunoassay of plasma enterolactone. *Anal Biochem* 2000; 284:153–157.

27. Zeleniuch-Jacquotte A, Adlercreutz H, Shore R, Koenig K, Kato I, Arslan A, Toniolo P. Circulating enterolactone and risk of breast cancer: a prospective study in New York. *Br J Cancer* 2004; 91:99–105.

28. Kilkkinen A, Virtamo J, Vartiainen E, Sankila R, Virtanen M, Adlercreutz H, Pietinen P. Serum enterolactone concentration is not associated with breast cancer risk in a nested case-control study. *Int J Cancer* 2004; 108:277–280.

29. Boccardo F, Lunardi G, Guglielmini P, Pardori M, Murialdo R, Schettini G, Rubagotti A. Serum enterolactone levels and risk of breast cancer in women with palpable cysts. *Eur J Cancer* 2004; 40:84–89.

30. Hausner H, Johnsen N, Hallund J, Tetens I. A single measurement is inadequate to estimate enterolactone levels in Danish postmenopausal women due to large intraindividual variation. *J Nutr* 2004; 134:1197–1200.

31. Russo J, Lynch H, Russo H. Mammary gland architecture as a determining factor in the susceptibility of the human breast to cancer. *Breast J* 2001; 7:278–291.

32. Tou J, Chen J, Thompson L. Flaxseed and its lignan precursor, secoisolariciresinol diglycoside, affect pregnancy outcome and reproductive development in rats. *J Nutr* 1998; 128:1861–1868.

33. Tou J, Thompson L. Exposure to flaxseed or its lignan component during different developmental stages influences rat mammary gland structures. *Carcinogenesis* 1999; 20:1831–1835.

34. Ward W, Jiang F, Thompson L. Exposure to flaxseed or purified lignan during lactation influences rat mammary gland structures. *Nutr Cancer* 2000; 37:187–192.

35. Tan K, Chen J, Ward W, Thompson L. Mammary gland morphogenesis is enhanced by exposure to flaxseed or its major lignan during suckling in rats. *Exp Biol Med* 2004; 229:147–157.

36. Tou J, Chen J, Thompson L. Flaxseed and its lignan precursor, secoisolariciresinol diglycoside, affect pregnancy outcome and reproductive development in rats. *J Nutr* 1998; 128:1861–1868.

37. Chen J, Tan K, Ward W, Thompson L. Exposure to flaxseed or its purified lignan during suckling inhibits chemically induced rat mammary tumorigenesis. *Exp Biol Med (Maywood)* 2003; 228:951–958.

38. Serraino M and Thompson L. The effect of flaxseed supplementation on early risk markers for mammary carcinogenesis. *Cancer Lett* 1991; 60:135–142.

39. Serraino M, Thompson L. The effect of flaxseed supplementation on the initiation and promotional stages of mammary tumorigenesis. *Nutr Cancer* 1992; 17:153–159.

40. Thompson L, Seidl M, Rickard S, Orcheson L, Fong H. Antitumorigenic effect of a mammalian lignan precursor from flaxseed. *Nutr Cancer* 1996; 26:159–165.

41. Rickard S, Yuan Y, Chen J, Thompson L. Dose effects of flaxseed and its lignan on N-methyl-N-nitrosourea-induced mammary tumorigenesis in rats. *Nutr Cancer* 1999; 35:50–57.

42. Thompson L, Rickard S, Orcheson L, Seidl M. Flaxseed and its lignan and oil components reduce mammary tumor growth at a late stage of carcinogenesis. *Carcinogenesis* 1996; 17:1373–1376.

43. Saarinen N, Huovinen R, Warri A, Makela S, Valentin-Blasini L, Sjoholm R, Ammala J, Lehtila R, Eckerman C, Collan Y, Santti R. Enterolactone inhibits the growth of 7,12-dimethylbenz(a)anthracene-induced mammary carcinomas in the rat. *Mol Cancer Ther* 2002; 1:869–876.

44. Chen J, Stavro P, Thompson L. Dietary flaxseed inhibits human breast cancer growth and metastasis and downregulates expression of insulin-like growth factor and epidermal growth factor receptor. *Nutr Cancer* 2002; 43:187–192.

45. Dabrosin C, Chen J, Wang L, Thompson L. Flaxseed inhibits metastasis and decreases extracellular vascular endothelial growth factor in human breast cancer xenografts. *Cancer Lett* 2002; 185:31–37.

46. Wang L, Chen J, Thompson L. The inhibitory effect of flaxseed on the growth and metastasis of estrogen receptor negative breast cancer xenografts is attributed to both its lignan and oil components. *Int J Cancer* 2005; in press.

47. Chen J, Wang L, Thompson L. Flaxseed and its components reduce metastasis after surgical excision of solid human breast tumors in nude mice. *Cancer Lett* 2005; in press.

48. Jordan C. Selective estrogen receptor modulation: concept and consequences in cancer. *Cancer Cell* 2004; 5:207–213.

49. Malinovszky K, Cameron D, Douglas S, Love C, Leonard T, Dixon J, Hopwood P, Leonard R. Breast cancer patients' experiences on endocrine therapy: monitoring with a checklist for patients on endocrine therapy (C-PET). *Breast* 2004; 13:363–368.

50. Chen J, Hui E, Ip T, Thompson L. Dietary flaxseed enhances the inhibitory effect of tamoxifen on the growth of estrogen dependent human breast cancer (MCF-7) in nude mice. *Clin Cancer Res* 2004; 10:7703–7711.

51. Power K, Saarinen N, Chen J, Thompson L. Lignans (enterolactone and enterodiol) negate the proliferative effect of isoflavone (genistein) on MCF-7 breast cancer cells *in vitro* and *in vivo*. *Am Assoc Cancer Res (AACR) Proc* 2004; 45:878.

52. Saarinen N, Power K, Chen J, Thompson L. Flaxseed attenuates the tumor promoting effect of soy in ovariectomized athymic mice with breast cancer xenografts. *Am Assoc Cancer Res (AACR) Proc* 2004; 45:878.

53. Sarkar F, Li Y. Soy isoflavones and cancer prevention. *Cancer Invest* 2003; 21:744–757.
54. Ju Y, Allred C, Allred K, Karko K, Doerge D, Helferich W. Physiological concentrations of dietary genistein dose-dependently stimulate growth of estrogen-dependent human breast cancer (MCF-7) tumors implanted in athymic nude mice. *J Nutr* 2001; 131:2957–2962.
55. Allred C, Ju Y, Allred K, Chang J, Helferich W. Dietary genistin stimulates growth of estrogen-dependent breast cancer tumors similar to that observed with genistein. *Carcinogenesis* 2001; 22:1667–1673.
56. Allred C, Allred K, Ju Y, Clausen L, Doerge D, Schantz S, Korol D, Wallig M, Helferich W. Dietary genistein results in larger MNU-induced, estrogen-dependent mammary tumors following ovariectomy of Sprague-Dawley rats. *Carcinogenesis* 2004; 25:211–218.
57. Thompson L, Chen J, Li T, Strasser-Weippl K, Goss P. Dietary flaxseed alters tumor biological markers in postmenopausal breast cancer. *Clin Cancer Res* 2005; 11:3828–3835.
58. Santen R, Yue W, Naftolin F, Mor G, Berstein L. The potential of aromatase inhibitors in breast cancer prevention. *Endocrine Related Cancer* 1999; 6:235–243.
59. Martin M, Haourigui M, Pelissero C, Benassayag C, Nunez E. Interactions between phytoestrogens and human sex steroid binding protein. *Life Sci* 1996; 58:429–436.
60. Phipps W, Martini M, Lampe J, Slavin J, Kurzer M. Effect of flax seed ingestion on the menstrual cycle. *J Clin Endocrinol Metab* 1993; 77:1215–1219.
61. Adlercreutz H, Mousavi Y, Clark J, Hockerstedt K, Hamalainen E, Wahala K, Makela T, Hase T. Dietary phytoestrogens and cancer: *in vitro* and *in vivo* studies. *J Steroid Biochem Mol Biol* 1992; 41:331–337.
62. Hutchins A, Martini M, Olson B, Thomas W, Slavin J. Flaxseed consumption influences endogenous hormone concentrations in postmenopausal women. *Nutr Cancer* 2001; 39:58–65.
63. Lu Q, Nakamura J, Savinov A, Yue W, Weisz J, Dabbs D, Wolz G, Brodie A. Expression of aromatase protein and messenger ribonucleic acid in tumor epithelial cells and evidence of functional significance of locally produced estrogen in human breast cancers. *Endocrinology* 1996; 137:3061–3077.
64. Pasqualini J, Chetrite G, Blacker C, Feinstein M, Delalonde L, Talbi M, Maloche C. Concentrations of estrone, estradiol, and estrone sulfate and evaluation of sulfatase and aromatase activities in pre- and postmenopausal breast cancer patients. *J Clin Endocrinol Metab* 1996; 81:1460–1464.
65. Adlercreutz H, Bannwart C, Wahala K, Makela T, Brunow G, Hase T, Arosemena P, Kellis J, Vickery L. Inhibition of human aromatase by mammalian lignans and isoflavonoid phytoestrogens. *J Steroid Biochem Mol Biol* 1993; 44:147–153.
66. Evans B, Griffiths K, Morton M. Inhibition of 5 alpha-reductase in genital skin fibroblasts and prostate tissue by dietary lignans and isoflavonoids. *J Endocrinol* 1995; 147:295–302.
67. Brooks J, Thompson L. Mammalian lignans and genistein decrease the activities of aromatase and 17β-hydroxysteroid dehydrogenase in MCF-7 cells. *J Steroid Biochem Mol Biol* 2005; 94:461–467.

68. Gupta M, McDougal A, Safe S. Estrogenic and antiestrogenic activities of 16α and 2-hydroxy metabolites of 17β-estradiol in MCF-7 and T47D human breast cancer cells. *J Steroid Biochem Mol Biol* 1998; 67:413–419.

69. Osborne M, Bradlow H, Wong G, Telang N. Upregulation of estradiol C16 alpha-hydroxylation in human breast tissue: a potential biomarker of breast cancer risk. *J Natl Cancer Inst* 1993; 85:1917–1920.

70. Brooks J, Ward W, Lewis J, Hilditch J, Nickell L, Wong E, Thompson L. Supplementation with flaxseed alters estrogen metabolism in postmenopausal women to a greater extent than does supplementation with an equal amount of soy. *Am J Clin Nutr* 2004; 79:318–325.

71. Haggans C, Travelli E, Thomas W, Martini M, Slavin J. The effect of flaxseed and wheat bran consumption on urinary estrogen metabolites in premenopausal women. *Cancer Epidemiol Biomarkers Prev* 2000; 9:719–725.

72. Welshons W, Murphy C, Koch R, Calaf G, Jordan V. Stimulation of breast cancer cells in vitro by the environmental estrogen enterolactone and the phytoestrogen equol. *Breast Cancer Res Treat* 1987; 10:169–175.

73. Wang C, Kurzer MS. Phytoestrogen concentration determines effects on DNA synthesis in human breast cancer cells. *Nutr Cancer* 1997; 28:236–247.

74. Tsai M, O'Malley B. Molecular mechanisms of action of steroid/thyroid receptor superfamily members. *Annu Rev Biochem* 1994; 63:451–486.

75. Pettersson K, Grandien K, Kuiper G, Gustafsson J. Mouse estrogen receptor beta forms estrogen response element-binding heterodimers with estrogen receptor alpha. *Mol Endocrinol* 1997; 11:1486–1496.

76. Ciocca D, Fanelli M. Estrogen receptors and cell proliferation in breast cancer. *Trends Endocrinol Metab* 1997; 8:313–321.

77. Kuiper G, Lemmen J, Carlsson B, Corton J, Safe S, van der Saag P, van der Burg B, Gustafsson J. Interaction of estrogenic chemicals and phytoestrogens with estrogen receptor beta. *Endocrinology* 1998; 139:4252–4563.

78. Mueller S, Simon S, Chae K, Metzler M, Korach K. Phytoestrogens and their human metabolites show distinct agonistic and antagonistic properties on estrogen receptor alpha (ERα) and ERβ in human cells. *Toxicol Sci* 2004; 80:14–25.

79. Saarinen N, Warri A, Makela S, Eckerman C, Reunanen M, Ahotupa M, Salmi S, Franke A, Kangas L, Santti R. Hydroxymatairesinol, a novel enterolactone precursor with antitumor properties from coniferous tree (*Picea abies*). *Nutr Cancer* 2000; 36:207–216.

80. Magee P, McGlynn H, Rowland I. Differential effects of isoflavones and lignans on invasiveness of MDA-MB-231 breast cancer cells in vitro. *Cancer Lett* 2004; 208:35–41.

81. Chen J, Thompson L. Lignans and tamoxifen, alone or in combination, reduce human breast cancer cell adhesion, invasion and migration *in vitro*. *Breast Cancer Res Treat* 2003; 80:163–170.

82. Lee AV, Cui X, Oesterreich S. Cross-talk among estrogen receptor, epidermal growth factor, and insulin-like growth factor signaling in breast cancer. *Clin Cancer Res* 2001; 7:4429–4435.

83. Osborne C, Schiff R. Growth factor receptor cross-talk with estrogen receptor as a mechanism for tamoxifen resistance in breast cancer. *Breast 2003*; 12:362–367.

84. Rickard S, Yuan Y, Thompson L. Plasma insulin-like growth factor I levels in rats are reduced by dietary supplementation of flaxseed or its lignan secoisolariciresinol diglycoside. *Cancer Lett* 2000; 161:47–55.

# 20 Anthocyanins and Cancer Prevention

*Colin D. Kay and Bruce J. Holub*

## CONTENTS

20.1 Introduction .................................................................................412
    20.1.1 Diet and Cancer ...............................................................412
    20.1.2 Flavonoids and Cancer ....................................................412
    20.1.3 Anthocyanins ..................................................................413
    20.1.4 Anthocyanins and Cancer................................................414
20.2 Antioxidant Activity ....................................................................416
    20.2.1 Structural Characteristics Effecting Antioxidant Activity ........416
    20.2.2 Glycosylation and Antioxidant Capacity .......................416
    20.2.3 Absorption, Metabolism, and Biological Antioxidant
           Activity ............................................................................417
    20.2.4 Effect of pH on Antioxidant Activity.............................418
    20.2.5 Compartmentalization and Antioxidant Activity ...........418
20.3 Beyond Radical Scavenging .......................................................419
    20.3.1 Direct Protection against DNA Damage.........................419
    20.3.2 Enzymatic Antioxidant Defense......................................419
    20.3.3 Cell Cycle and Tumor Development................................420
20.4 Hormone Activity ........................................................................421
20.5 Inflammation ................................................................................422
    20.5.1 Inflammation and Arachidonic Acid Metabolism..........422
    20.5.2 Inflammation, Oxidation, and Carcinogenesis...............424
20.6 Chemical-Induced Carcinogenesis .............................................424
    20.6.1 Phase I Xenobiotic Detoxification ..................................424
    20.6.2 Phase II Xenobiotic Detoxification .................................425
20.7 Conclusions..................................................................................425
References ..............................................................................................426

## 20.1 INTRODUCTION

### 20.1.1 DIET AND CANCER

Diet has been reported to play a role in the initiation and/or progression of between 35 and 70% of all cancers.[1-3] It is estimated that the quarter of the population with the lowest dietary intake of fruits and vegetables experiences twice the rate of lung, larynx, oral cavity, esophagus, stomach, colon, rectum, bladder, pancreas, cervix, and ovarian cancer.[2,4] In fact, more than 200 studies in the epidemiological literature have shown that a lack of adequate fruit and vegetable consumption results in increased cancer risk.[1,4,5]

Generally, dietary tocopherols (i.e., vitamin E), ascorbic acid (vitamin C), carotenoids (i.e., β-carotene), folate, selenium, and phenolic and polyphenolic phytochemicals are believed to account for much of the beneficial effects associated with fruit and vegetable consumption.[1,3,6-8] However, results of trials aimed at determining the link between the consumption of any one phytochemical/nutraceutical component and cancer have been inconsistent.[3] This chapter reviews evidence regarding the anticancer properties of the polyphenolic phytochemicals, collectively referred to as flavonoids, and focuses in particular on anthocyanins. As there is limited epidemiological data regarding an association between anthocyanins and cancer specifically, evidence from flavonoids, as a group of compounds including anthocyanins, is initially reviewed.

### 20.1.2 FLAVONOIDS AND CANCER

In recent years, numerous studies have suggested that the polyphenolic flavonoids present in fruits and vegetables may be protective against cancer. Knekt et al.[9] investigated a subset of nearly 10,000 cancer-free men and women from a Finnish survey conducted between the years of 1966 and 1975. Using dietary history and flavonoid intake estimates, the researchers found an inverse association between flavonoid intake and cancer incidence (all sites combined). It was determined that the association was primarily with lung cancer, and that the results were irrespective of the intake of antioxidant vitamins E, C, and β-carotene. Subsequently, Le Marchand et al.[10] conducted a population-based case-control study in Hawaii comprising more than 500 smokers and 500 matched controls. The researchers found an inverse association between the intake of flavonoids (quercetin and naringin) and lung cancer risk after adjusting for saturated fat and β-carotene intakes. It should also be noted that some well-designed studies have reported no association between flavonoid consumption and cancer incidence at various sites. In fact, in four other well-known investigations, no association was found between flavonoid intake and total cancer mortality.[6,11-13] It is also important to note that epidemiological, cohort, and case-control studies most often rely on indirect estimates of flavonoid intake. Generally, only a limited number of flavonoids from various foods are estimated (often fewer than five or six out of a class of thousands), usually with the exclusion of anthocyanins. This shortcoming makes it difficult to establish the magnitude of any effects that flavonoids, as individuals or as a group, may have on disease states of the populous. It is clear that there is a need for more controlled investigations concerning the associations between flavonoid intake and disease. For detailed reviews on the antimutagenic activity of flavonoids refer to Das et al.[14] and Middleton et al.[15]

### 20.1.3 ANTHOCYANINS

Flavonoids are a class of polyphenols comprising more than 4000 identified structures.[16] Flavonoids share a common C6–C3–C6 structure consisting of two aromatic rings linked by three carbons (Figure 20.1). As a result of the vast number of flavonoids identified, it will likely be many years before associations between flavonoids and cancer prevention and/or treatment will be thoroughly established. This chapter focuses on the available evidence for the anticancer properties of a group of flavonoids referred to collectively as anthocyanins.

Anthocyanins are a class of flavonoid prominent in many colored plants. The intense absorption of anthocyanins at visible wavelengths of light impart color (most commonly orange, red, and blue) to plant tissues including flowers, vegetables, and fruits. As a result of their intense colors, they have a history of use as dyeing agents and food additives. There are 18 common base anthocyanidin species, which differ in their patterns of hydroxylation and methylation (Figure 20.2). In addition, there are more than 300 glycoside derivatives of these common structures as well as a rapidly expanding list of identified acylated derivatives.[18,20] In plants, anthocyanins occur in glycosylated forms, generally linked with glucose, galactose, arabinose, rhamnose, xylose, or fructose. The sugar moiety is most often found on the 3 or 5 position, but can also occur at the 7, 3', or 5' positions (for an extensive list of glycosides refer to Mazza and Miniati[20]). Cyanidin, delphinidin, and pelargonidin are the most common anthocyanidins in nature,[18] with cyanidin glycosides reportedly present in nearly 90% of all fruits.[21] Anthocyanins are found in very high concentrations in berry fruits and can range from 10 to 600 mg/100 g fresh weight. A list of berry fruits containing high concentrations of anthocyanins is given in Table 20.1. It is estimated that the average daily consumption of anthocyanins is anywhere between 2 to 215 mg/day.[23]

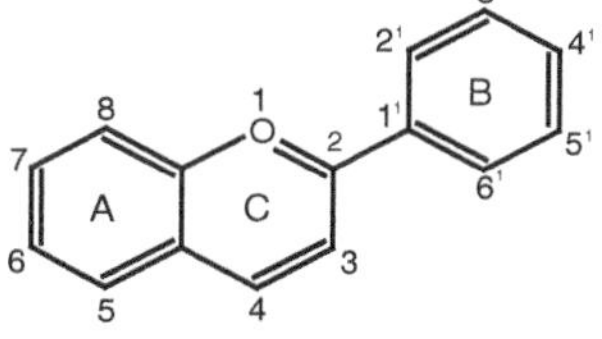

FIGURE 20.1 Basic flavan structure for common flavanoids. (Adapted from Spanos and Wrolstad.[17])

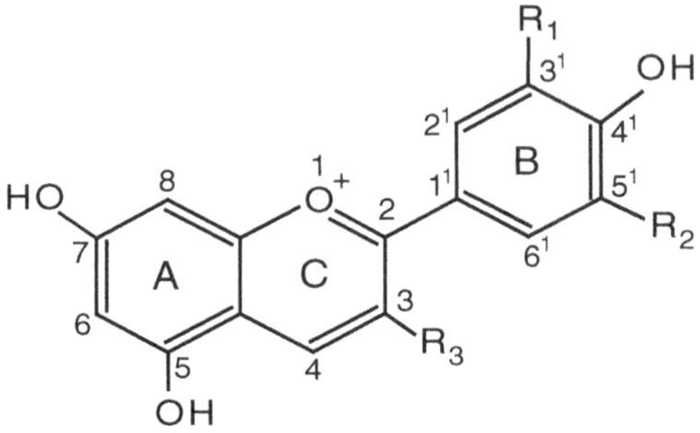

**FIGURE 20.2** Common anthocyanidin structures. (Adapted from Swain,[18] Kalt and Dufour,[19] Mazza and Miniati.[20] For a more complete list of anthocyanidins, refer to Swain.[18] For an extensive list of anthocyanosides, refer to Mazza and Miniati.[20])

| Anthocyanidin | | | |
|---|---|---|---|
| Aglycone | $R_1$ | $R_2$ | $R_3$ |
| Delphinidin | OH | OH | OH |
| Cyanidin | OH | H | OH |
| Petunidin | $OCH_3$ | OH | OH |
| Peonidin | $OCH_3$ | H | OH |
| Malvidin | $OCH_3$ | $OCH_3$ | OH |
| Pelargonidin | H | H | OH |
| Tricetinidin | OH | OH | H |
| Luteolinidin | OH | H | H |
| Apigenidin | H | H | H |

## 20.1.4 ANTHOCYANINS AND CANCER

Many of the perceived health effects associated with the consumption of anthocyanins have been attributed to their antioxidant capacities,[24–26] which often far exceed that of vitamin C and trolox.[27] In *in vitro* systems, anthocyanins have been associated with a variety of antioxidant properties including free radical scavenging, chelation of trace metals, and inhibition of lipid peroxidation and DNA oxidation.[27–33] Additionally, an extensive body of evidence has demonstrated that the consumption of anthocyanins from various sources (plant extracts, fruit juices, various berry species, and red wine) can increase the hydrophilic and lipophilic antioxidant capacity of the blood serum/plasma.[34–42] Recently, researchers have reported a correlation between increased *ex vivo* blood antioxidant status (serum TEAC analysis) and a reduced risk of breast cancer development.[43] As anthocyanins have been associated with increasing the antioxidant capacity of the

## TABLE 20.1
## Berry Fruits Containing High Concentrations of Anthocyanins

| Berry Fruit | Anthocyanins (mg/100 g fresh weight)[a] |
|---|---|
| Bilberry | 300–370 |
| Black currants | 110–430 |
| Black raspberry | 197–428 |
| Blackberry | 133–172 |
| Chokeberry | 305–631 |
| Cranberry | 78 |
| Grapes[b] | 0–603 |
| Highbush blueberry | 63–484 |
| Lingonberry | 174 |
| Lowbush (wild) blueberry | 91–255 |
| Strawberry | 8–79 |

[a] Concentrations represent data from specific investigations. Anthocyanin variability will depend on genus tested, maturity of fruit, size of fruit, and environmental conditions.

[b] The anthocyanin concentration is given for *Vitis vinifera* L. grapes. The high variability results from including both white and red varieties.

*Source:* Adapted from Skrede and Wrolstad.[22]

blood, future interventions involving anthocyanin supplementation as a possible strategy for cancer prevention may be warranted.

Cancer is generally believed to be initiated in part by oxidative mechanisms acting directly upon genetic material (i.e., DNA, RNA).[44,45] Additionally, the oxidation of macromolecules such as lipids and proteins may alter cellular processes associated with cancer development and progression. Many associate the anticancer actions of anthocyanins as simply preventing the oxidation of these biological structures (DNA, lipids, proteins). However, even though anthocyanins have been observed to prevent the oxidation of these structures *in vitro*, a large body of evidence now reveals a possible association between anthocyanins and cancer, which far exceeds their antioxidant properties. In animal and cell models, anthocyanins have been observed to prevent DNA damage, suppress lesion development, reduce the frequency of induced mutation, and inhibit tumor promotion.[27,33,46] The proposed anticarcinogenic mechanisms (as determined by *in vitro* and animal models) involve anthocyanin interactions with mammalian enzymes and receptors including direct protein binding capacities, anti-inflammatory effects, direct antimutagenic activity, inhibition of the metabolic activation of carcinogens, and the activation and induction of enzymes associated with xenobiotic metabolism.[15] Each of these mechanisms is discussed in detail in the following text.

## 20.2  ANTIOXIDANT ACTIVITY

Anthocyanins are highly reactive radical scavengers in various *in vitro* environments. Anthocyanins not only scavenge radicals, but through their ability to bind heavy metals such as iron, zinc, and copper, also prevent the formation of radicals.[47] Anthocyanins may also exert antioxidant abilities through the protection or enhancement of endogenous antioxidants (i.e., sparing effect), or through the induction of antioxidant enzymes such as glutathione-*S*-transferase (GST) and superoxide dismutase (SOD).[48,49] Also, there appears to be a synergism between anthocyanins, vitamin C, and other flavonoids which is similar to the reported recycling effect of vitamin E by vitamin C. This effect was observed in an investigation by Rossetto et al.[31] where the flavonoid catechin was observed to regenerate malvidin 3-glucosides thereby increasing their antioxidant capacity in a micellar system with induced linoleic acid peroxidation.

### 20.2.1  STRUCTURAL CHARACTERISTICS EFFECTING ANTIOXIDANT ACTIVITY

The structural characteristics responsible for the antioxidant effect of anthocyanins are generally associated with the number of free hydroxyls around the pyrone ring (greater number of hydroxyls = greater antioxidant capacity; refer to Figure 20.2); this is, however, an oversimplification. The antioxidant capacity of a polyphenolic compound is dictated not only by the number of free hydroxyls, but also by the basic structural orientation of the compound. The ring orientation will determine the ease of which a hydrogen atom from a hydroxyl group can be donated to a free radical and the ability of the compound to support an unpaired electron. The conjugation of the anthocyanin ring structure is also important. The C2–C3 double bound of the C-ring is consistently associated with a higher antioxidant capacity, having a stabilizing effect on the phenoxy radical.[15,50] The positioning of hydroxyls in relation to one another is also a very important determinant in the antioxidant capacity of anthocyanins. Hydroxyl groups in close proximity, such as the ortho-hydroxyls of the B-ring, appear to greatly enhance the antioxidant capacity of the compound[50,51] in experimental (*in vitro*) models; however, the availability of the highly reactive ortho-hydroxyls in a biological system (*in vivo*) has yet to be established. Conceptually, this site on the B-ring could form bonds with many compounds within biological fluids thus inhibiting the ability of this reactive site to participate in oxidation, metal chelation, or protein binding *in vivo*.

### 20.2.2  GLYCOSYLATION AND ANTIOXIDANT CAPACITY

Anthocyanins are found in plants in glycosylated forms. Glycosylation is reported to influence the antioxidant capacity of flavonoids/anthocyanins.[32,52,53] It is generally stated in the literature that glycosylation decreases the antioxidant capacity of anthocyanins by reducing free hydroxyls and metal chelation sites; however, contradictory results have been reported.[27,54,55] It is important to note that the effect of glycosylation on antioxidant capacity will depend on the environment in which oxidation is being assessed; i.e., aqueous-soluble or lipid-soluble phases.

Glycosylation diminishes the antioxidant capacity of the anthocyanin in an artificial membrane system by decreasing the number of free hydroxyls and metal chelation sites. More importantly, glycosylation will decrease the flavonoids accessibility to membranes as a result of the increased polarity (i.e., increased water solubility) associated with the sugar moiety. The physiological relevance of this effect has, however, not been sufficiently established *in vivo*. Aglycones are less water soluble and therefore have an increased partitioning into the lipid-soluble phase of the artificial membrane system. One would assume that the increased antioxidant capacity of anthocyanidins (aglycones) in this environment would therefore be partly as a result of the increased lipid solubility of the aglycones over the glycosides. Conversely, other assay systems such as the oxygen radical absorbance capacity (ORAC) assay,[54] the ferric reducing assay,[27] and certain lipid oxidation models[55] have found some glycosides to have higher antioxidant capacities than their respective aglycones. Therefore, the *in vitro* effect of glycosylation on antioxidant capacity will depend on the environment in which oxidation is being assessed (aqueous-soluble or lipid-soluble phase). Additionally, because anthocyanin aglycones have not been identified in the blood or urine, the physiological relevance of the antioxidant capacity of aglycones is questionable. This being said, as anthocyanin glycosides are generally believed to be cleaved by colonic microflora, the aglycones theoretically could have physiological relevance within the colon with the glycosides having more systemic relevance. It is clear that the respective *in vivo* antioxidant capabilities of the anthocyanin aglycones vs. their glycoside derivatives require further investigation.

### 20.2.3 ABSORPTION, METABOLISM, AND BIOLOGICAL ANTIOXIDANT ACTIVITY

The biological implications of an anthocyanins antioxidant activity will ultimately depend on the extent of its absorption and metabolism; unfortunately, the absorption and metabolism of anthocyanins are poorly understood. Originally, their absorption was speculated to only occur post-hydrolysis of the glycosidic bond; however, this has been proved incorrect as numerous studies have characterized anthocyanin glycosides in biological fluids. The limited pharmacokinetic data available suggest that the maximum plasma concentrations of 1 to 150 nmol/L are generally reached between 1 and 4 hours post-consumption of doses ranging between 0.1 to 1.0 g. Additionally, less than 1% of the initial dose is generally reported to be recovered in the urine.[21,42,56–60] Although the bioavailability of the parent anthocyanins appears to be low, concentrations of bioactive metabolites could contribute significantly to the anthocyanins bioactivity.

Anthocyanins were previously not believed to be significantly metabolized in humans; however, methylated and glucuronidated metabolites of anthocyanins have recently been reported.[60–62] Furthermore, a study by Felgines et al.[62] suggests that the excretion of anthocyanin metabolites may be as high as 2% of the initial ingested dose. Recent investigations in our laboratory have confirmed that the excretion of metabolites is higher than the excretion of total parent compounds.[62a] Although metabolism (methylation, sulfation, and glucuronidation) will affect the antioxidant capacity of these compounds, they will likely retain much of their bioactivity. Researchers administering quercetin and (–)-catechin to rats have observed an increased antioxidant capacity of the plasma/serum, even though the compounds were identified in the biological fluids as glucuronide and sulfate derivatives.[63] This suggests that conjugated metabolites of the parent compounds contribute to anthocyanin bioactivity.[49,60] Furthermore, researchers propose that the antioxidant activities of anthocyanins are maintained even after their degradation under physiological conditions. It is believed that a portion of absorbed anthocyanins are broken down into benzoic acid derivatives, either spontaneously or as a result of bacterial metabolism in the intestine. Protocatechuic acid is one of these breakdown products that have been characterized in human and animal models.[64] In cell culture experiments, the protocatechuic acid formed from cyanidin glycosides was observed to have antioxidant properties comparable to that of commercial antioxidants including BHT (butylated hydroxyanisole) and vitamin E.[65] This suggests that phenolic acid derivatives of the parent compounds may also play a role in the antioxidant defenses of the blood (serum/plasma) after the consumption of anthocyanins.[49]

### 20.2.4 EFFECT OF pH ON ANTIOXIDANT ACTIVITY

Anthocyanins exist in equilibrium in a variety of protonated, deprotonated, and hydrated forms. These range from colored quinonoid forms, to the flavylium ion, and to colorless hemiacetal forms.[55] The expression of the predominant form is generally pH dependent. There is little evidence regarding the effect of pH on the biological activity of these compounds. However, in spite of the loss of color of anthocyanins at physiological pH (i.e., pH 7), evidence presented by Narayan et al.[66] suggests that anthocyanin glycosides retain their antioxidant activity.

### 20.2.5 COMPARTMENTALIZATION AND ANTIOXIDANT ACTIVITY

Results of trials aimed at determining the link between antioxidant consumption, antioxidant status, and cancer have been inconsistent.[3] Although anthocyanins have shown promise in many *in vitro* antioxidant and anticancer models, it has not been established if these compounds can reach their target of suspected action and if high enough concentrations are reached to elicit an efficient response. Youdim et al.[67] were among the first to show evidence of the incorporation of anthocyanins into cells and cell membranes. In a cell culture experiment, using human aortic endothelial cells, cyanidin glycosides from the elderberry were observed to be incorporated into both the plasma membrane and cytosol. The cells were determined to have significant protection against oxidation induced by reactive oxygen species. Subsequently, Bagchi et al.[68] recently reported on the cellular uptake of berry anthocyanins by endothelial cells. Although absorption was indicated in these studies, the mechanism by which anthocyanins enter intracellular compartments, where genetic materials exist, has yet to be determined. If the antioxidant capacity exhibited by anthocyanins is associated with cancer prevention, their mechanisms likely extend beyond the prevention of DNA base oxidation and lesion formation alone.

## 20.3  BEYOND RADICAL SCAVENGING

### 20.3.1  Direct Protection against DNA Damage

Studies investigating hydrogen peroxide-induced toxicity in cell culture determined that the anthocyanins delphinidin and cyanidin (aglycones and glycosides) were protective against DNA strand breaks in human colon cells.[69,70] Furthermore, glycosides of cyanidin, petunidin, peonidin, and malvidin were observed to decrease the formation of oxidized DNA bases and lipid hydroperoxides in vitamin E–deficient rats.[71] Although the mechanisms mediating these effects have not been determined, pulse radiolysis studies utilizing *in vitro* plasmid environments have indicated that flavonoids may be protective against free radical–induced DNA damage through mechanisms independent of their antioxidant capabilities.[72] Additionally, an investigation by Sarma and Sharma[73] found cyanidin to complex with DNA, forming an anthocyanin-DNA co-pigment, which appeared to protect the DNA from oxidation when exposed to hydroxyl radicals. Unfortunately, the biological implications of such an interaction are at present unknown.

### 20.3.2  Enzymatic Antioxidant Defense

Anthocyanins, and other flavonoids such as quercetin, have been observed to have beneficial effects on endogenous enzymes associated with oxidative stress. In established models of oxidative stress, such as ischemia-reperfusion and hyperoxia, anthocyanins have been observed to inhibit xanthine oxidase, and complement superoxide dismutase, catalase, and glutathione peroxidase.[15,74] Ischemia-reperfusion is associated with the excessive production of reactive oxygen species and subsequent oxidative injury. During ischemia, the catabolism of the available ATP leads to an increased concentration of the purine metabolites xanthine and hypoxanthine. The conversion of xanthine-dehydrogenase to the free radical generating form, xanthine oxidase, occurs under the ischemic condition. Upon reperfusion, when oxygen is reintroduced suddenly, a massive "burst" of free radical generation results from the xanthine oxidase–catalyzed formation of superoxide. The ensuing free radical–mediated chain reaction results in extensive tissue injury at the site of reperfusion as a consequence of the increased leakage of superoxide from dysfunctional mitochondria, the accumulation of leukocytes, the accumulation of reduced catecholamines, flavines and quinines, and the release of iron from heme proteins. Ischemia-reperfusion injury is a major concern during organ transplantation and as result of vascular occlusion. Anthocyanins have been observed to have an inhibitory effect on xanthine oxidase and xanthine dehydrogenase activity under experimentally induced ischemic conditions.[15,74] Additionally, the chronic feeding of cyanidin 3-glucoside to rats resulted in a significant reduction in reactive oxygen radical production and prevented glutathione decline in a hepatic ischemia-reperfusion model of oxidative stress in rats. The resistance imposed by cyanidin-3-glucoside occurred without affecting levels of endogenous serum antioxidant enzymes.[33,75,76]

Hyperoxia is the result of an excess of oxygen in tissues or organs. Although hyperoxia is generally not experienced under normal/basal circumstances, it can be induced experimentally by increasing the level of atmospheric oxygen. Hyperoxia is an excepted model of oxidative stress and generally results in a significant increase in oxygen radical production followed by the induction of vast quantities of endogenous antioxidant defense enzymes including superoxide dismutase, catalase, and glutathione peroxidase. Supplementation of an anthocyanin-rich extract from blueberries was reported to impose resistance to hyperoxia-induced oxidative stress in rats without affecting endogenous serum antioxidant enzymes.[77]

### 20.3.3 CELL CYCLE AND TUMOR DEVELOPMENT

Anthocyanins isolated from various fruits have been observed to reduce the frequency of induced mutation and to display general inhibitory activity against carcinogenesis in numerous tissues and cancer cell lines. They have been shown to reduce hydrogen peroxide–induced DNA damage in primary human colon cells isolated from biopsies,[27] reduce the frequency of induced mutation by benzo(a)pyrene,[46] suppress lesion development and tumor promotion in human and animal models of colon carcinogenesis,[33,78,79] directly inhibit cell growth of human malignant carcinoma and lymphoma cultured cells,[80] impair angiogenesis,[68] and induce apoptosis in human leukemia cells (cell line HL-60; 33). Many of these reported activities appear to occur through mechanisms other than radical scavenging. By using cell culture models, many flavonoids, including anthocyanins, have been shown to reduce tumor development, inhibit proliferation, and prevent *in vitro* angiogenesis through nonradical scavenging mechanisms.[68,79,81] Some of the suggested properties of anthocyanins that mediate their action against tumor promotion and development include inhibition of the release of superoxide from stimulated human granulocytes,[46] direct cytostatic activity effecting cell proliferation and differentiation,[80] inhibition of epidermal growth factor receptor and vascular endothelial growth factor,[68,78] and direct inhibition of the kinase signaling pathways.[33,81]

Mechanistic studies using mouse epidermal cells suggest that the ortho-dihydroxyl phenyl (B-ring) portion of the anthocyanin is the component responsible for effects on lesion development. Researchers based this assumption on structure–activity relationship studies that have shown cyanidin, delphinidin, and petunidin to have significant antitumor promoting effects while, in this model, malvidin, peonidin, and pelargonidin had no effect.[33] Anthocyanins and their respective aglycones have also been observed to significantly reduce tumor development in cultured cells.[78,79] Researchers reported the aglycones to have a significantly higher activity over that of their respective glycosides; however, the glycosides were still active. Because anthocyanin aglycones have not been detected in the circulation, the effects of anthocyanin aglycones on the suppression of tumor development would presumably be achieved primarily in the colon while glycoside interactions may include systemic effects.

## 20.4  HORMONE ACTIVITY

The role of sex hormones in cancer development is well established and has been cited as a contributing factor in one third of all cancer incidences. Estrogens are known to increase the division of cells in hormone-dependent tissues such as the breast and ovaries.[1] It has been suggested that the spatial relationship between the phenolic hydroxyl groups of certain flavonoids is similar to that of estradiol allowing flavonoids to interact with estrogen receptors and to exhibit physiological effects similar to estrogens.[47] Because flavonoids share this structural similarity with steroids, retinoids, and thyroid hormones,[82] many classes of flavonoids, and particularly isoflavonoids, have been referred to as phytoestrogens. Phytoestrogens are known to bind estrogen receptors exerting both estrogenic and antiestrogenic effects depending on their concentration, the concentration of endogenous sex hormones present, and the receptor activity of the target tissue involved.

The majority of circulating hormones are bound to sex hormone-binding globulin (SHBG; also known as plasma sex steroid-binding protein, SBP). Free hormones, i.e., hormones not bound to SHBG, are available to migrate into cells and initiate hormonal responses. It is theorized that if there is a decrease in plasma concentrations of SHBG, a decrease in the SHBG rate of metabolism, or an increase in hormone production, there is an associated increase in risk of developing hormone-dependent cancers. Phytoestrogens are known to increase plasma levels of SHBG, thus decreasing the plasma concentration of free estrogen and testosterone. The reduced availability of free androgens and estrogens to the target cells would therefore reduce the risk of hormone-dependent cancers.[83] This relationship is based on evidence that high levels of circulating estrogen and low levels of SHBG appear to be associated with increased risk of hormone-dependent cancers involving estrogen such as breast and ovarian cancers.[1,83] This relationship also exists for hormone-dependent cancers involving testosterone such as prostate cancer.[84]

Recent evidence suggests that anthocyanins have weak estrogenic activities relative to other phytoestrogens in the flavonoid and isoflavonoid families. Anthocyanidins were tested for estrogenic activity in cell culture using an estrogen receptor-positive cell line (MCF-7). The anthocyanidins cyanidin, delphinidin, and pelargonidin (chloride forms) were found to exert estrogenic activity and to bind to estrogen receptor-α to activate estrogen-independent gene expression. Researchers suggested that these compounds may therefore play a role in altering the development of hormone-dependent cancers.[85] It was reported that the number of hydroxyl groups had a substantial effect on the estrogenic activity of these compounds. Increasing the number of hydroxyls on the B-ring appeared to reduce receptor affinity. Additionally, researchers concluded that the concentration of anthocyanins required to obtain the observed effects *in vivo* could be reached through normal dietary consumption.

## 20.5  INFLAMMATION

The immune system is an important source of reactive oxygen species (ROS) generation for cellular defense against invading microbes, viruses, and parasites. During this process, phagocytic cells produce oxidizing agents such as superoxide, nitric oxide, peroxynitrite, hydrogen peroxide, and hypochlorite. Subsequent inflammation can result in neutrophil and macrophage accumulation leading to further accumulation of ROS and subsequent oxidative stress. Under certain circumstances, many of these oxidizers can be mutagenic. A large body of clinical evidence suggests that chronic inflammation of certain tissues increases the risk of cancer development within those tissues. This is particularly evident for conditions of the colon such as ulcerative colitis.[1,86] Many studies have shown anthocyanins to have anti-inflammatory activity. Wang et al.[87] demonstrated that cyanidin and glycosides of cyanidin isolated from tart cherries exhibited anti-inflammatory activities *in vitro*. Additionally, a blackberry extract rich in anthocyanins was observed to act as a potent anti-inflammatory agent in a model of lung inflammation induced by carrageenan in rats.[88] Anthocyanins have been observed to suppress inflammatory mediators such as tumor necrosis factor alpha, interleukin-1, interleukin-6, and cytokine-induced neutrophil chemoattractant-1,[89] to prevent antioxidant enzyme decline, and to inhibit enzymatic radical production during inflammation.[33,75–77,87,89,90]

### 20.5.1  Inflammation and Arachidonic Acid Metabolism

Endothelial cells, smooth muscle cells, leukocytes, platelets, and parenchymal cells are all capable of producing a variety of reactive products as a result of arachidonic acid (AA) metabolism via oxygenase-mediated enzymatic activity and subsequent reactions. The metabolism of AA involves the formation of intermediate peroxy compounds and hydroxyl radicals, both of which may result in the initiation of lipid peroxidation chain reactions. Additionally, the damage caused by the resulting lipid hydroperoxides, in the presence of iron, results in the formation of alkoxyl radicals thus amplifying the lipid chain reaction. In a high lipid environment, such as in membranes, this effect can be devastating to cellular function. As anthocyanins are reported to be active against lipid peroxidation, one likely mechanism for their anti-inflammatory activity would be through their antioxidant activities against radicals produced as a result of AA metabolism.[90,91] Anthocyanins from dealcoholized red wine[92] and carrot cell extract[66] have been reported to inhibit enzymatic and non-enzymatic polyunsaturated fatty acid peroxidation induced by radicals *in vitro*. Furthermore, Tsuda et al.[28] demonstrated anthocyanins (glycosides and aglycones) to prevent lipid peroxidation induced by ultraviolet (UV) irradiation in a liposomal system. All pigments used (cyanidin-3-glucoside, delphinidin-3-glucoside, pelargonidin-3-glucoside, cyanidin, delphinidin, pelargonidin) in this investigation were reported to scavenge superoxide and hydroxyl radicals to varying extents. In addition to their capacity for scavenging radicals produced as a result of AA metabolism, anthocyanins also appear to have direct effects on cyclooxygenase (COX) and lipoxygenase; two enzymes involved in the metabolism of AA.

Specific prostaglandins and leukotrienes produced from the metabolism of AA, released from membrane phospholipids via phospholipases, are potent mediators of inflammation. COX is the enzyme responsible for the metabolism of AA thereby producing prostaglandins, and lipoxygenase is involved in the production of leukotrienes. Both cyclooxygenase- and lipoxygenase-mediated metabolism of AA involves the formation of intermediate peroxy compounds and hydroxyl radicals, which can result in the initiation of lipid peroxidation chain reactions.

There are two known COX isoforms, referred to as COX-1 and COX-2. COX-1 is commonly regarded as a "housekeeping enzyme" and is expressed in most cells, performing protective functions. COX-2 is highly inducible by inflammatory stimuli and is associated with deleterious effects when expressed at high levels. COX-2 is present in low concentrations under basal conditions; however, under inflammatory conditions it is subject to induction in the presence of mitogens and cytokines resulting in overexpression. The overexpression of COX-2 has been reported in neoplasms of the colorectum, prostate, gastric tissue, liver, lung, breast, and skin, thereby suggesting its role in tumorigenesis. COX-2 is therefore recognized as a potential enzyme to target for preventative interventions against cancer.[90,91]

Cyanidin and cyanidin-3-glycosides have been shown to have anti-inflammatory properties in various *in vitro* assays. Wang et al.[87] demonstrated cyanidin and glycosides of cyanidin isolated from tart cherries to exhibit *in vitro* anti-inflammatory activities when assaying cyclooxygenase activity. Interestingly, the isolated cyanidin was reported to have more anti-inflammatory activity than aspirin. Additionally, in a study conducted by Seeram et al.,[90] both cyanidin and malvidin showed significant COX inhibitory activities *in vitro* when compared to commercial anti-inflammatory drugs such as ibuprofen, naproxen, Vioxx®, and Celebrex™. The authors reported that the 3',4'-dihydroxyls of the B-ring were responsible for elevated COX inhibitory activity. Anthocyanins have also been shown to inhibit lipoxygenase activity in certain cell model systems.

Lipoxygenases are involved in the metabolism of AA forming various bioactive compounds referred to collectively as leukotrienes. Leukotrienes have multiple biological activities including chemo-attraction and vasoactivity. Many of these compounds are implicated in inflammatory processes.[15] The mechanism responsible for lipoxygenase inhibition by anthocyanins and flavonoids is believed to be a result of iron-reducing and iron-chelating properties;[15,66,93] however, the biological implications of the latter have yet to be determined.

## 20.5.2 INFLAMMATION, OXIDATION, AND CARCINOGENESIS

Nitrated compounds are recognized human carcinogens and are strongly associated with an increased risk of stomach and colorectal cancer.[94,95] Nitrogen oxides are produced in excess during host response to infection as a consequence of reactions involving nitric oxide and superoxide. The accumulation of nitrogen oxides (during immune cell-mediated oxidative burst) within inflamed tissues can result in the production of primary and secondary amines yielding nitrosamines.[86] Additionally, nitrosamines and nitrosamides can also be formed in cigarette smoke and in selected foods. Antioxidants are known to prevent nitrosation, and epidemiological evidence has suggested that they are protective against stomach cancer.[94] Although anthocyanins appear to affect nitric oxide production, the biological relevance of this activity is still unclear. A recent study revealed that anthocyanins and anthocyanidins exhibited strong inhibitory activity toward nitric oxide production in cell culture models using activated macrophages.[96] Furthermore, cyanidin 3-$O$-β-D-glucoside has been shown to inhibit nitric oxide synthase generation in cell culture.[89] Even though nitric oxide is associated with oxidation and inflammation, it is also a biological signal in smooth muscle relaxation and neurotransmission. The physiological consequence of interactions between anthocyanins and nitric oxide is inherently complicated and it will likely be many years before the biological implications of their actions in various cells and tissue are realized.

## 20.6 CHEMICAL-INDUCED CARCINOGENESIS

Nitrated compounds, polycyclic aromatic hydrocarbons, and carbon tetrachloride are established carcinogens used to assess mutagenicity in various experimental models. Anthocyanins have been reported to have antimutagenic activity toward these aforementioned compounds. Studies by Obi et al.[97] revealed that anthocyanins extracted from the petals of *Hibiscus rosasinensis* protected against carbon tetrachloride-induced liver damage in rats. Carbon tetrachloride, a hepatotoxin, is responsible for P450-induced trichloromethyl radical production and associated peroxidation of membrane lipids leading to extensive liver damage including liver cancer.[97] Additionally, studies of the antimutagenic activity of fruit juices high in anthocyanins using the Ames test revealed blueberry juice to have one of the highest antimutagenic activities observed against polycyclic aromatic hydrocarbons.[98] Furthermore, Tsuda et al.[99] observed that the anthocyanin pelargonidin prevented the formation of nitrated tyrosine *in vitro*. Unfortunately, the above investigations were unable to determine the extent to which anthocyanins acted directly as scavengers or indirectly on the enzymes involved with xenobiotic metabolism.[97]

### 20.6.1 PHASE I XENOBIOTIC DETOXIFICATION

Some flavonoids are potent inhibitors of the cytochrome P450 isozyme family CYP1A. CYP1A1 is responsible for the metabolic activation of carcinogens such as polycyclic aromatic hydrocarbons and nitrosamines.[100] Le Marchand et al.[10] determined an inverse association between the intake of flavonoids and lung cancer risk in a Hawaiian case-control study as mentioned above (Section 20.1.2, Flavonoids and Cancer). The researchers genotyped subjects for the P-450 enzyme variant allele CYP1A1 and suggested that the reduced risk of lung cancer was a result of a decreased bioactivation of carcinogens through the inhibition of the CYP1A1 isoform caused by flavonoids. Structure–activity relationship studies of anthocyanins suggest that the ortho-dihydroxyls of the B-ring play an important role in the antimutagenic activity of the anthocyanins.[101] Additionally, Tsyrlov et al.[102] speculated that the catechol moiety is likely responsible for the inhibition of cDNA-expression of the CYP1A P-450 family as a result of ligand-binding activity.

### 20.6.2 PHASE II XENOBIOTIC DETOXIFICATION

Bioactive extracts, high in anthocyanins, from the *Vaccinium* species may have the potential to inhibit the initiation and promotion stages of carcinogenesis under *in vitro* conditions. Quinone reductase is an enzyme responsible for inactivating electrophilic carcinogens and potentially preventing metabolic activation prior to DNA binding. Crude extracts of the lowbush blueberry, cranberry, lingonberry, and bilberry (*Vaccinium*) were shown to have the ability to induce the Phase II xenobiotic detoxification enzyme quinone reductase, thus displaying the capacity to inhibit the initiation of chemically induced carcinogenesis.[103,104] Extracts were further shown to actively inhibit ornithine decarboxylase, a rate-limiting enzyme in the synthesis of polyamines. Polyamine formation is believed to be associated with carcinogenesis as these compounds are formed in high quantities by rapidly proliferating cells.[103]

## 20.7 CONCLUSIONS

Anthocyanins have powerful antioxidant characteristics *in vitro*.[24–26] However, there is much that is not currently understood about their function within biological systems. In fact, there is much that is currently not understood about oxidation within biological systems in general. Studying oxidation *in vivo* is challenging as a result of the complexities involved in biological systems. Complications arise as a consequence of compartmentalization, variations in substrate and catalyst concentrations, surface properties of membranes, binding properties of macromolecules, electrical charges on molecules, and intracellular and extracellular environments, which consist of both aqueous-soluble and lipid-soluble phases. These complexities make it difficult to comprehend how anthocyanins and other flavonoids may reduce or prevent oxidation within the body. Therefore, it will likely be many years before a more thorough understanding of the exact contribution of anthocyanins to the body's antioxidant defense system is realized. If anthocyanins are indeed associated with cancer prevention, their mechanisms of action likely go beyond the prevention of oxidation and lesion formation.

The proposed biological activity of anthocyanins relating to their anticancer properties include direct antimutagenic activity, hormonal activity, inhibition of the metabolic activation of carcinogens, and anti-inflammatory activity. Much of these activities are related to the ability of anthocyanins to influence the activity and function of selected mammalian enzymes. Although anthocyanins have demonstrated a vast array of *in vitro* enzymatic activities, these have not been definitively established in humans (*in vivo*). Important questions still remain unanswered regarding the biological activity of anthocyanins and other flavonoids. For example, how do these compounds cross cellular membranes and partition intracellularly; and how are these compounds metabolized and distributed within tissues? Although anthocyanins have shown promise in many *in vitro* antioxidant and anticancer models, it has yet to be established if these compounds can reach their target of suspected action and if their concentrations are high enough to elicit an efficient response. Further dose-dependent studies on their bioavailability, pharmacokinetics, and *in vivo* bioactivity in controlled human trials are needed following their ingestion as nutraceuticals (supplements) or components of functional foods in varied food matrices. Even though our understanding of phytochemical interactions within human biology is still in its infancy, anthocyanins have demonstrated initial promise as anticancer compounds. Their inhibitory influence on cancer (initiation, progression/incidence) may be the result of direct or indirect antioxidant activity, hormonal activity, or the interaction with enzymes important in cancer initiation and/or progression. It is quite probable that their activity is the combined result of all of these reported effects. Regardless of their mechanism of action, the above evidence indicates the potential use of anthocyanins as a strategy for cancer prevention and perhaps the retardation of cancer progression and/or metastases in future interventions.

## REFERENCES

1. Ames BN, Gold LS, Willett WC. The causes and prevention of cancer. *Proc Natl Acad Sci USA* 1995; 92(12):5258–5265.
2. Steinmetz KA, Potter JD. Vegetables, fruit, and cancer prevention: a review. *J Am Diet Assoc* 1996; 96(10):1027–1039.
3. Willett WC. Diet and cancer. *Oncologist* 2000; 5(5):393–404.
4. Block G, Patterson B, Subar A. Fruit, vegetables, and cancer prevention: a review of the epidemiological evidence. *Nutr Cancer* 1992; 18(1):1–29.
5. van't Veer P, Jansen MC, Klerk M, Kok FJ. Fruits and vegetables in the prevention of cancer and cardiovascular disease. *Public Health Nutr* 2000; 3(1):103–107.
6. Hertog MG, Feskens EJ, Hollman PC, Katan MB, Kromhout D. Dietary antioxidant flavonoids and risk of coronary heart disease: the Zutphen Elderly Study. *Lancet* 1993; 342(8878):1007–1011.
7. Gey KF. Vitamins E plus C and interacting conutrients required for optimal health. A critical and constructive review of epidemiology and supplementation data regarding cardiovascular disease and cancer. *BioFactors* 1998; 7(1–2):113–174.

8. Shikany JM, White GL Jr. Dietary guidelines for chronic disease prevention. *South Med J* 2000; 93(12):1138–1151.

9. Knekt P, Jarvinen R, Seppanen R, Hellovaara M, Teppo L, Pukkala E. Dietary flavonoids and the risk of lung cancer and other malignant neoplasms. *Am J Epidemiol* 1997; 146(3):223–230.

10. Le Marchand L, Murphy SP, Hankin JH, Wilkens LR, Kolonel LN. Intake of flavonoids and lung cancer. *J Natl Cancer Inst* 2000; 92(2):154–160.

11. Hertog MG, Kromhout D, Aravanis C, Blackburn H, Buzina R, Fidanza F, Giampaoli S, Jansen A, Menotti A, Nedeljkovic S, Pekkarinen M, Simic BS, Toshima H, Feskens E, Hollman PCH, Katan MB. Flavonoid intake and long-term risk of coronary heart disease and cancer in the seven countries study. *Arch Intern Med* 1995; 155(4):381–386.

12. Goldbohm RA, Hertog MGL, Brants HAM, van Poppel G, van den Brandt PA. Intake of flavonoids and cancer risk: a prospective cohort study. In: Armado R, Anderson H, Bardóez S, Serra F, eds. *Polyphenols in Food.* Luxembourg: Official Publications of the European Communities; 1997:159–166.

13. Arts MJ, Haenen GR, Voss HP, Bast A. Masking of antioxidant capacity by the interaction of flavonoids with protein. *Food Chem Toxicol* 2001; 39(8):787–791.

14. Das A, Wang JH, Lien EJ. Carcinogenicity, mutagenicity and cancer preventing activities of flavonoids: a structure-system-activity relationship (SSAR) analysis. *Prog Drug Res* 1994; 42:133–166.

15. Middleton E Jr, Kandaswami C, Theoharides TC. The effects of plant flavonoids on mammalian cells: implications for inflammation, heart disease, and cancer. *Pharmacol Rev* 2000; 52(4):673–751.

16. Hollman PCH, van Trijp JMP, Mengelers JB, de Vries JHM, Katan MB. Bioavailability of the dietary antioxidant flavonol quercetin in man. *Cancer Lett* 1997; 114(1–2):139–140.

17. Spanos GA, Wrolstad RE. Phenolics of apple, pear, and white grape juices and their changes with processing and storage. *J Agric Food Chem* 1992; 40(9):1478–1487.

18. Swain T. Flavonoids. In: Goodwin TW, ed. *Chemistry and Biochemistry of Plant Pigments.* 2nd ed. Vol 1. New York: Academic Press; 1976:436–446.

19. Kalt W, Dufour D. Health functionality of blueberries. *Hort Technol* 1997; 7(3):216–221.

20. Mazza G, Miniati E. *Anthocyanins in Fruits, Vegetables, and Grains.* Boca Raton, FL: CRC Press; 1993.

21. Prior RL. Fruits and vegetables in the prevention of cellular oxidative damage. *Am J Clin Nutr* 2003; 78(suppl):570–578.

22. Skrede G, Wrolstad RE. Flavonoids from berries and grapes In: Shi J, Mazza G, eds. *Functional Foods: Vol. 2. Biochemical and Processing Aspects.* Boca Raton, FL: CRC Press; 2002:71–133.

23. Kuhnau J. The flavonoid, a class of semi essential food components, their role in human nutrition. *World Rev Nutr Diet* 1976; 24:117–120.

24. Georgopoulos A. Postprandial triglyceride metabolism in diabetes mellitus. *Clin Cardiol* 1999; 22(6 Suppl):28–33.

25. Kaplan M, Aviram M. Oxidized low density lipoprotein: atherogenic and proinflammatory characteristics during macrophage foam cell formation. An inhibitory role for nutritional antioxidants and serum paraoxonase. *Clin Chem Lab Med* 1999; 37(8):777–787.

26. Vendemiale G, Grattagliano I, Altomare, E. An update on the role of free radicals and antioxidant defense in human disease. *Int J Clin Lab Res* 1999; 29(2):49–55.

27. Pool-Zobel BL, Bub A, Schröder N, Rechkemmer G. Anthocyanins are potent antioxidants in model systems but do not reduce endogenous oxidative DNA damage in human colon cells. *Eur J Nutr* 1999; 38:227–234.

28. Tsuda T, Shiga K, Ohshima K, Kawakishi S, Osawa T. Inhibition of lipid peroxidation and the active oxygen radical scavenging effect of anthocyanin pigments isolated from *Phaseolus vulgaris* L. *Biochem Pharmacol* 1996; 52:1033–1039.

29. Sarma A, Sreelakshmi Y, Sharma R. Antioxidant ability of anthocyanins against ascorbic acid oxidation. *Phytochemistry* 1997; 45(4):671–674.

30. Wang SY, Jiao H. Scavenging capacity of berry crops on superoxide radicals, hydrogen peroxide, hydroxyl radicals, and singlet oxygen. *J Agric Food Chem* 2000; 48(11):5677–5684.

31. Rossetto M, Vanzani P, Mattivi F, Lunelli M, Scarpa M, Rigo A. Synergistic antioxidant effect of catechin and malvidin 3-glucoside on free radical-induced peroxidation of linoleic acid in micelles. *Arch Biochem Biophys* 2002; 408:239–245.

32. Seeram NP, Nair MG. Inhibition of lipid peroxidation and structure-activity-related studies of the dietary constituents anthocyanins, anthocyanidins, and catechins. *J Agric Food Chem* 2002; 50:5308–5312.

33. Hou D. Potential mechanisms of cancer chemoprevention by anthocyanins. *Curr Mol Med* 2003; 3:149–159.

34. Maxwell S, Cruickshank A, Thorpe, G. Red wine and antioxidant activity in serum. *Lancet* 1994; 344(8916):193–194.

35. Fuhrman B, Lavy A, Aviram M. Consumption of red wine with meals reduces the susceptibility of human plasma and low-density lipoprotein to lipid peroxidation. *Am J Clin Nutr* 1995; 61(3):549–554.

36. Whitehead TP, Robinson D, Allaway S, Syms J, Hale A. Effect of red wine ingestion on the antioxidant capacity of serum. *Clin Chem* 1995; 41(1):32–35.

37. Cao G, Booth SL, Sadowski JA, Prior R.L. Increases in human plasma antioxidant capacity after consumption of controlled diets high in fruit and vegetables. *Am J Clin Nutr* 1998; 68(5):1081–1087.

38. Serafini M, Maiani G, Ferro-Luzzi A. Alcohol-free red wine enhances plasma antioxidant capacity in humans. *J Nutr* 1998; 128(6):1003–1007.

39. Miyazawa T, Nakagawa K, Kudo M, Muraishi K, Someya K. Direct intestinal absorption of red fruit anthocyanins, cyanidin-3-glucoside and cyanidin-3,5-diglucoside, into rats and humans. *J Agric Food Chem* 1999; 47(3):1083–1091.

40. Young JF, Nielsen SE, Haraldsdottir J, Daneshvar B, Lauridsen ST, Knuthsen P, Crozier A, Sandstrom B, Dragsted LO. Effect of fruit juice intake on urinary quercetin excretion and biomarkers of antioxidative status. *Am J Clin Nutr* 1999; 69(1):87–94.

41. Kay CD, Holub BJ. The effect of wild blueberry (*Vaccinium angustifolium*) consumption on postprandial serum antioxidant status in human subjects. *Br J Nutr* 2002; 88(4):389–398.

42. Mazza G, Kay CD, Cottrell T, Holub BJ. Absorption of anthocyanins from blueberries and serum antioxidant status in human subjects. *J Agric Food Chem* 2002; 50(26):7731–7737.

43. Ching S, Ingram D, Hahnel R, Beilby J, Rossi E. Serum levels of micronutrients, antioxidants and total antioxidant status predict risk of breast cancer in a case control study. *J Nutr* 2002; 132(2):303–306.

44. Scandalios JG. *Molecular Biology of Free Radical Scavenging Systems*. New York: Cold Spring Harbor Laboratory Press; 1992.

45. Ross R. The pathogenesis of atherosclerosis: a perspective for the 1990s. *Nature* 1993; 362:801–809.

46. Gsiorowski K, Szyba K, Brokos B, Koaczyiska B, Jankowiak-Wodarczyk M, Oszmiaski J. Antimutagenic activity of anthocyanins isolated from *Aronia melanocarpa* fruits. *Cancer Lett* 1997; 119:37–46.

47. Havsteen B. Flavonoids, a class of natural products of high pharmacological potency. *Biochem Pharmacol* 1983; 32(7):1141–1148.

48. Fiander H, Schneider H. Dietary ortho phenols that induce glutathione *S*-transferase and increase the resistance of cells to hydrogen peroxide are potential cancer chemopreventives that act by two mechanisms: the alleviation of oxidative stress and the detoxification of mutagenic xenobiotics. *Cancer Lett* 2000; 156(2):117–124.

49. Ross JA, Kasum CM. Dietary flavonoids: bioavailability, metabolic effects, and safety. *Annu Rev Nutr* 2002; 22:19–34.

50. Zheng W, Wang SY. Oxygen radical absorbing capacity of phenolics in blueberries, cranberries, chokeberries, and lingonberries. *J Agric Food Chem* 2003; 51:502–509.

51. Lien EJ, Ren S, Bui HH, Wang R. Quantitative structure-activity relationship analysis of phenolic antioxidants. *Free Radical Biol Med* 1999; 26(3–4):285–294.

52. Ioku K, Tsushida T, Takei Y, Nakatani N, Terao J. Antioxidative activity of quercetin and quercetin monoglucosides in solution and phospholipid bilayers. *Biochim Biophys Acta* 1995; 1234(1):99–104.

53. Noroozi M, Angerson WJ, Lean ME. Effects of flavonoids and vitamin C on oxidative DNA damage to human lymphocytes. *Am J Clin Nutr* 1998; 67(6):1210–1218.

54. Wang H, Cao G, Prior R. Oxygen radical absorbing capacity of anthocyanins. *J Agric Food Chem* 1997; 45:304–309.

55. Kähkönen MP, Heinonen M. Antioxidant activity of anthocyanins and their aglycones. *J Agric Food Chem* 2003; 51:628–633.

56. Bub A, Watzl B, Heeb D, Rechkemmer G, Briviba K. Malvidin-3-glucoside bioavailability in humans after ingestion of red wine, dealcoholized red wine and red grape juice. *Eur J Nutr* 2001; 40(3):113–120.

57. Mülleder U, Murkovic M, Pfannhauser W. Urinary excretion of cyanidin glycosides. *J Biochem Biophys Methods*, 2002; 53(1–3):61–66.

58. Frank T, Netzel M, Strass G, Bitsch R, Bitsch I. Bioavailability of anthocyanidin-3-glucosides following consumption of red wine and red grape juice. *Can J Physiol Pharmacol* 2003; 81(5):423–435.

59. Nielsen IL, Dragsted LO, Ravn-Haren G, Freese R, Rasmussen SE. Absorption and excretion of black currant anthocyanins in humans and watanabe heritable hyperlipidemic rabbits. *J Agric Food Chem* 2003; 51(9):2813–2820.

60. Kay CD, Mazza G, Holub BJ, Wang J. Anthocyanin metabolites in human urine and serum. *Br J Nutr* 2004; 91(6):933–942.

61. Wu X, Cao G, Prior RL. Absorption and metabolism of anthocyanins in elderly women after consumption of elderberry or blueberry. *J Nutr* 2002; 132(7):1865–1871.

62. Felgines C, Talavera S, Gonthier MP, Texier O, Scalbert A, Lamaison JL, Remesy C. Strawberry anthocyanins are recovered in urine as glucuro- and sulfoconjugates in humans. *J Nutr* 2003; 133(5):1296–1301.

62a. Kay CD, et al. 2005; unpublished.

63. Terao J. Dietary flavonoids as antioxidants in vivo: conjugated metabolites of (–)-epicatechin and quercetin participate in antioxidative defence in blood plasma. *J Med Invest* 1999; 46(3–4):159–168.

64. Tsuda T, Horio F, Osawa T. Absorption and metabolism of cyanidin 3-*O*-beta-D-glucoside in rats. *FEBS Lett* 1999; 449:179–182.

65. Seeram NP, Bourquin LD, Nair MG. Degradation products of cyanidin glycosides from tart cherries and their bioactivities. *J Agric Food Chem* 2001; 49(10):4924–4929.

66. Narayan MS, Naidu KA, Ravishankar GA, Srinivas L, Venkataraman LV. Anti-oxidant effect of anthocyanin on enzymatic and non-enzymatic lipid peroxidation. *Prostag Leukotr Ess Fatty Acids* 1999; 60(1):1–4.

67. Youdim KA, Martin A, Joseph JA. Incorporation of the elderberry anthocyanins by endothelial cells increases protection against oxidative stress. *Free Radical Biol Med* 2000; 29(1):51–60.

68. Bagchi D, Sen CK, Bagchi M, Atalay M. Anti-angiogenic, antioxidant, and anti-carcinogenic properties of a novel anthocyanin-rich berry extract formula. *Bio-chemistry (Moscow)* 2004; 69(1):75–80.

69. Glei M, Matuschek M, Steiner C, Böhm V, Persin C, Pool-Zobel BL. Initial *in vitro* toxicity testing of functional foods rich in catechins and anthocyanins in human cells. *Toxicol Vitro* 2003; 17:723–729.

70. Lazzé MC, Pizzala R, Savio M, Stivala LA, Prosperi E. Anthocyanins protect against DNA damage induced by tert-butyl-hydroperoxide in rat smooth muscle and hepatoma cells. *Mutat Res* 2003; 535(1):103–115.

71. Ramirez-Tortosa, Anderson ØM, Gardner PT, Morrice PC, Wood SG, Duthie SJ, Collins AR, Duthie GG. Anthocyanin-rich extract decreases indices of lipid per-oxidation and DNA damage in vitamin E-depleted rats. *Free Radical Biol Med* 2001; 31(9):1033–1037.

72. Anderson RF, Amarasinghe C, Fisher LJ, Mak WB, Parker JE. Reduction in free-radical-induced DNA strand breaks and base damage through fast chemical repair by flavonoids. *Free Radical Res* 2000; 33:91–103.

73. Sarma AD, Sharma R. Anthocyanin-DNA copigmentation complex: mutual pro-tection against oxidative damage. *Phytochemistry* 1999; 52:1313–1318.

74. Costantino L, Albasini A, Rastelli G, Benvenuti S. Activity of polyphenolic crude extracts as scavengers of superoxide radicals and inhibitors of xanthine oxidase. *Planta Med* 1992; 58(4):342–344.

75. Tsuda T, Horio F, Kitoh J, Osawa T. Protective effects of dietary cyanidin 3-*O*-β-D-glucoside on liver ischemia-reperfusion injury in rats. *Arch Biochem Biophys* 1999; 368(2):361–366.

76. Tsuda T, Horio F, Osawa T. The role of anthocyanins as an antioxidant under oxidative stress in rats. *BioFactors* 2000; 31(1–4):133–139.

77. Cao G, Shukitt-Hale B, Bickford PC, Joseph JA, McEwen J, Prior RL. Hyperoxia-induced changes in antioxidant capacity and the effect of dietary antioxidants. *J Appl Physiol* 1999; 86(6):1817–1822.

78. Meiers S, Kemény M, Weyand U, Gastpar R, Angerer E, Marko D. The anthocyanidins cyanidin and delphinidin are potent inhibitors of the epidermal growth-factor receptor. *J Agric Food Chem* 2001; 49:958–962.

79. Kang S, Seeram NP, Nair MG, Bourquin LD. Tart cherry anthocyanins inhibit tumor development in ApcMin mice and reduce proliferation of human colon cancer cells. *Cancer Lett* 2003; 194:13–19.

80. Kamei H, Kojima T, Hasegawa M, Koide T, Umeda T, Yukawa T, Terabe K. Suppression of tumor cell growth by anthocyanins *in vitro*. *Cancer Invest* 1995; 13(6):590–594.

81. Fotsis T, Pepper MS, Aktas E, Breit S, Rasku S, Adlercreutz H, Wahala K, Montesano R, Schweigerer L. Flavonoids, dietary-derived inhibitors of cell proliferation and *in vitro* angiogenesis. *Cancer Res* 1997; 57(14):2916–2921.

82. Baker, Michael E. Flavonoids as hormones — a perspective from an analysis of molecular fossils. In: Manthey JA, Buslig BS, eds. *Flavonoids in the Living System*. New York: Plenum Press; 1998:249–267.

83. Martin ME, Haourigui M, Pelissero C, Benassayag C, Nunez EA. Interactions between phytoestrogens and human sex steroid binding protein. *Life Sci* 1996; 58(5):429–436.

84. Gann PH, Hennekens CH, Ma J, Longcope C, Stampfer MJ. Prospective study of sex hormone levels and risk of prostate cancer. *J Natl Cancer Inst* 1996; 88(16):1118–1126.

85. Schmitt E, Stopper H. Estrogenic activity of naturally occurring anthocyanidins. *Nutr Cancer* 2001; 41(1&2):154.

86. Jourd'heuil D, Kang D, Grisham MB. Interactions between superoxide and nitric oxide: implications in DNA damage and mutagenesis. *Front Biosci* 2 1997; 189–196.

87. Wang H, Nair MG, Strasburg GM, Chang Y, Booren AM. Antioxidant and anti-inflammatory activities of anthocyanins and their aglycone, cyanidin, from tart cherries. *J Nat Prod* 1999; 62:294–296.

88. Antonietta R, Ivana S, Paola D, Rosanna D, Luigi M, Tiziana G, Domenica M, Giovanni D, Lidia S, Achille C, Salvatore C. Protective effects of anthocyanins from blackberry in a rat model of acute lung inflammation. *Free Radical Res* 2003; 37(8):891–900.

89. Tsuda T, Horio F, Kato Y, Osawa T. Cyanidin 3-O-beta-D-glucoside attenuates the hepatic ischemia-reperfusion injury through a decrease in the neutrophil chemoattractant production in rats. *J Nutr Sci Vitaminol* 2002; 48(2):134–141.

90. Seeram N, Zhang Y, Nair MG. Inhibition of proliferation of human cancer cells and cyclooxygenase enzymes by anthocyanins and catechins. *Nutr Cancer* 2003; 46(1):101–106.

91. Umar A, Viner JL, Hawk ET. The future of colon cancer prevention. *Ann NY Acad Sci* 2001; 952:88–108.

92. Ghiselli A, Nardini M, Baldi A, Scaccini C. Antioxidant activity of different phenolic fractions separated from an Italian red wine. *J Agric Food Chem* 1998; 46(2):361–367.

93. Waladkhani A, Clemens MR. Effect of dietary phytochemicals on cancer development. *Int J Mol Med* 1998; 1:747–753.

94. Block G. The data support a role for antioxidants in reducing cancer risk. *Nutr Rev* 1992; 50(7):207–213.

95. Branca F, Hanley AB, Pool-Zobel B, Verhagen H. Biomarkers in disease and health. *Br J Nutr* 2001; 86(Suppl 1):55–92.

96. Wang J, Mazza G. Inhibitory effects of anthocyanins and other phenolic compounds on nitric oxide production in LPS/IFN-γ-activated RAW 264.7 macrophages. *J Agric Food Chem* 2002; 50:850–857.

97. Obi FO, Usenu IA, Osayande JO. Prevention of carbon tetrachloride-induced hepatotoxicity in the rat by *H. rosasinensis* anthocyanin extract administered in ethanol. *Toxicology* 1998; 131:93–98.

98. Camire ME. Bilberries and blueberries as functional foods and nutraceuticals. In: Mazza G, Oomah D, eds. *Herbs, Botanicals, & Teas.* Lancaster, PA: Technomic; 2000:289–319.

99. Tsuda T, Kato Y, Osawa T. Mechanism for the peroxynitrite scavenging activity by anthocyanins. *FEBS Lett* 2000; 484:207–210.

100. Zhai S, Dai, R, Friedman FK, Vestal RE. Comparative inhibition of human cytochromes P450 1A1 and 1A2 by flavonoids. *Drug Metab Dispos* 1998; 26(10):989–992.

101. Yoshimoto M, Okuno S, Yamaguchi M, Yamakawa O. Antimutagenicity of deacylated anthocyanins in purple-fleshed sweetpotato. *Biosci Biotechnol Biochem* 2001; 65(7):1652–1655.

102. Tsyrlov IB, Mikhailenko VM, Gelboin HV. Isozyme- and species-specific susceptibility of cDNA-expressed CYP1A P-450s to different flavonoids. *Biochim Biophys Acta* 1994; 1205:325–335.

103. Bomser J, Madhavi DL, Singletary K, Smith MA. *In vitro* anticancer activity of fruit extracts from *Vaccinium* species. *Planta Med* 1996; 62(3):212–216.

104. Smith MAL, Marley KA, Seigler D, Singletary KW, Meline B. Bioactive properties of wild blueberry fruits. *J Food Sci* 2000; 65(2):352–356.

# Part VI

Dietary Components That
Protect from Cancer:
Isothiocyanates

# 21 Isothiocyanates and Cancer Prevention

*Marilyn E. Morris and Urvi Telang*

## CONTENTS

21.1 Introduction .................................................................................................435
21.2 Bioavailability and Pharmacokinetics of ITCs ...................................437
21.3 *In Vitro* Studies .........................................................................................439
21.4 *In Vivo* Studies with Animal Cancer Models....................................441
21.5 Clinical Studies............................................................................................442
21.6 Mechanisms of Action of Isothiocyanates ..........................................444
    21.6.1 Inhibition of Phase I Enzymes...............................................444
    21.6.2 Induction of Phase II Enzymes...............................................446
    21.6.3 Apoptosis and Cell Cycle Regulation....................................447
21.7 Conclusions...................................................................................................448
Acknowledgments ..................................................................................................448
References .................................................................................................................448

## 21.1 INTRODUCTION

Extensive epidemiological evidence supports the contention that high fruit and vegetable consumption is associated with a reduction in the incidence of cancer. Moreover, it is well established that consumption of cruciferous vegetables is inversely associated with the risk of cancer of the lung, colon, stomach, and prostate.[1-3] In the mid-1980s, studies in rats demonstrated that isothiocyanates (ITCs) (Figure 21.1), which occur widely as conjugates in *Brassica* and other vegetables of the family Cruciferae (e.g., cabbage, cauliflower, Brussels sprouts, watercress, broccoli, kale) and the genus *Raphanus* (radishes and daikons), inhibit the metabolic activation of a variety of carcinogens that occur in tobacco products and the diet, suggesting chemopreventive effects of ITCs.[4,5] Organic ITCs (R–NCS) occur in plants as thioglycoside conjugates known as glucosinolates. Damage to plant cells, such as from cutting and chewing, releases myrosinase (β-thioglucoside glucohydrolase) that catalyzes the hydrolysis of glucosinolates and the formation of ITCs by a Lossen rearrangement (Figure 21.2). The microflora in the intestinal tract also acts as a source for the hydrolysis of glucosinolates to ITCs in humans.[6]

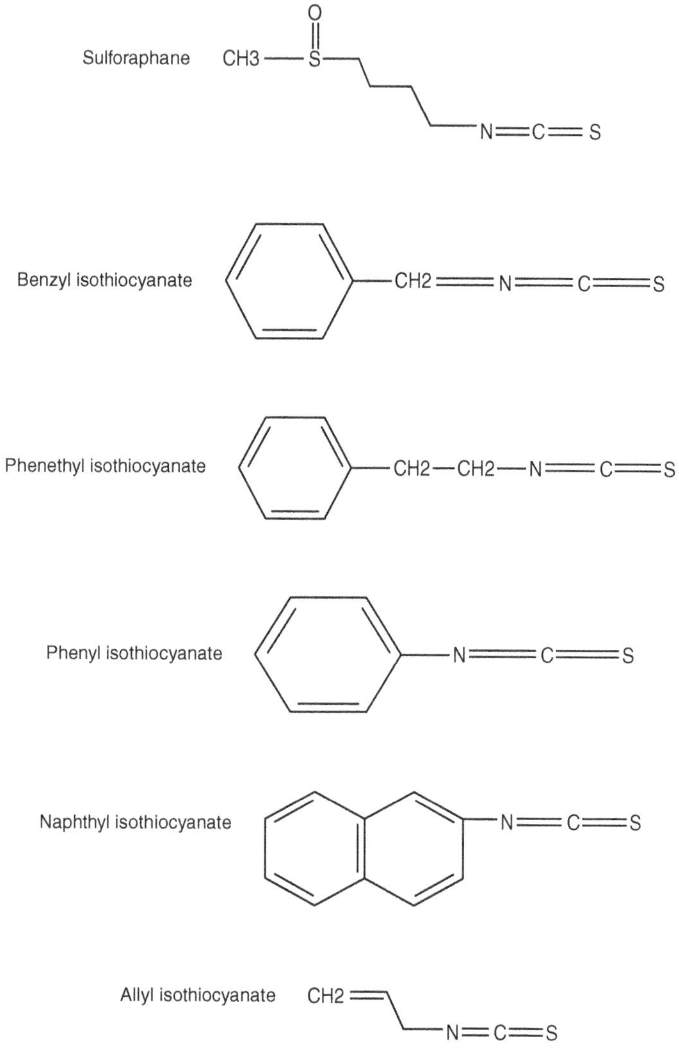

**FIGURE 21.1** Chemical structures of common ITCs.

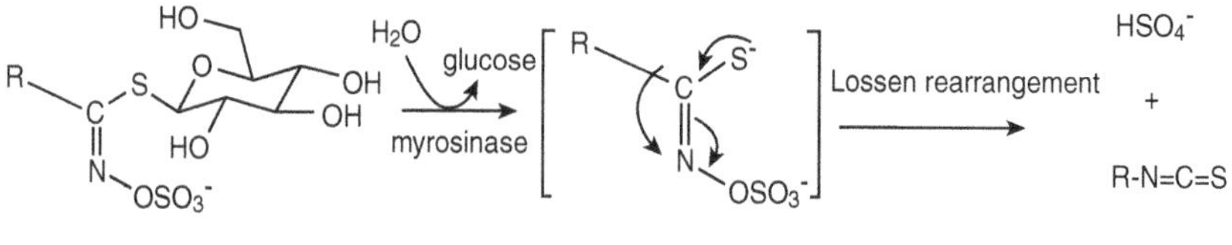

**FIGURE 21.2** Hydrolysis of glucosinolates and the formation of ITCs by a Lossen rearrangement.

**TABLE 21.1**
**ITC Content in the Diet**

| Vegetable | Glucosinolate (GL) or ITC Content | Ref. |
|---|---|---|
| Raw cabbage | 0.108 μmol/g (PEITC) | 56 |
| Mustard | 10.8 μmol/g (AITC) | 56 |
| | 3.2 μmol/g (PEITC) | |
| Broccoli sprouts | 8 μmol/g ITCs | 57 |
| Watercress | 6.5 μmol/g ITC | 58 |
| Brussels sprouts | 15.84 mol/g (total glucosinolate) | 59 |
| | 8.7 mol/g (sinigrin) | |

Consuming normal amounts of vegetables such as watercress or broccoli releases tens of milligram amounts of ITCs.[7] Glucosinolate levels have been estimated to be as high as 180 mg/g in some vegetables.[7] High levels of sulforaphane (SF) and phenethyl isothiocyanate (PEITC), the two most common ITCs in the diet, are detected in plasma following the consumption of broccoli and watercress, respectively.[8,9] The estimated ITC/glucosinolate levels in common cruciferous vegetables are given in Table 21.1. It has been estimated that the consumption of 100 g of broccoli could release 40 μmol of the ITC SF,[10] while consumption of about 30 g of watercress releases about 46.5 μmol of PEITC.[11] Additionally, ITCs are constituents of numerous herbal supplements including Daily Cruciferous Plus®, Broccoli Sprouts®, BioBasics®, Fruit and Veggie Tabs®, and NutriHealth MultiPlus®.

More than 20 natural and synthetic ITCs have been shown to block carcinogenesis. The capacity for organic isothiocyanates to block chemical carcinogenesis was first recognized more than 30 years ago with naphthyl ITC (NITC). Recent studies describing the effect of ITCs *in vitro*, *in vivo*, and in clinical studies are described later in this chapter. Current mechanisms proposed for the anticarcinogenic effects of ITCs include (1) inhibition of Phase I enzymes converting procarcinogens to highly reactive electrophilic carcinogens; (2) induction of Phase II enzymes inactivating carcinogens and promoting their excretion; and (3) induction of apoptosis of cancer cells.[12,13]

## 21.2 BIOAVAILABILITY AND PHARMACOKINETICS OF ITCs

Absorption of ITCs is rapid, and the parent compound can be detected in the blood minutes after administration. The pharmacokinetics of PEITC both in rats and humans have been evaluated in our laboratory: PEITC has high oral bioavailability and low clearance ($0.70 \pm 0.17$ L/h/kg at the lowest dose of 2 μmol/kg) in rats (Ji, Y and Morris, ME, unpublished). Nonlinear elimination and distribution were evident at high doses. In humans, following ingestion of the vegetable

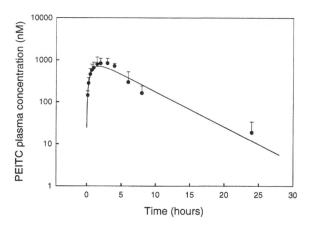

**FIGURE 21.3** Plasma concentration vs. time profile of PEITC in humans following the consumption of 100 g watercress. Data are expressed as mean ± SD, $n = 4$; closed circles represent the measured concentration and the line represents the predicted concentration fitted by compartmental model analysis using WinNonlin Version 2.1 (Pharsight, Mountainview, CA). (From Ji Y, Morris ME. *Anal Biochem* 2003; 323(1):39–47. Reproduced with permission.)

watercress at a 100 g dose, the mean $C_{max}$ value was 928 n$M$ and the half-life was 4.9 h (Figure 21.3). Average oral clearance (clearance/availability) was 490 ml/min, suggesting a low clearance.[9] A recent evaluation of a high dose of SF (50 µmol) in rats reported high concentrations in plasma ($C_{max}$ of 20 µ$M$) and a half-life of about 2.2 h.[14] Therefore, in contrast to dietary components such as the flavonoids, oral clearance of these ITCs is low and bioavailability is excellent, indicating greater exposure to the parent compound in the intestine, liver, and systemically, than observed with other dietary chemicals.

In humans, the conjugation and excretion of ITCs is mainly catalyzed by glutathione-$S$-transferase M1 (GSTM1) and GSTT1,[15] although a variety of other GSTs, including GST A1, P1, M2, and M4 are also involved to a minor extent. GSTM1 and GSTT1 exhibit significant polymorphisms in humans: the incidence of homozygous null deletion is approximately 50% for GSTM1 in white subjects in the U.S., as well as in Japanese and Chinese subjects; for GSTT1 the incidence is 12 to 16% in German and English subjects and 60 to 64% in Chinese and Korean subjects.[16] Studies examining the correlation of ITC intake obtained through vegetable consumption and GSTM1 and GSTT1 genotypes among various populations have also suggested that lung cancer risk and colorectal adenomas were decreased among persons genetically deficient in GSTM1 and/or GSTT1, although GSTM1 deficiency appears to be more important.[1,17–19] In those subjects with detectable levels of ITCs in their urine and a GSTM1 deficiency, there was a 64% decrease in the risk of developing lung cancer.[19] These studies suggest the importance of the polymorphic expression of GSTs in determining the systemic concentrations and efficacy of ITCs.

## TABLE 21.2
### *In Vitro* Cytotoxic Effects of Isothiocyanates

| ITC Treatment | Cell Type Cell Line | Cell Density/Survival Inhibition | Apoptosis Induction | Ref. |
|---|---|---|---|---|
| Sulforaphane | | | | |
| 24 h, 50 μ*M* | Human prostate cancer LNCaP | 50% | 50% | 60 |
| 24 h, 15 μ*M* | Human colon carcinoma HT29 | 25% | 75% | 61 |
| 48 h | Mouse breast cancer F3II | IC$_{50}$: 8 μ*M* | | 62 |
| 48 h | Human breast cancer MCF-7 | IC$_{50}$: 13.7 μ*M* | | 23 |
| BITC | | | | |
| 48 h | Human breast cancer MCF-7 | 5.95 μ*M* | | 23 |
| 24 h | Human pancreatic cancer BxPC-3 | IC$_{50}$: 8 μ*M* | Threefold (5 μ*M*) | 63 |
| 24 h | Human leukemia Jurkat T | IC$_{50}$: 6 μ*M* | Sixfold (5 μ*M*) | 64 |
| PEITC | | | | |
| 24 h, 5 μ*M* | Human prostate cancer PC-3 | 75% | Threefold | 80 |
| 3 h | Human bladder carcinoma | IC$_{50}$: 22.0 μ*M* | | 81 |
| 24 h | UM-UC-3 | | 5.9 fold (15 μ*M*) | 81 |
| 48 h | Human breast cancer MCF-7 | IC$_{50}$: 7.32 μ*M* | | 23 |
| MBITC | | | | |
| 24 h, 10 μ*M* | Human leukemia Jurkat T | +2.8 fold G2 phase cell arrest | 2.4 fold | 26 |
| AITC | | | | |
| 24 h, 40 μ*M* | Human prostate cancer LNCaP | 40% IC$_{50}$: 15–17 μ*M* | Threefold | 27 |
| 3 h | Human colon cancer HT-29 | IC$_{50}$: 5.9 μ*M* | | 22 |

## 21.3 *IN VITRO* STUDIES

Inhibition of cell growth and modulation of the cell cycle have been reported for allyl ITC (AITC) (10 μ*M*), benzyl ITC (BITC) (5 μ*M*), and PEITC (2.5 μ*M*) in HeLa cells,[20] and similar effects have been reported for SF (15 μ*M*) in HT-29 cells. Similar results have been reported in other cell lines including human leukemia HL60 and prostate cancer cell lines LNCaP and DU-145 (reviewed by Reference 21). A comprehensive study of the effect of ITCs on the growth of different cancer cells reported that AITC, BITC, and PEITC were able to inhibit cell growth.[22] The results of some recent studies are summarized in Table 21.2.

The cytotoxicity of PEITC, BITC, NITC, and SF, as well as the cytotoxicity of the chemotherapeutic agents daunomycin (DNM) and vinblastine (VBL), have been evaluated in human breast cancer MCF-7 and human mammary epithelial

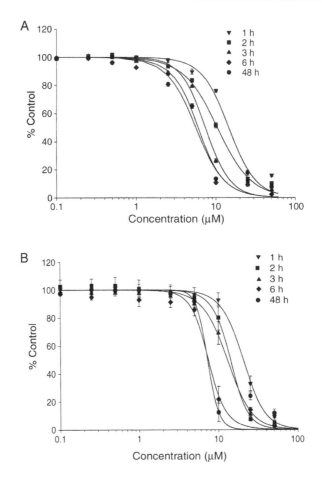

**FIGURE 21.4** Cytotoxicity in human breast cancer MCF-7 cells. The effect of varying concentrations of (A) BITC, (B) PEITC, and (C) SF on cell growth of MCF-7/Adr cells following exposure times of (▼) 1 h, (■) 2 h, (▲) 3 h, (♦) 6 h, and (●) 48 h. Each data point represents mean ± SE from four wells in one representative study. The study was repeated two to four times. (From Tseng E, Scott-Ramsay EA, Morris ME. *Biol Med* (Maywood) 2004; 229(8):835–842. Reproduced with permission of the Society for Experimental Biology and Medicine.)

MCF-12A cells[23] (Figure 21.4). $IC_{50}$ values for BITC, PEITC, NITC, and SF were 5.95 ± 0.10, 7.32 ± 0.25, 77.9 ± 8.03, and 13.71 ± 0.82 $\mu M$ in MCF-7 cells. The corresponding $IC_{50}$ values for DNM and VBL in MCF-7 cells were 7.12 ± 0.42 $\mu M$ and 0.106 ± 0.004 $\mu M$ (mean ± SE). Values for BITC, PEITC, NITC, and SF in MCF-12A cells were 8.07 ± 0.29, 7.71 ± 0.07, 33.63 ± 1.69, and 40.45 ± 1.25 $\mu M$, respectively. BITC and PEITC can inhibit the growth of human breast cancer cells as well as human mammary epithelium cells, at concentrations similar to the chemotherapeutic drug DNM. SF and NITC exhibited higher $IC_{50}$ values. These concentrations are four- to sixfold lower than the $IC_{50}$ for the isoflavonoid,

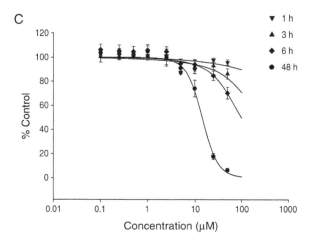

**FIGURE 21.4 (CONTINUED)**

genistein, a compound that has also been studied in MCF-7 cells. Genistein has been reported to have the lowest $IC_{50}$ among the dietary flavonoids tested in MCF-7 cells.[24]

While some studies have demonstrated similar cytotoxicity in cancer and normal cells,[23,25] others have reported differences. A synthetic ITC 4-(methylthio) butyl ITC has shown selective action against human leukemia cells, and almost no effect on lymphocytes.[26] AITC also has an inhibitory effect in the human prostate cancer cell lines, while normal cell line PrEC remained unaffected by the same exposure.[27]

The cytotoxic effects of ITCs are apparent even after shorter exposures. Comprehensive time-dependent studies of the effect of ITCs on the growth of different cell lines reported that a number of ITCs, including AITC, BITC, PEITC, and NITC, were able to inhibit cell growth after 2- or 3-h exposures, producing $IC_{50}$ values similar to those for exposure for 48 to 72 h, indicating that short-term exposure is sufficient to produce an observable effect *in vitro*.[22,23]

## 21.4 *IN VIVO* STUDIES WITH ANIMAL CANCER MODELS

The anticarcinogenic activities of ITCs have been demonstrated in a number of carcinogen-induced cancer models *in vivo*. More than 20 natural and synthetic ITCs have demonstrated cancer preventive properties in animals treated with chemical carcinogens, including polycyclic aromatic hydrocarbons and nitrosamines. For example, ITCs can inhibit 4-(methylnitrosamino)-1-(3-pyridyl)-butanone (NNK)-induced carcinogenesis by inhibiting the microsomal metabolism of NNK to reactive species that form methyl and pyridyloxobutyl adducts in DNA.[28–30] Carcinogen inhibition was seen in a number of different organs such as lung, liver, fore-stomach, mammary gland, and colon. BITC has shown effectiveness in mammary gland cancer, while PEITC has been effective in carcinogen-induced models of mammary, lung, oral, as well as esophageal cancer in rats and mice.[31,32] Studies have shown that SF is effective in prevention of azoxymethane-induced colonic cancer.[5] Table 21.3 summarizes the results of recent studies on carcinogen-induced cancer models in rodents.

## 21.5  CLINICAL STUDIES

Several epidemiological studies have reported a correlation between the intake of *Brassica* vegetables and the risk of cancers in humans. Although this inverse correlation cannot be attributed solely to ITCs, as other constituents such as vitamins, folic acid, and fiber may also play a role in the reduction of cancer risk, newer studies quantifying the amount of ITCs in the biological samples have provided evidence that ITCs are important in cancer prevention.

Epidemiological studies in lung cancer risk have shown associations between consumption of ITCs and reduced risk after the smoking status of the subject is taken into account. A case-control study in Chinese women reported an odds ratio (OR) of 0.31 for smokers with high ITC intake, and an OR of 0.70 for nonsmokers with comparable ITC intake.[33]

A breast cancer study with 720 cases and 810 controls reported that the consumption of broccoli, a vegetable rich in SF, is inversely associated with breast cancer risk in premenopausal women and that the association was not significant in postmenopausal women. When they measured cancer risk and total cruciferous vegetable intake, the correlation was not significant.[34] A study in Chinese women evaluated the correlation between urinary ITC levels (determined by a cyclocondensation derivatization of the total ITCs and dithiocarbamates in the urine[35]) to breast cancer risk. The study, performed on 337 cases and matched controls, reported a 50% reduction in the cancer risk for the highest quartile of ITC consumption.[36]

A prospective case-control study in male subjects reported that the section of the population with the highest intake of cruciferous vegetables had a lower incidence of bladder cancer. Detailed studies into the risks associated with individual cruciferous vegetables showed that cabbage and broccoli were able to reduce the risk, independent of the intake of other crucifers.[37]

A case-control study on Chinese subjects compared the dietary intake of cruciferous vegetables in 213 cases of colorectal cancer with 1194 controls. When their data were categorized by ITC consumption, a nonsignificant association was seen between high intake and colorectal cancer risk. However, there was a significant inverse correlation seen between colorectal cancer risk and high intake for individuals with null genotypes for GSTM1 and T1,[38] suggesting that the higher plasma concentrations of ITCs that would be expected in individuals with null genotypes may be responsible for this significant effect.

Thus, while some studies have reported that the association between crucifer consumption and cancer risk was not significant, other studies have shown strong associations after adjustments for lifestyle practices such as smoking and for

**TABLE 21.3**
**Effects of ITCs on Carcinogen-Induced Cancer in Animal Studies**

| ITC Treatment | Animal | Model | Carcinogen (dose) | Dosing | % Rats with Tumors (test vs. control) | Ref. |
|---|---|---|---|---|---|---|
| **BITC** | | | | | | |
| 50 mg | Sprague-Dawley rats F | Mammary | DMBA (12 mg) | Oral: Single dose 4 h before DMBA | 8/77 | 65 |
| 0.017 mmol/g diet | | | | Diet: DMBA + BITC 10 weeks | 63/100 | 65 |
| 5.0 mg/g diet | ICR/Ha mice F | Forestomach | DMBA (0.05 mg/g diet) | Diet: DMBA + BITC 4 weeks | 5/87 | 65 |
| **PEITC** | | | | | | |
| 55 mg | Sprague-Dawley rats F | Mammary | DMBA (12 mg) | Oral: Single dose 4 h before DMBA | 43/100 | 65 |
| 5.5 mg/g diet | ICR/Ha mice F | Forestomach | DMBA (12 mg) | Diet: DMBA + PEITC 4 weeks | 12/93 | 65 |
| 3 µmol/g diet | F344 rats M | Lung | NNK (1.76 mg/kg body wt) | Diet: PEITC 21 weeks + s.c. NNK at end of week 1 | 43/80 | 31 |
| 5 µmol | A/J mice F | Lung | NNK (10 mmol) | Oral: PEITC 2 hours before NNK i.p. | 62/100 (tumor multiplicity in each rat) | 66 |
| 50 m$M$ | Syrian hamster M | Buccal pouch | NMBA (50 m$M$) | Topical 24 weeks | 6% | 67 |
| **SF** | | | | | | |
| 20 µmol | F344 rats M | Colon | AM (15 mg/kg body wt) | Oral: 3 times a week for 8 weeks, weekly s.c. azoxymethane weekly for 2 weeks | 40/100 | 5 |
| 5 µmol | | | | | 42/100 | 5 |

Note: M: male; F: Female; DMBA: 7,12-dimethyl-benz[a]anthracene; NNK: 4-(methylnitrosamino)-1-(3-pyridyl)-butanone; AM: axozymethane; NMBA: N-nitrosomethylbenzylamine.

**TABLE 21.4**
**Clinical Studies of Highest Crucifer Intake Groups**

| Cancer Investigated | Population | Study Design | OR or RR for High Intake Groups | Comment | Ref. |
|---|---|---|---|---|---|
| Lung cancer | Chinese women | 223 cases 187 controls | 0.31 (smokers) 0.70 (non-smokers) | | 18 |
| | American | 503 cases 465 controls | 1.09 (smokers) 1.08 (former smokers) | Data in column are for subjects null for GST T1 and M1; these showed least OR | 19 |
| Breast cancer | American | 740 cases 810 controls | 0.6 (premeno-pausal) | Broccoli intake measured; no significant associations for GST polymorphs or post-menopausal women | 34 |
| | Chinese | 1459 cases 1556 controls | 0.5 | Reports that association was seen in pre- and postmenopausal women | 36 |
| Bladder cancer | Males | 47909 subjects | RR 0.49 | Lowest incidence of cancer observed in the group with highest intake of cruciferous vegetables | 37 |

*Note:* OR: odds ratio; RR: risk ratio; GST: glutathione-*S*-transferase.

genotypes of glutathione-*S*-transferase. Varying results of epidemiological studies can be a consequence of methodological differences. Most studies categorize the subjects by crucifer intake levels, and Table 21.4 includes recent studies containing data for the highest crucifer intake groups. The incorporation of indicators of ITC consumption (such as the quantitation of total dithiocarbamates in urine) has resulted in the demonstration of significant inverse correlations between diet and cancer risk even with smaller studies, indicating the importance of verifying ITC exposure.[36]

## 21.6 MECHANISMS OF ACTION OF ISOTHIOCYANATES

### 21.6.1 INHIBITION OF PHASE I ENZYMES

ITCs have been shown to inhibit rat and human cytochrome P-450 (CYP) iso-forms, important for the activation of procarcinogens. CYPs 1A1, 1A2, 2B1, 2E1,

**TABLE 21.5**
**Phase I Enzyme Modulation by ITCs**

| ITC | System | Enzyme | Reaction Monitored | Result | Ref. |
|---|---|---|---|---|---|
| PEITC | RLM | CYP2E1 | NDMA demethylation | $IC_{50}$: 8.3 $\mu M$ | 68 |
| | | CYP1A2 | MROD | $IC_{50}$: 54 $\mu M$ | 69 |
| | | CYP2B1/2 | PROD | $IC_{50}$: 1.2 $\mu M$ | |
| | HLM | CYP1A2 | NNK keto-alcohol formation | $IC_{50}$: 4.6 $\mu M$ | 70 |
| | R-CYP (human) | CYP1A2 | Phenacetin-$o$-deethylase | Ki: 4.5 $\mu M$ | 39 |
| SF 10 $\mu M$ | HH | CYP3A4 | Changes in mRNA expression | −2.5-fold | 71 |
| 5 $\mu M$ for 24 h | RH | CYP1A1 | EROD | −80% | 71 |
| Red cabbage juice | Rat (oral; RLM activity measured) | CYP1A2 | MROD | +2.61-fold | 72 |

*Note:* NDMA: *N*-dimethylnitrosamino, NNK: 4-(methylnitrosamino)-1-(3-pyridyl)-1-butanone; MROD: methoxyresorufin dealkylation, EROD: ethoxyresorufin dealkylation, PROD: pentoxyresorufin dealkylation; RLM: rat liver microsomes; HLM: human liver microsomes: RH: rat hepatocytes; HH: human hepatocytes; R-CYP: recombinant cytochrome P-450. Positive sign indicates induction and negative sign indicates inhibition.

and 3A4 are inhibited by ITCs, through competitive, noncompetitive, or mixed inhibition.[39] Of these isoforms, 1A1 and 2E1 play the most important role in the activation of carcinogens. Table 21.5 presents studies in which ITCs have shown to exert inhibitory actions on CYPs. Structure–activity relationship studies have shown that arylalkyl ITCs with 6-carbon chains can cause maximum inhibition of CYP enzymes in rat liver microsomes.[40]

Human and rodent studies have demonstrated that PEITC blocks metabolic activation of 4-(methylnitrosamino)-1-(3-pyridyl)1-butanone (NNK) and benzo(*a*)pyrene (BaP), major lung carcinogens in tobacco smoke, via CYPs, resulting in increased urinary excretion of detoxified metabolites, suggesting inhibitory effects on CYP1A1, 1A2, and 2B1.[28,30,40] In humans, watercress ingestion resulted in a reduction in the levels of oxidative metabolites of acetaminophen, which was attributed to inhibition of oxidative metabolism by CYP2E1,[41] and enhancement in the area under the plasma concentration–time curve (AUC) of chlorzoxazone, a clinical probe for CYP2E1.[42] Watercress consumption in humans was shown to inhibit the metabolism of the tobacco specific carcinogen NNK (4-methylnitrosamino)-1-(3-pyridyl)-1-butanone), possibly by the inhibition of Phase I enzymes like CYP1A2.[43]

Recently, using microsomes from baculovirus-infected insect cells expressing human CYP isoforms, PEITC was found to competitively inhibit CYP1A2 and

**TABLE 21.6**
**Phase II Enzyme Induction by ITCs**

| ITC Treatment | Cell Line/Tissue | Enzyme in System | Induction Effect | Ref. |
|---|---|---|---|---|
| PEITC (5 μ$M$) | Human colon cell line | NQO1 | +140% | 48 |
| SF | | | | |
| 10 μ$M$ | Caco2 cells | UGT1A1, GST1A | +2-fold | 74 |
| 10 μ$M$ | Human prostate cancer cell | GST1A | +1.7-fold | 75 |
| 1 μ$M$ | Human lymphoblastoid cells | NQO1 | +2-fold | 76 |
| 40 μmol/kg/day | Rat duodenum | GST | +2.48-fold | 77 |
| 7-Methylsulfinylheptyl ITC (0.2 μ$M$) | Hepa 1c1c7 cells | NQO1 | +2-fold | 47 |
| 6-Methylsulfinylhexyl ITC (15 μmol/day) | ICR mice (liver) | GST | +2-fold | 78 |
| AITC (40 μmol/kg/day) | Rats (forestomach) | NQO1 | +1.5-fold | 77 |
| BITC (10 μ$M$) | RL34 rat liver cells | GSTP1 | +2.3-fold | 44 |

*Note:* NQO1: NAD(P)H quinone oxidoreductase 1; GST: glutathione-*S*-transferase.

2A6, noncompetitively inhibit CYP2B6, 2C9, 2C19, 2D6, and 2E1, and inhibit CYP3A4 following a mixed-type of competitive and noncompetitive inhibition.[39,44] However, controversial data exist. After PEITC administration to mice, CYP2E1 level increased in liver and lung microsomes.[30] Administration of PEITC to rats has been found to cause modest induction of CYP1A1 and 1A2 both in protein expression and metabolic activity,[45] different from the observation in baculovirus systems. A human study failed to show alteration of coumarin metabolism, a substrate for CYP2D6, after watercress consumption.[46]

### 21.6.2 INDUCTION OF PHASE II ENZYMES

Phase II enzymes are generally referred to as detoxifying enzymes, transferring hydrophilic endogenous substances such as glucuronic acid, sulfate, or glutathione to Phase I metabolites, or parent molecules. The hydrophilic molecules thus formed are more easily cleared from the body than their lipophilic parent compounds. ITCs have been classified as monofunctional inducers of Phase II enzymes; i.e., they induce Phase II enzymes without inducing Phase I enzymes.

A number of studies have demonstrated the Phase II inducing properties of ITCs both *in vivo* and *in vitro* (Table 21.6). An *in vivo* study of a mixture indole-3-carbinol, PEITC, and 1-isothiocyanato-3-(methylsulfinyl)-propane (a glucosinolate breakdown product) in F344 mice at dietary doses showed increase in the pancreatic mRNA levels for the enzymes NAD(P)H quinone oxidoreductase 1 (NQO1) and glutathione-$S$-transferase (GST) by 3.1- and 7.1-fold, respectively. Another comprehensive *in vivo* study of seven ITCs was conducted by Munday and compared the levels of induction of NQO1 and GST of the ITCs.[77]

SF has been reported to be the most potent Phase II enzyme inducer, while others like PEITC and AITC also showed significant induction of the enzymes. SF induced the transcription of UGT1A1 and GSTA1 in Caco2 cells and produced a synergistic induction effect on UTG1A1 with apigenin.[74] SF induced the Phase II enzyme GSTA1 at the transcriptional levels in human prostate cancer cell lines, HepG2, HT29, and enterocytes. In HepG2 and HT29 cells, concentrations of 0.3 to 30 $\mu M$ of SF significantly induce the transcription of GSTA1 and UDP glucuronosyl transferase, and exhibit a 2.8-fold increase in the formation of bilirubin glucuronide, indicating increased activity of the UDP enzyme. A human study on jejunum enterocytes has also reported that there was an increase in the induction of these enzymes 2.0- and 2.4-fold, respectively.[79]

Other ITCs, 7-methylsulfinylheptyl ITC and 8-methylsulfinyloctyl ITC, present in watercress have also been reported to have potent inducing activity toward quinone reductase.[47] BITC induced GSTP1 isoform in rat liver epithelial cells RL34 cells and increased in NQO1 activity in LS-174 human colon cell line.[44] PEITC increases the activities of UDP-glucuronosyltransferase (UGT), GST, and NQO1.[47] PEITC treatment of LS-174 human colon cells produced an increased protein expression of NQO1 and $\gamma$-glutamylcysteine synthetase.[48] Following watercress ingestion in smokers, there was an increased urinary elimination of the glucuronides of cotinine, suggesting an increased glucuronidation.[28]

Recent studies have suggested that ITCs induce glutathione-$S$-transferase, NQO1, and $\gamma$-glutamylcysteine through activating genes via the antioxidant/electrophile response element (ARE/EpRE), located upstream of genes that code for these enzymes. ITCs dissociate the cytoplasmic-anchoring protein Kelch-like ECH-associated protein 1 (Keap I) from the transcription factor Nrf2, allowing the latter to translocate to the nucleus and to form Nrf2/Maf heterodimers, which bind ARE/EpRE and activate transcription of genes coding the enzyme.[12,49] One proposed mechanism for the ITC-mediated effect on Keap I is ITC binding to the ATP binding domain present in Keap I. Keap I is a 624 amino acid protein that contains 25 cysteine residues, 9 of which are expected to have highly reactive sulfhydryl groups because they are close to 1 or more basic amino groups.[50]

### 21.6.3 Apoptosis and Cell Cycle Regulation

Most ITCs inhibit cell growth by arresting the $G_2/M$ or the $G_1$ cycle. The induction of apoptosis occurs via the activation of intracellular signaling pathways such as the MAPK and the caspase pathway. The MAPKs (ERK, JNK, and p38) convert various extracellular signals to intracellular responses through a series of phosphorylation pathways. Caspases are cysteine proteases, which are activated as a result of binding of death ligands to death receptors. The balance of anti-apoptotic

(Bcl-2 and Bcl-XL) vs. pro-apoptotic (Bad and Bax) proteins on the cell is also an important determinant of stress required to initiate apoptosis.

Studies into the mechanism of *in vitro* apoptosis induction have shown that while the action of SF and AITC is linked to an increase in caspase activity and the expression of pro-apoptotic proteins in the Bcl-2 family,[27,51] PEITC may cause the activation of the MAPK pathways, with JNK strongly activated. Components such as p53-dependent pathways have also been reported to be involved in the process.[52,53] In prostate cancer cell lines, PEITC has been shown to increase apoptosis by the reduced expression of BcL-2 and BcL-XL, and an increase in caspase activity.[27] A proposed sequence of events in apoptosis induced by ITCs is illustrated in a review by Thornalley.[13]

## 21.7  CONCLUSIONS

ITCs are widely present in the human diet. Epidemiological as well as experimental data have shown that ITCs have the potential to reduce the risk of cancer. ITCs modulate enzyme activity *in vivo* as well as *in vitro* and have also been shown to induce apoptosis and inhibit cell growth *in vitro* in a number of human cancer cell lines. Their chemopreventive properties have made the compounds attractive candidates for development as drugs. PEITC has entered a Phase I clinical trial for the compound in its ability to prevent lung cancer in smokers.[54] Development of more potent synthetic analogues of ITCs as drugs has also been undertaken.[55] As ITCs enter clinical use, the influence of the genetic polymorphism of GST on the chemopreventive properties of ITCs needs to be further studied.

## ACKNOWLEDGMENTS

The research was supported in part by U.S. Army Contracts DAMD17-00-1-0376 and DAMD 17-03-1-0527 and grants from the Susan G. Komen Breast Cancer Foundation and the Kapoor Charitable Foundation, University at Buffalo, State University of New York.

## REFERENCES

1. Lin HJ, Probst-Hensch NM, Louie AD, et al. Glutathione transferase null genotype, broccoli, and lower prevalence of colorectal adenomas [comment]. *Cancer Epidemiol Biomarkers Prev* 1998; 7(8):647–652.
2. van Poppel G, Verhoeven DT, Verhagen H, Goldbohm RA. *Brassica* vegetables and cancer prevention. Epidemiology and mechanisms. *Adv Exp Med Biol* 1999; 472:159–168.
3. Kristal AR, Lampe JW. *Brassica* vegetables and prostate cancer risk: a review of the epidemiological evidence. *Nutr Cancer* 2002; 42(1):1–9.

4. Morse MA, Lu J, Gopalakrishnan R, et al. Mechanism of enhancement of esophageal tumorigenesis by 6-phenylhexyl isothiocyanate. *Cancer Lett* 1997; 112(1):119–125.

5. Chung FL, Conaway CC, Rao CV, Reddy BS. Chemoprevention of colonic aberrant crypt foci in Fischer rats by sulforaphane and phenethyl isothiocyanate. *Carcinogenesis* 2000; 21(12):2287–2291.

6. Liebes L, Hochster H, Conaway CC, et al. Thirty day multiple dose administration of PEITC: a phase I study with steady state pharmacokinetics. *Proc of the 11th NCI-EORTC-AACR Symposium*; 2000.

7. Talalay P, Zhang Y. Chemoprotection against cancer by isothiocyanates and glucosinolates. *Biochem Soc Trans* 1996; 24(3):806–810.

8. Fahey JW, Zhang Y, Talalay P. Broccoli sprouts: an exceptionally rich source of inducers of enzymes that protect against chemical carcinogens. *Proc Natl Acad Sci USA* 1997; 94(19):10367–10372.

9. Ji Y, Morris ME. Determination of phenethyl isothiocyanate in human plasma and urine by ammonia derivatization and liquid chromatography-tandem mass spectrometry. *Anal Biochem* 2003; 323(1):39–47.

10. Hecht SS. Chemoprevention by isothiocyanates. *J Cell Biochem Suppl* 1995; 22:195–209.

11. Chung FL, Morse MA, Eklind KI, Lewis J. Quantitation of human uptake of the anticarcinogen phenethyl isothiocyanate after a watercress meal. *Cancer Epidemiol Biomarkers Prev* 1992; 1(5):383–388.

12. Talalay P, Fahey JW. Phytochemicals from cruciferous plants protect against cancer by modulating carcinogen metabolism. *J Nutr* 2001; 131(11 Suppl):3027S–3033S.

13. Thornalley PJ. Isothiocyanates: mechanism of cancer chemopreventive action. *Anticancer Drugs* 2002; 13(4):331–338.

14. Hu R, Hebbar V, Kim BR, et al. *In vivo* pharmacokinetics and regulation of gene expression profiles by isothiocyanate sulforaphane in the rat. *J Pharmacol Exp Ther* 2004; 310(1):263–271. Epub 2004 Feb 26.

15. Ketterer B. Dietary isothiocyanates as confounding factors in the molecular epidemiology of colon cancer [comment]. *Cancer Epidemiol Biomarkers Prev* 1998; 7(8):645–646.

16. Lin HJ, Han CY, Bernstein DA, Hsiao W, Lin BK, Hardy S. Ethnic distribution of the glutathione transferase Mu 1-1 (GSTM1) null genotype in 1473 individuals and application to bladder cancer susceptibility. *Carcinogenesis* 1994; 15(5):1077–1081.

17. London SJ, Yuan JM, Chung FL, et al. Isothiocyanates, glutathione S-transferase M1 and T1 polymorphisms, and lung-cancer risk: a prospective study of men in Shanghai, China. *Lancet* 2000; 356(9231):724–729.

18. Zhao B, Seow A, Lee EJ, et al. Dietary isothiocyanates, glutathione S-transferase -M1, -T1 polymorphisms and lung cancer risk among Chinese women in Singapore. *Cancer Epidemiol Biomarkers Prev* 2001; 10(10):1063–1067.

19. Spitz MR, Duphorne CM, Detry MA, et al. Dietary intake of isothiocyanates: evidence of a joint effect with glutathione S-transferase polymorphisms in lung cancer risk. *Cancer Epidemiol Biomarkers Prev* 2000; 9(10):1017–1020.

20. Hasegawa T, Nishino H, Iwashima A. Isothiocyanates inhibit cell cycle progression of HeLa cells at G2/M phase. *Anticancer Drugs* 1993; 4(2):273–279.

21. Conaway CC, Yang YM, Chung FL. Isothiocyanates as cancer chemopreventive agents: their biological activities and metabolism in rodents and humans. *Curr Drug Metab* 2002; 3(3):233–255.

22. Zhang Y, Tang L, Gonzalez V. Selected isothiocyanates rapidly induce growth inhibition of cancer cells. *Mol Cancer Ther* 2003; 2(10):1045–1052.

23. Tseng E, Scott-Ramsay EA, Morris ME. Dietary organic isothiocyanates are cytotoxic in human breast cancer MCF-7 and mammary epithelial MCF-12A cell lines. *Exp Biol Med (Maywood)* 2004; 229(8):835–842.

24. Peterson G, Barnes S. Genistein inhibition of the growth of human breast cancer cells: independence from estrogen receptors and the multi-drug resistance gene. *Biochem Biophys Res Commun* 1991; 179(1):661–667.

25. Fimognari C, Nusse M, Berti F, Iori R, Cantelli-Forti G, Hrelia P. Sulforaphane modulates cell cycle and apoptosis in transformed and non-transformed human T lymphocytes. *Ann NY Acad Sci* 2003; 1010:393–398.

26. Fimognari C, Nusse M, Iori R, Cantelli-Forti G, Hrelia P. The new isothiocyanate 4-(methylthio)butylisothiocyanate selectively affects cell-cycle progression and apoptosis induction of human leukemia cells. *Invest New Drugs* 2004; 22(2):119–129.

27. Xiao D, Srivastava SK, Lew KL, et al. Allyl isothiocyanate, a constituent of cruciferous vegetables, inhibits proliferation of human prostate cancer cells by causing G2/M arrest and inducing apoptosis. *Carcinogenesis* 2003; 24(5):891–897.

28. Hecht SS. Chemoprevention of cancer by isothiocyanates, modifiers of carcinogen metabolism. *J Nutr* 1999; 129(3):768S–774S.

29. Guo Z, Smith TJ, Wang E, et al. Effects of phenethyl isothiocyanate, a carcinogenesis inhibitor, on xenobiotic-metabolizing enzymes and nitrosamine metabolism in rats. *Carcinogenesis* 1992; 13(12):2205–2210.

30. Smith TJ, Guo Z, Li C, Ning SM, Thomas PE, Yang CS. Mechanisms of inhibition of 4-(methylnitrosamino)-1-(3-pyridyl)-1-butanone bioactivation in mouse by dietary phenethyl isothiocyanate. *Cancer Res* 1993; 53(14):3276–3282.

31. Morse MA, Wang CX, Stoner GD, et al. Inhibition of 4-(methylnitrosamino)-1-(3-pyridyl)-1-butanone-induced DNA adduct formation and tumorigenicity in the lung of F344 rats by dietary phenethyl isothiocyanate. *Cancer Res* 1989; 49(3):549–553.

32. Stoner GD, Morrissey DT, Heur YH, Daniel EM, Galati AJ, Wagner SA. Inhibitory effects of phenethyl isothiocyanate on N-nitrosobenzylmethylamine carcinogenesis in the rat esophagus. *Cancer Res* 1991; 51(8):2063–2068.

33. Zhao B, Seow A, Lee EJ, et al. Dietary isothiocyanates, glutathione S-transferase -M1, -T1 polymorphisms and lung cancer risk among Chinese women in Singapore. *Cancer Epidemiol Biomarkers Prev* 2001; 10(10):1063–1067.

34. Ambrosone CB, McCann SE, Freudenheim JL, Marshall JR, Zhang Y, Shields PG. Breast cancer risk in premenopausal women is inversely associated with consumption of broccoli, a source of isothiocyanates, but is not modified by GST genotype. *J Nutr* 2004; 134(5):1134–1138.

35. Liebes L, Conaway CC, Hochster H, et al. High-performance liquid chromatography-based determination of total isothiocyanate levels in human plasma: application to studies with 2-phenethyl isothiocyanate. *Anal Biochem* 2001; 291(2):279–289.

36. Fowke JH, Chung FL, Jin F, et al. Urinary isothiocyanate levels, brassica, and human breast cancer. *Cancer Res* 2003; 63(14):3980–3986.

37. Michaud DS, Spiegelman D, Clinton SK, Rimm EB, Willett WC, Giovannucci EL. Fruit and vegetable intake and incidence of bladder cancer in a male prospective cohort. *J Natl Cancer Inst* 1999; 91(7):605–613.

38. Seow A, Yuan JM, Sun CL, Van Den Berg D, Lee HP, Yu MC. Dietary isothiocyanates, glutathione S-transferase polymorphisms and colorectal cancer risk in the Singapore Chinese Health Study. *Carcinogenesis* 2002; 23(12):2055–2061.

39. Nakajima M, Yoshida R, Shimada N, Yamazaki H, Yokoi T. Inhibition and inactivation of human cytochrome P450 isoforms by phenethyl isothiocyanate. *Drug Metab Dispos* 2001; 29(8):1110–1113.

40. Conaway CC, Jiao D, Chung FL. Inhibition of rat liver cytochrome P450 isozymes by isothiocyanates and their conjugates: a structure–activity relationship study. *Carcinogenesis* 1996; 17(11):2423–2427.

41. Chen L, Mohr SN, Yang CS. Decrease of plasma and urinary oxidative metabolites of acetaminophen after consumption of watercress by human volunteers. *Clin Pharmacol Ther* 1996; 60(6):651–660.

42. Leclercq I, Desager JP, Horsmans Y. Inhibition of chlorzoxazone metabolism, a clinical probe for CYP2E1, by a single ingestion of watercress. *Clin Pharmacol Ther* 1998; 64(2):144–149.

43. Hecht SS, Chung FL, Richie JP, Jr, et al. Effects of watercress consumption on metabolism of a tobacco-specific lung carcinogen in smokers. *Cancer Epidemiol Biomarkers Prev* 1995; 4(8):877–884.

44. Nakamura Y, Ohigashi H, Masuda S, et al. Redox regulation of glutathione S-transferase induction by benzyl isothiocyanate: correlation of enzyme induction with the formation of reactive oxygen intermediates. *Cancer Res* 2000; 60(2):219–225.

45. Manson MM, Ball HW, Barrett MC, et al. Mechanism of action of dietary chemoprotective agents in rat liver: induction of phase I and II drug metabolizing enzymes and aflatoxin B1 metabolism. *Carcinogenesis* 1997; 18(9):1729–1738.

46. Murphy SE, Johnson LM, Losey LM, Carmella SG, Hecht SS. Consumption of watercress fails to alter coumarin metabolism in humans. *Drug Metab Dispos* 2001; 29(6):786–788.

47. Rose P, Faulkner K, Williamson G, Mithen R. 7-Methylsulfinylheptyl and 8-methylsulfinyloctyl isothiocyanates from watercress are potent inducers of phase II enzymes. *Carcinogenesis* 2000; 21(11):1983–1988.

48. Bonnesen C, Eggleston IM, Hayes JD. Dietary indoles and isothiocyanates that are generated from cruciferous vegetables can both stimulate apoptosis and confer protection against DNA damage in human colon cell lines. *Cancer Res* 2001; 61(16):6120–6130.

49. Lampe JW, Peterson S. *Brassica*, biotransformation and cancer risk: genetic polymorphisms alter the preventive effects of cruciferous vegetables. *J Nutr* 2002; 132(10):2991–2994.

50. Dinkova-Kostova AT, Massiah MA, Bozak RE, Hicks RJ, Talalay P. Potency of Michael reaction acceptors as inducers of enzymes that protect against carcinogenesis depends on their reactivity with sulfhydryl groups. *Proc Natl Acad Sci USA* 2001; 98(6):3404–3409.

51. Singh AV, Xiao D, Lew KL, Dhir R, Singh SV. Sulforaphane induces caspase-mediated apoptosis in cultured PC-3 human prostate cancer cells and retards growth of PC-3 xenografts *in vivo*. *Carcinogenesis* 2004; 25(1):83–90. Epub 2003 Sep 26.

52. Chen YR, Wang W, Kong AN, Tan TH. Molecular mechanisms of c-Jun N-terminal kinase-mediated apoptosis induced by anticarcinogenic isothiocyanates. *J Biol Chem* 1998; 273(3):1769–1775.

53. Huang C MW-y. Essential role of p53 in phenethyl isothiocyanate-induced apoptosis. *Cancer Res* 1998; 58:4102–4106.

54. Accessed at http://cancer.gov/clinicaltrials/NYU-9905.

55. Gerhauser C, You M, Liu J, et al. Cancer chemopreventive potential of sulforamate, a novel analogue of sulforaphane that induces phase 2 drug-metabolizing enzymes. *Cancer Res* 1997; 57(2):272–278.

56. Rouzaud G, Young SA, Duncan AJ. Hydrolysis of glucosinolates to isothiocyanates after ingestion of raw or microwaved cabbage by human volunteers. *Cancer Epidemiol Biomarkers Prev* 2004; 13(1):125–131.

57. Shapiro TA, Fahey JW, Wade KL, Stephenson KK, Talalay P. Chemoprotective glucosinolates and isothiocyanates of broccoli sprouts: metabolism and excretion in humans. *Cancer Epidemiol Biomarkers Prev* 2001; 10(5):501–508.

58. Getahun SM, Chung FL. Conversion of glucosinolates to isothiocyanates in humans after ingestion of cooked watercress. *Cancer Epidemiol Biomarkers Prev* 1999; 8(5):447–451.

59. Hwang ES, Jeffery EH. Evaluation of urinary N-acetyl cysteinyl allyl isothiocyanate as a biomarker for intake and bioactivity of Brussels sprouts. *Food Chem Toxicol* 2003; 41(12):1817–1825.

60. Chiao JW, Chung FL, Kancherla R, Ahmed T, Mittelman A, Conaway CC. Sulforaphane and its metabolite mediate growth arrest and apoptosis in human prostate cancer cells. *Int J Oncol* 2002; 20(3):631–636.

61. Gamet-Payrastre L, Li P, Lumeau S, et al. Sulforaphane, a naturally occurring isothiocyanate, induces cell cycle arrest and apoptosis in HT29 human colon cancer cells. *Cancer Res* 2000; 60(5):1426–1433.

62. Jackson SJ, Singletary KW. Sulforaphane: a naturally occurring mammary carcinoma mitotic inhibitor, which disrupts tubulin polymerization. *Carcinogenesis* 2004; 25(2):219–227.

63. Srivastava SK, Singh SV. Cell cycle arrest, apoptosis induction and inhibition of nuclear factor kappa B activation in anti-proliferative activity of benzyl isothiocyanate against human pancreatic cancer cells. *Carcinogenesis* 2004; 25(9):1701–1709.

64. Miyoshi N, Uchida K, Osawa T, Nakamura Y. A link between benzyl isothiocyanate-induced cell cycle arrest and apoptosis: involvement of mitogen-activated protein kinases in the Bcl-2 phosphorylation. *Cancer Res* 2004; 64(6):2134–2142.

65. Wattenberg LW. Inhibition of carcinogenic effects of polycyclic hydrocarbons by benzyl isothiocyanate and related compounds. *J Natl Cancer Inst* 1977; 58(2):395–398.

66. Jiao D, Eklind KI, Choi CI, Desai DH, Amin SG, Chung FL. Structure–activity relationships of isothiocyanates as mechanism-based inhibitors of 4-(methylnitrosamino)-1-(3-pyridyl)-1-butanone-induced lung tumorigenesis in A/J mice. *Cancer Res* 1994; 54(16):4327–4333.

67. Solt DB, Chang K, Helenowski I, Rademaker AW. Phenethyl isothiocyanate inhibits nitrosamine carcinogenesis in a model for study of oral cancer chemoprevention. *Cancer Lett* 2003; 202(2):147–152.

68. Jiao D, Conaway CC, Wang MH, Yang CS, Koehl W, Chung FL. Inhibition of *N*-nitrosodimethylamine demethylase in rat and human liver microsomes by isothiocyanates and their glutathione, L-cysteine, and *N*-acetyl-L-cysteine conjugates. *Chem Res Toxicol* 1996; 9(6):932–938.

69. Thapliyal R, Maru GB. Inhibition of cytochrome P450 isozymes by curcumins *in vitro* and *in vivo*. *Food Chem Toxicol* 2001; 39(6):541–547.

70. Smith TJ, Guo Z, Guengerich FP, Yang CS. Metabolism of 4-(methylnitrosamino)-1-(3-pyridyl)-1-butanone (NNK) by human cytochrome P450 1A2 and its inhibition by phenethyl isothiocyanate. *Carcinogenesis* 1996; 17(4):809–813.

71. Maheo K, Morel F, Langouet S, et al. Inhibition of cytochromes P-450 and induction of glutathione S-transferases by sulforaphane in primary human and rat hepatocytes. *Cancer Res* 1997; 57(17):3649–3652.

72. Kassie F, Uhl M, Rabot S, et al. Chemoprevention of 2-amino-3-methylimidazo[4,5-f]quinoline (IQ)-induced colonic and hepatic preneoplastic lesions in the F344 rat by cruciferous vegetables administered simultaneously with the carcinogen. *Carcinogenesis* 2003; 24(2):255–261.

73. Basten GP, Bao Y, Williamson G. Sulforaphane and its glutathione conjugate but not sulforaphane nitrile induce UDP-glucuronosyl transferase (UGT1A1) and glutathione transferase (GSTA1) in cultured cells. *Carcinogenesis* 2002; 23(8):1399–1404.

74. Svehlikova V, Wang S, Jakubikova J, Williamson G, Mithen R, Bao Y. Interactions between sulforaphane and apigenin in the induction of UGT1A1 and GSTA1 in CaCo-2 cells. *Carcinogenesis* 2004; 25(9):1629–1637.

75. Brooks JD, Paton VG, Vidanes G. Potent induction of phase 2 enzymes in human prostate cells by sulforaphane. *Cancer Epidemiol Biomarkers Prev* 2001; 10(9):949–954.

76. Misiewicz I, Skupinska K, Kowalska E, Lubinski J, Kasprzycka-Guttman T. Sulforaphane-mediated induction of a phase 2 detoxifying enzyme NAD(P)H:quinone reductase and apoptosis in human lymphoblastoid cells. *Acta Biochim Pol* 2004; 51(3):711–721.

77. Munday R, Munday CM. Induction of phase II detoxification enzymes in rats by plant-derived isothiocyanates: comparison of allyl isothiocyanate with sulforaphane and related compounds. *J Agric Food Chem* 2004; 52(7):1867–1871.

78. Morimitsu Y, Nakagawa Y, Hayashi K, et al. A sulforaphane analogue that potently activates the Nrf2-dependent detoxification pathway. *J Biol Chem* 2002; 277(5):3456–3463.

79. Petri N, Tannergren C, Holst B, Mellon FA, Bao Y, Plumb GW, Bacon J, O'Leary KA, Kroon PA, Knutson L, Forsell P, Eriksson T, Lennernas H, Williamson G. Absorption/metabolism of sulforaphane and quercetin, and regulation of phase II enzymes, in human jejunum in vivo. *Drug Metab Disp* 2003; 31(6):805–813.

80. Xiao D, Johnson CS, Trump DL, Singh SV. Proteasome-mediated degradation of cell division cycle 25C and cyclin-dependent kinase I in phenethyl isothiocyanate-induced G2-M-phase cell cycle arrest in PC-3 human prostate cancer cells. *Mol Cancer Ther* 2004; 3(5):567–575.

81. Tang L, Zhang Y. Dietary isothiocyanates inhibit the growth of human bladder carcinoma cells. *J Nutr* 2004; 134(8):2004–2010.

# Part VII

*Dietary Components That
Protect from Cancer: Saponins*

# 22 Anticancer Activity of Ginseng and Soy Saponins

*David G. Popovich and David D. Kitts*

## CONTENTS

22.1   Introduction .................................................................................................458
22.2   Saponins ......................................................................................................458
22.3   Saponin Functions and Formation in Plants .............................................459
22.4   Cancer Preventative Properties of Ginseng and Ginsenosides ...........459
      22.4.1   Antioxidant Properties of Ginseng .............................................460
      22.4.2   Immune-Stimulating Properties of Ginseng ..............................461
      22.4.3   Anticancer Activity of Ginseng and Ginsenosides .................462
      22.4.4   Effect on Cultured Cancer Cells .................................................463
      22.4.5   Effect on Cellular Membranes .....................................................467
      22.4.6   Effect of Ginseng and Ginsenosides on Membrane
               Hemolysis .......................................................................................467
      22.4.7   Effect of Ginsenoside Structure on Bioactivity ......................468
      22.4.8   Potential Synergy, Multidrug-Resistant Cancer ......................469
      22.4.9   *In Vivo* Animal Cancer Models ...............................................470
      22.4.10 Human Anticancer Evidence ....................................................471
22.5   Cancer Preventative Properties of Soyasaponins ...................................471
      22.5.1   Bioavailability of Soyasaponins .................................................472
      22.5.2   Antioxidant Activity ......................................................................472
      22.5.3   Immune System ..............................................................................474
      22.5.4   Cultured Cell Experiments ...........................................................474
      22.5.5   Hepatoprotective Effects of Soyasaponins ...............................476
      22.5.6   Soysaponins and Animal Colon Cancer Model ........................476
22.6   Conclusion ..................................................................................................476
References .............................................................................................................477

## 22.1  INTRODUCTION

Saponins are triterpenoid glycosides that have long been a focus of tradition and herbal folklore.[1] The South American soap-bark tree, *Quillaja saponaria,* is probably the best-known source of saponins and has a history of use by aboriginal inhabitants of the Central Andes in South America. Other sources of saponins include ginseng, one of the most-studied traditional herbal ingredient,[2] and soy, one of the primary food sources for saponins.[3] Traditional oriental medicinal practitioners have used ginseng as part of their treatment regime for more than 5000 years.[4] Soy also has a long traditional use as a staple food in Asian countries. Recently, there has been considerable focus on soy constituents, especially in Western countries, for their potential health-promoting functions such as estrogen-like activity of phytoestrogens, and cholesterol-lowering abilities associated with soy proteins. Soy, as well as ginseng, also contains bioactive saponins. The focus of this chapter is on the bioactive properties of saponins derived from ginseng and soy with emphasis on their potential anticarcinogenicity.

## 22.2  SAPONINS

Saponins are characterized by the property of producing a soapy lather and are usually found as a sugar glycoside linked to a hydrophobic steroid-like aglycone. The primary active components of ginseng are generally recognized to be a group of 30 different triterpene saponins, also referred to as ginsenosides or dammarane triterpenoids. Ginsenosides share a similar basic structure consisting of a gonane steroid nucleus having 17 carbon atoms arranged in four rings (Figure 22.1). Differences in ginsenoside structure, which determines the classification of ginsenosides, include the type, position, and number of sugar moieties attached by glycosidic bonds at positions C-3 and C-6. Two main aglycone structures in ginseng have been identified. Ginsenosides unit sugar moieties attached at C-3 and C-6 are referred to as protopanaxadiol ginsenosides and protopanaxatriol ginsenosides, respectively. Only one oleanolic acid type saponin, ginsenoside-Ro, has been identified from ginseng.[5]

Soyasaponins are triterpenoid glycosides with four common rings. Three main aglycone soyasaponins have been identified and labeled as soyasaponin A, B, E. (Figure 22.5). Many different combinations of sugar moieties attached at positions C-3, C-21, and C-22 of the ring structure have been characterized. At least six difference saponin glycosides have been identified as belonging to group A saponins[6] and five saponin glycoside compounds have been identified as belonging to group B saponins.[7] Furthermore, unnatural saponins can be generated after storage[8] and extraction conditions.

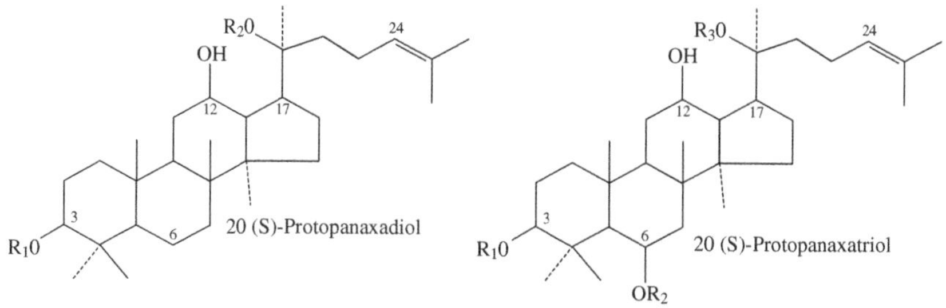

20 (S)-Protopanaxadiol

| 20 (S)-Protopanaxadiol | | |
|---|---|---|
| | R1 | R2 |
| Rb1 | O-G-G | O-G-G |
| Rb2 | O-G-G | O-G-Ap |
| Rb3 | O-G-G | O-G-X |
| Rc | O-G-G | O-G-Af |
| Rd | O-G-G | O-G |
| Rg3 | O-G-G | O-H |
| Rh2 | O-G | O-H |
| | | |
| Aglycone (PD) | O-H | O-H |

| 20 (S)-Protopanaxadiol | | | |
|---|---|---|---|
| | R1 | R2 | R3 |
| Re | O-H | O-G-R | O-G |
| Rf | O-H | O-G-G | O-H |
| Rg1 | O-H | O-G | O-G |
| Rg2 | O-H | O-G-R | O-H |
| Rh1 | O-H | O-G | O-H |
| | | | |
| Aglycone (PT) | O-H | O-H | O-H |

**FIGURE 22.1** A selection of the ginsenosides of 20(S)-protopanaxadiol and 20(S)-protopanaxatriol classifications. Ginsenoside basic structure consists of gonane steroid nucleus having 17 carbon atoms arranged in four rings. Individual ginsenosides differ by attachments of molecules at regions R1–R3, respectively. Ap = arabinopyranose, Af = arabinofuranose, G = glucopyranose, R = rhamnopyranose, X = xylopyranose.[118]

## 22.3 SAPONIN FUNCTIONS AND FORMATION IN PLANTS

Saponins function to provide plants with a defensive system against predator attack.[9] Many saponins have been suggested to have multiple adverse effects on animal health, fungi and bacteria viability, and mold growth.[10] Ginsenosides, like many other saponins, are synthesized from the central isoprenoid pathway, where squalene synthase catalyzes the first step in the overall formation.[11] The initial pathway eventually leads to 2,3-oxidosqualene products, which are further modified to plant sterols, dammarane-type triterpene saponins (ginsenosides) or oleanane-type triterpene saponins[11] and a host of different compounds. There is growing interest in developing antineoplastic agents from plant-derived triterpenoids and a number of different compounds have shown promise.[12]

## 22.4 CANCER PREVENTATIVE PROPERTIES OF GINSENG AND GINSENOSIDES

Cancer preventative strategies generally include enhancing the overall antioxidant status, thereby reducing damaging effects of free radicals and reducing overall

DNA damage and mutant cell formation. Furthermore, immune stimulation is also part of an overall cancer preventative and defensive strategy by priming the system to recognize and eliminate mutated, damaged, or infected cells. Ginseng is a general term recognized to encompass herbs from the family *Araliaceae* and the genus *Panax*. The word *Panax* is derived from the Greek word meaning "cure-all." A majority of scientific studies have focused on two species of ginseng: *P. ginseng* C.A. Meyer (Asian ginseng) and *P. quinquefolius* (North American ginseng). Siberian or Russian ginseng (*Eleutherococcus senticosus*) is derived from an entirely different plant than ginseng and contains different active components and should not be confused with true ginseng.

Typically, roots from Asian ginseng (*P. ginseng* C.A. Meyer) are commonly divided into either white or red ginseng based on the drying technique used to ensure preservation. Asian ginseng usually refers to the root of *P. ginseng* C.A. Meyer that has been air-dried. Red ginseng usually refers to Korean red ginseng that has been subjected to a steam-heating process before drying and processing; steaming ginseng will produce a red tinge due to caramelization of sugars when compared to the beige color of air-dried root. However, red ginseng is not solely a product of Korea; it is also produced in China. Compositional studies indicate that there are minor differences in content between red and white ginseng, with red ginseng typically believed to have the stronger potency.[13] North American ginseng (*P. quinquefolius*) is virtually identical in shape and physical characteristics to Asian ginseng. North American ginseng is typically grown in the eastern United States and in the Canadian provinces of Ontario and British Columbia. Furthermore, ginseng root has historically been a valuable agricultural commodity, especially in Hong Kong, China, and Korea. However, recent interest has focused on developing herbal extracts from alternative plant materials such as the ginseng leaf[14,15] and berry.[16]

### 22.4.1 ANTIOXIDANT PROPERTIES OF GINSENG

Antioxidant properties such as free radical scavenging activity of ginseng extracts have been demonstrated from a number of *in vitro* studies but antioxidant properties attributed to specific ginsenosides have not been clearly established. These reports showed activity of ginseng extracts in scavenging stable free radical (e.g., 1,1-diphenyl-2-picrylhydrazyl, DPPH)[17,18] and carbon-centered free radicals (2,2′-azobis(2-amindinopropane) dihydrochloride, AAPH).[17,19] North American ginseng extracts have been shown to be effective at both chelation of metal ion and scavenging of free radicals in lipid and aqueous mediums.[18] North American ginseng was reported to have higher affinity to scavenge free radicals compared with Asian ginseng.[19] Both Asian and North American ginseng can protect low-density lipoproteins and supercoiled DNA against cupric ion inducting oxidation and DNA breakage, respectively.[19] Alternatively, aqueous extracts from Korean red ginseng, prepared both with and without heat, did not significantly differ in free radical scavenging ability and were overall not strong scavengers.[17] Methanol extracts of heat-treated Asian ginseng reduced lipid peroxidation in rat brain homogenates, which was induced with ferric ion and ferric ion plus ascorbic acid, and the extract protected against supercoiled DNA strand scission.[20] In transfected hepatoma cells, ginsenosides Rb2 induced the transcription of Cu, Zn-superoxide dismutase gene (*SOD1*) to a greater extent than ginsenoside Rb1 and total saponins did not have an effect.[21] Superoxide dismutase is a key enzyme involved in the removal of superoxide radicals. Ginseng extracts have also been shown to affect the antioxidant defense mechanism by increasing hepatic glutathione peroxidase activity and superoxide dismutase in rats receiving a ginseng extract for 3 months.[22]

Pretreatment of endothelial cells with ginsenosides of Korean red ginseng, reduced NADPH-driven superoxide generation.[23] Artificial digestion (*in vitro*) of the standardized ginseng extract (G115) modified the ginsenoside composition and resulted in a greater effect on pulmonary vasodilation and protection from free radical injury compared to ginsenoside standards Rb1 and Rg1.[24] This effect on vasodilation and protection from free radicals is mediated through nitric oxide (NO) production. The antioxidant potential of individual ginsenosides were ranked by the affinity to induced free radical (AAPH) hemolysis of human erythrocytes,[25] with the relative order of antioxidant activity in the following decreasing order: Rc, Rb1, Re, Rd, Rg1, and Rb3.[25] Rg3, Rd, and Rh2 were suggested to possess pro-oxidant characteristics in this erythrocyte hemolysis model;[26] these results tend to suggest that larger ginsenosides, those with more attached sugar molecules such as Rc and Rb1, have greater antioxidant potential compared to relative smaller ginsenosides, such as Rh2.

## 22.4.2 Immune-Stimulating Properties of Ginseng

The immune-stimulating properties of ginseng have long been touted as one of the main biological effects of ginseng.[27] The results from *in vitro* immune stimulation studies are varied. For example, a North American ginseng extract (200 μg/ml) has been reported to stimulate human polymorphonuclear leukocytes *in vitro* and treatment stimulated human tumor necrosis factor-α (TNF-α) release after 6 h.[28] TNF-α is an important marker in early immune response. Specific ginsenosides Rb1, Rb2, and Rc were found to inhibit TNF-α dose dependently after lipopolysaccharide (LPS) stimulation of murine macrophage cells (RAWE264.7) and differentiated human macrophage cells (U937).[29] Asian ginseng increased cytokine (interleukin-12, IL-12) release from mouse macrophage cells (J774A.1) but no change was reported for IL-1β, IL-15, TNF-α.[30] Cellular immunity was enhanced in individuals exposed to ginseng extracts in normal, chronic fatigue syndrome, and in AIDS subjects according to *in vitro* natural killer function activity of isolated peripheral blood mononuclear cells.[31] In a rat model of cystic fibrosis lung infection, subcutaneous injection of ginseng improved bacterial clearance from the lungs, improved lung pathology, and lowered lung abscess incidence.[32]

The effect of ginseng extracts in healthy human volunteers is reported to enhance cellular immunity.[33] Capsules of the ginseng extract (100 mg) taken for

12 weeks with an influenza vaccination reduced the frequency of influenza from 42 cases for the placebo group (vaccination only) to 15 for the ginseng-treated group.[27] A similar immunomodulatory activity toward influenza has been reported using a proprietary extract.[34] Administration of Korean red ginseng to patients infected with HIV-1 was reported to delay the resistance to active antiretroviral drug therapy.[35] Treatment with Korean red ginseng in combination with zidovudine (ZDV, also known as AZT) therapy resulted in a significantly longer time (e.g., 34 months) to develop drug-resistant mutant strains compared to control patients. IL-8, a cytokine that exerts chemotaxis on neutrophils, T-cells, and basophils, was also induced by ginseng root, an induction that is accompanied by increased IL-8 mRNA expression.[36]

Human bacteria collected from fecal material have been reported to hydrolyze ginsenosides Rb1 and Rb2 to specific 20-β-$O$-glucopyranosy-20(S)-protopanaxadiol metabolites, referred to as IH-901 or compound K.[37] Ginsenosides Rb1 and Rb2 are transformed to Rg3 under mildly acidic conditions common to the stomach environment; after which Rg3 is further metabolized by intestinal bacteria fusobacterium K-60, bacteriodes HJ-15, and bifidobacterium K-506 and transformed to Rh2.[38] Compound K transformed from ginseng saponins has reported antitumor activity.[39] The general efficacy of saponins to stimulate the immune system may in part be explained by the affinity to affect the cells of the gastrointestinal tract and alter permeability. Enhanced gastrointestinal permeability to nutrients or xenobiotic agents creates an environment that facilitates increased uptake of antigens[10] and thus a broad stimulation of the immune system. Oral administration of a boiled Asian ginseng extract to mice has been reported to enhance the antibody formation to either a primary or a secondary challenge with sheep red cells, in a dose-dependent manner. Specifically, at a dose of 250 mg/kg, the primary IgM response was increased by 50% and the secondary IgG and IgM responses were increased by 50 and 100%, respectively.[40] Although the precise mechanisms for saponins- or ginsenosides-induced change on gastrointestinal tract cell membrane permeability have not been fully clarified, they are, however, able to interact with the gastrointestinal cell environment[10] by influencing microbial growth and function.

### 22.4.3 ANTICANCER ACTIVITY OF GINSENG AND GINSENOSIDES

By far the most comprehensive data on ginsenoside anticancer activity were derived from culture cancer cell experiments utilizing a variety of different cancer cell lines. The main focus of many of these cancer model experiments was on determination of the cytotoxic effect and ability to influence cellular proliferation. Furthermore, determination of the mode of cell death, either by apoptotic or necrotic cell death pathways, has produced a number of reports that associated individual ginsenosides, usually the hydrophobic ones, with specific cellular death signals such as activation of caspase-3. Alternatively, there are also many reports on the ability of specific ginsenosides to influence cultured cell membrane integrity and hemolysis, resulting in altered membrane channel and ion activation. The extent to which ginsenosides or other saponin compounds are able to induce membrane injury, hemolysis, and activation of membrane channel may be linked to an ability to influence multidrug resistance cancer cells through modulation of the membrane bound P-glycoprotein (P-gp) pump.

## 22.4.4 Effect on Cultured Cancer Cells

In recent years, the diverse effect of ginseng and individual ginsenosides has been studied using cultured cancer cell lines. The cell lines include human liver,[41] leukemia,[42,43] prostate,[44] breast,[45] intestinal,[14,46] and a variety of mouse and other cell types. Different ginsenosides do not inhibit cultured cancer cell proliferation equally. Only the more hydrophobic ginsenosides, such as Rg3, Rh2, Rh1, and both of the aglycones of the protopanaxadiol and protopanaxadiol groups, have been reported to have an impact on cell proliferation. A summary of the $LC_{50}$ determined from cultured cancer cell cytotoxicity experiments using leukemia and intestinal cells conducted in our laboratory is shown in Figure 22.2. Generally, ginsenosides aglycones PD and PT and ginsenosides Rh2 reduce cultured cell viability within a measurable $LC_{50}$, whereas more common ginsenosides, such as Rb1, Rc, Rd, Re, and Rg1, do not reduce the growth of intestinal cell lines[46] and other cultured cancer cells.[41] Furthermore, ginseng extracts do not normally inhibit the growth of cultured cells because of the variable composition of individual ginsenosides, and the low concentration of the hydrophobic ginsenosides. Specifically, ginsenoside Rh2 has an effect on cell proliferation reported by a variety of different research groups;[14,42,45,47] however, the extent to which Rh2 affects the genomic regulation of the cell impacting protein expression, or acts specially on the cellular membrane is unclear at present.

Ginsenosides Rh2, PD, and PT have been reported to induce apoptosis or programmed cell death detected either by DNA ladder pattern by electrophoresis[47] or by a buildup of sub-$G_1$ cells measured by flow cytometry.[42,46] In our laboratory we found that when ginsenosides Rh2, PD, and PT were applied to cells at their respective $LC_{50}$, the build-up of sub-$G_1$ cells was greatest for Rh2-treated intestinal cells (Caco-2, Int-407), whereas PD produced greater number sub-$G_1$ cell for leukemia cells (THP-1) (Figure 22.3, below). The apoptotic cell death pathway is distinguished from necrotic cell death as an active death program guided by distinct cellular events. Further specific markers of apoptosis, such as caspase-3 or proteins involved in arresting or progression of the cell cycle have been measured after exposure to ginsenoside Rh2. Rh2 increased activation of caspase-3 in transfected SK-HEP-1 cells,[48] and both caspase-3 and 8 in human melanoma (A375-S2) cells.[47] Furthermore, Rh2 has been reported to decrease cyclin-dependent kinase2 (cdk2) in three of four mouse cell lines,[49] increased p27 kip1 activity,[49] increased p21 WAF1, and cyclin D, but decreased cdk2 and cyclin E in breast cancer cells.[45]

The genomic effects of ginsenosides measured by protein expression, such as the cell cycle regulators, have been associated with the composition of the culture media. The protein content or other serum component of media (BSA, or

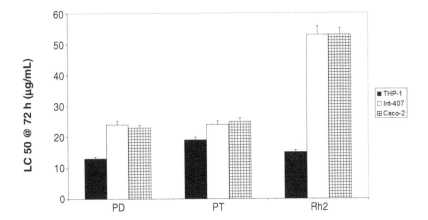

**FIGURE 22.2** $LC_{50}$ determined in three distinct culture cancer cells THP-1 (monocyte leukemia[42]), Caco-2 (adenocarcinoma colon cells), and Int-407 (transformed embryonic intestinal cells[46]) after 72-h exposure to cytotoxic ginsenosides (PD, PT, Rh2). Other ginsenosides such as fingerprint ginsenosides (Rb1, Rb2, Rc, Rd, Re, Rg1) were not found to be cytotoxic and thus to not have a measurable $LC_{50}$. Data are expressed as mean ± standard deviation.

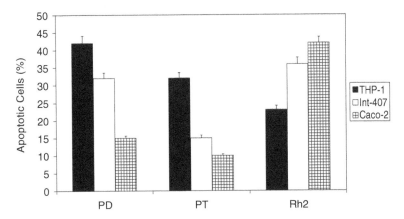

**FIGURE 22.3** Sub-$G_1$ cell buildup from ginsenosides PD, PT, Rh2 exposure in Caco-2, Int-407, and THP-1 measured by flow cytometry. Ginsenosides were applied to cells at their respective $LC_{50}$ concentrations.

cholesterol) may influence the effect of ginsenosides in cell culture experiments[50] and reduce or prevent the effects of ginsenosides, especially Rh2,[51] when compared to the aglycone. Serum-free media conditions resulted in a greater cellular concentration of PD compared to Rh2 at the same dose, and the cellular uptake of Rh2 and PD were reduced as the concentration of serum increased.[50] Cellular PD uptake was rapid and at least partially incorporated in the inner region of the membrane.[50] The growth inhibition of PD (1.3 $\mu M$) is stronger than Rh2 (2.0 $\mu M$) in serum-free media.[50] PD is also stronger than Rh2 in 10% serum media but at much greater concentration.[42] A reduction in the serum concentration of the media has an effect in cell systems and may enhance the biological activity of ginsenosides. The effects of specific ginsenosides on cultured cancer cells as a function of serum concentration are listed in Tables 22.1 and 22.2, respectively.

**TABLE 22.1**

**Cell Culture Studies Using Specific Ginsenoside Tested with Serum Media Concentration of 5% or Less**

| Compounds | Cells | Major Finding | Ref. |
|---|---|---|---|
| Rh2 | SK-HEP-1 and transfected bcl-2 cells | Activation of caspase-3 | 104 |
| Rh2 | A375-S2 | Dose- and time-dependent inhibition; sub-$G_1$ buildup between 0 and 40 $\mu$mol/L but at 60 $\mu$mol/L declines; ↑ caspase 8 and 3 | 47 |
| Rh2 | B16, Meth-A, A31-1-1, A-31-1-13 | ↓ cdk2 in 3 of 4 cell lines Rh2 incorporated into cells | 49 |
| Rh2 | SK-HEP-1, HeLA, Chang liver, COS7, FT02B | ↑ p27 kip1 no effect on cyclin E, cdk2, p21 WAF1 | 105 |
| Rh2 | Rat C6 gliomal cells (transfected) | Rh2 cell death related to ROS generation, ↑ caspase, no Bcl-XL | 106 |
| Rh1, Rh2 | B16 (mouse) | Rh2 inhibit growth, stimulate melonogenesis, ↑ adhesiveness, ↑ agglutinability; cell surface membrane and composition were changed, Rh2 incorporated into membranes, changed lipid organization, ↑ polarization = more rigid cell; Rh2 does not | 107 |
| Rg3, Rg5, Rk1, Rs5, Rs4 | SK-HEP-1 | Rg3, Rg5, Rk1, Rs5, Rs4 are cytotoxic, whereas Rb1, Rc, Rb2, Rd are not | 41 |
| Panaxadiol | SK-HEP-1 | Depolarization of mitochondria membrane. ↑ caspase 9, 3, not 8, ↑ cytochrome c, ↑ cdk2 | 108 |
| Rs4 | SK-HEP-1 (hepatoma cells) | ↑ p53 and p21 WAF1 | 109 |
| Rb1, M1 (intestinal metabolite) | B16-Bl6 | Rb1 no effect, M1 dose and time dependent, inside cell after 15 min; ↑ p27 kip1, ↓ c-Myc and cyclin-D1 | 110 |
| PD, Rh2, Rg3, Compound K (intestinal metabolite) | L1210, Ehrlich ascite tumor cells | Rg3, Rh2, K, ↑ liposome permeability without cholesterol, Rh2, Rg3, ↓ cytotoxicity as cholesterol level of cells ↑ | 69 |

**TABLE 22.2**
**Cell Culture Studies Using Specific Ginsenoside Tested with a Serum**
**Medium Concentration of 10%**

| Compounds | Cells | Major Finding | Ref. |
|---|---|---|---|
| Rd2, Re, Rf, Rg1-3, Ro | LNCaP, L929 | ↓ PSA (prostate specific antigen) ↓ AR (androgen receptor) ↓ 5α reductase, ↑ bcl-2 and caspase-3 | 44 |
| Rh2 | MCF-7 | Dose-dependent inhibition, cytostatic not cytotoxic; ↑ p21WAF1 and cyclin D, ↓ cdk2 and cyclin E | 45 |
| Rh1, Rh2, Rh3, Rh4 | HL-60 | Rh2 and Rh3 ↓ cells, induced differentiation | 111 |
| PD, PT | HT 1080 | PD and PT reduced tumor invasion seem to be related to glucocorticoid receptor | 112 |
| PD, PT | NIH 3T3 | No effect on viability needed methanesulfonate (alkylating agent); ↑ p53, p21, ↓ cdk2, cyclin E, D1 | 113 |
| Rb1, Rg3, Rh2, PD | L1210, P388, A549, Me180 | Rg3 is converted to Rh2 and PD by human fecal flora; Rh2 and PD cytotoxic | 114 |
| IH-901, Rb1 | HL-60, PC-14, Hep G2, MKN-45 | Rb1 no effect, ↑ caspase-3, no Bcl-2 change, ↑ cytochrome c | 43 |
| Rg3 | KB, KBV20C, P388, P388/DOX (mouse) | Rg3 restored sensitivity to cancer drugs in resistant cells (KBV20C), but not in drug sensitive (KB); serum in medium affects sensitivity | 73 |
| Rh1 | MCF-7 | Weak phytoestrogen, no glucocorticoid activity | 115 |
| Rh1, Rh2 | NIH 3T3 (mouse) | ↓ phospholipase C, ↓ intracellular diacylglycerol | 116 |
| IH-901, Rb1 | PC-14 PC/DDP (resistant), HL-60 MKN-45, HepG2 | Rb1 has no cytotoxic effect IH-901 threefold more effective in CDDP (cisplatin) resistant cells | 117 |
| PD, PT, Rh2, Rh1, Rg3 | THP-1 | PD, PT, Rh2, Rh1 are cytotoxic; Rg3 is not cytotoxic, ↑ Sub-$G_1$, ↑ LDH | 42 |
| PD, PT, Rh2, Rh1 | Caco-2, Int-407 | PD, PT, Rh2 are cytotoxic ↑ Sub-$G_1$, ↑ LDH; Rh2 ↑ Sub-$G_1$ greatest at $LC_{50}$ | 46 |
| Rh2, PD, PT, Rh2-enriched extract | Caco-2 | Rh2 greatest buildup of necrotic cells and Rh2, PT, extract ↑ caspase-3 activity; Rh2 extract is cytotoxic influence apoptotic and necrotic cells | 14 |

## 22.4.5　Effect on Cellular Membranes

Saponins, such as ginsenosides, exert a nonspecific effect on membrane function,[14,52] which is targeted directly at the membrane composition or function. Steroids have similar structural characteristics to ginsenosides, and ginsenosides have been reported to be a functional ligand of the glucocorticoid receptor,[53] potentially producing steroid-like effects. A classical view of steroid activity involves inducing protein synthesis, which requires time to relocate in the cell.[54] However, rapid effects of steroids have been reported and these effects are likely not genomic. Steroids have been reported to affect cells in a nonspecific, nongenomic way, as a result of a change in membrane physiochemical properties.[55] Two mechanisms proposed for nongenomic effects include an interaction with specific receptors (membrane) and an interaction with membrane lipids.[56] Ginsenosides such as Rh2 and Rg3 can influence cellular viability but the mechanism of action remains unclear. Two types of mechanisms have been proposed in the literature for the effect of ginseng on cultured cells: the first mechanism is a genomic one that modulates the cell cycle, and the second mechanism involves an effect on the cellular membrane. It is not clear if ginsenosides are effective at first modulating membrane properties, followed by a genomic effect; or in fact they may have a combined effect.

## 22.4.6　Effect of Ginseng and Ginsenosides on Membrane Hemolysis

The hemolytic activity of saponins has been known for some time and is commonly measured by the degree of rupture of erythrocytes.[57] Using a free radical–induced human erythrocyte hemolysis model, ginsenosides exhibit different hemolytic effects. The majority of ginsenosides have a protective effect on hemolysis even after exposure to free radical–induced hemolysis; however, certain ginsenoside such as Rg3 and Rh2 increased the extent of free radical–induced hemolysis.[26] These effects were based on structural classifications. For example, Rg3, Rh2, and Rg2 have sugar moieties in common that are attached at position C-3 of the triterpene ring (see Figure 22.1) and all exhibit increased hemolytic activity,[25] compared to those which have sugar attachment at position C-6. Furthermore, the aglycone protopanaxadiol and Rg3 exhibit strong hemolytic activity even in the absence of free radical initiators and the percentage of hemolytic activity increased as concentration increased.[25] Hence, one of the reported biological effects of ginseng concerns membrane modifying properties.[58] Likewise, dammarane triterpenoids isolated from birch leaf share similar structural characteristics to the aglycone protopanaxadiol from ginseng, and were found to be cytotoxic to Ehrlich ascite carcinoma cells.[58] An increase in the membrane permeability of cells was measured by the release of ultraviolet (UV)-absorbing substances from the cell and a decrease in thymidine ($^3$H) incorporation. A dose-dependent increase in membrane permeability occurred along with an increase in microviscosity.[58]

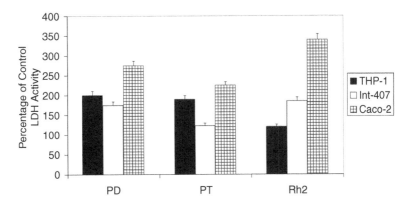

**FIGURE 22.4** LDH activity measure after a 72-h exposure to cytotoxic ginsenosides (PD, PT, Rh2) in two cultured intestinal cancer cell lines (Caco-2, Int-407) and leukemia cells (THP-1) at their respective $LC_{50}$ values (see Figure 22.1).

Saponins from *P. notoginseng* have also been shown to alter lipid fluidity of platelet membranes in male Wistar rats, receiving an intraperitoneal (200 mg/kg) injection of ginsenosides that inhibited platelet aggregation and adhesiveness after permanent occlusion of the middle cerebral artery.[59] Ginsenoside Rg1 inhibited adrenaline- and thrombin-induced platelet aggregation in human platelets analyzed *in vitro* and reduced the elevation of cytosolic free calcium concentration.[60] Rg2 was reported to inhibit intracellular calcium mobilization from rabbit plasma.[61]

Rg3 has been reported to reduce plasma membrane fluidity in bovine adrenal chromaffin cells.[62] Similarly, an increase in the concentration of cholesterol in cells resulted in the stiffening of the plasma membrane, and a reduction in the motion of the membrane.[63] A reduction of membrane fluidity has also been reported in cells treated with 17β-estradiol and the anticancer drug tamoxifen. It is speculated that these compounds possibly associate with the hydrophobic portions inside the membrane.[64]

In our laboratory we found the ginsenosides PD, PT, and Rh2 tested at respective $LC_{50}$ values resulted in an increased release of lactate dehydrogenase (LDH) from cultured intestinal and leukemia cells (Figure 22.4). LDH leakage is a useful cytoplasmic marker of membrane integrity.[65] Membrane protein function is also dependent on structure with alterations in membrane composition affecting fluidity.[66,67] For example, 17α-hydroxyprogesterone decreases fluidity and increases membrane aggregation and permeability.[56] It is unclear if ginsenosides can interact with cells and function as steroids, or are associated with steroid-like effects on the membrane by interaction with other components.

### 22.4.7 EFFECT OF GINSENOSIDE STRUCTURE ON BIOACTIVITY

The membrane effects of ginseng triterpene saponins have been suggested to be a function of the attachment of sugar moieties located on the triterpene ring structure. Cytotoxic effects of protopanaxadiol ginsenosides have been reported to decrease as sugar moieties are attached to position C-3; protopanaxadiol was reported to have lower $LC_{50}$ compared to Rh2 and Rg3 in cultured cell experiments.[42,68] Monoglucosides, such as Rh2 and Rg3 and compound K (intestinal metabolite), are cytotoxic and exert membrane-altering properties in Ehrlich ascite carcinoma cells and in a liposome model.[69] The effect on the membrane was a function of the culture media on the cholesterol content. By increasing the cholesterol content, at neutral pH, the cytotoxic effect was reduced. Furthermore, pre-incubation of Rh2 and Rg3 with cholesterol-free liposomes was reported to neutralize cytotoxicity.[69] The addition of glucose functional groups to the aglycone PD and PT of ginseng reduced apoptotic potential and lowered the potency to alter membrane integrity, as measured by the release of lactate dehydrogenase from cells.[42] Similarity, different saponins have different effects on the membrane. Glycoalkaloids have the tendency to form complexes with plant sterols,[70] and sea cucumber saponins have the strongest effect on cholesterol-containing membranes.[69] Structural characteristics of the saponins thus have a role in this effect. Ginsenosides such as Rb1, Re, Rg2, Rg1, Rd, Rf, and Ro, which have two sugar attachments at positions C-3 or C-6 and C-20, do not affect the cell membrane or exhibit cytotoxicity. The attachment of the functional groups possibly prevents the penetration of saponin into the membrane by altering cell surface conformation[69] or by changing the polarity of the active compound.

## 22.4.8 POTENTIAL SYNERGY, MULTIDRUG-RESISTANT CANCER

By far the most promising aspect of ginsenosides affinity to influence cultured cancer cell proliferation is the potential to modulate multidrug-resistant cancer cell metabolism. It seems that certain cells (intestinal, kidney, liver, etc.) have evolved a specific way to excrete cytotoxic plant constituents. Many novel cancer cell inhibitors, such as Taxol, are indeed derived from plant sources and therefore cells will eventually confer a cellular resistance to the agent on prolonged exposure.

P-glycoprotein (P-gp) is a glycoprotein membrane constituent encoded by the *MDR1* gene that is associated with resistance to anticancer drugs.[68] P-gp is an energy-dependent drug efflux pump, which is involved in both intrinsic and acquired drug resistance. Expression of this transporter plays a role in resistance to chemotherapy,[71] effectively pumping chemotherapy drugs from the cell and thereby lowering the effective concentration. Furthermore, resistance is often encountered from drugs that are amphipathic and have been isolated from plants and microorganisms.[71] Future studies with bioactive ginsenosides and Rh2-enriched extract should be evaluated on the potential effect to stimulate the P-gp efflux pump. P-gp transporter has been purposed to be an evolutionary adaptation to remove toxic compounds from the bile or intestine.[71] Higher levels of *MDR1* expression is found in colon, kidney, liver, adrenal, pancreas, and in leukemia cells. Expression of *MDR1* after chemotherapy was found to be increased in leukemia, breast cancer, and lymphomas, among others cells.[71] Identifying agents that will slow or stop the efflux pump is a valuable addition to chemotherapy and certain ginsenosides have been tested in combination with resistant drugs. Dauno-mycin (DAU) and vinblastine (VBL) resistant leukemia cells (P388 ADM) were treated with 20(S)-Rh2, 20(S)-PT, and compound K, an intestinal biotransformed metabolite of Rb1, to effectively reverse both DAU and VBL drug resistant cells. Ginsenosides have been suggested to inhibit the efflux pump according to struc-tural characteristics related to the attachment of bulky side changes at position C-3 of the triterpene ring.[72] Bulky side chains of certain ginsenosides (Rb1, Rc, Rd, Re) may not have adequate conformation to exert an effect on the glycoprotein or membrane structures. Furthermore, ginsenoside Rg3 was effective at increasing the sensitivity of vincristine (VCR)-resistant cells (KBV20C); Rg3 competitively inhibited binding to P-gp[73] and increased survival time of mice transplanted with multidrug-resistant P388 leukemia tumor compared to adriamycin treatment.[73] With these findings taken into consideration, future studies should be planned to establish whether bioactive ginsenosides (PD, PT, Rh2) directly influence the P-gp membrane pump or generally alter the conformation or composition of the cellular membrane.

### 22.4.9 IN VIVO ANIMAL CANCER MODELS

A red ginseng extract was reported to inhibit the incidence of lung tumors in benzo($a$)pyrene-induced newborn mice to a greater extent than white fresh gin-seng.[74] Using the aberrant crypt foci (ACF) assay, a model of colorectal cancer, red ginseng powder (0.5 g/kg, 2 mg/kg) was reported to be cytostatic as evidenced by the progressive inhibition of established ACF, induced by azoxymethane in Sprague-Dawley rat (F344).[75] Further reports indicated that dietary red ginseng powder, when fed to F344 rats, had an inhibitory effect on the initiation stage of 1,2-dimethylhydrazine-induced ACF, and that this inhibition was greater for red ginseng than for white ginseng.[76] Red ginseng was also found to inhibit the development of liver cancer induced by diethylnitrosamine in Wistar white rats. Red ginseng (5.6 g/kg/week) administered with water via a gastric tube reduced the rate of liver cancer (14.3%) in the later stage, compared to an untreated control group (100%).[77] It is noteworthy that ginseng has been reported to have a non-organ-specific effect on cancer.[78] Studies with white ginseng from plant culture showed an inhibitory effect toward the development of tumors of the mammary gland, nervous system, kidney, uterine cervix, and vagina after chemical induction of tumors, in a variety of experimental animals.[78]

In mice that lack a thymus (nude mice), oral administration of Rh2 by cannula after inoculation with human ovarian cancer cells resulted in a significant reduc-tion in tumor volumes in all groups treated with Rh2, compared to ethanol-treated and cisplatin-treated groups. Furthermore, tumor growth was also reported to be significantly reduced compared to a cisplatin-treated group. Cisplatin is a chemo-therapy that is given as treatment for cancer and also referred to as *cis*-diam-minedichloroplatinum (II) (CDDP). The survival rates of nude mice given cancer cells and treated with either 15 or 120 $\mu M$ Rh2 were increased compared to ethanol- and cisplatin-treated groups.[79] Tode et al.[79] suggested that Rh2 may function *in vivo* to improve survival of mice by altering the membrane cell surfaces. Red ginseng saponins, such as structurally related Rg3, inhibit lung metastasis in mouse models. Lung metastasis was produced by metastatic tumor cells, B16-BL6 melanoma and colon 26-M3.1 carcinoma, in syngeneic (genetically identical) mice. Red ginseng saponins were suggested to inhibit the adhesion and invasion of these metastatic cells and significantly decreased the number of blood vessels oriented toward the tumor mass (e.g., antiangiogenesis).[80] Furthermore, nude mice inoculated with human ovarian cancer cells produced greater tumor growth retardation with daily oral administration of Rh2 (0.4 mg/kg) than with an intraperitoneal administration of CDDP (2 mg/kg), a potent antitumor agent. It is important to note, however, that a dose-dependent relationship between Rh2 and antitumorigenicity was not obtained.[81]

### 22.4.10 HUMAN ANTICANCER EVIDENCE

A case-control study of ginseng intake and association with cancer risk from a Korean population showed that the odds ratio for ginseng consumers to develop cancer was 0.56, and that ginseng prepared as an extract or powder was more effective than fresh ginseng[82] in reducing cancers. Further case-control evidence showed that odds ratios were 0.56 in relation to ginseng intake and variable for different ginseng preparations such as fresh ginseng extract (0.57), white ginseng extract (0.33), and lowest odds ratio for red ginseng users (0.20)[83] Yun and Choi[84] reported from a prospective cohort study of 4634 people over 40 years of age that Korean ginseng consumers had a relative risk of 0.40 (95% confidence interval) compared to nonconsumers to develop cancer. The relative risk of consumers given fresh ginseng (0.31) and for multiple and overlapping ginseng extract consumers were similar (0.34), and in a small subset of ginseng consumers no death was reported in 24 consumers of red ginseng.[84] Furthermore, a dose–response relationship was reported and the risk ratios of gastric (0.33) and lung cancer (0.30) development were reduced even though these cancers have different mechanisms of carcinogenesis and etiology, again indicating that ginseng has a non-organ-specific preventative effect against cancer.[84] Red ginseng increased disease-free survival (68%) in the ginseng consumption group compared to the group that did not consume red ginseng (33%). Furthermore, an increase in overall survival (76%) was noted for ginseng intake groups compared to control group (39%) for postoperative chemotherapy (stage III gastric cancer). This effect was attributed to red ginseng.[85]

### 22.5 CANCER PREVENTATIVE PROPERTIES OF SOYASAPONINS

There are many more in-depth reports on the potential anticancer activity of ginseng saponins compared to soyasaponins. Most of the anticancer activity of soybeans has been associated with their phytoestrogen activity; however, as with ginseng saponins, evidence is mounting outlining a specific effect of soyasaponins on antioxidant activity, immune system modulation, and an ability to inhibit the growth of cultured cancer cells. Generally, the saponin content of soybean and processed soy products ranges between 0.2 and 2%. The variability depends on the source of the soybean, the part of the soybean plant, and the choice of analytical method.[86] The basic structure of soyasaponins can be divided into three main groups with varying combination of sugar moieties attached to the chemical backbone (Figure 22.5). Similar to ginsenosides, soyasaponin anticancer properties generally are characterized according to chemical structure-related properties, such as hydrophobic–hydrophilic balance. However, one of the limiting factors in future research into the soyasaponin bioactive properties is the availability of purified saponins. Most reports have focused on the extraction of soyasaponins from soybean and soybean flour and have not specifically analyzed or characterized all the individual saponins contained in the extracts. It is hoped that purified soyasaponins will be commercially available so an effective characterization of individual saponins will be achieved.

### 22.5.1 BIOAVAILABILITY OF SOYASAPONINS

In a small human trial to assess the bioavailability of group B soy saponins in women ($n = 8$), no recovery of soy saponins after an invested single dose of 434 $\mu M$ was observed in the urine, whereas a fecal metabolite of group B saponins (Soyasapogenol B) was found after a 5-day fecal collection.[87] In a Caco-2 cell model of the gastrointestinal absorption, soy saponins tended to have low absorption ability after 4 h of exposure. Soyasaponin I was found to be absorbed between 0.5 and 2.9% and soyasapogenol between B 0.2 and 0.8%. At a concentration up to 3 mmol/L Soyasaponin I did not induce cytotoxicity whereas soyasapogenol B showed some cytotoxic effect at 1 mmol/L.[87]

### 22.5.2 ANTIOXIDANT ACTIVITY

Soyasaponins have been shown to possess some antioxidant activity. For example, hydrogen peroxide damage to mouse fibroblast cells was found to be inhibited by soyasaponin Bg, soyasaponin I, and soyasaponin Ab; these compounds may be involved in reducing cellular and DNA damage. These effects were similar to glycyrrhizin saponins; the authors suggest that water-soluble soybean saponins may help protect cells from hydrogen peroxide–induced damage.[88] A further report suggested that soyasaponin Bg has a concentration-dependent *in vitro* scavenging activity toward superoxide ($O^-_2$) and to DPPH radical-inhibition and that the scavenging activity was similar to a synthetic antioxidant *tert*-butyl hydroxyl toluene (BHT). Specifically soyasaponin Bg showed a 21% inhibition and an $IC_{50}$ of 63.8 $\mu M$ compared to BHT 21% with an $IC_{50}$ of 67.5 $\mu M$.[89]

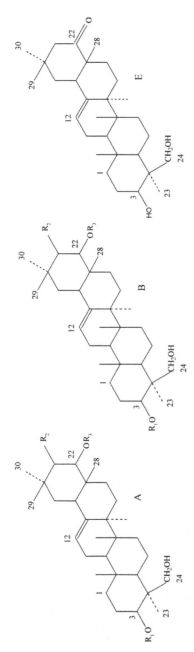

| Group A | | |
|---|---|---|
| Soyasapongen A aglyocone | $R_1 = H$ | |
| Soyasapongen $A_1$ | $R1 = GlcA^2-Gal^2-Glc$, $R2 = OH$, $R3 = Ara^3-Glc$ | |
| Soyasapongen $A_2$ | $R1 = GlcA^2-Gal^2$, $R2 = OH$, $R3 = Ara^3-Glc$ | |

| Group B | | |
|---|---|---|
| Soyasapongen B aglyocone | $R_1 = H$ | |
| Soyasapongen I | $R1 = GlcA^2-Gal^2-Rha$ | |
| Soyasapongen II | $R1 = GlcA^2-Ara^2-Rha$ | |
| Soyasapongen III | $R1 = GlcA^2-Gal$ | |

**FIGURE 22.5** The main soyasaponins aglycones (A, B, E) and selection of groups A and B soy saponins. (Adapted from Gurfinkel and Rao.[100])

### 22.5.3 Immune System

Eight soyasaponins were tested for a relationship between adjuvant activities. A number of soyasaponins were tested in mice against a chicken ovalbumin antibody (OVA) challenge to determine if chemical structural differences are related to activity. Saponins with glycosidic attached sugar moieties showed adjuvanticity stimulating anti-OVA total IgG and IgG1 antibody responses. The aglycone soyasapogenol A and B did not produce the same response.[90] The additions of a sugar moiety to soyasaponin $A_1$ when compared to soyasaponin $A_2$ increased the total IgG and IgG1 antibody responses, both of which were greater than soyasaponins I–III. Furthermore, among soyasaponin I–III, soyasaponin I produced the greatest antibody response followed by soyasaponin II and III.[90] Glycosidic attachment of side chains seems, at least in part, related to an antibody response and is based on the hydrophobic–hydrophilic nature of the compound.

One report of soyasaponins isolated from soybean seeds were found to completely inhibit an HIV-induced cytophatic effect and a virus-specific antigen at a concentration of 0.5 mg/ml.[91] An *in vitro* study of soyasaponin I and II affinity to inhibit herpes simplex virus type I (HSV-1) reported that soyasaponin II reduced HSV-1 virus production to a greater degree than soyasaponin I. The authors also showed evidence that soyasaponin II inhibited human cytomegalovirus, influenza virus, and HIV-1 expressed in a variety of host cells; these virus effects were found not to be a function of soyasaponin inhibition of virus penetration or protein synthesis but were likely acting as a viricidal.[91] It is likely that soyasaponins, like ginsenosides, act in a general nonspecific way.

### 22.5.4 Cultured Cell Experiments

Soy saponins extracted from soybean were reported to interact with colonic epithelial carcinoma (HCT-15) cell membranes, assessed by scanning electron microscopy. Soyasaponins also increased the hemolysis of red blood cells, but the hemolysis was not as pronounced when compared to gypsophila saponin,[92] a structurally similar saponin. In another report, soy saponins inhibited the growth of HCT-15 cells in a dose-dependent manner and showed minor morphological alterations on cell surface membranes. These morphological changes and growth inhibition were not found to be related to an increased membrane permeability measured by lactate dehydrogenase (LDH) leakage from cells, whereas gypsophila saponin exposure was related to LDH release.[93]

Soy saponins have been screened for an affinity to suppress the growth of human colorectal adenocarcinoma cell line (HT-29). Soyasaponins $A_1$, $A_2$, I, B, and deacetylated and acetylated group A saponins failed to produce an effect on cell growth up to a concentration of 50 ppm (50 µg/ml); soyasaponin III and soyasapogenol B monoglucuronide showed a marginal effect on cell growth at 50 ppm. However, aglycones, soyasapogenol A and B reduced cell growth starting at concentration of 6 ppm (6 µg/ml), while almost completely suppressing growth at 50 ppm.[94] Gurfinkel and Rao[94] suggest the lipophilic saponin aglycones were more bioactive compared to saponin glycosides, a hypothesis that may relate to an ability to penetrate cellular membranes. It is noteworthy that a similar finding was reported for ginseng saponins.[42]

Soy saponin extract, prepared from soybean flour, was reported to decrease human colorectal adenocarcinoma cell line (HT-29) growth; the growth inhibition was found to be both dose and time dependent.[20,95,96] A saponin extract (150 ppm) increased alkaline phosphatase activity of HT-29 cells, a marker of cellular differentiation, by 1.5-fold compared to control cells.[96] Greater amounts of alkaline phosphatase were measured as the concentration of the soy extract increased. A soy saponin extract suppressed the degradation of IκBα, which is involved in the NF-κB inflammatory signal transduction cascaded and also downregulated cyclooxygenase-2 (COX-2) and protein kinase C (PKC) activities.[96]

Soyasapogenol A and soyasapogenol B, two aglycones of soyasaponins, also inhibit cell proliferation at a concentration of 10 $\mu M$ in estrogen-insensitive human breast cancer cells (MDA-MB-231).[97] In MCF-7 cells, an estrogen-dependent breast cancer cell line, soyasapogenol B reduced cellular proliferation at 10 $\mu M$, whereas soyasapogenol A was reported to increase cellular proliferation 2.5-fold. The different effects of soyasapogenol A and B have been suggested to be a result of estrogenic activity of soyasapogenol A.[97]

Soyasapogenol B prepared from commercial soybean by-product (soybean molasses) exhibits antimutagenic activity in CHO cells (Chinese hamster ovary).[98] Similarly, soyasapogenol B protects CHO cells against 2 acetoxyactyl-aminofluorene (2AAAF) damage, which is a direct-acting mutagen. In Hep G2 cells (human hepatocellular carcinoma) a soy saponin extract was found to protect against aflatoxin $B_1$ (AFB$_1$)-induced mutagenicity and AFB$_1$-DNA adduct formation. At a concentration of 30 µg/ml, soy saponins inhibited adduct formation by 50% compared to L-ascorbic acid (38%) and butylated hydroxytoluene (33%), respectively.

Soyasaponin I prepared from a crude soybean saponin mixture has been reported to be a specific inhibitor of sialytransferase activity, which was expressed in COS-7 cells (*Cercopithecus aethiops*, African green monkey).[99] Increased sialytransferase activity has been associated with oncogenic transformation, tumor metastasis, invasion,[99] and poor prognosis among patients with cancer.

In a recently published report, saponins isolated from soybeans were evaluated for their effect on colon cancer cell proliferation. In HCT-15 colon cancer cells, group B saponins reduced cell viability between 25 and 500 ppm (µg/ml) and the inhibition was time dependent.[100] An LC$_{50}$ was determined to be 100 ppm. An increase in the accumulations of cell cycle cells in the S-phase (DNA synthesis phase) at concentrations of 25 and 100 ppm was reported to start 6 h after exposure. This accumulation of S-phase cells was associated with an inhibition of cyclin-dependent kinase-2 (CDK-2) activity, a cell cycle regulatory protein. Furthermore, an induction of macroautophagy (morphological alterations) in colonic cells was observed and was not related to traditional apoptosis morphology. It is possible that macroautophagy characteristics, such as reduced cytoplasmic density and vacuolization, eventually leads to Type II programmed cell death.[100]

### 22.5.5 HEPATOPROTECTIVE EFFECTS OF SOYASAPONINS

In primary cultured rat hepatocytes, group B soy saponins (soyasaponins I, II, III, IV) were found to possess varying hepatoprotective actions toward liver injury.[101,102] Soyasaponin III and IV expressed the greatest hepatoprotective effect in cells after exposure to antiserum raised against rat liver plasma membrane. Soyasaponin III started to offer protection at a concentration of 10 µM; alternatively, soyasaponins I and II showed little protection.[101] The authors suggested the difference in hepatoprotection is related to structural characteristics of the soyasaponins. For example, attachment of sugar moieties to position C-3 of the group B saponins was related to the effect. Disaccharide attachment (soyasaponin III and IV) generally showed greater effects compared to trisaccharide sugar attachment (soyasaponin I and II).

### 22.5.6 SOYSAPONINS AND ANIMAL COLON CANCER MODEL

Soy saponin extract isolated from soy flour was tested in male CF1 mice for the incidence of aberrant crypt foci induced by azoxymethane exposure in mice colon.[103] Aberrant crypt foci are related to the development of colon cancer. After exposure to azoxymethane for 4 weeks, a test diet was given with 3% soy saponins and the intake of saponins reduced the incidence of aberrant crypt foci. It was further determined that the soy saponins intake alone did not show adverse effects on animal growth.[103]

## 22.6 CONCLUSION

The role of saponins in soy and ginseng in reducing the risk of certain cancers has been demonstrated in culture, experimental animals, and humans. Plants of the genus *Panax* are known for production of steroid ginsenosides, which have a multitude of nonspecific effects that target membrane function and subsequent signal transduction activity. Similarly, soyasaponins are bioactive triterpenoid glycosides, which have antimutagenic, hepatoprotective, and immune sensitive responses, and anticarcinogenic activities. Many of the bioactive functions of both ginseng and soyasaponins have a structure–activity relationship, in particular as it relates to cytotoxic activity in culture cancer cells. This chapter details the anticarcinogenic activities of both ginseng and soyasaponin and suggests that special consideration be given to steroid saponins in biological and pharmacological studies of ginseng and soy preparation for potential nutraceutical, pharmaceutical, or functional food use.

# REFERENCES

1. Estrada A, Katselis GS, Laarveld B, Barl B. Isolation and evaluation of immunological adjuvant activities of saponins from *Polygala senega* L. *Comp Immunol Microbiol Infect Dis* 2000; 23:27–43.
2. Popovich DG, Kitts DD. Bioactive properties of ginseng and ginsenosides constituents. *Recent Res Dev Mol Cell Biochem* 2003; 1:137–149.
3. Rao AV, Sung MK. Saponins as anticarcinogens. *J Nutr* 1995; 125:717S–724S.
4. Yun TK. Brief introduction of *Panax ginseng* C.A. Meyer. *J Korean Med Sci* 2001; 16 Suppl:S3–S5.
5. Tang W, Eisenbran G. *Panax ginseng* C.A. Meyer. In: Tang W, Eisenbrand G, eds. *Chinese Drugs of Plant Origin: Chemistry, Pharmacology, and Use in Traditional and Modern Medicine*. Berlin: Springer-Verlag; 1992:710–737.
6. Shiraiwa M, Kudo S, Shimoyamada M, Harada K, Okubo K. Composition and structure of "group A saponin" in soybean seed. *Agric Biol Chem* 1991; 55:315–322.
7. Shiraiwa M, Harada K, Okubo K. Composition and structure of "group B saponin" in soybean seed. *Agric Biol Chem* 1991; 55:911–917.
8. Tava A, Mella M, Bialy Z, Jurzysta M. Stability of saponins in alcoholic solutions: ester formation as artifacts. *J Agric Food Chem* 2003; 51:1797–1800.
9. Sen S, Makkar HP, Becker K. Alfalfa saponins and their implication in animal nutrition. *J Agric Food Chem* 1998; 46:131–140.
10. Francis G, Kerem Z, Makkar HP, Becker K. The biological action of saponins in animal systems: a review. *Br J Nutr* 2002; 88:587–605.
11. Lee MH, Jeong JH, Seo JW et al. Enhanced triterpene and phytosterol biosynthesis in *Panax ginseng* overexpressing squalene synthase gene. *Plant Cell Physiol* 2004; 45:976–984.
12. Setzer WN, Setzer MC. Plant-derived triterpenoids as potential antineoplastic agents. *Mini Rev Med Chem* 2003; 3:540–556.
13. Kim WY, Kim JM, Han SB et al. Steaming of ginseng at high temperature enhances biological activity. *J Nat Prod* 2000; 63:1702–1704.
14. Popovich DG, Kitts DD. Mechanistic studies on protopanaxadiol, Rh2 and ginseng (*Panax quinquefolius*) extract induced cytotoxicity in intestinal Caco-2 cells. *J Biochem Mol Toxicol* 2004; 18:143–149.
15. Popovich DG, Kitts DD. Generation of ginsenosides Rg3 and Rh2 from North American ginseng. *Phytochemistry* 2004; 65:337–344.
16. Attele AS, Zhou YP, Xie JT et al. Antidiabetic effects of Panax ginseng berry extract and the identification of an effective component. *Diabetes* 2002; 51:1851–1858.
17. Kim YK, Guo Q, Packer L. Free radical scavenging activity of red ginseng aqueous extracts. *Toxicology* 2002; 172:149–156.
18. Kitts DD, Wijewickreme AN, Hu C. Antioxidant properties of a North American ginseng extract. *Mol Cell Biochem* 2000; 203:1–10.
19. Hu C, Kitts DD. Free radical scavenging capacity as related to antioxidant activity and ginsenoside composition of Asian and North American ginseng extracts. *J Am Oil Chem Soc* 2001; 78:249–255.
20. Keum YS, Park KK, Lee JM et al. Antioxidant and anti-tumor promoting activities of the methanol extract of heat-processed ginseng. *Cancer Lett* 2000; 150:41–48.

21. Kim YH, Park KH, Rho HM. Transcriptional activation of the Cu,Zn-superoxide dismutase gene through the AP2 site by ginsenoside Rb2 extracted from a medicinal plant, *Panax ginseng*. *J Biol Chem* 1996; 271:24539–24543.

22. Voces J, Alvarez AI, Vila L, Ferrando A, Cabral DO, Prieto JG. Effects of administration of the standardized *Panax ginseng* extract G115 on hepatic antioxidant function after exhaustive exercise. *Comp Biochem Physiol C Pharmacol Toxicol Endocrinol* 1999; 123:175–184.

23. Kim CS, Park JB, Kim KJ, Chang SJ, Ryoo SW, Jeon BH. Effect of Korea red ginseng on cerebral blood flow and superoxide production. *Acta Pharmacol Sin* 2002; 23:1152–1156.

24. Rimar S, Lee-Mengel M, Gillis CN. Pulmonary protective and vasodilator effects of a standardized *Panax ginseng* preparation following artificial gastric digestion. *Pulm Pharmacol* 1996; 9:205–209.

25. Liu ZQ, Luo XY, Liu GZ, Chen YP, Wang ZC, Sun YX. *In vitro* study of the relationship between the structure of ginsenoside and its antioxidative or prooxidative activity in free radical induced hemolysis of human erythrocytes. *J Agric Food Chem* 2003; 51:2555–2558.

26. Liu ZQ, Luo XY, Sun YX, Chen YP, Wang ZC. Can ginsenosides protect human erythrocytes against free-radical-induced hemolysis? *Biochim Biophys Acta* 2002; 1572:58–66.

27. Scaglione F, Cattaneo G, Alessandria M, Cogo R. Efficacy and safety of the standardised ginseng extract G115 for potentiating vaccination against the influenza syndrome and protection against the common cold. *Drugs Exp Clin Res* 1996; 22:65–72.

28. Zhou DL, Kitts DD. Peripheral blood mononuclear cell production of TNF-alpha in response to North American ginseng stimulation. *Can J Physiol Pharmacol* 2002; 80:1030–1033.

29. Cho JY, Yoo ES, Baik KU, Park MH, Han BH. *In vitro* inhibitory effect of protopanaxadiol ginsenosides on tumor necrosis factor (TNF)-alpha production and its modulation by known TNF-alpha antagonists. *Planta Med* 2001; 67:213–218.

30. Wang H, Actor JK, Indrigo J, Olsen M, Dasgupta A. Asian and Siberian ginseng as a potential modulator of immune function: an in vitro cytokine study using mouse macrophages. *Clin Chim Acta* 2003; 327:123–128.

31. See DM, Broumand N, Sahl L, Tilles JG. *In vitro* effects of echinacea and ginseng on natural killer and antibody-dependent cell cytotoxicity in healthy subjects and chronic fatigue syndrome or acquired immunodeficiency syndrome patients. *Immunopharmacology* 1997; 35:229–235.

32. Song Z, Johansen HK, Faber V et al. Ginseng treatment reduces bacterial load and lung pathology in chronic *Pseudomonas aeruginosa* pneumonia in rats. *Antimicrob Agents Chemother* 1997; 41:961–964.

33. Scaglione F, Ferrara F, Dugnani S, Falchi M, Santoro G, Fraschini F. Immunomodulatory effects of two extracts of *Panax ginseng* C.A. Meyer. *Drugs Exp Clin Res* 1990; 16:537–542.

34. Wang M, Guilbert LJ, Ling L et al. Immunomodulating activity of CVT-E002, a proprietary extract from North American ginseng (*Panax quinquefolium*). *J Pharm Pharmacol* 2001; 53:1515–1523.

35. Cho YK, Sung H, Lee HJ, Joo CH, Cho GJ. Long-term intake of Korean red ginseng in HIV-1-infected patients: development of resistance mutation to zidovudine is delayed. *Int Immunopharmacol* 2001; 1:1295–1305.

36. Sonoda Y, Kasahara T, Mukaida N, Shimizu N, Tomoda M, Takeda T. Stimulation of interleukin-8 production by acidic polysaccharides from the root of *Panax ginseng*. *Immunopharmacology* 1998; 38:287–294.

37. Hasegawa H, Sung JH, Benno Y. Role of human intestinal *Prevotella oris* in hydrolyzing ginseng saponins. *Planta Med* 1997; 63:436–440.

38. Bae EA, Han MJ, Choo MK, Park SY, Kim DH. Metabolism of 20(S)- and 20(R)-ginsenoside Rg3 by human intestinal bacteria and its relation to in vitro biological activities. *Biol Pharm Bull* 2002; 25:58–63.

39. Bae EA, Choo MK, Park EK, Park SY, Shin HY, Kim DH. Metabolism of ginsenoside R(c) by human intestinal bacteria and its related antiallergic activity. *Biol Pharm Bull* 2002; 25:743–747.

40. Jie YH, Cammisuli S, Baggiolini M. Immunomodulatory effects of *Panax ginseng* C.A. Meyer in the mouse. *Agents Actions* 1984; 15:386–391.

41. Park IH, Piao LZ, Kwon SW et al. Cytotoxic dammarane glycosides from processed ginseng. *Chem Pharm Bull* 2002; 50:538–540.

42. Popovich DG, Kitts DD. Structure-function relationship exists for ginsenosides in reducing cell proliferation and inducing apoptosis in the human leukemia (THP-1) cell line. *Arch Biochem Biophys* 2002; 406:1–8.

43. Lee SJ, Ko WG, Kim JH, Sung JH, Moon CK, Lee BH. Induction of apoptosis by a novel intestinal metabolite of ginseng saponin via cytochrome c-mediated activation of caspase-3 protease. *Biochem Pharmacol* 2000; 60:677–685.

44. Liu WK, Xu SX, Che CT. Anti-proliferative effect of ginseng saponins on human prostate cancer cell line. *Life Sci* 2000; 67:1297–1306.

45. Oh M, Choi YH, Choi S et al. Anti-proliferating effects of ginsenoside Rh2 on MCF-7 human breast cancer cells. *Int J Oncol* 1999; 14:869–875.

46. Popovich DG, Kitts DD. Ginsenosides 20(S)-protopanaxadiol and Rh2 reduce cell proliferation and increase sub-G1 cells in two cultured intestinal cell lines (Int-407 and Caco-2). *Can J Physiol Pharmacol* 2004; 82:183–190.

47. Fei XF, Wang BX, Tashiro S, Li TJ, Ma JS, Ikejima T. Apoptotic effects of ginsenoside Rh2 on human malignant melanoma A375-S2 cells. *Acta Pharmacol Sin* 2002; 23:315–322.

48. Jin YH, Yoo KJ, Lee YH, Lee SK. Caspase 3-mediated cleavage of p21WAF1/CIP1 associated with the cyclin A-cyclin-dependent kinase 2 complex is a prerequisite for apoptosis in SK-HEP-1 cells. *J Biol Chem* 2000; 275:30256–30263.

49. Ota T, Maeda M, Odashima S, Ninomiya-Tsuji J, Tatsuka M. $G_1$ phase-specific suppression of the Cdk2 activity by ginsenoside Rh2 in cultured murine cells. *Life Sci* 1997; 60:L39–L44.

50. Ota T, Maeda M, Odashima S. Mechanism of action of ginsenoside Rh2: uptake and metabolism of ginsenoside Rh2 by cultured B16 melanoma cells. *J Pharm Sci* 1991; 80:1141–1146.

51. Odashima S, Ohta T, Kohno H et al. Control of phenotypic expression of cultured B16 melanoma cells by plant glycosides. *Cancer Res* 1985; 45:2781–2784.

52. Foulkes EC. Toxic effects on membrane structure and function. In: Foulkes EC, ed. *Biological Membranes in Toxicology*. Ann Arbor, MI: Taylor & Francis; 1998:59–88.

53. Lee YJ, Chung E, Lee KY, Lee YH, Huh B, Lee SK. Ginsenoside-Rg1, one of the major active molecules from *Panax ginseng*, is a functional ligand of glucocorticoid receptor. *Mol Cell Endocrinol* 1997; 133:135–140.

54. Wehling M. Specific, nongenomic actions of steroid hormones. *Annu Rev Physiol* 1997; 59:365–393.

55. Falkenstein E, Norman AW, Wehling M. Mannheim classification of nongenomically initiated (rapid) steroid action(s). *J Clin Endocrinol Metab* 2000; 85:2072–2075.

56. Shivaji S, Jagannadham MV. Steroid-induced perturbations of membranes and its relevance to sperm acrosome reaction. *Biochim Biophys Acta* 1992; 1108:99–109.

57. Hostettman K. Analysis and isolation. In: Hostettmann K, Marston A, eds. *Chemistry and Pharmacology of Natural Products*. New York: Cambridge University Press; 1995:122–174.

58. Prokof'eva NG, Anisimov MM, Kiseleva MI, Rebachuk NM, Pokhilo ND. Cytotoxic activity of dammarane triterpenoids from birch leaves. *Izv Akad Nauk Ser Biol* 2002; 645–649.

59. Ma LY, Xiao PG. Effects of panax notoginseng saponins on platelet aggregation in rats with middle cerebral artery occlusion or *in vitro* and on lipid fluidity of platelet membrane. *Phytother Res* 1998; 12:138–140.

60. Kimura Y, Okuda H, Arichi S. Effects of various ginseng saponins on 5-hydroxytryptamine release and aggregation in human platelets. *J Pharm Pharmacol* 1988; 40:838–843.

61. Teng CM, Kuo SC, Ko FN et al. Antiplatelet actions of panaxynol and ginsenosides isolated from ginseng. *Biochim Biophys Acta* 1989; 990:315–320.

62. Tachikawa E, Kudo K, Nunokawa M, Kashimoto T, Takahashi E, Kitagawa S. Characterization of ginseng saponin ginsenoside-Rg(3) inhibition of catecholamine secretion in bovine adrenal chromaffin cells. *Biochem Pharmacol* 2001; 62:943–951.

63. Burns M, Duff K. Use of *in vivo* models to study the role of cholesterol in the etiology of Alzheimer's disease. *Neurochem Res* 2003; 28:979–986.

64. Clarke R, van den Berg HW, Murphy RF. Reduction of the membrane fluidity of human breast cancer cells by tamoxifen and 17 beta-estradiol. *J Natl Cancer Inst* 1990; 82:1702–1705.

65. Sung M, Kendall C, Koo M, Rao A. Effect of soybean saponins and gypsophilla saponin on growth and viability of colon carcinoma cells in culture. *Nutr Cancer* 1995; 23:259–269.

66. Burns CP, Luttenegger DG, Dudley DT, Buettner GR, Spector AA. Effect of modification of plasma membrane fatty acid composition on fluidity and methotrexate transport in L1210 murine leukemia cells. *Cancer Res* 1979; 39:1726–1732.

67. Willmer EN. Steroids and cell surface. *Biol Rev* 1962; 36:368–398.

68. Hasegawa H, Sung JH, Matsumiya S et al. Reversal of daunomycin and vinblastine resistance in multidrug-resistant P388 leukemia *in vitro* through enhanced cytotoxicity by triterpenoids. *Planta Med* 1995; 61:409–413.

69. Popov AM. Comparative study of cytotoxic and hemolytic effects of triterpenoids isolated from ginseng and sea cucumber. *Izv Akad Nauk Ser Biol* 2002; 155–164.

70. Keukens EA, de Vrije T, van den BC et al. Molecular basis of glycoalkaloid induced membrane disruption. *Biochim Biophys Acta* 1995; 1240:216–228.

71. Pastan I, Gottesman MM. Multidrug resistance. *Annu Rev Med* 1991; 42:277–286.

72. Molnar J, Szabo D, Pusztai R et al. Membrane associated antitumor effects of crocine-, ginseno. *Anticancer Res.* 2000; 20:861–867.
73. Kim SW, Kwon HY, Chi DW et al. Reversal of P-glycoprotein-mediated multidrug resistance by ginsenoside Rg(3). *Biochem Pharmacol* 2003; 65:75–82.
74. Yun TK, Kim SH, Lee YS. Trial of a new medium-term model using benzo(a)pyrene induced lung tumor in newborn mice. *Anticancer Res* 1995; 15:839–845.
75. Wargovich MJ. Colon cancer chemoprevention with ginseng and other botanicals. *J Korean Med Sci* 2001; 16:S81–S86.
76. Fukushima S, Wanibuchi H, Li W. Inhibition by ginseng of colon carcinogenesis in rats. *J Korean Med Sci* 2001; 16 Suppl:S75–S80.
77. Wu XG, Zhu DH, Li X. Anticarcinogenic effect of red ginseng on the development of liver cancer induced by diethylnitrosamine in rats. *J Korean Med Sci* 2001; 16:S61–S65.
78. Bespalov VG, Alexandrov VA, Limarenko AY et al. Chemoprevention of mammary, cervix and nervous system carcinogenesis in animals using cultured *Panax ginseng* drugs and preliminary clinical trials in patients with precancerous lesions of the esophagus and endometrium. *J Korean Med Sci* 2001; 16:S42–S53.
79. Tode T, Kikuchi Y, Kita T, Hirata J, Imaizumi E, Nagata I. Inhibitory effects by oral administration of ginsenoside Rh2 on the growth of human ovarian cancer cells in nude mice. *J Cancer Res Clin Oncol* 1993; 120:24–26.
80. Mochizuki M, Yoo YC, Matsuzawa K et al. Inhibitory effect of tumor metastasis in mice by saponins, ginsenoside-Rb2, 20(R)- and 20(S)-ginsenoside-Rg3, of red ginseng. *Biol Pharm Bull* 1995; 18:1197–1202.
81. Nakata H, Kikuchi Y, Tode T et al. Inhibitory effects of ginsenoside Rh2 on tumor growth in nude mice bearing human ovarian cancer cells. *Jpn J Cancer Res* 1998; 89:733–740.
82. Yun TK, Choi SY. A case-control study of ginseng intake and cancer. *Int J Epidemiol* 1990; 19:871–876.
83. Yun TK, Choi SY, Yun HY. Epidemiological study on cancer prevention by ginseng: are all kinds of cancers preventable by ginseng? *J Korean Med Sci* 2001; 16 Suppl:S19–S27.
84. Yun TK, Choi SY. Non-organ specific cancer prevention of ginseng: a prospective study in Korea. *Int J Epidemiol* 1998; 27:359–364.
85. Suh SO, Kroh M, Kim NR, Joh YG, Cho MY. Effects of red ginseng upon postoperative immunity and survival in patients with stage III gastric cancer. *Am J Chin Med* 2002; 30:483–494.
86. Anderson RL, Wolf WJ. Compositional changes in trypsin inhibitors, phytic acid, saponins and isoflavones related to soybean processing. *J Nutr* 1995; 125:581S–588S.
87. Hu J, Reddy MB, Hendrich S, Murphy PA. Soyasaponin I and sapongenol B have limited absorption by Caco-2 intestinal cells and limited bioavailability in women. *J Nutr* 2004; 134:1867–1873.
88. Yoshikoshi M, Yoshiki Y, Okubo K, Seto J, Sasaki Y. Prevention of hydrogen peroxide damage by soybean saponins to mouse fibroblasts. *Planta Med* 1996; 62:252–255.
89. Yoshiki Y, Kahara T, Okubo K, Sakabe T, Yamasaki T. Superoxide- and 1,1-diphenyl-2-picrylhydrazyl radical-scavenging activities of soyasaponin beta g related to gallic acid. *Biosci Biotechnol Biochem* 2001; 65:2162–2165.

90. Oda K, Matsuda H, Murakami T, Katayama S, Ohgitani T, Yoshikawa M. Relationship between adjuvant activity and amphipathic structure of soyasaponins. *Vaccine* 2003; 21:2145–2151.

91. Nakashima H, Okubo K, Honda Y, Tamura T, Matsuda S, Yamamoto N. Inhibitory effect of glycosides like saponin from soybean on the infectivity of HIV *in vitro*. *AIDS* 1989; 3:655–658.

92. Sung MK, Kendall CW, Rao AV. Effect of soybean saponins and gypsophila saponin on morphology of colon carcinoma cells in culture. *Food Chem Toxicol* 1995; 33:357–366.

93. Sung MK, Kendall CW, Koo MM, Rao AV. Effect of soybean saponins and gypsophilla saponin on growth and viability of colon carcinoma cells in culture. *Nutr Cancer* 1995; 23:259–270.

94. Gurfinkel DM, Rao AV. Soyasaponins: the relationship between chemical structure and colon anticarcinogenic activity. *Nutr Cancer* 2003; 47:24–33.

95. Oh YJ, Sung MK. Soybean saponins inhibit cell proliferation by suppressing PKC activation and induce differentiation of HT-29 human colon adenocarcinoma cells. *Nutr Cancer* 2001; 39:132–138.

96. Kim HY, Yu R, Kim JS, Kim YK, Sung MK. Antiproliferative crude soy saponin extract modulates the expression of IkappaBalpha, protein kinase C, and cyclooxygenase-2 in human colon cancer cells. *Cancer Lett* 2004; 210:1–6.

97. Rowlands JC, Berhow MA, Badger TM. Estrogenic and antiproliferative properties of soy sapogenols in human breast cancer cells *in vitro*. *Food Chem Toxicol* 2002; 40:1767–1774.

98. Berhow MA, Wagner ED, Vaughn SF, Plewa MJ. Characterization and antimutagenic activity of soybean saponins. *Mutat Res* 2000; 448:11–22.

99. Wu CY, Hsu CC, Chen ST, Tsai YC. Soyasaponin I, a potent and specific sialyltransferase inhibitor. *Biochem Biophys Res Commun* 2001; 284:466–469.

100. Gurfinkel DM, Rao AV. Determination of saponins in legumes by direct densitometry. *J Agric Food Chem* 2002; 50:426–430.

101. Kinjo J, Imagire M, Udayama M, Arao T, Nohara T. Structure-hepatoprotective relationships study of soyasaponins I-IV having soyasapogenol B as aglycone. *Planta Med* 1998; 64:233–236.

102. Ikeda T, Udayama M, Okawa M, Arao T, Kinjo J, Nohara T. Partial hydrolysis of soyasaponin I and the hepatoprotective effects of the hydrolytic products. Study of the structure-hepatoprotective relationship of soyasapogenol B analogs. *Chem Pharm Bull* (Tokyo) 1998; 46:359–361.

103. Koratkar R, Rao AV. Effect of soya bean saponins on azoxymethane-induced preneoplastic lesions in the colon of mice. *Nutr Cancer* 1997; 27:206–209.

104. Park JA, Lee KY, Oh YJ, Kim KW, Lee SK. Activation of caspase-3 protease via a Bcl-2-insensitive pathway during the process of ginsenoside Rh2-induced apoptosis. *Cancer Lett* 1997; 121:73–81.

105. Lee KY, Park JA, Chung E, Lee YH, Kim SI, Lee SK. Ginsenoside-Rh2 blocks the cell cycle of SK-HEP-1 cells at the $G_1$/S boundary by selectively inducing the protein expression of p27kip1. *Cancer Lett* 1996; 110:193–200.

106. Kim HE, Oh JH, Lee SK, Oh YJ. Ginsenoside RH-2 induces apoptotic cell death in rat C6 glioma via a reactive ox. *Life Sci* 1999; 65:L33–L40.

107. Ota T, Fujikawa-yamamoto K, Zong ZP et al. Plant-glycoside modulation of cell surface related to control of differentiation in cultured B16 melanoma cells. *Cancer Res* 1987; 47:3863–3867.

108. Jin YH, Yim H, Park JH, Lee SK. Cdk2 activity is associated with depolarization of mitochondrial membrane potential during apoptosis. *Biochem Biophys Res Commun* 2003; 305:974–980.

109. Kim SE, Lee YH, Park JH, Lee SK. Ginsenoside-Rs4, a new type of ginseng saponin concurrently induces apoptosis and selectively elevates protein levels of p53 and p21WAF1 in human hepatoma SK-HEP-1 cells. *Eur J Cancer* 1999; 35:507–511.

110. Wakabayashi C, Murakami K, Hasegawa H, Murata J, Saiki I. An intestinal bacterial metabolite of ginseng protopanaxadiol saponins has the ability to induce apoptosis in tumor cells. *Biochem Biophys Res Commun* 1998; 246:725–730.

111. Kim YS, Kim DS, Kim SI. Ginsenoside Rh2 and Rh3 induce differentiation of HL-60 cells into granulocytes: modulation of protein kinase C isoforms during differentiation by ginsenoside Rh2. *Int J Biochem Cell Biol* 1998; 30:327–338.

112. Park MT, Cha HJ, Jeong JW et al. Glucocorticoid receptor-induced down-regulation of MMP-9 by ginseng components, PD and PT contributes to inhibition of the invasive capacity of HT1080 human fibrosarcoma cells. *Mol Cells* 1999; 9:476–483.

113. Hwang SJ, Cha JY, Park SG et al. Diol- and triol-type ginseng saponins potentiate the apoptosis of NIH3T3 cells exposed to methyl methanesulfonate. *Toxicol Appl Pharmacol* 2002; 181:192–202.

114. Bae EA, Han MJ, Choo MK, Park SY, Kim DH. Metabolism of 20(S)- and 20(R)-ginsenoside Rg3 by human intestinal bacteria and its relation to in vitro biological activities. *Biol Pharm Bull* 2002; 25:58–63.

115. Lee Y, Jin Y, Lim W et al. A ginsenoside-Rh1, a component of ginseng saponin, activates estrogen receptor in human breast carcinoma MCF-7 cells. *J Steroid Biochem Mol Biol* 2003; 84:463–468.

116. Byun BH, Shin I, Yoon YS, Kim SI, Joe CO. Modulation of protein kinase C activity in NIH 3T3 cells by plant glycosides from *Panax ginseng. Planta Med* 1997; 63:389–392.

117. Lee SJ, Sung JH, Lee SJ, Moon CK, Lee BH. Antitumor activity of a novel ginseng saponin metabolite in human pulmonary adenocarcinoma cells resistant to cisplatin. *Cancer Lett* 1999; 144:39–43.

118. Kitts DD, Popovich DG. Ginseng. In: Watson D, ed. *Performance Functional Foods*. New York: Woodhead; 2003:78–88.

# Part VIII

## Dietary Components That Protect from Cancer: Specialized Lipids

# 23 Omega-3 Fatty Acids and Cancer Prevention

*Bandaru S. Reddy*

## CONTENTS

23.1 Introduction ........................................................................................487
23.2 Evidence from Epidemiological Studies ...........................................488
23.3 Evidence from Preclinical Efficacy Studies ......................................489
23.4 Mode of Action of Types of Dietary Fats against Colon Cancer .........492
23.5 Summary and Conclusions ...............................................................495
23.6 Future Directions ..............................................................................496
Acknowledgments ........................................................................................497
References ....................................................................................................497

## 23.1 INTRODUCTION

Cancer of the large bowel is the fourth most common cancer in the world. More than 945,000 colon cancer cases and 492,000 colon cancer-related deaths were reported in the year 2000. Colon cancer is one of the leading causes of cancer death in both men and women in Western countries including the U.S., Canada, Northern and Western Europe, Australia, and New Zealand; however, colon cancer is markedly less frequent in Asia, Africa, and South America.[1,2] In the U.S. about 147,000 new cases of this cancer and 57,000 related deaths were estimated for the year 2004.[2] Marked international differences in the incidence and mortality of colon cancer and the increase of risk in populations migrating from low- to high-risk areas such as from Japan to the U.S. within one or two generations suggest that environmental factors, specifically dietary habits rather than the genetic factors, play an important role in the etiology of this cancer. It is noteworthy that there is an upward trend in colon cancer risk in Japan, which cannot be attributed to genetic differences.[3] Nutritional epidemiologic studies conducted in Japan point to the fact that this upward trend in colon risk has been attributed to westernization of Japanese food habits.[4] The failure to control cancer deaths from colorectal cancer and other types of cancer provides the rationale to develop strategies for prevention. The logical approach to control colorectal cancer is to prevent it before it progresses to invasive and metastatic malignancy. Dietary fats have been implicated in the development of several types of cancer including the

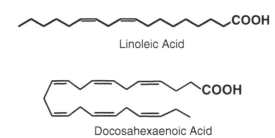

FIGURE 23.1 Chemical structures of omega-3 and omega-6 fatty acids.

cancer of the colon in humans. These observations led to experimental studies in preclinical models designed to assess the effect of types of dietary fat including saturated fat, omega-6 polyunsaturated fatty acids (n-6 PUFAs) and n-3 PUFAs (Figure 23.1).

The purpose of this chapter is to provide a brief overview of epidemiological, preclinical, and mechanistic studies thus far conducted on the relationship between the n-3 PUFAs and colon cancer development. Future directions are also discussed regarding primary and secondary prevention of colon cancer by n-3 PUFA-rich diets.

## 23.2 EVIDENCE FROM EPIDEMIOLOGICAL STUDIES

Fish oils are unique because they contain high levels of n-3 PUFAs that are relatively low in vegetable oils and animal fats. n-3 PUFAs that are present in fish oil include docosahexaenoic acid (C22:6, DHA), eicosapentaenoic acid (C20:5, EPA), and docosapentaenoic acid (C22:5, DPA). Vegetable oils including corn oil and safflower oil contain high levels of n-6 PUFAs including linoleic acid (C18:2, LA). International epidemiological studies have provided evidence that dietary factors are important determinants of large bowel cancer in different populations worldwide. Cancer statistics in Japan for 2001 published by the Foundation for Promotion of Cancer Research indicate that there is an upward trend in age-adjusted mortality rates for colon cancer from 1955 to 1999.[3] According to this report, the death rates due to colon cancer in Japanese men and women in 1955 were 2.9 and 3.0, respectively, whereas they increased to 14.7 and 9.8, respectively, in men and women in 1999. Interestingly, animal fat consumption in 1960 was about 25 g/day (per capita), whereas in 1999 it increased to about 58 g/day. Meat intake was increased from 19 to 78 g/day (per capita), whereas grain consumption decreased from 453 g to 245 g/day during these years.[3] In fact, meat consumption has been found to be associated with an increased risk for the development of colon adenomas in Japan. The change in dietary habits in Japan may, in part, explain the time trend in colon cancer mortality.

The importance of types of dietary fat differing in fatty acid composition rather than total fat cannot be discounted. A recent report by an expert panel assembled by the American Institute for Cancer Research and the World Cancer

Research Fund came to a scientific consensus that evidence for an association between the intake of saturated fat and/or animal fat and colon cancer risk is very strong.[5] Continuing population studies reveal that mortality data for colorectal cancer in 22 European countries, the U.S., and Canada correlate with the consumption of animal fat.[6]

Eating a diet rich in n-3 PUFAs, as present fish and fish oils, may decrease the risk of colorectal cancer. Caygill et al.[7] reported an inverse correlation between fish and fish oil consumption and colorectal cancer. This inverse relationship was significant for both male and female patients with colorectal cancer, whether the intakes were in the current period or 10 years or 23 years before cancer mortality.[7] It is noteworthy that these effects were only observed in countries with a high (>85 g/day) animal fat intake. Also, the Mediterranean diet, which is rich in olive oil and fish, is associated with a low risk of colorectal cancer.[8] The results of these epidemiological studies suggest that diets high in saturated fats increase the risk of colorectal cancer, whereas diets high in n-3 PUFAs reduce the risk.

## 23.3  EVIDENCE FROM PRECLINICAL EFFICACY STUDIES

The development of strategies for colorectal cancer prevention by use of chemopreventive agents and dietary modification has been markedly facilitated by the use of relevant animal models including carcinogen-induced colon cancer mimicking the neoplastic processes that occur in humans.[9] These animal models include induction of colon tumors in rats by administration of azoxymethane (AOM), which is a potent inducer of carcinomas of the large intestine in various strains of male and female rats. AOM has been used extensively by many investigators to induce colon tumors and to study the effects of nutritional factors and chemopreventive agents in colon carcinogenesis.[9–16] Biological behavior of AOM-induced rat colon carcinomas is similar to that of human colon carcinomas.[9] Characteristics of the human disease process reflected in the AOM-Fischer rat model (F344) are the occurrence of both adenomas and adenocarcinomas.[9] Also, aberrant crypt foci (ACF), which are recognized as early appearing preneoplastic lesions, develop in experimentally induced colon carcinogenesis in laboratory rodents as well as in the colonic mucosa of patients with colon cancer.[17,18] Recently, β-catenin-accumulated crypts were identified in the colonic mucosa at the early stages of AOM-induced colon carcinogenesis and are considered early-appearing preneoplastic lesions.[19,20] AOM treatment also induces oncogene mutations at codon 12 of K- and H-*ras* and increases in the expression of the *ras* family of proto-oncogenes. Such increases have been causally associated with colon tumor development.[21,22] Enhanced *ras* oncogene expression has been observed in a variety of human colon tumors.[23] AOM-induced colon tumors also demonstrate enhanced cyclooxygenase-2 (COX-2) and inducible nitric oxide synthase (iNOS) expression similar to human colon tumors.[12,24] It has been increasingly apparent that the β-catenin signaling pathway is closely associated with the development of colon cancer.[25] Also, frequent mutations in the β-catenin gene are confirmed in AOM-induced colon tumors in rodent models.[26]

Ample and consistent experimental evidence from preclinical efficacy studies conducted earlier have provided convincing evidence that not only the amounts but also types of dietary fat differing in fatty acid composition are important factors in determining the modulatory effect of fatty acids in colon tumor development.[27–30] Studies conducted in our laboratory and those of others have consistently demonstrated that the diets high in beef tallow and lard, which are high in saturated fats and corn oil (high in n-6 PUFAs; 20 to 23% in the diet), significantly increased chemically induced colon carcinogenesis in F344 and Sprague-Dawley rats as compared to diets low (5%) in these fats.[10,27–32] Deschner et al.[33] demonstrated that dietary n-3 PUFA (fish oil), inhibits methylazoxymethanol (metabolite of azoxymethane)-induced focal areas of dysplasia and colon tumors, whereas n-6 PUFAs (corn oil) enhance colon tumorigenesis in rats. In a recent study, Chang et al.[10] reported that high dietary fish oil significantly inhibited colon tumors as compared to high corn oil diets. In addition, colon tumor inhibition by fish oil diet was associated with lower levels of DNA damage in the distal colon compared with corn oil diet.[10,34] These studies provided evidence in preclinical models that high dietary saturated fats of animal origin or n-6 PUFAs had a greater colon tumor-enhancing effect than the diets low in such fatty acids; whereas high dietary n-3 PUFAs had no such enhancing effect.

We also have evaluated the modulatory effects of diets high in corn oil and safflower oil (rich in n-6 PUFAs), high in olive oil (rich in monounsaturated fatty acid, such as oleic acid), and high in fish oil during the postinitiation stage of AOM-induced colon carcinogenesis in male F344 rats.[13,31,32,35] Animals fed the diets containing high corn oil or safflower oil (23.5%) had a higher incidence of colon tumors than did those fed the diets low in fat (5%). By contrast, diets high in olive oil or menhaden fish oil had no such colon tumor-enhancing effect. The varied effects of different types of fat on colon carcinogenesis during postinitiation stage suggest that fatty acid composition is one of the determining factors in colon tumor promotion by dietary fat and that the influence of the types and amounts of dietary fat is exerted mostly during the postinitiation phase of carcinogenesis.[28,35,36] In this connection it is interesting to note that in a Phase II clinical trial of patients with colonic polyps, dietary fish oil supplements had in fact inhibited cell proliferation in the colonic mucosa.[37]

Studies conducted thus far clearly indicate tumor-promoting effects of diets rich in n-6 PUFAs and saturated fatty acids, and lack of such effects by n-3 PUFAs. Dietary fat intake in the U.S., Canada, and other Western countries, where the colon cancer rates are high, consists predominantly of a mixture of saturated, monounsaturated, and polyunsaturated fats.[5,38] Also, the typical Western diet contains about ten times more n-6 PUFAs than n-3 PUFAs. It is noteworthy that a recent assay in mice demonstrated that high dietary fat simulating mixed lipid composition of the average Western-style diet produced dysplastic lesions in the colon, indicative of tumorigenesis.[38,39]

**TABLE 23.1**
**Effect of Types and Amount of Dietary Fat on Azoxymethane-Induced Colon Carcinomas in Male F344 Rats[a]**

| Study No. | Amount and Types of Dietary Fat | % Animals with Colon Tumors |
|---|---|---|
| 1 | 5% Corn oil (LFCO) | 54[b] |
| | 23.5% Corn oil (HFCO) | 92 |
| | 4% Fish oil + 1% Corn oil (LFFO) | 50[b] |
| | 22.5% Fish oil + 1% Corn oil (HFFO) | 33[b] |
| 2 | 5% Corn oil (LFCO) | 58[c] |
| | 20% Mixed lipids (HFML) | 100 |
| | 17% Fish oil + 5% Corn oil (HFFO) | 62[c] |

[a] Animals were fed the experimental diets containing types of dietary fat beginning 1 day or 1 week after carcinogen treatment (postinitiation stage of colon carcinogenesis) until termination of the study.
[b] Significantly different from HFCO diet, $p < 0.05$.
[c] Significantly different from HFML diet, $p < 0.01$.

*Source:* Modified from Reddy.[31]

In a recent study we examined the effects of high-fat diets containing mixed lipids rich in saturated fatty acids or fish oil during the different stages of colon carcinogenesis in male F344 rats (Table 23.1).[12] Colonic preneoplastic lesions, ACF, were assessed in animals fed the experimental diets for 8, 23, and 38 weeks. Rats fed the high-fat mixed lipids (HFML) diet showed a significantly greater number of ACF/colon and multicrypt aberrant foci compared with those fed the low-fat, corn oil (LFCO), or high-fat fish oil (HFFO) diet at all time points. Also, rats fed the HFML diet showed a 100% incidence of colonic adenocarcinomas compared with incidences of 58 and 62% in rats fed the LFCO and HFFO diets, respectively. Also, the multiplicity of adenocarcinomas was significantly higher in animals fed the HFML diet (about fourfold increase) as compared to those fed the LFCO diet.

The efficacy of dietary n-3 PUFAs including docosahexaenoic acid (DHA) and eicosapentaenoic acid (EPA) and n-6 PUFA, linoleic acid (LA) against colon carcinogenesis has also been investigated in rodent models.[42] Intragastric administration of 0.7 ml of DHA twice a week for 4 and 12 weeks significantly suppressed AOM-induced ACF in the colon. Intragastric administration of 1 ml of DHA five times a week for 36 weeks significantly suppressed AOM-induced colon tumor multiplicity, specifically moderately differentiated adenocarcinomas in the middle and distal colon of male F344 rats.[43] Minoura et al.[11] reported that the rats fed EPA at 4.7% plus LA at 0.3% had a significantly lower colon tumor incidence and multiplicity than those fed the LA diet. Rats on the EPA diet had fewer well-differentiated adenocarcinomas and more mucinous adenocarcinomas than those on the LA diet. In general, overall evidence from preclinical studies is consistent with the epidemiological data.

## 23.4 MODE OF ACTION OF TYPES OF DIETARY FATS AGAINST COLON CANCER

Successful approach for implementation of preventive strategies depends on a mechanistic understanding of carcinogenesis at the tissue, cellular, and molecular levels. Carcinogenesis is typically a slow, chronic process and the development of invasive disease is characterized by molecular derangements. Although the molecular mechanisms by which n-3 PUFAs inhibit colon carcinogenesis have not been fully elucidated, several putative mechanisms of action have been proposed for colon cancer preventive activity of types of dietary fat (Figure 23.2). As discussed in detail by Hong et al.,[44] dietary n-3 PUFAs may protect against colon carcinogenesis by either decreasing DNA adduct formation and/or by enhancing DNA repair. Lower levels of AOM-induced DNA adducts were detected in fish oil–fed rats as compared to those fed corn oil, rich in n-6 PUFAs. Also, fish oil supplementation caused an increase in apoptosis in the colon compared with corn oil–fed rats.[44,45] It is therefore reasonable to conclude that one of the mechanisms by which n-3 PUFAs protect against colon carcinogenesis is in part by reducing the level of DNA-adducts and by enhancing the deletion of colonic cells through apoptosis.[44]

Metabolic epidemiological studies demonstrated that populations who are on a typical Western diet and at high risk for colon cancer excrete high levels of secondary bile acids.[46,47] Several preclinical studies indicate that diets high in saturated fatty acids (beef tallow and lard) and n-6 PUFAs (corn oil or safflower oil) increase the concentration of colonic luminal secondary bile acids including deoxycholic acid and lithocholic acid, whereas dietary fish oil had no such enhancing effect.[31] Secondary bile acids have been shown to stimulate protein kinase C (PKC) in a manner similar to phorbol esters, to induce cell proliferation, to increase ornithine decarboxylase activity, a rate-limiting enzyme in polyamine biosynthesis, and to act as promoters in colon carcinogenesis.[48–53] Collectively, these observations suggest that secondary bile acids that are modulated by types of dietary fat may be important for inducing cellular response in relation to colon tumor promotion.

There are studies to indicate that inducible nitric oxide (NO) synthase (iNOS), which is regulated primarily at the transcriptional levels is overexpressed in human colon adenomas[54] and in colon tumors of laboratory animal models.[55] Overproduction of NO by iNOS is critical to carcinogenesis process and induces deaminated DNA lesions, thus resulting in DNA damage.[56] Both NO and peroxinitrate produced in the tissues by NOS also activate cyclooxygenase (COX)-2. These data clearly suggest a key role for NO in tumor initiation, promotion, and progression. Studies conducted in our laboratory indicate that deoxycholic acid

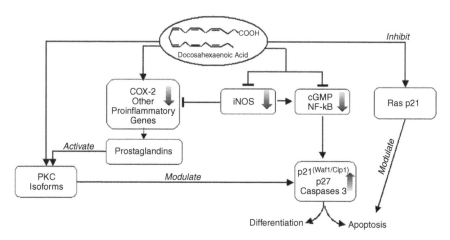

**FIGURE 23.2** Mechanisms by which n-3 PUFAs inhibit colon carcinogenesis. The schematic diagram illustrates potential cellular and molecular events mediated by n-3 PUFAs against colon carcinogenesis. The cascade of molecular events modulated by n-3 PUFAs includes proinflammatory genes such as COX-2 and iNOS, activated ras, specific PKC isoforms, and differentiating factors including RXR that modulate cell differentiation and apoptosis. High dietary n-3 PUFAs exert antitumor activity by interfering with the post-translational modification and membrane localization of ras-p21 through modulation of farnesyl protein transferase, thus inhibiting ras-p21 function.

induces iNOS activity in intestinal cells suggesting that one of the mechanisms by which tumor promoters including secondary bile acids may involve an increase in expression of iNOS through an activation pathway that enhances colon carcinogenesis.[57]

It is known that the fatty acid composition of cells is sensitive to diet. Studies conducted in our laboratory indicate that increasing levels of dietary fish oil in rats increased the omega-3 fatty acids, namely, DHA and EPA, in the colonic mucosal membrane phospholipid fractions at the expense of omega-6 PUFAs such as linoleic acid and arachidonic acid. This suggests that the DHA and EPA of fish oil can modulate the activity of membrane-bound enzymes by partially replacing arachidonic acid and linoleic acid in the phospholipid pool.[58] It is well established that arachidonic acid and some of its metabolites including prostaglandins (PGs) play an important role in the intracellular signaling pathway associated with cell proliferation and gene expression. PGs increase cell proliferation, promote angiogenesis, and inhibit immune surveillance, all of which are involved in tumor growth.

It has been shown that inhibition of colon carcinogenesis by DHA is mediated through the activation of retinoid X receptors (RXR), an obligatory component of a large number of nuclear receptors.[59] This observation suggests that n-3 PUFAs mediate growth inhibitory effects in the colon through the RXR subunit of nuclear receptor heterodimers. Members of the nuclear-receptor superfamily are transcription factors that selectively regulate cell differentiation and proliferation, many of which are important sites for carcinogenesis making their ligands an ideal target for prevention.[60]

Overexpression of COX-2 plays an important role in colon carcinogenesis.[61] Tsujii and DuBois[62] have shown that overexpression of COX-2 can lead to the suppression of apoptosis. High intake of saturated fat and n-6 PUFAs alters membrane phospholipid turnover, releasing membrane arachidonic acid from phospholipids, and affecting prostaglandin synthesis via COX enzyme.[28,35] Elevated levels of COX-2 have been observed in human colon tumors and chemically induced colon tumors in rodents.[63,64] Recent reports have shown a link between the tumorigenic potential of APC mutations and arachidonic metabolism by the observation that deletion of the COX-2 gene reduces the number of tumors in mice heterozygous for an APC[716] by more than sixfold.[65] Of some interest, additional evidence supporting a role for COX-2 comes from our studies, which showed a marked reduction in colon tumors in rodents treated with a highly selective COX-2 inhibitor, celecoxib.[24] Our recent laboratory results have provided convincing evidence that a high-fat mixed lipid (HFML) diet enhances AOM-induced expression of COX-2 and eicosanoid formation from arachidonic acid in colon tumors of rats whereas the high-fat fish oil (HFFO) diet inhibits the levels of COX-2. These results suggest that inhibition of eicosanoid production through the modulation of COX-2 activity may be important for ability of n-3 PUFAs to inhibit colon tumorigenesis.[12] Also, colon tumors of animals fed the HFML diet showed a nearly 50% lower apoptotic index than was observed in the colon tumors of rats fed the HFFO diet. These results suggest that the overexpression of COX-2 in the tumors of animals fed the HFML diet in contrast to HFFO diet inhibits apoptosis and the consequent tumor burden. These results also support the contention that overexpression of COX-2 can lead to the suppression of apoptosis. A major question that remains to be answered is which signaling pathways are involved downstream of the COX-2 enzyme. These could provide not only a key link between dietary fatty acids, eicosanoids, COX-2, and transcriptional regulation of colon carcinogenesis, but also provide additional molecular targets for colon cancer prevention strategies.

Recent studies from our laboratory have shown that high dietary n-6 PUFAs enhance activities of diverse enzymes including protein kinases (PKC) whereas high-fat diet containing n-3 PUFAs appears to suppress the activities of these enzymes.[65] Members of PKCs include several isoenzymes with unique functions. Specific PKC isoenzymes translocate to the membrane from the cytosol upon activation.[66,67] Jiang et al.[68] reported that chemopreventive efficacy of dietary fish oil is associated with the alterations in colonic PKC expression that is activated upon stimulation by growth factors. PUFAs may influence the activity of the EGF receptor/mitogen-activated protein kinase pathway, which could alter the expression of a number of oncogenes. It is interesting that several kinases have been shown to participate in *ras*-mediated growth-promoting signal transduction pathways.[69] The *ras*-p21, a guanine nucleotide-binding 21-kDa protein product of *ras* genes, is anchored to the cytoplasmic face of plasma membrane and functions in the regulation of cell proliferation. Mutational versions of *ras*-p21 are implicated in the etiology of human colon cancer.[70] It is also known that trafficking of pro-*ras* from cytosol to plasma membrane is facilitated by a series of closely linked post-translational modifications including farnesylation, which is catalyzed by farnesyl protein transferase (FPTase). It appears that inhibition of ras farnesylation blocks membrane association of *ras*-p21 and prevents neoplastic transformation of cells. Studies conducted in our laboratory have provided data to indicate that high dietary n-6 PUFAs increase *ras*-p21 expression in colonic tumors, whereas high dietary n-3 PUFAs interfere with post-translational modification and membrane localization of *ras*-p21 through the modulation of FPTase activity, thus inhibiting *ras*-p21 function.[71]

Additional studies conducted in our laboratory have demonstrated that DHA inhibits growth of CaCo-2 colon cancer cells *in vitro* and induces apoptosis.[72] The effects of DHA on the genetic precursors of human colon cancer were also analyzed in CaCo-2 cells using DNA oligonucleotide arrays.[73] DHA treatment modulated multiple signaling pathways involved in the regulation of cell cycle regulatory genes, COX-2 target genes, lipoxygenases, and peroxisome proliferators. Effects of DHA on cell cycle progression and induction of apoptosis were directly paralleled by an increase in the activation of several proapoptotic caspases, inactivation of antiapoptotic Bcl-2 family of genes and activation of cyclin-dependent kinase inhibitors such as p21[waf1/cip1] and p27. Comprehensive evaluation of the role of the apoptosis-related genes in colon cancer continues as the protein products of these genes suggest themselves as molecular targets for effective intervention by selective chemopreventive agents including nutritional factors.

## 23.5 SUMMARY AND CONCLUSIONS

In conclusion, both epidemiological and preclinical studies provide evidence for the beneficial effects of diets rich in n-3 PUFA in the prevention of colorectal cancer. Preclinical studies have provided convincing evidence that the colon tumor–promoting effect of dietary fat depends on its fatty acid composition. Preclinical studies also demonstrate that a Western-style diet rich in mixed lipids including saturated fats of animal origin as well as n-6 PUFAs has a greater potential to promote colon tumorigenesis compared to diets containing equivalent amounts of fat but rich in n-3 PUFAs. Although the mechanisms by which diets high in saturated fats (such as those in Western diets) and n-6 PUFAs promote colon carcinogenesis are not fully known, the studies conducted thus far indicate that increased levels of colonic luminal secondary bile acids, modulation of *ras*-p21 activity, eicosanoid production *via* the influence on COX activity, and the expression of apoptosis by the types of dietary fat especially n-6 PUFAs may play a key role in colon carcinogenesis.

The goal of prevention is to decrease the morbidity and mortality from colorectal cancer. It should be recognized that nutritional prevention has the potential to be a major component of colorectal cancer control, especially through primary prevention in the general population. Although there are no clear-cut data to indicate how much and how long n-3 PUFAs should be consumed in order to promote primary prevention of colorectal cancer, the levels of dietary n-3 PUFAs should be consistent with the recommendations based on epidemiological studies of coronary heart disease as discussed by several nutritionists.[74–78] These studies suggest that one to two fish meals per week or as little as 30 to 35 g/day of fish throughout life decreases the risk of coronary heart disease. Lands et al.[75] have suggested that the ratio of n-6 PUFAs to n-3 PUFAs may be important for health. Based on preclinical and epidemiological studies on arteriosclerosis and coronary heart disease, Okuyama et al.[78] recommended a reduction in the intake of linoleic acid and an increase in the intake of n-3 PUFAs so that an n-6/n-3 ratio of 2 could be achieved for effective prevention of atherosclerosis and related diseases. This recommendation may well be applied for the effective primary prevention of colorectal cancer in the general population. Importantly, consumption of fibrous foods, fruits, and vegetables is necessary for those in Western countries to reduce the risk of colorectal cancer.

## 23.6 FUTURE DIRECTIONS

Colon cancer control in high-risk patients such as those with hereditary polyposis and sporadic colon polyps is of growing importance as therapy modalities alone have not been fully effective in countering either the high incidence or low survival rate of colorectal cancer. The development of chemopreventive agents to prevent intraepithelial neoplasia such as benign adenomas and early neoplastic lesions represents a significant advance in clinical cancer prevention research.[79] Clinical trials are the best means to identify the most-promising preventive agents for secondary prevention of colorectal cancer. Development of combination chemoprevention will be essential, just as combination chemotherapy has been so important in the treatment of invasive disease.[60] It should be recognized, however, that intervention with nutritional supplements or diet modification alone might not be sufficient for secondary prevention of colorectal cancer. However, intervention by diet modification as recommended to the general population along with chemopreventive agents that have been shown to possess anticancer properties against colon carcinogenesis in preclinical models is an ideal strategy for secondary prevention of colon cancer in these high-risk individuals. One such modification is a series of logically arranged comprehensive studies to elucidate the efficacy of potential chemopreventive agents administered in conjuncture with a diet rich in n-3 PUFAs. This approach is extremely important when promising chemopreventive agents demonstrate significant efficacy but may produce toxic effects at higher doses. Clear delineation of the synergistic effects in laboratory studies will allow rational design of mechanistically driven combination therapies for optimal clinical effects. This is a promising area for future prevention studies in high-risk individuals.

## ACKNOWLEDGMENTS

Current and past studies on n-3 PUFAs in colon cancer prevention are supported by U.S. National Cancer Institute Grants CA-17613 and CA-37663. I thank Ms. Laura McDermott for preparation of the manuscript.

## REFERENCES

1. Stewart BW, Kleihuas P, eds. *World Cancer Report*. World Health Organization. International Agency for Cancer Research on Cancer. Lyon, France: IARC Press; 2003.
2. Jamal A, Tiwari RC, Murray T, Samuels A, Ghafoor A, Ward E, Feuer EJ, Thun, M. Cancer statistics, 2004. *CA Cancer J Clin* 2004; 54:8–29.
3. Kakizoe T, Yamaguchi N, Mitsuhashi F, Koshiji M, Oshima A, Ohtaka M. Cancer statistics in Japan–2001, Foundation for Promotion of Cancer Research in Japan; 2001.
4. Tominaga S, Kati I. Diet, nutrition and cancer in Japan. *Nutr Health* 1992; 8:125–132.
5. World Cancer Research Fund and American Institute for Cancer research. Panel on Food. Nutrition and the Prevention of Cancer. Washington, DC: American Institute for Cancer Research; 1997.
6. Caygill CP, Hill MJ. Fish, n-3 fatty acids and human colorectal and breast cancer mortality. *Eur J Cancer Prev* 1995; 4:329–332.
7. Caygill CPJ, Charland SL, Lippin JA. Fat, fish, fish oil, and cancer. *Br J Cancer* 1996; 74:159–164.
8. Gerber M. Olive oil and cancer. In: Hill MJ, Giacosa A., Caygill CPJ, eds. *Epidemiology of Diet and Cancer*. London: Ellis Horwood; 1994:263–275.
9. Reddy BS. Carcinogen-induced colon cancer models for chemoprevention and nutritional studies. In: Teicher BA, ed. *Tumor Models in Cancer Research*. Totowa, NJ: Humana Press; 2002:183–191.
10. Chang W-CL, Chapkin RS, Lupton JR. Fish oil blocks azoxymethane-induced rat colon tumorigenesis by increasing cell differentiation and apoptosis rather than decreasing cell proliferation. *J Nutr* 1998; 128:491–497.
11. Minoura T, Takata T, Sakaguchi M, Takada H, Yamamura M, Yamamoto M. Effect of dietary eicosapentaenoic acid on azoxymethane-induced colon carcinogenesis. *Cancer Res* 1988; 48:4790–4794.
12. Rao CV, Hirose Y, Indranie C, Reddy BS. Modulation of experimental colon tumorigenesis by types and amounts of dietary fatty acids. *Cancer Res* 2001; 61:1927–1933.
13. Reddy BS, Maruyama H. Effect of dietary fish oil on azoxymethane-induced colon carcinogenesis in male F 344 rats. *Cancer Res* 1986; 46:3367–3370.
14. Periera, MA, Grubs CJ, Barnes LH, Li H, Olson GR, Eto I, Juliana M, Whitaker LM, Kelloff GJ, Steele VE, Lubet RA. Effects of the phytochemicals, curcumin and quercetin, upon azoxymethane-induced colon cancer and 7,12-dimethyl-benz[α]anthracene-induced mammary caner in rats. *Carcinogenesis* 1996; 17:1305–1311.

15. Zhang J, Wu G, Chapkin RS, Lupton JR. Energy metabolism of colonocytes changes during tumorigenesis process and is dependent on diet and carcinogen. *J Nutr* 1998; 128:1262–1269.

16. Zeng Y, Kramer P, Olsen G, Lubet RA, Steele V, Kelloff GJ. Prevention by retinoids of azoxymethane-induced tumors and aberrant crypt foci and their modulation of cell proliferation in the colon of rats. *Carcinogenesis* 1997; 18:2119–2121.

17. Bird RP. Observation and quantification of aberrant crypt in the murine colon treated with a colon carcinogen: preliminary finding. *Cancer Lett* 1987; 37:147–151.

18. Pretlow TP, Oriordan MA, Pretlow TG, Stellato TA. Aberrant crypts in human colonic mucosa: putative preneoplastic lesions. *J Cell Biochem* 1992; 16G:55–62.

19. Yamada Y, Mori H. Precancerous lesions for colorectal cancers in rodents: a new concept. *Carcinogenesis* 2003; 24:1015–1019.

20. Wargovich MJ, Chen CD, Jimerez A, Steele VE, Velasco M, Stephen LC. Aberrant crypts as biomarkers for colon cancer: evaluation of potential chemopreventive agents in the rat. *Cancer Epidemiol Biomarkers Prev* 1996; 5:355–360.

21. Singh J, Kulkarni N, Kelloff G, Reddy BS. Modulation of azoxymethane-induced mutational activation of *ras* protooncogenes by chemopreventive agents in colon carcinogenesis. *Carcinogenesis* 1994; 15:1317.

22. Singh J, Rivenson A, Tomita M, Shimamura S, Ishibasi N, Reddy BS. *Bifidobacterium longum,* a lactic acid-producing intestinal bacterium inhibits colon cancer and modulates the intermediate biomarkers of colon carcinogenesis. *Carcinogenesis* 1997; 18:833.

23. Forrester K, Almoguera C, Han K, Grizzle ME, Perucho M. Detection of high incidence of K-ras oncogenes during human colon tumorigenesis. *Nature* 1987; 327:298–303.

24. Kawamori T, Rao CV, Seibert K, Reddy BS. Chemopreventive activity of celecoxib, a specific cyclooxygenase-2 inhibitor, against colon carcinogenesis. *Cancer Res* 1998; 58:409–412.

25. Takahashi M, Fukuda K, Sugimura T, Wakabayashi K. β-Catenin is frequently mutated and demonstrates altered cellular location in azoxymethane-induced rat colon tumors. *Cancer Res* 1998; 58:42–46.

26. Brabletz T, Herrmann K, Jung A, Faller G, Kirchner T. Expression of nuclear β-catenin and c-myc is correlated with tumor size but not with proliferative activity of colorectal adenomas. *Am J Pathol* 2000; 156:865–870.

27. Bull AW, Soullier BK, Wilson PS, Hayden MT, Nigro ND. Promotion of azoxymethane-induced intestinal cancer by high fat diets in rats. *Cancer Res* 1979; 39:4956–4959.

28. Reddy BS, Maeura Y. Tumor promotion by dietary fat in azoxymethane-induced colon carcinogenesis in female F344 rats: influence of amount and sources of dietary fat. *J Natl Cancer Inst* 1984; 72:745.

29. Reddy BS, Maruyama H. Effect of different levels of dietary corn oil and lard during the initiation phase of colon carcinogenesis in male F344 rats. *J Natl Cancer Inst* 1986; 77:815–822.

30. Nigro ND, Singh DV, Campbell RL, Pak MS. Effect of dietary beef fat on the intestinal tumor formation by azoxymethane in rats. *J Natl Cancer Inst* 1975; 54:439.

31. Reddy BS. Nutritional factors and colon cancer. *Crit Rev Food Sci Nutr* 1995; 35:175–190.
32. Reddy BS, Narisawa T, Vukusich D, Weisburger JH, Wynder EL. Effect of quality and quantity of dietary fat and dimethylhydrazine in colon carcinogenesis in rats. *Proc Soc Exp Biol Med* 1976; 151:237.
33. Deschner EE, Lytle JS, Wong G, Ruperto JF, Newmark HL. The effect of dietary omega-3 fatty acids (fish oil) on azoxymethane-induced focal areas of dysplasia and colon tumor incidence. *Cancer* 1990; 66:2350–2356.
34. Hong MY, Chapkin RS, Morris JS, Wang N, Carroll RJ, Turner ND, Chung WCL, Lupton RL. Anatomical site-specific response to DNA damage is related to later tumor development in the rat azoxymethane colon carcinogenesis model. *Carcinogenesis* 2001; 22:1831–1835.
35. Reddy BS, Burill C, Rigotty J. Effect of diets high in omega-3 and omega-6 fatty acids on initiation and postinitiation stages of colon carcinogenesis. *Cancer Res* 1991; 51:487–491.
36. Reddy BS, Sugie S. Effect of different levels of omega-3 and omega-6 fatty acids on azoxymethane-induced colon carcinogenesis in F344 rats. *Cancer Res* 1988; 48:6642–6647.
37. Anti M, Armelao F, Marra G. Effect of different doses of fish oil on rectal cell proliferation in patients with sporadic colonic adenomas. *Gastroenterology* 1994; 107:1709–1718.
38. Yang K, Fan K, Newmark H, Leung D, Lipkin M, Steele VE, Kelloff GJ. Cytokeratin, lectin, and acidic mucin modulation in differentiating colonic epithelial cells of mice after feeding Western-style diets. *Cancer Res* 1996; 56:4644–4648.
39. Risio M, Lipkin M, Newmark H, Yang K, Rossini FP, Steele VE, Boon CW, Kelloff GJ. Apoptosis, cell proliferation, and Western-style diet-induced tumorigenesis in mouse colon. *Cancer Res* 1996; 56: 4910–4916.
40. Pretlow TP, Barrow BJ, Ashton WS, O'Riordan MA, Pretlow TG, Jurcisek JA, Stellato TA. Aberrant crypts: putative preneoplastic foci in human colonic mucosa. *Cancer Res* 1991; 51:1564–1567.
41. Wargovich MJ, Chen DC, Harris C, Yang E, Velasco M. Inhibition of aberrant crypt growth by nonsteroidal antiinflammatory agents and differentiating agents in the rat colon. *Int J Cancer* 1995; 60:515–519.
42. Takahashi M, Minamoto T, Yamashita N, Yawaza K, Sugimura T, Esumi H. Reduction in formation and growth of 1,2-dimethylhydrazine-induced aberrant crypt foci in rat colon by docosahexaenoic acid. *Cancer Res* 1993; 53:2786–2789.
43. Takahashi M, Minamoto T, Yamashita N, Kato T, Yazowa K, Esumi H. Effect of docosahexaenoic acid on azoxymethane-induced colon carcinogenesis in rats. *Cancer Lett* 1994; 83:177–184.
44. Hong MY, Lupton JR, Morris JS, Wang N, Carroll RJ, Davidson LA, Elder RH, Chapkin RS. Dietary fish oil reduces $O^6$-methylguanine DNA adduct levels in rat colon in part by increasing apoptosis during tumor initiation. *Cancer Epidemiol Biomarkers Prev* 2000; 9:819–826.
45. Chang W-C, Chapkin RS, Lupton JR. Fish oil blocks azoxymethane-induced colon tumorigenesis by increasing cell differentiation and apoptosis rather than decreasing cell proliferation. *J Nutr* 1998; 128:491–497.
46. Reddy BS, Wynder EL. Large bowel cancer. Fecal constituents of populations with diverse incidence of colon cancer. *J Natl Cancer Inst* 1973; 50:1437–1442.

47. Reddy BS, Hedges A, Laakso K, Wynder EL. Metabolic epidemiology of large bowel cancer: fecal bulk and constituents of high-risk North American and low-risk Finnish population. *Cancer* 1978; 42:2832–2838.

48. Reddy BS, Watanabe K, Weisburger JH, Wynder EL. Promoting effect of bile acids in colon carcinogenesis in germ-free and conventional F344 rats. *Cancer Res* 1977; 37:3238–3242.

49. Craven RA, Pfanstial J, DeRubertis FR. Role of activation of protein kinase C in the stimulation of colonic epithelial proliferation and reactive oxygen formation by bile acids. *J Clin Invest* 1987; 79:532–541.

50. Davidson LA, Jiang YH, Derr JN, Aukema HM, Lupton JR, Chapkin RS. Protein kinase C isoforms in human and rat colonic mucosa. *Arch Biochem Biophys* 1994; 312:547–553.

51. Rao CV, Reddy BS. Modulating effect of amount and types of dietary fat on ornithine decarboxylase, tyrosine protein kinase, and prostaglandins production during colon carcinogenesis. *Carcinogenesis* 1993; 14:1327–1333.

52. Rao CV, Simi B, Wynn T-T, Garr K, Reddy BS. Modulating effect of amount and types of dietary fat on colonic mucosal phospholipase A2, phosphatidylinositol-specific phospholipase C activities, and cyclooxygenase metabolite formation during different stages of colon tumor promotion in male F344 rats. *Cancer Res* 1996; 56: 532–537.

53. Bull AW, Marnett LJ, Dawe EJ, Nigro ND. Stimulation of deoxythymidine incorporation in the colon of rats treated intrarectally with bile acids and fats. *Carcinogenesis* 1993; 4:207–210.

54. Ambs S, Merriam WG, Bennett WP, Felley-Bosco E, Ogunfusika MO, Oser SM, Slein S, Shields PG, Billair TR, Harris CC. Frequent nitric oxide synthase-2 expression in human colon adenomas: implication for tumor angiogenesis and colon cancer progression. *Cancer Res* 1998; 58:334–341.

55. Takahashi M, Fukuda K, Ohata T, Sugimura T, Wakabayashi K. Increased expression of inducible and endothelial constitutive nitric oxide synthase in rat colon tumors induced by azoxymethane. *Cancer Res* 1997; 57:1233–1237.

56. De Rojas-Walker T, Tamir S, Ji H, Wishnok JS, Tannenbaum SR. Nitric oxide induces oxidative damage in addition to deamination in macrophage DNA. *Chem Res Toxicol* 1995; 8:473.

57. Hirose Y, Rao CV, Reddy BS. Modulation of inducible nitric oxide synthase expression in rat intestinal cells by colon tumor promoters. *Int J Oncol* 2001; 18:141–146.

58. Reddy BS, Sugie S. Effect of different levels of omega-3 and omega-6 fatty acids on azoxymethane-induced colon carcinogenesis in F 344 rats. *Cancer Res* 1988; 48:6642–6847.

59. Fan Y-Y, Spencer TE, Wang N, Moyer MP, Chapkin RS. Chemopreventive n-3 fatty acids activate RXRα in colonocytes. *Carcinogenesis* 2003; 24:1541–1548.

60. Sporn MB, Suh N. Chemoprevention: an essential approach to controlling cancer. *Nature Rev* 2002; 2:537–543.

61. Eberhart CE, Coffey RJ, Radhika A, Giardiello FM, Ferrenbach S, DuBois RN. Up-regulation of cyclooxygenase-2 gene expression in human colorectal adenomas and adenocarcinomas. *Gastroenterology* 1994; 107:1183–1188.

62. Tsujii M, DuBois RN. Alterations in cellular adhesion and apoptosis in epithelial cells overexpressing prostaglandin endoperoxide synthase 2. *Cell* 1995; 83:493–501.

63. Kargman SL, O'Neil GP, Vickers PJ, Evens JF, Mancini JA, Jothy S. Expression of prostaglandin G/H-1 and -2 protein in human colon cancer. *Cancer Res* 1995; 55:2556–2559.

64. DuBois RN, Radhika A, Reddy BS, Entingh AJ. Increased cyclooxygenase-2 levels in carcinogen-induced rat colonic tumors. *Gastroenterology* 1996; 110:1259–1262.

65. Oshima M, Dinchuck JE, Kargman SL, Oshima H, Hancock B, Kwong E. Suppression of intestinal polyposis in APC[716] knockout mice by inhibition of cyclooxygenase (COX-2). *Cell* 1996; 87:803–809.

65a. Reddy BS, Simi B, Patel N, Aliaga C, Rao CV. Effect of amount and types of dietary fat on intestinal bacterial 7-dehydroxylase and phosphatidylinositol-specific phospholipase C and colonic mucosal diacylglycerol kinase and PKC activities during different stages of colon tumor promotion. *Cancer Res* 1996; 56:2314–2320.

66. Dakker LV, Parker PJ. Protein kinase C: a question of specificity. *Trends Biochem Sci* 1994; 19:73–77.

67. Kazanietz MG, Blumberg PM. Protein kinase C and signal transduction in normal and neoplastic cells. In: Sirica EA, ed. *Cellular and Molecular Pathogenesis.* Philadelphia: Lippincott-Raven; 1996:389–402.

68. Jiang Y-H, Lupton JR, Chapkin RS. Dietary fat and fiber modulate the effect of carcinogen on colon kinase Cλ expression in rats. *J Nutr* 1993; 127:1938–1943.

69. Egan SE, Weinberg RA. The pathway to signal achievement. *Nature* (London) 1993; 365: 781–783.

70. Barbacid M. Ras oncogenes: their role in neoplasia. *Eur J Clin Invest* 1990; 20:225.

71. Singh J, Hamid R, Reddy BS. Modulating effect of types and amount of dietary fat on *ras*-p21 function during promotion and progression stages of colon cancer. *Cancer Res* 1997; 57:253–258.

72. Fearon KCH. The anticancer and anticachectic effects of n-3 fatty acids. *Clin Nutr* 2002; 21 Suppl 2:69–73.

73. Narayanan BA, Narayanan NK, Reddy BS. Docosahexaenoic acid regulated genes and transcription factor inducing apoptosis in human colon cancer cells. *Int J Oncol* 2001; 19:1255–1262.

74. Tokudome S, Nagaya T, Tokudome S et al. Japanese versus Mediterranean diets and cancer. *Pacific J Cancer Prev* 2000; 1:61–66.

75. Lands WCM, Hamazaki T, Okuyama H, Sakai K, Goto Y, Hubbard VS. Changing dietary patterns. *Am J Clin Nutr* 1990; 51:991–993.

76. Simopoulos AP. Omega-3 fatty acids and cardiovascular disease: the epidemiologic evidence. *Environ Heath Prev Med* 2002; 6:203–208.

77. Siscovick DS, Raghunathan TE, King I, Weinmann S, Wicklund KG, Albright J, Bovberg V, Arbogast P, Smith H, Kushi LH, Cobb LA. Dietary intake and cell membrane levels of long chain n-3 polyunsaturated fatty acids and the risk of primary cardiac arrest. *J Am Med Assoc* 1995; 274:1363–1367.

78. Okuyama H, Fujii Y, Ikemoto A. N-6/n-3 ratio of dietary fatty acids rather than hypercholesterolemia as the major risk factor for atherosclerosis and coronary heart disease. *J Health Sci* 2000; 46:157–177.

79. Hawk ET, Umar A, Viner JL. Colorectal cancer chemoprevention — an overview. *Gastroenterology* 2004; 126:1423–1447.

# 24 Conjugated Linoleic Acid and Cancer

*Yongsoon Park*

## CONTENTS

24.1    Introduction ..................................................................................503
24.2    Tumor Model and Tissue Specificity ..............................................504
    24.2.1    *In Vitro* Cell Culture Model ..............................................504
    24.2.2    *In Vivo* Animal Model .....................................................505
24.3    Inhibitory Mechanisms of CLA on the Stages of Carcinogenesis .......506
    24.3.1    Initiation ..........................................................................506
    24.3.2    Promotion .........................................................................507
    24.3.3    Progression .......................................................................509
24.4    CLA Modulation of Lipid Metabolism and Gene Expression ............509
24.5    CLA Intake and Cancer in Humans .................................................511
24.6    Conclusion .....................................................................................511
References .................................................................................................512

## 24.1    INTRODUCTION

Conjugated linoleic acid (CLA) refers to a group of polyunsaturated fatty acids that exist as positional isomers and stereoisomers of conjugated dienoic octadec-adienoate (C18:2). The double bonds of CLA are in the positions of 7,9; 8,10; 9,11; 10,12; 11,13 and the three-dimensional geometric combinations of *cis* and/or *trans* configurations.[1,2] CLA is found in foods such as beef, lamb, and dairy products derived from these ruminant sources[3-6] and ranges from 2.9 to 8.9 mg/g fat.[7] The isomers in foods are, in descending order: c9,t11-CLA (also called rumenic acid); t7,c9-CLA; 11,13-CLA (c/t); 8,10-CLA (c/t); t10,c12-CLA; and other, minor isomers.[4,8,9] In addition, CLA is present in human blood, tissues, and milk, and is derived from a diet including certain fat-containing foods of ruminant origin.[10] Studies showed that increasing dietary CLA led to increases in the CLA content of plasma,[11,12] adipose tissue,[13] and milk fat[14] in humans.

Synthetically prepared CLA is an isomeric composition somewhat different from isomers found naturally in foods. Synthetic CLA preparation has tradition-ally relied on an alkaline-catalyzed reaction using linoleate as substrate. The isomeric composition of synthetic CLA oil is primarily c9,t11-CLA and t10,c12-

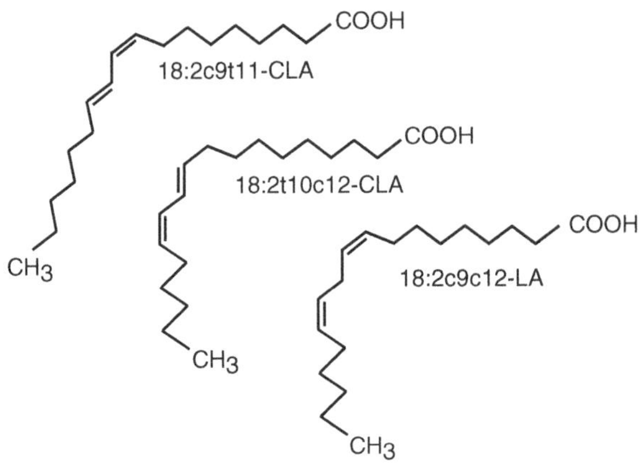

**FIGURE 24.1** Structure of c9,t11-CLA, t10,c12-CLA, and linoleic acid (18:2c9c12). (From Belury MA. *Annu Rev Nutr* 2002; 22:505–531. With permission.)

CLA (Figure 24.1).[15] As a result of high cost or lack of availability, most studies conducted in experimental animals, humans, and in cultures to demonstrate the physiological effect of CLA use the synthetic mixture of isomers. Numerous physiological properties have been attributed to CLA, including action as an antiadipogenic, antidiabetogenic, anticarcinogenic, and antiatherosclerotic agent.[15–18]

## 24.2 TUMOR MODEL AND TISSUE SPECIFICITY

### 24.2.1 In Vitro Cell Culture Model

Studies show dose- and time-dependent anticancer activity of CLA *in vitro*. CLA inhibited the growth of human hepatoma cells, HepG2[19] and 7800NJ;[20] lung adenocarcinoma cells, A-247, SK-LU-1 and A549;[21] human colon cancer cells, SW480;[22] human glioblastoma cells;[23] and human breast cancer cells, MCF-7[24] and T47D.[20] Although both c9,t11 and t10,c12-CLA can inhibit the proliferation, they may have separate mechanisms and different targets of actions.[24] Furthermore, CLA inhibited proliferation of estrogen-receptor-positive MCF-7 cells,[22,24–30] but not of estrogen-receptor-negative MDA-MB-231 cells.[21] In these studies, CLA inhibited the expression of the proto-oncogene c-myc in estrogen-responsive MCF-7 cells. Because expression of c-myc is known to be modulated by estrogens among other factors, the reduction in c-myc expression may relate to a CLA involvement in an estrogen-regulated or some other growth factor-regulated mechanisms.

Whereas CLA in the form of free fatty acid exerts an *in vitro* antiproliferative effect, milk fat enriched with CLA appears to have even greater *in vitro* activity.[31] Bovine milk fat enriched with CLA was more effective in inhibiting human MCF-7 breast cancer cells than were isolated CLA isomers.[23]

**TABLE 24.1**
**Anticarcinogenic Properties of CLA *In Vivo***

| Tissue | Physiological Function | Ref. |
|---|---|---|
| Mammary | ↓ chemically induced carcinogenesis in rats | 35, 39, 58 |
| | ↓ chemically induced carcinogenesis in rats by c9t11-CLA or synthetic CLA | 34, 59 |
| | ↓ chemically induced carcinogenesis in rats regardless of level of fat or esterification of CLA in triglyceride or free fatty acid | 40, 41 |
| | ↓ growth of transplantable cancer tumor cells in nude mice | 42, 43 |
| | ↔ growth of transplanted cancer tumor cell in mice | 47 |
| Prostate | ↓ growth of transplantable cancer tumor cells in nude mice | 44 |
| | ↔ growth of transplanted cancer tumor cell | 46 |
| Skin | ↓ stages of chemically induced tumorigenesis in mice | 32, 37 |
| Colon | ↓ chemically induced carcinogenesis in rats | 38, 57, 87 |
| | ↔ carcinogenesis in Min mice and rats | 2, 48 |
| Forestomach | ↓ chemically induced forestomach | 36 |

*Note:* ↓, decreases; ↑, increases; ↔, no effect.

## 24.2.2 IN VIVO ANIMAL MODEL

Dietary CLA inhibits numerous cancer models in experimental animals (Table 24.1). The role of CLA in modulating carcinogenesis has been understood by determining the effects on the stages of carcinogenesis known as initiation, promotion, and progression. The anticarcinogenic property of CLA was first identified during the initiation stage of the mouse skin multistage carcinogenesis model,[32] where the stages of initiation, promotion, and progression are operationally separable.[33] In this initial study a lipid fraction extracted from fried ground beef was topically applied to mouse skin prior to initiation of 7,12-dimethylbenz(*a*)anthracene.[32] CLA (0.5 and 1%) reduces terminal end bud density and methylnitrosourea-induced rat mammary tumor yields in a dose-dependent manner.[34] In addition, CLA inhibited dimethylbenz(*a*)anthracene-induced tumorigenesis of mammary tumors[35] and forestomach neoplasia.[36]

Independent from anti-initiator activity, CLA inhibits carcinogenesis postinitiation. The synthetic mixture of CLA isomers inhibits chemically induced skin tumor promotion as well as mammary and colon tumorigenesis when added to semisynthetic diet.[34,35,37–39] Skin tumor yield (average number of tumors per mouse) after 16 weeks of promotion with phorbol ester was inhibited by approximately 45% in CLA-fed mice.[32] When mice were fed semipurified diets containing various levels of synthetically prepared CLA (5% corn oil plus 0, 0.5, 1, or 1.5% CLA) after initiation and for the duration of promotion with the phorbol ester, 12-*O*-tetradecanolyphorbol-13-acetate for 35 weeks, skin tumor yield was also inhibited 30% in mice fed 1.5% CLA as compared with mice fed no CLA.[37] Although in chemically induced rat mammary carcinogenesis the stages of initiation and promotion are not readily separable, CLA inhibited carcinogenesis when fed before or after carcinogen treatment.[40,41] Consistent with *in vitro* studies, the inhibitory effect of CLA on mammary carcinogenesis is independent of type or level of fat in the diet and occurs in a dose-dependent manner.[35,40]

A great deal of evidence demonstrates that dietary CLA inhibits the initiation and promotion stages of carcinogenesis, but the role of CLA in the progression stage is not well understood. The growth of mammary[42,43] and prostate[44] cancer cell lines after transplantation into nude mice was significantly reduced if animals were fed a diet with CLA. The inhibition of chemically induced mammary carcinogenesis occurred whether CLA was fed as a free fatty acid or triglyceride,[41] and 9,11-CLA and 10,12-CLA isomers appear to be equally active.[45] In addition, the CLA-responsive chemically induced mammary carcinogenesis model[35] is a model for human cancer ductal carcinomas *in situ*. This tumorigenesis model is consistent with the possibility that CLA reduces metastasis resulting from breast cancer. It is important to investigate how CLA modulates malignant tumor formation and metastasis because the growth of secondary tumors is the major cause of morbidity and mortality in patients with cancer. Although there is no study reporting that CLA enhances tumorigenesis, CLA was unable to alter the growth of transplanted prostate[46] and breast[47] cancer cells in some studies and did not reduce tumorigenesis in an intestinal model of colon carcinogenesis using the Apc Min mouse model.[48] In contrast to the effect of CLA on carcinogenesis, the n-6 and n-3 fatty acids have differential effects (from no effects to potent enhancing or inhibitory effects) depending on the tumor model and tissue studies.[15,49] Thus, CLA's inhibition of multiple models of carcinogenesis appears to be unique.

## 24.3 INHIBITORY MECHANISMS OF CLA ON THE STAGES OF CARCINOGENESIS

### 24.3.1 INITIATION

Early studies focused on initiation stages of anticarcinogenic effects of CLA. As an anti-initiator, CLA may modulate events such as free radical-induced oxidation, carcinogen metabolism, and/or carcinogen-DNA adduct formation in some tumor models.[50] CLA increases the activity of antioxidant-enzymes (superoxide dismutase, catalase, and glutathione peroxidase) in human breast cancer cells (MCF-7) and colon cancer cells (SW480), suggesting that CLA may shift the pro-oxidant/antioxidant balance.[22,27] It has been postulated that, due to the conjugated structure of CLA, there is more efficient trapping of electrons in its double bonds than in methylene-interrupted double bonds, and that antioxidant enzymes are induced as an adaptation of oxidant exposure.[50]

Isomers and metabolites of CLA are readily incorporated into phospholipid and neutral lipid fractions of numerous tissues.[35,36,40,51,52] When radiolabeled tracers were used to study the kinetics of $^{14}$C-CLA uptake into keratinocytes or hepatoma cells, $^{14}$C-CLA was incorporated to the same extent and at a similar rate as $^{14}$C-linoleate, and the levels of incorporation of $^{14}$C-CLA and $^{14}$C-linoleate into epidermal phospholipids and neutral lipid fractions were similar.[53] As the CLA content in the diet increased over a range of 0.5 to 2%, there was a progressive increase in the CLA content of rat mammary and peritoneal fat pads, liver, and plasma, and in the level of CLA metabolites represented by 18:3 and 20:3, and a decrease in the linoleic acid metabolites, in particular arachidonic acid.[34] However, another study of rats fed a diet containing CLA-rich butter (and linoleate) showed that CLA preferentially accumulated in neutral lipids (~79%) with less incorporation into phosphatidylcholine (~10%), the major phospholipids of lever cells, while linoleate preferentially accumulated in phosphatidylcholine (~50%), with less in neutral lipids (~17%).[54] This led to the conclusion that CLA may attenuate lipid peroxidation in neutral lipid-rich tissues by interfering with the formation of linoleic acid-derived arachidonic acid, a fatty acid that is most susceptible to lipid oxidation and formation of malondialdehyde. The ability of CLA to decrease malondialdehyde formation in skeletal muscle and liver microsomes was recently shown to be a reflection of its ability to decrease levels of polyenoic fatty acid such as arachidonic acid.[55] In addition, adding 1% CLA to the diet of female rats exposed to dimethylbenz[a]anthracene results in lower levels of mammary tissue malondialdehyde (an end product of lipid peroxidation), but fails to change the levels of 8-hydroxydeoxyguanosine (a marker of oxidatively damaged DNA),[18] Although CLA does not appear to act directly as an antioxidant, it is not known if a decrease in lipid peroxidation contributes to the cancer-protective effect of CLA seen in the mammary gland.[55] The data suggest that CLA may have some antioxidant function *in vivo* in suppressing lipid peroxidation, but its anticarcinogenic activity cannot be accounted for by protecting the target cell DNA against oxidative damage.[40] To further weaken the hypothesis that CLA exerts anticancer effects as a result of lipid peroxidation, dietary CLA does not increase lipid peroxidation in mice with transplanted metastatic murine mammary tumors.[48] These studies dealing with oxidation have not identified any oxidation products of CLA. While no definitive conclusions can be made, it is unlikely that CLA-inducing lipid peroxidation is the sole mechanism of action.[19,21,44]

### 24.3.2 PROMOTION

On the promotion stage, recent studies of the anticarcinogenic mechanisms of CLA have focused particularly in the mammary and skin carcinogenesis models.[41] This stage of carcinogenesis represents a premalignant state in which tumors arise from cells that have increased cell proliferation, reduced programmed cell death (or apoptosis), and/or dysregulated differentiation. In cultured cells, CLA reduced proliferation of mammary tumor cells *in vitro*[25,56] and *in vivo*.[57] Rats initiated with methylnitrosourea and then fed a diet with CLA (1%) exhibited reduced proliferation of terminal end bud and lobuloalveolar bud structures of mammary epithelium.[58] The terminal end bud is the site of tumor formation for both rat and human breast cancer and CLA inhibits proliferation by a reduction in density of the terminal end bud.[58] Ip and colleagues[59] demonstrated that CLA- or c9,t11-CLA-rich butter fat reduces the incorporation of bromodeoxyuridine and the expression of cyclins A and D.[59] Because these two cyclins regulate the conversion of the $G_1 \rightarrow S$ phase of the cell cycle,[59,60] CLA reduces cell proliferation in terminal end bud structures by regulating the cell cycle in the rat mammary epithelium[59] and in the SGC-7901 cell, with reduced expressions of cyclin A, B, and D and enhanced expressions of cyclin-dependent kinase inhibitors and p21.[61] Furthermore, mammary adenocarcinomas induced by PhIP contained significantly fewer proliferating cell nuclear antigen-positive cells in rats fed dietary CLA (0.1 g/100 g).[62] Both studies showed that CLA moderately increased levels of p16 and p27 proteins.[59,62] In MCF-7 breast cancer cells, CLA also inhibited cell proliferation and enhanced the accumulation of p53 and pRb, although t10,c12-CLA isomer was more effective than c9,t11-CLA.[63] These studies suggest that CLA modulates molecular signaling events and blocks DNA synthesis that affects the cell cycle, ultimately regulating cell proliferation.

However, there was no relationship between dietary CLA and markers of cell proliferation of other models. CLA had no effect on phorbol ester-induced hyperplasia, ornithine decarboxylase activity, or c-myc mRNA expression in the mouse epidermis,[64] but increased cell proliferation in diethylnitrosamine-induced focal lesions in rat livers.[15] These data demonstrate that the ability of CLA to reduce cell proliferation may be tissue-specific and/or tumor-model-specific.

In contrast to proliferation, CLA induced apoptosis in numerous tissues including mammary,[60] liver,[15] colon,[65] and adipose[66] tissues, and in cultured mammary epithelial cells,[67] human breast,[68] SGC-7901,[69,70] and HT-29[71] tumor cells. Although most studies used a mixture of isomers, a 50:50 mixture of c9,t11-CLA and t10,c12-CLA was more effective than individual isomers at inducing apoptosis in breast cancer cell lines.[68] In mammary tissue initiated with methylnitrosourea, CLA (64 $\mu M$) or c9,t11-CLA (128 $\mu M$) induced apoptosis of cells in the terminal end bud and premalignant lesions.[60] In these studies, CLA induction of apoptosis was associated with a reduction of Bcl-2. The Bcl-2 gene family is a signaling protein and has differential effects on apoptosis; for example, Bcl-2 and Bcl-$x_L$ suppress apoptosis, whereas others, such as Bax and Bak, promote apoptosis. Because CLA reduces Bcl-2 and moderately induces Bax, it appears that CLA elevates apoptosis primarily by reducing the suppressor of apoptosis, Bcl-2. In 1,2-dimethylhydrazine-treated colon mucosa, CLA decreases the incidence of colon cancer by decreasing cellular proliferation and inducing apoptosis of the colonic mucosa by decreased prostaglandin $E_2$ (PGE$_2$) levels and increased Bax/Bcl-2 ratios.[72]

CLA has been shown to modulate the protein kinase C (PKC) abundance/activity in membranes from prostate cancer cells (LNCaP) to produce an apoptotic profile with increased PKC-$\delta$, -$\alpha$, and -$\zeta$ and a decreased PKC-$\iota$,[73] but Ip and colleagues[60] did not observe any changes in the isoforms in mammary tissue for rats in the study. On the other hand, CLA downregulated ErbB3 signaling, the phosphoinositide 3-kinase, and the Akt pathway in human colon cell line,[71] and inhibited the expression of extracellular-mitogen-activated protein kinase phosphatase-1 protein in a rodent model of forestomach neoplasia.[74] These data suggest that CLA inhibits tumor promotion by inducing signaling events leading to enhanced apoptosis.

CLA induces markers of differentiation in the noncancer model adipose tissue;[75,76] it is possible that CLA inhibits carcinogenesis by induction of differentiation. CLA fed during the time of mammary gland development and maturation has long-lasting protective effects on mammary carcinogenesis,[41,58] likely by this very means.

### 24.3.3 Progression

Cell adhesion molecules are important ingredients in maintaining cell–cell adhesion and cell–matrix interactions. The abnormality of cell adhesion molecules closely correlates with neoplastic transformation and metastasis.[77] Recent study has shown that c9,t11-CLA increased the level of expression of E-cadherin and alpha-catenin, while decreasing the level of intercellular adhesion molecule-1 (ICAM-1) and vascular cell adhesion molecule-1 in human gastric carcinoma cell line SGC-7901.[78] The levels of the adhesion molecules ICAM-1 and E-selection also were reduced by 50% in human umbilical vein endothelial cells when incubated with 10 m$M$ CLA.[79] These studies suggest that CLA is involved in metastatic processes and the invasion of tumor cells.

## 24.4 CLA MODULATION OF LIPID METABOLISM AND GENE EXPRESSION

As previously discussed, diets with CLA result in an accumulation of CLA, especially the 9,11-CLA isomer in phospholipids of tissues, and modify subsequent eicosanoid production (Figure 24.2).[1] The role of CLA in reducing cyclooxygenase products (e.g., $PGE_2$, $PGF_{2\alpha}$) has been shown in bone and macrophages,[80,81] the epidermis of mice,[64] rat colons,[65] and keratinocytes,[82] but not small intestine tissue of Min mice,[48] spleen of rats,[81] and MCF-7 cells.[26] CLA also reduced accumulation of the lipoxygenase products leukotriene-B4 and -C4 in spleen and lung[81] but not $^{14}C$-hydroxyeicosatetraenoic acid ($^{14}C$-12-HETE) in cultured human platelets.[83] It suggests that CLA modulation of eicosanoid production may be tissue specific, and its inhibition of carcinogenesis in some tissues may involve the reduction of arachidonate-derived eicosanoids by one of three mechanisms.

First, CLA may displace arachidonate incorporation into phospholipids as shown in cultured keratocytes[82] and colonic mucosa of rats.[65] Dietary CLA displaces the arachidonate precursor, linoleate, in a dose-responsive manner in livers of mice fed various doses of CLA (0.5 to 1.5 g/100 g) in one study[51] but not others.[52,82]

A second explanation for the reduction of arachidonate-derived eicosanoids by CLA may be through inhibition of the constitutive enzymes, cyclooxygenases (COX)-1, and/or the inducible form, COX-2, at the level of mRNA, protein, or activity.[84,85] CLA or elongated and desaturated products from CLA (e.g., conjugates

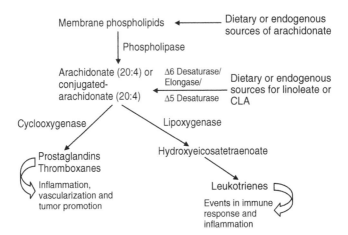

**FIGURE 24.2** General schematic pathway for eicosanoid synthesis from arachidonic acid. (From Belury MA. *Annu Rev Nutr* 2002; 22:505–531. With permission.)

of either arachidonate or eicosatetraenoate) may act as antagonists for COX thereby reducing available enzymes (at the level of expression or activity) for arachidonate. Using an *in vitro* activity assay, CLA or individual isomers inhibited the rate of oxygenation of arachidonate in the presence of COX-1[84] and COX-2 at the levels of mRNA and protein in a cultured macrophage cell line.[85]

CLA may modulate lipid metabolism in part by a third mechanism dependent on the activation of the nuclear hormone receptors, peroxisome proliferator-activated receptors (PPARs).[1] It has been shown that CLA moderates affinity for binding to and activating PPARγ,[86,87] and modulates transcription of genes responsive to PPARγ in adipose tissue *in vivo*[15] and *in vitro*.[85] PPARγ is found in extrahepatic tissues such as adipose, prostate, colon, and mammary gland, and is a required factor in adipose tissue differentiation.[88] In addition to evidence showing that CLA may induce PPARγ-responsive genes *in vivo*, CLA may increase the level of PPARγ itself.[89] Because activators of PPARγ are protective against cancers arising in the mammary gland, colon, and prostate,[18,90] it is possible that some of the molecular mechanisms of action of CLA on carcinogenesis are mediated by PPARγ. The ability of PPARγ to mediate effects of CLA is through increased levels of PPARγ protein[89] or through activation of PPARγ by downstream metabolites of CLA, such as desaturase and elongase products.[86] By blocking Δ6 desaturase using synthetic inhibitor SC-26196,[91] the ability of CLA isomers to activate PPARγ was significantly reduced.[1] These data suggest that activation of PPARγ by CLA is increased by the formation of the Δ6 desaturated products from CLA, c6,c9,t11-CLA, or c6,t10,c12-CLA, but the activation of PPARγ by these products is yet to be determined.

## 24.5  CLA INTAKE AND CANCER IN HUMANS

There is limited evidence for a direct association between CLA intake and cancer in humans. An inverse relationship has been found between milk consumption and breast cancer risk in women, suggesting that some of this protective effect may be due to CLA in milk.[92] Typical CLA intake has been estimated to be 52 mg/day among young men,[93] 137 mg/day among women,[94] and 227 mg/day among lactating women[14] in the U.S., and 430 and 350 mg/day for German men and women.[95] It has been shown that CLA level in breast adipose tissue was lower in patients who had localized breast cancer ($n = 261$, cases) than in those treated for a benign breast tumor ($n = 99$, controls; 96). The majority of CLA was in sn-1 and sn-3 position within the triacylglycerol molecule in both the case and control population, but the difference was greater in the control than in the case.[96] Because the isomers of CLA in breast adipose tissue were similar to those found in many food items, differences in the dietary intake of CLA at least partially explain the differences in breast adipose tissue CLA content between the cases and controls.[96] However, in the Netherlands Cohort Study, estimated CLA intake was reported to demonstrate a positive (albeit weak) relation with breast cancer incidence in postmenopausal women.[97] Thus, there is insufficient evidence from epidemiologic studies in humans; future studies are warranted on the relationship between blood levels of CLA isomers and their metabolites and breast cancer risk.

## 24.6  CONCLUSION

CLA inhibits carcinogenesis in numerous animal models and cell cultures at multiple stages, offering the possibility that several types of cancer in humans may be prevented with a diet rich in CLA. Extrapolation of dietary CLA concentrations that are effective in animal models indicates that equivalent CLA concentrations in a 70-kg human would be on the order of 3.5 g/day, which is significantly higher than the estimated consumption in the U.S.

Before any dietary recommendation can be made, limitations of the available evidence must be recognized. First, there is insufficient evidence based on human epidemiological data and it is difficult to evaluate from such data the impact of CLA alone because of its high correlation with fat intake. While case-control studies implicate a high-fat diet as a risk factor for breast cancer, cohort studies often show a negative association. Second, although c9,t11-isomer is postulated as the most biological form of CLA, it is difficult to predict which isomer of CLA is the putative candidate. Third, the kinetics of CLA incorporation in the phospholipids and the mechanisms whereby CLA exerts its effects are not well understood. These three limitations warrant further work to understand the implications of dietary CLA and the possibility of lowering the risk from human cancer development.

## REFERENCES

1. Belury MA. Inhibition of carcinogenesis by conjugated linoleic acid: potential mechanisms of action. *J Nutr* 2002; 132:2995–2998.
2. Pariza MW. Perspective on the safety and effectiveness of conjugated linoleic acid. *Am J Clin Nutr* 2004; 79:1132S–1136S.
3. Chin SF, Liu W, Storkson JM, Ha YL, Pariza MW. Dietary sources of conjugated dienoic isomers of linoleic acid, a newly recognized class of anticarcinogens. *J Food Compos Anal* 1992; 5:185–197.
4. Ma DW, Wierzbicki AA, Field CJ, Clandinin MT. Conjugated linoleic acid in Canadian dairy and beef products. *J Agric Food Chem* 1999; 47:1956–1960.
5. Lin H, Boylston TD, Chang MJ, Luedecke LO, Shultz TD. Survey of the conjugated linoleic acid contents of dairy products. *J Dairy Sci* 1995; 78:2358–2365.
6. McGuire MK, Park YS, Harrison LY, Shultz TD, McGuire MA. Conjugated linoleic acid concentration of human milk and infant formulae. *Nutr Res* 1997; 17:1277–1283.
7. MacDonald HB. Conjugated linoleic acid and disease prevention: a review of current knowledge. *J Am Coll Nutr* 2000; 19:111S–118S.
8. Fritsche J, Rickert R, Steinhart H. Formation, contents, and estimation of daily intake of conjugated linoleic acid isomers and trans-fatty acids in foods. In: Yurawecz, MP, Mossoba MM, Kramer JKG, Pariza MW, Nelson GJ, eds. *Advances in Conjugated Linoleic Acid Research*. Vol. 1. Champaign, IL: AOCS Press; 1999:378–396.
9. Kramer JK, Parodi PW, Jensen RG, Mossobo MM, Yurawecz, MP, Adlof RO. Rumenic acid: a proposed common name for the major conjugated linoleic acid isomer found in natural products. *Lipids* 1998; 33:835.
10. Devery R, Miller A, Stanton C. Conjugated linoleic acid and oxidative behaviour in cancer cells. *Biochem Soc Trans* 2001; 29:341–344.
11. Huang YC, Ludecke LO, Shultz TD. Effect of cheddar cheese consumption on plasma conjugated linoleic acid concentrations in men. *Nutr Res* 1994; 14:373–386.
12. Britton M, Fong C, Wickens D, Yudkin J. Diet as a source of phospholipid esterified 9,11-octadecadienoic acid in humans. *Clin Sci* 1992; 83:97–101.
13. Jiang J, Wolk A, Vessby B. Relation between the intake of milk fat and the occurrence of conjugated linoleic acid in human adipose tissue. *Am Soc Clin Nutr* 1999; 7:21–27.
14. Park Y, McGuire MK, Behr R, McGuire MA, Evans MA, Shultz TD. High-fat dairy product consumption increases delta 9c,11t-18:2 (rumenic acid) and total lipid concentrations of human milk. *Lipids* 1999; 34:543–549.
15. Belury MA. Dietary conjugated linoleic acid in health: physiological effects and mechanisms of action. *Annu Rev Nutr* 2002; 22:505–531.
16. Pariza MW, Park Y, Cook ME. Conjugated linoleic acid and the control of cancer and obesity. *Toxicol Sci* 1999; 52:107–110S.
17. Brown JM, McIntosh MK. Conjugated linoleic acid in human: regulation of adiposity and insulin sensitivity. *J Nutr* 2003; 133:3041–3046.
18. Field CJ, Schley PD. Evidence for potential mechanisms for the effect of conjugated linoleic acid on tumor metabolism and immune function: lessons from n-3 fatty acid. *Am J Clin Nutr* 2004; 79:1190S–1198S.

19. Igarash M, Miyazawa T. The growth inhibitory effect of conjugated linoleic acid on a human hepatoma cell line, HepG2, is induced by a change in fatty acid metabolism, but not the facilitation of lipid peroxidation in the cells. *Biochim Biophys Acta* 2001; 1530:132–171.

20. Desbordes C, Lea MA. Effects of C18 fatty acid isomers on DNA synthesis in hepatoma and breast cancer cells. *Anticancer Res* 1995; 15: 2017–2021.

21. Schonberg S, Krokan HE. The inhibitory effect of conjugated dienoic derivatives (CLA) of linoleic acid on the growth of human tumor cell lines is in part due to increased lipid peroxidation. *Anticancer Res* 1995; 15:1241–1246.

22. O'Shea M, Stanton C, Devery R. Antioxidant enzyme defense responses of human MCF-7 and SW480 cancer cells to conjugated linoleic acid. *Anticancer Res* 1999; 19:1953–1959.

23. Kelly GS. Conjugated linoleic acid: a review. *Altern Med Rev* 2001; 6:367–382.

24. Chujo H, Yamasaki M, Nou S, Koyanagi N, Tachibana H, Yamada K. Effect of conjugated linoleic acid isomers on growth factor-induced proliferation of human breast cancer cells. *Cancer Lett* 2003; 202:81–87.

25. Durgam VR, Fernandes G. The growth inhibitory effect of conjugated linoleic acid on MCF-7 cells is regulated to estrogen response system. *Cancer Lett* 1997; 116:121–130.

26. Park Y, Allen KG, Shultz TD. Modulation of MCF-7 breast cancer cell signal transduction by linoleic acid and conjugated linoleic acid in culture. *Anticancer Res* 2000; 20:669–676.

27. O'Shea M, Devery R, Lawless F, Murphy J, Stanton C. Milk fat conjugated linoleic acid (CLA) inhibits growth of human mammary MCF-7 cancer cells. *Anticancer Res* 2000; 20:3591–3601.

28. Shultz TD, Chew BP, Seaman WR. Differential stimulatory and inhibitory responses of human MCF-7 breast cancer cells to linoleic acid and conjugated linoleic acid in culture. *Anticancer Res* 1992; 12:2143–2145.

29. Cunningham DC, Harrison LY, Shultz TD. Proliferative responses of normal human mammary and MCF-7 breast cancer cells to linoleic acid, conjugated linoleic acid and eicosanoid synthesis inhibitors in culture. *Anticancer Res* 1997; 17:197–203.

30. Tanmahasamut P, Liu J, Hendry LB, Sidell N. Conjugated linoleic acid blocks estrogen signaling in human breast cancer cells. *J Nutr* 2004; 134:674–680.

31. Miller A, Stanton C, Murphy J, Devery R. Conjugated linoleic acid (CLA)-enriched milk fat inhibits growth and modulates CLA-responsive biomarkers in MCF-7 and SW480 human cancer cell lines. *Br J Nutr* 2003; 90:877–885.

32. Ha YL, Grimm NK, Pariza MW. Anticarcinogens from fried ground beef heat-altered derivatives of linoleic acid. *Carcinogenesis* 1987; 8:1881–1887.

33. DiGiovanni J. Multistage carcinogenesis in mouse skin. In: Grunberger D, ed. *Pharmaceutical Therapy.* New York: Pergamon Press; 1992:63–128.

34. Banni S, Angioni E, Casu V, Melis MP, Carta G, Corongiu FP, Thompson H, Ip C. Decrease in linoleic acid metabolites as a potential mechanism in cancer risk reduction by conjugated linoleic acid. *Carcinogenesis* 1999; 20:1019–1024.

35. Ip C, Chin SF, Scimeca JA, Pariza MW. Mammary cancer prevention by conjugated dienoic derivative of linoleic acid. *Cancer Res* 1991; 51:6118–6124.

36. Ha YL. Storkson JM, Pariza MW. Inhibition of benzo(a)pyrene-induced mouse of forestomach neoplasia by conjugated dienoic derivatives of linoleic acid. *Cancer Res* 1990; 50:1097–1101.

37. Belury MA, Nickel K, Bird CE, Wu Y. Dietary conjugated linoleic acid modulation of phorbol ester skin tumor promotion. *Nutr Cancer* 1996; 26:149–157.
38. Liew C, Schut HAJ, Chin SF, Pariza MW, Dashwood RH. Protection of conjugated linoleic acid against 2-amino-3-methylimidazol[4,5-f]quinoline-induced colon carcinogenesis in the F344 rat: a study of inhibitory mechanisms. *Carcinogenesis* 1995; 16:3037–3043.
39. Ip C, Jiang C, Thompson HJ, Scimeca JA. Retention of conjugated linoleic acid in the mammary gland is associated with tumor inhibition during the post-initiation phase of carcinogenesis. *Carcinogenesis* 1997; 18:755–759.
40. Ip C, Briggs SP, Haegels AD, Thompson HJ, Storkson J, Scimeca JA. The efficacy of conjugated linoleic acid in mammary cancer prevention is independent of the level or type of fat in the diet. *Carcinogenesis* 1996; 17:1045–1050.
41. Ip C, Scimeca JA, Thompson HJ. Effect of timing and duration of dietary conjugated linoleic acid on mammary cancer prevention. *Nutr Cancer* 1995; 24:241–247.
42. Hubbard NE, Lim D, Summers L, Ericson KL. Reduction of murine mammary tumor metastasis by conjugated linoleic acid. *Cancer Lett* 2000; 150:93–100.
43. Visonneau S, Cesano A, Tepper SA, Scimeca JA, Santoli D, Kritchevsky D. Conjugated linoleic acid suppresses the growth of human breast adenocarcinoma cells in SCID mice. *Anticancer Res* 1997; 17:969–974.
44. Cesano A, Visonneau S, Scimeca JA, Kritchevsky D, Santoli D. Opposite effect of linoleic acid and conjugated linoleic acid on human prostatic cancer in SCID mice. *Anticancer Res* 1998; 18:833–838.
45. Ip C, Dong Y, Ip MM, Banni S, Carta G, Angioni E, Murru E, Spada S, Melis MP, Saebo A. Conjugated linoleic acid isomers and mammary cancer prevention. *Nutr Cancer* 2002; 43:52–58.
46. Scimeca JA. Cancer inhibition in animals. In: Yurawecz, MP, Mossoba MM, Kramer JKG, Pariza MW, Nelson GJ, eds. *Advances in Conjugated Linoleic Acid Research*. Vol. 1. Champaign, IL: AOCS Press; 1999:420–443.
47. Wong MW, Chew BP, Wong TS, Hosick HL, Boylston TD, Shultz TD. Effects of dietary conjugated linoleic acid on lymphocyte function and growth of mammary tumors in mice. *Anticancer Res* 1997; 17:987–993.
48. Petrick MBH, McEntee MF, Johnson BT, Obukowicz MG, Whelan J. Highly unsaturated (n-3) fatty acids, but not α-linolenic, conjugated linoleic or γ-linolenic acids, reduce tumorigenesis in APC[Min/+] mice. *J Nutr* 2000; 130:2434–2443.
49. Fischer SM, Leyton J, Lee ML, Locniskar M, Belury MA, Maldve RE, Slaga TJ, Bechtel DH. Differential effects of dietary linoleic acid on mouse skin-tumor promotion and mammary carcinogenesis. *Cancer Res* 1992; 52:2049–2054S.
50. Belury MA. Conjugated linoleate: a polyunsaturated fatty acid with unique chemoprotective properties. *Nutr Rev* 1995; 53:83–89.
51. Belury MA, Kempa-Steczko A. Conjugated linoleic acid modulates hepatic lipid composition in mice. *Lipids* 1977; 32:199–204.
52. Moya-Camarena Sy, Vanden Heuvel JP, Belury MA. Conjugated linoleic acid activates peroxisome proliferators-activated receptor α and β subtypes but does not induce hepatic peroxisome proliferation in Sprague-Dawley rats. *Biochim Biophys Acta* 1999; 1436:331–341.
53. Liu KL, Belury MA. Conjugated linoleic acid modulation of phorbol ester-induced events in murine keratinocytes. *Lipids* 1997; 32:725–730.

54. Banni S, Carta G, Angioni E, Murru E, Scanu P, Melis MP, Bauman DE, Fischer SM, Ip C. Distribution of conjugated linoleic acid and metabolites in different lipid fractions in the rat liver. *J Lipid Res* 2001; 42:1056–1061.

55. Livisay SA, Zhou S, Ip C, Decker EA. Impact of dietary conjugated linoleic acid on the oxidative stability of rat liver microsomes and skeletal muscle homogenates. *J Agric Food Chem* 2000; 48:4162–4167.

56. Shultz TD, Chew BP, Seaman WR, Luedecke LO. Inhibitory effect of conjugated dienoic derivatives of linoleic acid and β-carotene on the *in vitro* growth of human cancer cells. *Cancer Lett* 1992; 63:125–133.

57. Ip C, Singh M, Thompson HJ, Scimeca JA. Conjugated linoleic acid suppresses mammary carcinogenesis and proliferative activity of the mammary gland in the rat. *Cancer Res* 1994; 54:1212–1215.

58. Thompson H, Zhu Z, Banni S, Darcy K, Loftus T, Ip C. Morphological and biochemical status of the mammary gland as influenced by conjugated linoleic acid: implication for a reduction in mammary cancer risk. *Cancer Res* 1997; 57:5067–5072.

59. Ip C, Dong Y, Thompson HJ, Bauman DE. Ip MM. Control of rat mammary epithelium proliferation by conjugated linoleic acid. *Nutr Cancer* 2001; 39:233–238.

60. Ip C, Ip MM, Loftus T, Shoemaker SF, Shea-Eaton W. Induction of apoptosis by conjugated linoleic acid in cultured mammary tumor cells and premalignant lesions of the rat mammary gland. *Cancer Epidemiol Biomarkers Prev* 2000; 9:689–696.

61. Liu JR, Li BX, Chen BQ, Han XH, Xue YB, Yang YM, Zheng YM, Liu RH. Effect of *cis*-9, *trans*-11-conjugated linoleic acid on cell cycle of gastric adenocarcinoma cell line (SGC-7901). *World J Gastroenterol* 2002; 8:224–229.

62. Futakuchi M, Cheng JL, Hirose M, Kimoto N, Cho YM, Iwata T, Kasai M, Tokudome S, Shirai T. Inhibition of conjugated fatty acids derived from safflower or perilla oil of induction and development of mammary tumors in rats induced by 2-amino-1-methy-6-phenylimidazo[4,5-b]pyridine (PhIP). *Cancer Lett* 2002; 178:131–139.

63. Kemp MQ, Jeffy BD, Romagnolo DF. Conjugated linoleic acid inhibits cell proliferation through a p53-dependent mechanism: effects on the expression of $G_1$-restriction points in breast and colon cancer cells. *J Nutr* 2003; 133:3670–3677.

64. Kavanaugh CJ, Liu KL, Belury MA. Effect of dietary conjugated linoleic acid on phorbol ester-induced PGE2 production and hyperplasia in mouse epidermis. *Nutr Cancer* 1999; 33:132–138.

65. Park HS, Ryu JH, Ha, YL, Park JHY. Dietary conjugated linoleic acid (CLA) induces apoptosis of colonic mucosa in 1,2-dimethylhydrazine-treated rats: a possible mechanism of the anticarcinogenic effect of CLA. *Br J Nutr* 2001; 86:549–555.

66. Tsuboyama-Kasaoka N, Takahashi M, Tanemura K, Kim HJ, Tange T, Okuyama H, Kasai M, Ikemoto S, Ezaki O. Conjugated linoleic acid supplementation reduces adipose tissue by apoptosis and develops lipodystrophy in mice. *Diabetes* 2000; 49:1534–1542.

67. Ip MM, Masso-Welch PA, Shoemaker SF, Shea-Eaton WK, Ip C. Conjugated linoleic acid inhibits proliferation and induces apoptosis of normal rat mammary epithelial cells in primary culture. *Exp Cell Res* 1999; 250:22–34.

68. Majumder B, Wahle KW, Moir S, Schofield A, Choe SN, Farquharson A, Grant I, Heys SD. Conjugated linoleic acids (CLAs) regulate the expression of key apoptotic genes in human breast cancer cells. *FASEB J* 2002; 16:1447–1449.

69. Chen BQ, Yang YM, Gao YH, Liu JR, Xue YB, Wang XL, Zheng YM, Zhang JS, Liu RH. Inhibitory effects of c9, t11-conjugated linoleic acid on invasion of human gastric carcinoma cell line SGC-7901. *World J Gastroenterol* 2003; 9:1909–1914.

70. Liu JR, Chen BQ, Yang YM, Wang XL, Xue YB, Zheng YM, Liu RH. Effect of apoptosis on gastric adenocarcinoma cell line SGC-7901 induced by *cis*-9, *trans*-11-conjugated linoleic acid. *World J Gastroenterol* 2002; 8:999–1004.

71. Cho HJ, Kim WK, Kim EJ, Jung KC, Park S, Lee HS, Tyner AL, Park JH. Conjugated linoleic acid inhibits cell proliferation and ErbB3 signaling in HT-29 human colon cell line. *Am J Physiol Gastrointest Liver Physiol* 2003; 284:G996–1005.

72. Park HS, Cho HY, Ha YL, Park JH. Dietary conjugated linoleic acid increases the mRNA ratio of Bax/Bcl-2 in the colonic mucosa of rats. *J Nutr Biochem* 2004; 15:229–235.

73. Wahle KWJ, Heys SD. Cell signal mechanisms, conjugated linoleic acids (CLAs) and anti-tumorigenesis. *Prostag Leukotr Ess Fatty Acids* 2002; 67:183–186.

74. Chen BQ, Xue YB, Liu JR, Yang YM, Zheng YM, Wang XL, Liu RH. Inhibition of conjugated linoleic acid on mouse forestomach neoplasia induced by benzo(a)pyrene and chemopreventive mechanisms. *World J Gastroenterol* 2003; 9:44–49.

75. Houseknecht KL, Vanden Heuvel JP, Moya-Camarena SY, Portocarrero CP, Peck LW, Nickel KP, Belury MA. Dietary conjugated linoleic acid normalizes impaired glucose tolerance in the Zucker diabetic fatty fa/fa rat. *Biochem Biophys Res Commun* 1998; 244:678–682.

76. Satory DL, Smith SB. Conjugated linoleic acid inhibits proliferation but stimulates lipid filling of murine 3T3-L1 preadipocytes. *J Nutr* 1998; 129:92–97.

77. Sebedio JL, Gnaedig S, Chardigny JM. Recent advances in conjugated linoleic acid research. *Curr Opin Clin Nutr Metab Care* 1999; 2:499–506.

78. Chen BQ, Yang YM, Wang Q, Gao YH, Liu JR, Zhang JS, Wang XL, Liu RH. Effects of c9,t11-conjugated linoleic acid on adhesion of human gastric carcinoma cell line SGC-7901. *World J Gastroenterol* 2004; 10:1392–1396.

79. Kritchevsky D. Antimutagenic and some other effects of conjugated linoleic acid. *Br J Nutr* 2000; 85:459–465.

80. Li Y, Watkins BA. Conjugated linoleic acids alter bone fatty acid composition and reduce ex vivo prostaglandin E2 biosynthesis in rats fed n-6 or n-3 fatty acids. *Lipids* 1998; 33:417–425.

81. Sugano M, Tsujita A, Yamasaki M, Noguchi M, Yamada K. Conjugated linoleic acid modulates tissue levels of chemical mediators and immunoglobulins in rats. *Lipids* 1998; 33:521–527.

82. Liu KL, Belury MA. Conjugated linoleic acid reduces arachidonic acid content and PGE2 synthesis in murine keratinocytes. *Cancer Lett* 1998; 124:1–8.

83. Truitt A, McNeill G, Vanderhoek JY. Antiplatelet effects of conjugated linoleic acid isomers. *Biochim Biophys Acta* 1999; 1438:239–246.

84. Bulgarella J, Patton D, Bull A. Modulation of prostaglandin H synthase activity by conjugated linoleic acid (CLA) and specific CLA isomers. *Lipids* 2001; 36:407–412.

85. Yu Y, Correll PH, Vanden Heuvel JP. Conjugated linoleic acid decreases production of pro-inflammatory products in macrophages: evidence for a PPAR gamma-dependent mechanism. *Biochim Biophys Acta* 2002; 1581:89–99.

86. Belury MA, Moya-Camarena SY, Lu M, Shi L, Leesnitzer LM, Blanchard SG. Conjugated linoleic acid is an activator and ligand for peroxisome proliferators-activated receptor-γ (PPARγ). *Nutr Res* 2002; 22:817–824.

87. Kohno H, Suzuki R, Yasui Y, Hosokawa M, Miyashita K, Tanaka T. Pomegranate seed oil rich in conjugated linoleic acid suppresses chemically induced colon carcinogenesis in rats. *Cancer Sci* 2004; 95:481–486.

88. Ntambi JM, Kim YC. Adipocyte differentiation and gene expression. *J Nutr* 2000; 130:3122S–3126S.

89. Evans M, Pariza M, Park Y, Curtis L, Kuebler B, McIntosh M. *trans*-10-*cis*-12 Conjugated linoleic acid reduces triglyceride content while differentially affecting peroxisome proliferators activated receptor-γ2 and aP2 expression. *Lipids* 2000; 36:1223–1232.

90. Sporn MB, Suh N, Mangelsdorf DJ. Prospects for prevention and treatment if cancer with selective PPARγ modulators (SPARMS). *Trends Mol Med* 2001; 7:395–400.

91. Obukowicz MG, Raz A, Pyla PD, Rico JD, Wendling JM, Needleman P. Identification and characterization of a novel Δ6/Δ5 fatty acid desaturase inhibitor as a potential anti-inflammatory agent. *Biochem Pharm* 1998; 55:1045–1058.

92. Knekt P, Jarvinen R, Seppanen R, Pukkala E, Aromaa A. Intake of dairy products and the risk of breast cancer. *Br J Cancer* 1996; 73:687–691.

93. Herbel BK, McGuire MK, McGuire MA, Shultz TD. Safflower oil consumption does not increase plasma conjugated linoleic acid concentrations in humans. *Am J Clin Nutr* 1998; 67:332–337.

94. Ritzenthaler KL, McGuire MK, Falen R, Shultz TD, Dasgupta N, McGuire MA. Estimation of conjugated linoleic acid intake by written dietary assessment methodologies underestimates actual intake evaluated by food duplicate methodology. *J Nutr* 2001; 131:1548–1554.

95. Fritsche J, Steinhart H. Amounts of conjugated linoleic acid (CLA) in German foods and evaluation of daily intake. *Z Lebensm Unters Forsch A* 1998; 2065:77–82.

96. Lavillonniere F, Bougnoux P. Conjugated linoleic acid (CLA) and the risk of breast cancer. In: Yurawecz, MP, Mossoba MM, Kramer JKG, Pariza MW, Nelson GJ, eds. *Advances in Conjugated Linoleic Acid Research*. Vol. 1. Champaign, IL: AOCS Press; 1999:378–396.

97. Voorrips LE, Brants HA, Kardinaal AF, Hiddink GJ, van den Brandt PA, Goldbohm RA. Intake of conjugated linoleic acid, fat, and other fatty acids in relation to postmenopausal breast cancer: the Netherlands Cohort Study on Diet and Cancer. *Am J Clin Nutr* 2002; 76:873–882.

# 25 Sphingolipids as Chemopreventive Agents

*Eva M. Schmelz*

## CONTENTS

25.1 Introduction.................................................................................519
25.2 Sphingolipid Biochemistry .........................................................520
    25.2.1 Sphingolipid Metabolism ..............................................520
    25.2.2 Sphingolipid Metabolism in Cancer Cells.....................521
25.3 Routes of Administration of Exogenous Sphingolipids to Prevent
    Cancer *In Vivo*...........................................................................523
    25.3.1 Topical Administration ..................................................523
    25.3.2 Administration of Sphingolipids via Injection...............523
        25.3.2.1 Intraperitoneal Injection.................................523
        25.3.2.2 Intravenous Injection......................................524
    25.3.3 Oral Administration .......................................................524
        25.3.3.1 Natural Sphingolipids .....................................524
        25.3.3.2 Synthetic Sphingolipids ..................................527
25.4 Combinatorial Treatment.............................................................528
    25.4.1 Combinatorial Treatment — Oral Administration..........529
    25.4.2 Sphingolipids in Combination with Chemotherapy.......529
25.5 Mechanisms of Cancer Prevention by Exogenous Sphingolipids.......530
25.6 Future Directions of Sphingolipids in Cancer Prevention and
    Treatment ....................................................................................531
Acknowledgments..................................................................................532
References ..............................................................................................533

## 25.1 INTRODUCTION

In the past decades, tremendous efforts have been devoted to the development of cancer treatment strategies. Although some approaches were successful in treating some types of cancers, the incidence and mortality of other cancers have not changed accordingly. Therefore, many researchers have focused on strategies to *prevent* cancer. The ideal chemopreventive agent would target tumor cells specifically, eliciting a different response from transformed than from normal cells. However, many agents are also highly cytotoxic to nontransformed cells, and cause severe side effects that limit their application. Because chemopreventive compounds may have to be administered over long periods of time to high-risk groups, the administration also needs to be effective, easy, and cost-efficient. Unlimited cancer cell growth is a result of unlimited proliferation, a reduction of apoptosis or a combination of both, and reduced differentiation. Sphingolipids are prominent candidates that warrant investigation as chemopreventive agents because as lipid second messengers, they regulate processes that are deregulated in cancer: cell growth, differentiation, and death. Sphingolipids are often growth inhibitory, cytotoxic to most cancer cell lines, and can induce apoptosis or differentiation. Furthermore, they have been shown to inhibit or circumvent multidrug resistance, inhibit cell motility, and inhibit angiogenesis. This has been documented in numerous *in vitro* studies (reviewed in References 1 to 4). Here, we summarize reports that identify sphingolipids as potential chemopreventive agents *in vivo* and explore the mechanisms of this prevention and possible differences between prevention and treatment strategies with sphingolipids.

## 25.2 SPHINGOLIPID BIOCHEMISTRY

### 25.2.1 SPHINGOLIPID METABOLISM

Sphingolipids are ubiquitous components of all eukaryotic cells. They are composed of a sphingoid base, which is mostly sphingosine in mammalian cells but sphingoid bases without double bonds, or double bonds in other positions, or hydroxylation are often found in sphingolipids of plant or yeast origin. Ceramide is generated by acylation of the sphingoid base with long-chain fatty acids that are mostly saturated. A headgroup on position 1 forms more complex sphingolipids (Figure 25.1). Variations in these components make sphingolipids the structurally most diverse class of membrane lipids. Sphingolipids were first described more than 100 years ago by the physician Thudicum, and for the longest time it was believed that sphingolipids are only structural components because of their localization in cell membranes. In 1989, a new concept of sphingolipid metabolites as lipid second messengers mediating the response of cells to exogenous compounds and events was introduced with the description of the sphingomyelin cycle.[5,6] Today, the generation of ceramide has been demonstrated in many other cell lines in response to growth factors, cytokines, and stresses such as ultraviolet (UV) light, γ-irradiation, serum deprivation, hypoxia, and heat (see recent reviews[7–9]). The generation of sphingolipid metabolites is also a common event after treatment of cancer cells with anticancer drugs such as vincristine, daunorubicin, taxol, doxorubicin, and cisplatin to induce apoptosis in cancer cells. Some agents generate ceramide by activating the *de novo* sphingolipid biosynthesis, or both pathways. Ceramides generated via these two distinctly different pathways accumulate in the cells and trigger the cellular response that includes growth

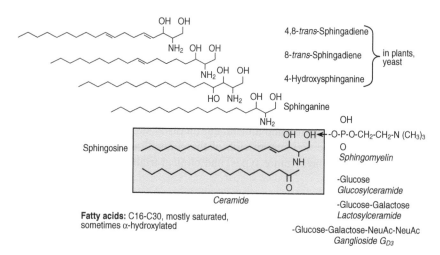

**FIGURE 25.1** Structure of sphingolipids.

inhibition, induction of senescence, cell death via apoptosis and necrosis, inhibition of migration and induction of differentiation. However, multiple other enzymes of the sphingolipid metabolism now have been identified as targets and, accordingly, other sphingolipids and sphingolipid metabolites have been implicated in the regulation of cell behavior. These include sphingosine, several gangliosides, glucosylceramide, lactosylceramide, ceramide-1-phosphate, and sphingosine-1-phosphate. The different metabolites may have opposing effects, such as sphingosine-1-phosphate, which in contrast to ceramides and sphingoid bases stimulates cell growth, increases the survival of cells, suppresses apoptosis, affects cell differentiation, and modulates cytoskeleton organization, adhesion, and cell motility.[10–15] The effects of metabolites such as octadecane-1,2-diol are also discussed.[16] The differential activation of enzymes of sphingolipid metabolism, and the amount and species of bioactive sphingolipid metabolites — and their intracellular localization — are therefore crucial determinants of the cellular response and, thus, may be targets for regulation.

## 25.2.2 SPHINGOLIPID METABOLISM IN CANCER CELLS

Changes in the sphingolipid metabolism in cancer cells may generate "wrong" metabolites or cause the depletion of appropriate metabolites, and thereby create conditions that support unlimited cell growth and that prevent regulation by exogenous agents. Aberrant enzyme activity or expression that affects sphingolipid metabolism has been reported in several cancer systems. A reduced activity and expression of sphingomyelinases in colonocytes of carcinogen-treated rats[17,18] and in human tumors,[19] may result in the failure to generate ceramide in response to extracellular stimuli, and protect cells from undergoing apoptosis. This is also the underlying mechanism of the resistance of some tumor cells to γ-irradiation[20,21] and chemotherapeutic agents.[22,23] An overexpression of acid ceramidase in tumor cells has been shown to protect against TNF-α-induced apoptosis,[24] removing cytotoxic ceramide and releasing sphingosine as substrate for sphingosine kinase. An increase in sphingosine kinase activity with the subsequent accumulation of sphingosine-1-phosphate has been correlated with hyperproliferation, transformation, and development of a malignant tumor phenotype.[25] Ovarian tumors not only show a significant elevation of sphingosine-1-phosphate in tumor tissue itself,[26] but also secrete sphingosine-1-phosphate into ascites fluid, affecting cell dissemination and attachment on distal sites.[27] Thus, the inhibition of sphingosine kinase and suppression of the generation of mitotic metabolites may be effective in these tumor types, and clinical trials testing this hypothesis are already ongoing.

Another pathway in cancer cells to reduce ceramide accumulation is to upregulate synthesis of complex sphingolipids, glucosylceramide, and, to a lesser extent, sphingomyelin. This has been shown to be a critical event in some multidrug-resistant cells,[28] and inhibition of glucosylceramide synthase activity, the enzyme responsible for the transfer of glucose to the ceramide moiety, has been the subject of extended investigations; drugs inhibiting this enzyme are being tested in patients. However, more recent reports demonstrated that transfection of melanoma cells with a functioning glucosylceramide synthase did not reverse the multidrug-resistant phenotype.[29] Furthermore, the use of more selective glucosylceramide synthase inhibitors did not reverse multidrug resistance, and the authors hypothesize that the previously used inhibitor PDMP may have effects in addition to inhibition of glucosylceramide synthase that affect multidrug resistance.[30] Given the importance of targeting specific enzymes in cancer cells to avoid side effects, the role of glucosylceramide synthase in the chemoresistance of cancer cells clearly needs to be clarified.

The changes in the activity of enzymes in sphingolipid metabolism can modify the intracellular composition of bioactive sphingolipids. The levels of ceramide are reportedly reduced in head and neck squamous cell carcinomas, (specifically C18-ceramide[31]), colon cancer,[32] larynx carcinoma,[33] and astrocytomas.[34] These low levels were associated with unlimited proliferation, resistance to apoptosis, and a poor outcome for the patients. A low ceramide content was also associated with chemoresistance of leukemia cells *in vitro* and *in vivo*.[35] A decrease in lactosylceramide, but elevation of glucosylceramide, galactosylceramide, and gangliosides were observed in tumor cells.[29,34,36,37] Reversal of these changes lowered the resistance of cells to treatment[38,39] and enhanced vincristine, doxorubicin, and taxol toxicity[35,40–42] and the efficiency of radiation treatment.[43] Decreased ganglioside levels suppressed tumor formation and metastasis in a syngeneic melanoma model.[44] In contrast, other laboratories found increases in the ceramide and dihydroceramide (which lacks the 4,5-*trans* double bond required for its biological activity) content in sarcomas, melanomas, and Lewis lung carcinomas[45] and transformed fibroblasts,[46] possibly a requisite for the survival of these tumors.

The changes in the sphingolipid composition in cancer cells may be used for diagnosis purposes and for treatment decisions and prediction of drug efficacy.

For example, human glioma cell lines (LN18, LN229, LN319, and T98G) were analyzed for their sphingolipid composition using a combination of liquid chromatography and tandem mass spectrometry. Several cell lines contained elevated sphingosine-1-phosphate levels[47] and may therefore be candidates for treatment with sphingosine kinase inhibitors.

## 25.3 ROUTES OF ADMINISTRATION OF EXOGENOUS SPHINGOLIPIDS TO PREVENT CANCER *IN VIVO*

The amphiphilic nature of sphingolipid metabolites and their inherent toxicity makes their site-directed administration *in vivo* a challenge. However, topical, intraperitoneal, and intravenous injections and oral administration of complex sphingolipids and sphingolipid metabolites have been reported.

### 25.3.1 TOPICAL ADMINISTRATION

Sencar mice were treated with dimethylbenz-[*a*]-anthracene to induce skin cancer. Topical application of sphingosine, methylsphingosine, and *N*-acetylsphingosine did not inhibit the development of papillomas, and at high doses, the formation of papillomas was even enhanced.[48,49] This was also seen in a follow-up study measuring the efficacy of sphingosine, *N*-methylsphingosine, and *N*-acetylsphingosine; again, the sphingolipids did not change papilloma incidence,[50] but both *N*-methylsphingosine and *N*-acetylsphingosine increased cancer-free survival. Furthermore, weekly application of sphingosine and *N*-acetylsphingosine for 10 weeks after treatment with phorbol esters suppressed tumor progression.[50]

Another sphingolipid derivative, safingol, the L-threo isomer of sphinganine, a potent inhibitor of protein kinase C, was developed to treat dermatoses and cancer. Topical application of safingol, however, caused liver damage that was more pronounced in female than in male rats possibly due to insufficient clearance of safingol by cytochrome P450 isozymes.[51]

Topical application of a 1% mixture of short-chain ceramides twice per day to patients with cutaneous breast cancer resulted in a partial response in only 1 of 26 patients, which was found to be not promising enough to conduct further studies using this approach.[52]

### 25.3.2 ADMINISTRATION OF SPHINGOLIPIDS VIA INJECTION

#### 25.3.2.1 Intraperitoneal Injection

To the best of our knowledge, chemopreventive studies with sphingolipids administered via intraperitoneal (i.p.) injection have not been reported. Some chemotherapeutic studies used ceramide analogs that induced apoptosis *in vitro* also induced apoptosis *in vivo* in human colon cancer xenografts, and significantly reduced their tumor size.[53] However, this study did not mention the toxic side effects of the successful dose.

### 25.3.2.2 Intravenous Injection

The systemic delivery of sphingolipids is hindered by their hydrophobicity, their possible degradation by enzymes, and their toxicity. Single doses of safingol (L-threo-sphinganine, see above) up to 5 mg/kg body weight did not cause adverse effects in rats or dogs,[54] but repeated injections increased its plasma concentration, and caused hemolysis and marked renal and hepatoxicity at higher dosages. Furthermore, safingol caused degeneration and necrosis of the intima of the venes at the injection sites. In contrast, injection of sphingosine, dimethylsphingosine, or trimethylsphingosine in mice that have been inoculated with MKN74 human gastric cancer cells showed a pronounced and sustained inhibition of tumor growth by the methylated sphingosine derivatives that did not cause side effects.[55] The delivery of sphingolipids via liposomes has been shown to be very effective in cell culture[56] and was intended to protect ceramide from degradation or pre-cipitation, and generate a maximum ceramide increase in cancer cells. Repeated injections of ceramide-containing liposomes into mice carrying breast tumors resulted in a significant decrease of tumor size without causing severe toxic side effects.[57] Ceramide liposomes also suppressed ovarian cancer cell dissemination.[58] Ceramides dissolved in soybean oil reduced pulmonary metastases derived from Meth A-T tumor cells.[59] However, these are again chemotherapeutic approaches; whether there are chemopreventive applications of these methods is not known.

### 25.3.3 ORAL ADMINISTRATION

Topical administration appears to be effective in inhibiting skin cancer progres-sion, and either route of injection is not ideal for long-term cancer prevention strategies and, thus, likely is more important in treatment strategies. In contrast, oral administration is a convenient way to deliver sphingolipids and, therefore, appears to be a more relevant route in the prevention of colon cancer and possibly other sites.

### 25.3.3.1 Natural Sphingolipids

Sphingolipids are minor components of food, but milk and meat products, eggs, and soybeans are rich in sphingolipids.[60] In animal products, the major sphin-golipid is sphingomyelin, containing a sphingosine backbone and amid-bound fatty acids that are mostly saturated and contain 16, or 22 to 24 carbons. In plants, the prominent sphingolipids are cerebrosides, containing a variety of different sugar headgroups (glucose, galactose, mannose), sphingoid bases, and fatty acids (see Figure 25.1). Intestinal cells are constantly exposed to bioactive sphingolipid metabolites when dietary complex sphingolipids are hydrolyzed to ceramide and sphingosine by intestinal enzymes. Ceramides and sphingoid bases are efficiently absorbed by small intestinal cells,[61] and it seems unlikely that orally administered sphingosine could reach the colon in appreciable amounts. However, about 10% of complex sphingolipids reach the colon intact and can be hydrolyzed by the colonic microflora to ceramides and sphingoid bases.[61] Due to a limited digestion of complex sphingolipids to ceramide and sphingoid bases,[62] even high amounts of sphingolipids (1% of the diet by weight or 50 to 100 times more than the estimated average consumption) did not cause side effects in mature rats or their offspring.[63] This indicates that oral administration of complex sphingolipids is a safe route of delivering bioactive molecules to colonic cells. To test if this is sufficient to prevent colon tumor formation, complex sphingolipids isolated from buttermilk (sphingomyelin, glucosylceramide, lactosylceramide, and ganglioside $G_{D3}$) were mixed into an essentially sphingolipid-free AIN 76A diet at 0.1% and fed to carcinogen-treated CF1 mice (Figure 25.2A). The end point of these studies was the appearance of early morphological changes in colon tumorigenesis, the aberrant crypt foci (ACF), precursors of adenomas, and adenocarcinomas. All the tested complex sphingolipids reduced ACF formation by 50 to 70%[64–66] (Figure 25.3). This was not unexpected because the same metabolites are released in the intestinal tract from these complex sphingolipids.[66] By using the same study design, ganglioside $G_{M1}$ extracted from brain[64] or glucosylceramide derived from soy that contains a sphingoid base with an 8.9-*trans* double bond also prevented ACF formation.[67] These studies demonstrate that the beneficial effects of orally administered natural sphingolipids are not specific for those containing certain headgroups or sphingoid bases, and also not specific for the mouse model since sphingolipids (sphingomyelin) also reduced chemically induced ACF in rats.[68]

To confirm that the suppression of early stages of colon cancer indeed translates into a suppression of colon tumors, CF1 mice were fed sphingomyelin for 52 weeks, beginning before tumor initiation. This reduced the tumor formation by more than 70%[69] (Figure 25.4A). However, administration of sphingolipids only after tumor initiation, e.g., when the damage to the colonic cells already has occurred, yielded in the same suppression of tumor formation, suggesting that there is a "window of opportunity" for the prevention of colon cancer with orally administered sphingolipids that includes predisposed and premalignant cells. How long carcinogen-treated cells respond to these doses of sphingolipids, i.e., if this effect is limited to pre-neoplastic cells (chemopreventive approach) or if the regulation of already more progressed cells is also possible with these doses (chemotherapeutic approach) remains to be determined.

Rodent models are available that closely resemble the human disease to assess the efficacy of orally administered sphingolipids on human colon cancer. C57/B6J$^{Min/+}$ mice (*m*ultiple *i*ntestinal *n*eoplasia, Min mice) carry mutations in the APC (*a*denomatous *p*olyposis *c*oli) gene that is found in almost all patients with familial adenomatous polyposis and 40 to 80% of sporadic colon cancer.[70,71] Feeding Min mice with a mixture of complex sphingolipids (70% sphingomyelin, 5% lactosylceramide, 7.5% glucosylceramide, and 7.5% ganglioside $G_{D3}$) at 0.1% of the diet for 65 days reduced tumor formation throughout the intestinal tract by 40%. Adding ceramide to this mixture but maintaining sphingolipids at 0.1% of the diet increased tumor suppression to 50%.[72] Similar results were observed

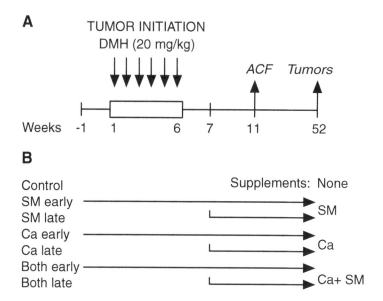

**FIGURE 25.2** Initiation of colon tumors in CF1 mice. Mice are injected with dimethyl-hydrazine (DMH) to induce colon tumors. (A) After 4 weeks of feeding the control diet or sphingolipid supplements, the number of early stages in colon carcinogenesis, the ACF are evaluated. (B) After 46 weeks, the effect of sphingomyelin or combinations with calcium on tumor incidence is evaluated.

after feeding glucosylceramide from soy.[67] Because there were no mice that were completely tumor free, it is possible that orally administered sphingolipids prevent the tumor formation comparably to the chemically induced colon cancer model, but were not effective or less effective against tumors that the Min mice already had developed when they are 5 weeks old.

Although there is no constant elevation of bioactive sphingolipid metabolites in whole blood after administration of complex sphingolipids over several weeks,[72] sphingolipid metabolites derived from orally administered complex sphingolipids are absorbed into the intestinal cells and transported into the body. A recent study demonstrated that sphingolipid supplements to the diet significantly reduced number and size of diethylnitrosamine-induced enzyme-altered foci, pre-neoplastic lesions in the liver in Sprague-Dawley rats,[73] indicating that sufficient amounts of sphingolipids are indeed reaching the liver to prevent early stages of carcinogen-induced liver cancer. If this is also true for other sites is currently unknown. It may depend on the structure of the sphingolipids, as not the uptake of metabolites *per se* but their fate in the intestinal cells and, thus, the availability for transport are altered by structural changes in the sphingoid base.[74,75] The use of synthetic or semisynthetic analogs may therefore be more successful in the prevention of cancer at distant sites; however, studies to confirm this have yet to be reported.

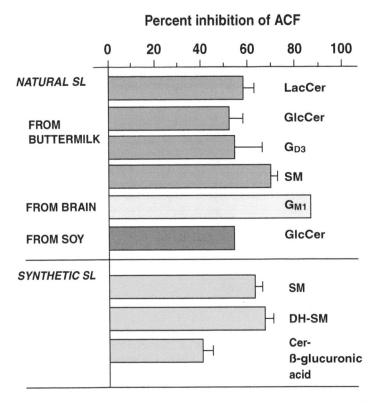

**FIGURE 25.3** Reduction of chemically induced ACF in CF1 by orally administered natural and synthetic sphingolipids.[63–67]

## 25.3.3.2 Synthetic Sphingolipids

Changes in the sphingolipid structure can alter their physicochemical properties, thereby the metabolism in the cells, and their release into the body. It also can affect their signaling capacity. There are many reports on sphingolipid analogs, tested mostly in cell culture. Because these are intended for treatment of cancer, these reports are not included here.

The use of natural compounds gives rise to the risk that co-isolated contaminants alter the response to the treatment. However, synthetic sphingomyelin administered in the same fashion as the natural compounds (Figure 25.2A) lowered the number of ACF to the same degree as sphingomyelin extracted from buttermilk (Figure 25.3) demonstrating that the chemopreventive effect of the natural preparation was indeed due to the sphingomyelin in the diet and not altered by a co-purified contaminant.[76] Synthetic sphingomyelin containing a sphinganine rather than a sphingosine base (lacks the 4,5-*trans* double bond) showed a comparable reduction. As ceramides that contain sphinganine (termed dihydroceramides) are inactive in most biological systems,[77] this study suggests that the most important bioactive metabolites in ACF suppression may be the free

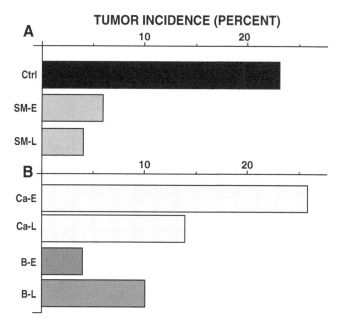

**FIGURE 25.4** Suppression of carcinogen-induced colon tumors by (A) sphingomyelin administered orally either before (SM-E) or after (SM-L) tumor initiation or (B) in combination with calcium also administered before (B-E) or after (B-L) tumor initiation.

sphingoid bases rather than ceramide because there is no difference in the biological activity of sphingosine and sphinganine. Still, because intracellular sphingolipids are easily interconvertible, an introduction of the double bond after the uptake of dihydroceramide by a desaturase and an effect of the intracellularly generated ceramide cannot be ruled out.

Alterations of the sphingolipid components were chosen to design a compound that can specifically target colon cancer. Introduction of a β-glucuronic acid as headgroup on position 1 of the ceramide moiety was intended to eliminate hydrolysis and uptake in the small intestine, thereby increasing the amount of lipids entering the colon and increasing the amount of released bioactive metabolites and their beneficial effects. This compound also reduced ACF in carcinogen-treated CF1 mice (Figure 25.3);[78] however, the comparable fast passage through the mouse colon may have been a limiting factor, and the requirement for hydrolysis should be addressed for the use of "designer sphingolipids" in rodent models.

## 25.4 COMBINATORIAL TREATMENT

Combinatorial treatment has often shown a higher efficacy against tumor development than using a single agent or a single treatment regimen, and is often used in the treatment of patients. Although some the following studies cannot be categorized as chemopreventive studies, they nonetheless can inspire and direct further research.

### 25.4.1 COMBINATORIAL TREATMENT — ORAL ADMINISTRATION

The consumption of milk and milk products has been associated with a decreased risk in colon cancer in some human studies,[79] while other studies found no association.[80,81] It is not entirely clear if the protective effects of foods such as milk and milk products result from the activity of one compound, or are due to the combination of bioactive compounds in the same food. Milk and milk products are rich in complex sphingolipids,[82] but another major compound in milk, calcium, has often been implied as effective ingredient in milk to prevent colon cancer. Therefore, calcium supplements were tested to determine if they enhance the preventive effect of sphingomyelin supplements on chemically induced colon cancer in CF1 mice using the same tumor initiation and feeding protocol as shown in Figure 25.2B. Calcium alone (70 μmol/g diet representing 50% above the recommended daily allowance, the amount shown to have a protective effect against colon cancer in humans[83]) administered orally either before or after tumor initiation did not significantly reduce ACF formation (Figure 25.4B). The combination of both sphingomyelin at 0.05% and calcium did not enhance the effects of sphingomyelin alone (Figure 25.4B). A combination of sphingomyelin with either conjugated linoleic acid or butyrate (also anticancer compounds found in milk) did not increase the suppression of ACF by sphingomyelin alone.[84] It is not known if this is due to this model and that combinations in other rodent models may be effective; however, the sphingolipid content in foods needs to be taken into account for the evaluation of the association of diet and cancer incidence.

### 25.4.2 SPHINGOLIPIDS IN COMBINATION WITH CHEMOTHERAPY

Immunodeficient nude mice are a widely used model to study the effect of drugs and treatment regimens on human cancer cells. Xenografts of prostate cancer cells were grown in nude mice to a volume of 500 mm². Then, the mice were injected subcutaneously every 3 days for 28 days with a ceramide analog that induced apoptosis *in vitro*. This reduced the growth of the tumors when compared to untreated controls, but the combination with γ-irradiation completely blocked tumor growth but did not induce tumor shrinkage.[85] In another study, injection of sphingomyelin (i.v.) alone did not affect the growth of human colon cancer xenografts; however, in combination with 5FU, a drug often used to treat colon cancer, there was a significant reduction of tumor size, which may be associated with the increase of apoptosis in the xenografts.[86]

Interestingly, a combination of short-chain sphingomyelin in nontoxic doses with doxorubicin enhanced the uptake of the drug and its toxicity in cancer cells, but less in primary endothelial cells.[87] Although it is not known if this is possible in *vivo*, it is a potential important concept for cancer therapy that needs to be explored further.

## 25.5 MECHANISMS OF CANCER PREVENTION BY EXOGENOUS SPHINGOLIPIDS

The effects of exogenous sphingolipids have been well documented in many *in vitro* studies, but the mechanisms of how sphingolipid metabolites suppress tumor formation *in vivo* are less defined. A somewhat simplified concept of chemoprevention with sphingolipids is the hypothesis that exogenous sphingolipids can provide the bioactive sphingolipid metabolites lacking in cancer cells that have a defect in the generation of bioactive metabolites due to reduced sphingomyelinase activity or enhanced removal of bioactive metabolites. This is based on many *in vitro* observations demonstrating that cell-permeable sphingolipid metabolites mimic the effect of endogenously generated metabolites and therefore could reverse the unlimited growth capacity of cancer cells. However, the molecular diversity of tumor cells even in the same patient and the number of already identified intracellular targets of sphingolipids that are involved in some aspects of carcinogenesis suggest that there are likely more pathways of how exogenous sphingolipids prevent tumor formation.

In our studies using orally administered sphingolipids to prevent chemically induced colon cancer in CF1 mice, we found that a reversal of carcinogen-induced increase of proliferation and reduced rate of apoptosis rather than the induction of apoptosis per se may be the important event.[66,67,72] This reversal was not limited to a specific structure of sphingolipids but was seen after administration of all complex sphingolipids from milk and soy. To determine how sphingolipids cause this "growth normalization," we evaluated the effect of sphingolipids on one of the earliest events in colon carcinogenesis, the dysregulation of β-catenin. β-Catenin is a cell adhesion protein that connects E-cadherin or other membrane proteins to the actin cytoskeleton via α-catenin.[88] β-Catenin also functions as a signaling molecule in developmental systems,[89] and in the cellular response to growth stimulation through the Wnt pathway or activated growth factor receptors.[88,90] Stabilized β-catenin accumulates in the cytosol, translocates to the nucleus, and activates transcription of genes that are involved in proliferation, adhesion, and migration such as cyclin $D_1$, c-myc, and E-cadherin (see www.stanford.edu/~rnusse/wntwindow.html for an updated list of targets). β-Catenin metabolism is regulated by the adenomatous polyposis coli (APC) gene product that is mutated in 40 to 80% of sporadic colon cancer.[70,71] *APC* mutations seem to be crucial for the development of dysplastic ACF that will progress toward adenoma and adenocarcinoma both in humans and in chemically induced colon cancer in rodents,[91] rather than regress as most of the hyperplastic ACF. All cells in Min mice are heterozygous for *APC* and tumor formation is preceded by the loss of the *APC* wild-type allele, and the deregulation of β-catenin. The dysregulation of β-catenin is therefore a critical early event, common in all our rodent models, and also important in human colon cancer, identifying β-catenin as target for chemopreventive drugs. However, β-catenin may not necessarily be critical in later stages after the addition of further mutations render β-catenin superfluous.

In Min mice that were fed the control AIN 76A diet alone and developed a large number of intestinal tumors, we found a high expression of cytosolic β-catenin in intestinal sections as determined by fluorescence immunohisto-chemistry. Min mice that were fed sphingolipid supplements and that had developed only a small number of tumors displayed mostly membrane-associated β-catenin. This is the localization found in the genetic background mice, suggesting a reversal of aberrant β-catenin expression by sphingolipids.[72] The same effect of exogenous sphingolipids could be seen *in vitro* in human colon cancer cell lines that also carry an *APC* mutation, and stably overexpress cytosolic β-catenin. Both sphingosine and ceramides in nontoxic concentrations reduced cytosolic and nuclear β-catenin.[72] This is a critical step in cancer prevention because removal of cytosolic and nuclear β-catenin has been shown to reverse the trans-formed properties of cells[92] and suggests that the reversal of critical early changes in colon carcinogenesis may be the key event in cancer prevention. In Figure 25.5, the central role for β-catenin and its regulation are depicted. Interestingly, key proteins that regulate β-catenin metabolism such as Akt, GSK-3β, EGFR, and PKC isozymes are directly or indirectly regulated by sphingolipid metabo-lites. Although it is possible, even likely, that this is not the only mechanism by which sphingolipids prevent cancer, given the importance of increased cytosolic β-catenin not only in the etiology of colon cancer but also in breast, skin, prostate, and kidney cancer, the determination of the mechanisms how sphingolipids reg-ulate β-catenin and its role in cancer prevention and possible use as a marker for sphingolipid efficacy both *in vitro* and *in vivo* is warranted.

## 25.6 FUTURE DIRECTIONS OF SPHINGOLIPIDS IN CANCER PREVENTION AND TREATMENT

The efficacy of sphingolipids in cancer treatment is evaluated by their capacity to induce apoptosis in cancer cells. Because nontransformed cells also undergo apoptosis after treatment with sphingolipids, this seems not to be the mechanism of choice for prevention strategies. The serious side effects not only will limit the beneficial effects, but also reduce the compliance with the treatment, and the quality of life for the patients. The regulation of aberrant signaling pathways to remove growth advantages and inhibit progression of cancer cells rather than to directly induce apoptosis is a challenging concept of prevention that may require different concentrations of bioactive metabolites and exposure times than treat-ment of cancer. The targets of nontoxic doses of sphingolipids in the prevention of cancer in addition to β-catenin — such as cell cycle regulators, adhesion molecules, growth factor receptors, etc. — in colon cancer have to be identified and evaluated as marker for sphingolipid efficacy and for their impact on the outcome of the prevention regimen. Nonetheless, the *in vivo* studies conducted

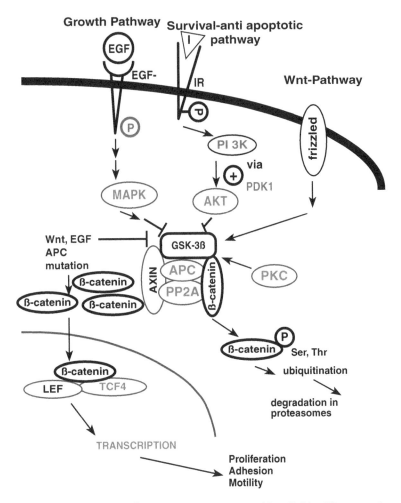

**FIGURE 25.5** Regulation of β-catenin by exogenous sphingolipids. All targets that can be regulated by sphingolipids are in gray.

in our laboratories and others show clearly a beneficial effect of orally administered sphingolipids in the prevention of colon cancer without toxic side effects. However, more research is necessary to determine the effective *in vivo* doses, delivery methods to distant sites, limitations of usefulness, and possible interactions with other drugs to design a safe and effective prevention strategy with sphingolipids.

## ACKNOWLEDGMENTS

The prevention studies using sphingolipids in combination with calcium were funded by the National Dairy Council.

## REFERENCES

1. Merrill AH Jr, Schmelz EM, Dillehay DL, Spiegel S, Shayman JA, Schroeder JJ, Riley RT, Voss KA, Wang E. Sphingolipids — the enigmatic lipid class: biochemistry, physiology, and pathophysiology. *Toxicol Appl Pharmacol* 1997; 142:208–225.
2. Reynolds CP, Maurer BJ, Kolesnick RN. Ceramide synthesis and metabolism as a target for cancer therapy. *Cancer Lett* 2004; 206:169–180.
3. Kok JW, Sietama H. Sphingolipid metabolism enzymes as targets for anticancer therapy. *Curr Drug Targets* 2004; 5:375–382.
4. Ogretmen B, Hannun YA. Biologically active sphingolipids in cancer pathogenesis and treatment. *Nat Rev Cancer* 2004; 4:604–616.
5. Okazaki T, Bell RM, Hannun YA. Sphingomyelin turnover induced by vitamin D3 in HL-60 cells. Role in cell differentiation. *J Biol Chem* 1989; 264:19076–19080.
6. Hannun YA, Bell RM. Functions of sphingolipids and sphingolipid breakdown products in cellular regulation. *Science* 1989; 243:500–507.
7. Andrieu-Abadie N, Levade T. Sphingomyelin hydrolysis during apoptosis. *Biochim Biophys Acta* 2002; 1585:126–134.
8. Pettus BJ, Chalfant CE, Hannun YA. Ceramide in apoptosis: an overview and current perspectives. *Biochim Biophys Acta* 2002; 1585:114–125.
9. Cuvillier O, Levade T. Sphingomyelin hydrolysis during apoptosis. *Biochim Biophys Acta* 2002; 1585:126–134.
10. Van Brocklyn JR, Lee MJ, Menzeleev R, Olivera A, Edsall L, Cuvillier O, Thomas DM, Coopman PJ, Thangada S, Liu CH, Hla T, Spiegel S. Dual actions of sphingosine-1-phosphate:extracellular through the Gi-coupled receptor Edg-1 and intracellular to regulate proliferation and survival. *J Cell Biol* 1998; 142:229–240.
11. Bornfeldt KE, Graves LM, Raines EW, Igarashi Y, Wayman G, Yamamura S, Yatomi Y, Sidhu JS, Krebs EG, Hakomori S, Ross, R. Sphingosine-1-phosphate inhibits PDGF-induced chemotaxis of human arterial smooth muscle cells: spatial and temporal modulation of PDGF chemotactic signal transduction. *J Cell Biol* 1995; 130:193–206.
12. Xia P, Gamble JR, Rye KA, Wang L, Hi CS, Cockerill P, Khew-Goodall Y, Bert AG, Barter PJ, Vadas MA. Tumor necrosis factor-alpha induces adhesion molecule expression through the sphingosine kinase pathway. *Proc Natl Acad Sci USA* 1998; 95:14196–14201.
13. Wang F, Van Brocklyn JR, Edsall L, Nava VE, Spiegel S. Sphingosine-1phosphate inhibits motility of human breast cancer cells independently of cell surface receptors. *Cancer Res* 1999; 59:6185–6191.
14. Hobson JP, Rosenfeldt HM, Barak LS, Olivera A, Poulton S, Caron MG, Milstien S, Spiegel S. Role of the sphingosine-1-phosphate receptor EDG-1 in PDGF-induced cell motility. *Science* 2001; 291:1800–1803.
15. Edsall LC, Pirianov GG, Spiegel S. Involvement of sphingosine 1-phosphate in nerve growth factor-mediated neuronal survival and differentiation. *J Neurosci* 1997; 17:6952–6960.
16. Tserng K-Y, Griffin RL. Ceramide metabolite, not intact ceramide molecule, may be responsible for cellular toxicity. *Biochem J* 2004; 380:715–722.

17. Dudeja PK, Dahiya R, Brasitus TA. The role of sphingomyelin synthase and sphingomyelinase in 1,2-dimethylhydrazine-induced lipid alterations of rat colonic membranes. *Biochim Biophys Acta* 1986; 863:309–312.

18. Notterman DR, Alon U, Sierk AJ, Levine AJ. Transcriptional gene expression profiles of colorectal adenoma, adenocarcinoma, and normal tissue examined by oligonucleotide arrays. *Cancer Res* 2001; 61:3124–3130.

19. Hertervig E, Nilsson Å, Nyberg L, Duan RD. Alkaline sphingomyelinase activity is decreased in human colorectal carcinoma. *Cancer* 1997; 79:448–453.

20. Michael JM, Lavin MF, Watters DJ. Resistance to radiation-induced apoptosis in Burkitt's lymphoma cells is associated with defective ceramide signaling. *Cancer Res* 1997; 57:3600–3605.

21. Chmura SJ, Nodzenski E, Beckett MA, Kufe DW, Quintans J, Weichselbaum RR. Loss of ceramide production confers resistance to radiation-induced apoptosis. *Cancer Res* 1997; 57:1270–1275.

22. Cai Z, Bettaieb A, Mahdani NE, Legres LG, Stancou R, Masliah J, Chouaib S. Alteration of the sphingomyelin/ceramide pathway is associated with resistance of human breast carcinoma MCF7 cells to tumor necrosis factor-alpha-mediated cytotoxicity. *J Biol Chem* 1997; 272:6918–6926.

23. Wang XZ, Beebe JR, Pwiti L, Bielawska A, Smyth MJ. Aberrant sphingolipid signaling is involved in the resistance of prostate cancer cell lines to chemotherapy. *Cancer Res* 1999; 59:5842–5848.

24. Strelow A, Bernardo K, Adam-Klages S, Linke T, Sandhoff K, Kronke M, Adam D. Overexpression of acid ceramidase protects from tumor necrosis factor-induced cell death. *J Exp Med* 2000; 192:601–612.

25. Xia P, Gamble JR, Wang L, Pitson SM, Moretti PA, Wattenberg BW, D'Andrea RJ, Vadas MA An oncogenic role of sphingosine kinase. *Curr Biol* 2000; 10:1527–1530.

26. Sutphen R, Xu Y, Wilbanks GD, Fiorica J, Grendys EC, LaPolla JP, Arango H, Hoffman MS, Martino M, Wakely K, Griffin D, Blanco RW, Cantor AB, Xiao YJ, Krischer JP. Lysophospholipids are potential biomarkers of ovarian cancer. *Cancer Epidemiol Biomarkers Prev* 2004; 13:1185–1191.

27. Hong G, Baudhuin LM, Xu Y. Sphingosine-1-phosphate modulates cell growth and adhesion of ovarian cancer cells. *FEBS Lett* 1999; 460:513–518.

28. Lavie Y, Cao H, Bursten SL, Giuliano AE, Cabot MC. Accumulation of glucosylceramides in multi-drug resistant cancer cells. *J Biol Chem* 1996; 27:19530–19536.

29. Veldman RJ, Klappe K, Hinrichs J, Hummel I, van der Schaaf G, Sietsma H, Kok JW. Altered sphingolipid metabolism in multidrug-resistant ovarian cancer cells is due to uncoupling of glycolipid biosynthesis in the Golgi apparatus. *FASEB J* 2002; 16:1111–1113.

30. Norris-Cervetto E, Callaghan R, Platt F, Dwek RA, Butters TD. Inhibition of glucosylceramide synthase does not reverse drug resistance in cancer cells. *J Biol Chem* 2004; 279:40412–40418.

31. Koybasi S, Senkal CE, Sundararaj K, Spassieva S, Bialewski J, Osta W, Day TA, Jiang JC, Jazwinski SM, Hannun YA, Obeid LM, Ogretmen, B. Defects in cell growth regulation by C18:0-ceramide and longevity assurance gene 1 (LAG1) in human head and neck squamous cell carcinomas (HNSCC). *J Biol Chem* 2004; 279:44311–44319.

32. Selzner M, Bielawska A, Morse MA, Rudiger HA, Sindram D, Hannun YA, Clavien PA. Induction of apoptotic cell death and prevention of tumor growth by ceramide analogues in metastatic human colon cancer. *Cancer Res* 2001; 61:1233–1240.

33. Chi FL, Yuan YS, Wang SY, Wang ZM. Study on ceramide expression and DNA content in patients with healthy mucosa, leukoplakia, and carcinoma of the larynx. *Arch Otolaryngol Head Neck Surg* 2004; 130:307–310.

34. Riboni I, Campanella R, Bassi R, Villani R, Gaini SM, Martinelli-Boneschi F, Viani P, Tettamanti G. Ceramide levels are inversely associated with malignant progression of glial tumors. *Glia* 2002; 39:105–113.

35. Itoh M, Kitano T, Watanabe M, Kondo T, Yabu T, Taguchi Y, Iwai K, Tashima M, Uchiyama T, Okazaki T. Possible role of ceramide as an indicator of chemoresistance: decrease of ceramide content via activation of glucosylceramide synthase and sphingomyelin synthase in chemoresistant leukemia. *Clin Cancer Res* 2003; 8:415–423.

36. Kok JW, Veldman RJ, Klappe K, Koning H, Filipeanu CM, Muller M. Differential expression of sphingolipids in MRP1 overexpressing HT29 cells. *Int J Cancer* 2000; 87:172–178.

37. Prinetti A, Basso L, Appierto V, Villani MG, Valsecchi M, Loberto N, Prioni S, Chigorno V, Cavadini E, Formelli F, Sonnino S. Altered sphingolipid metabolism in *N*-(4-hydroxyphenyl) retinamide-resistant A2780 human ovarian carcinoma cells. *J Biol Chem* 2003; 278:5574–5583.

38. Sjöblom T, Shimizu A, O'Brien KP, Pietras K, Dal Cin P, Buchdunger E, Dumanski JP, Ostman A, Heldin CH. Growth inhibition of dermatofibrosarcoma protuberans tumors by the platelet-derived growth factor receptor antagonist STI571 through induction of apoptosis. *Cancer Res* 2001; 61:5778–5783.

39. Rodriguez-Lafrasse C, Alphonse G, Aloy MT, Ardail D, Gerard JP, Louisot P, Rousson R. Increasing endogenous ceramide using inhibitors of sphingolipid metabolism maximizes ionizing radiation-induced mitochondrial injury and apoptotic cell killing. *Int J Cancer* 2002; 101:589–598.

40. Cabot MC, Giuliano AE, Han TY, Liu YY. SDZ PSC 833, the cyclosporine A analogue and multidrug resistance modulator, activates ceramide synthesis and increases vinblastine sensitivity in drug-sensitive and drug-resistant cancer cells. *Cancer Res* 1999; 59:880–885.

41. Sietsma H, Veldman RJ, Kolk D, Ausema B, Nijhof W, Kamps W, Vellenga E, Kok JW. 1-Phenyl-2-decanoylamino-3-morpholino-1-propanol chemosensitizes neuroblastoma cells for taxol and vincristine. *Clin Cancer Res* 2000; 6:942–948.

42. Olshefski RS, Ladisch S. Glucosylceramide synthase inhibition enhances vincristine-induced cytotoxicity. *Int J Cancer* 2001; 93:131–138.

43. Alphonse G, Bionda C, Aloy MT, Ardail D, Rousson R, Rodrigues-Lafrasse C. Overcoming resistance to g-rays in squamous carcinoma cells by poly-drug elevation of ceramide levels. *Oncogene* 2004; 23:2703–2715.

44. Deng W, Li R, Ladisch S. Influence of cellular ganglioside depletion on tumor formation. *J Natl Cancer Inst* 2000; 92:912–917.

45. Koyanagi S, Kuga M, Soeda S, Hosoda Y, Yokomatsu T, Takechi H, Akiyama T, Shibuya S, Shimeno H. Elevation of de novo ceramide synthesis in tumor masses and the role of microsomal dihydroceramide synthase. *Int J Cancer* 2003; 105:1–6.

46. Martin A, Duffy PA, Liossis C, Gomez-Munoz A, O'Brien L, Stone JC, Brindley DN. Increased concentrations of phosphatidate, diacylglycerol and ceramide in ras- and tyrosine kinase (fps)-transformed fibroblasts. *Oncogene* 1997; 14:1571–1580.

47. Sullards MC, Wang E, Peng Q, Merrill AH Jr. Metabolomic profiling of sphingolipids in human glioma cell lines by liquid chromatography tandem mass spectrometry. *Cell Mol Biol* 2003; 49:789–797.

48. Enkvetchakul B, Merrill AH Jr, Birt DF. Inhibition of the induction of ornithine decarboxylase activity by 12-*O*-tetradecanoylphorbol-13-acetate in the mouse skin by sphingosine sulfate. *Carcinogenesis* 1989; 10:379–381.

49. Enkvetchakul B, Barnett T, Liotta DC, Geisler V, Menaldino DS, Merrill AH Jr, Birt DF. Influences of sphingosine on two-stage skin tumorigenesis in SENCAR mice. *Cancer Lett* 1992; 62:35–42.

50. Birt DF, Merrill AH Jr, Barnett T, Enkvetchakul B, Pour PM, Liotta DC, Geisler V, Menaldino DS, Schwartzbauer J. Inhibition of skin papillomas by sphingosine, *N*-methyl sphingosine, and *N*-acetyl sphingosine. *Nutr Cancer* 1998; 31:119–126.

51. Carfagna MA, Young KM, Susick RL. Sex differences in rat hepatic cytolethality of the protein kinase C inhibitor safingol: role of biotransformation. *Toxicol Appl Pharmacol* 1996; 137:173–181.

52. Jatoi A, Suman VJ, Schaefer P, Block M, Loprinzi C, Roche P, Garneau S, Morton R, Stella PJ, Alberts SR, Pittelkow M, Sloan J, Pagano R. A phase II study of topical ceramides for cutaneous breast cancer. *Breast Cancer Res Treat* 2003; 80:99–104.

53. Macchia M, Barontini S, Bertini S, Di Bussolo V, Fogli S, Giovannetti E, Grossi E, Minutolo F, Danesi R. Design, synthesis, and characterization of the antitumor activity of novel ceramide analogues. *J Med Chem* 2001; 44:3994–4000.

54. Kedderis LB, Bozigan HP, Kleeman JM, Hall RL, Palmer TE, Harrison SD Jr, Susick RL Jr. Toxicity of the protein kinase C inhibitor safingol administered alone and in combination with chemotherapeutic agents. *Fund Appl Toxicol* 1995; 25:201–217.

55. Endo K, Igarashi Y, Nisar M, Zhou Q, Hakomori S-I. Cell membrane signaling as target in cancer therapy: inhibitory effect of *N,N*-dimethyl and *N,N,N*-trimethyl sphingosine derivatives on *in vitro* and *in vivo* growth of human tumor cells in nude mice. *Cancer Res* 1991; 51:1613–1618.

56. Stover TC, Kester M. Liposomal delivery enhances short-chain ceramide-induced apoptosis of breast cancer cells. *J Pharmacol Exp Ther* 2003; 307:468–475.

57. Stover, TC, Sharma, A, Robertson, GP, Kester, M. Systemic delivery of liposomal short-chain ceramide limits solid tumor growth in murine models of breast adenocarcinoma. *Clin Cancer Res* 2005; 11:3465–3474.

58. Shabbits JA, Mayer LD. High ceramide content liposomes with in vivo antitumor activity. *Anticancer Res* 2003; 23:3663–3669.

59. Takenaga M, Igarashi R, Matsumoto K, Takeuchi J, Mizushima N, Nakayama T, Morizawa Y, Mizushima, Y. Lipid microsphere preparation of a lipophilic ceramide derivative suppresses colony formation in a murine experimental metastasis model. *J Drug Target* 1999; 7:187–195.

60. Vesper H, Schmelz EM, Nikolova-Karakashian M., Dillehay DL, Lynch DV, Merrill AH Jr. Sphingolipids in food and the emerging importance of sphingolipids to nutrition. *J Nutr* 1999; 129:1239–1250.

61. Schmelz EM, Crall KL, LaRocque R, Dillehay DL, Merrill AH Jr. Uptake and metabolism of sphingolipids in isolated intestinal loops of mice. *J Nutr* 1994; 124:702–712.

62. Nyberg L, Nilsson Å, Lundgren P, Duan R-D. Localization and capacity of sphingomyelin digestion in the rat intestinal tract. *J Nutr Biochem* 1997; 8:112–118.

63. Kobayashi T, Shimizugawa T, Osakabe T, Watanabe S, Okuyama H. A long-term feeding of sphingolipids affected the level of plasma cholesterol and hepatic triacylglycerol but not tissue phospholipids and sphingolipids. *Nutr Res* 1997; 17:111–114.

64. Dillehay DL, Webb SK, Schmelz EM, Merrill AH Jr. Dietary sphingomyelin inhibits 1,2-dimethylhydrazine-induced colon cancer in CF1 mice. *J Nutr* 1994; 124:615–620.

65. Schmelz EM, Dillehay DL, Webb SK, Reiter A, Adams J, Merrill AH Jr. Sphingomyelin consumption suppresses aberrant colonic crypt foci and increases the proportion of adenomas versus adenocarcinomas in CF1 mice treated with 1,2-dimethylhydrazine:implications for dietary sphingolipids and colon carcinogenesis. *Cancer Res* 1996; 56:4936–4941.

66. Schmelz E., Sullards M., Dillehay DL, Merrill AH Jr. Inhibition of colonic cell proliferation and aberrant crypt foci formation by dairy glycosphingolipids in 1,2-dimethylhydrazine-treated CF1 mice. *J Nutr* 2000; 130:522–527.

67. Symolon H, Schmelz EM, Dillehay DL, Merrill AH Jr. Dietary soy sphingolipids suppress tumorigenesis and gene expression in 1,2-dimethylhydrazine-treated CF1 mice and ApcMin/+ mice. *J Nutr* 2004; 134:1157–1161.

68. Exon JH, South EH. Effects of sphingomyelin on aberrant colonic crypt foci development, colon crypt cell proliferation and immune function in an aging rat tumor model. *Food Chem Toxicol* 2003; 41:471–476.

69. Lemonnier LA, Dillehay DL, Vespremi MJ, Abrams J, Brody E, Schmelz EM. Sphingomyelin in the suppression of colon tumors: prevention versus intervention. *Arch Biochem Biophys* 2003; 419:129–138.

70. Nagase H, Nakamura Y. Mutations of the APC (adenomatous polyposis coli) gene. *Hum Mutat* 1993; 2:425–434.

71. Sparks AB, Morin PJ, Kinzler KW. Mutational analysis of the APC/β-catenin/TCF pathway in colorectal cancer. *Cancer Res* 1998; 58:1130–1134.

72. Schmelz EM. Roberts PC, Kustin EM, Lemonnier LA, Sullards MC, Dillehay DL, Merrill AH Jr. Modulation of β-catenin localization and intestinal tumorigenesis *in vitro* and *in vivo* by sphingolipids. *Cancer Res* 2001; 61:6723–6729.

73. Silins I, Nordstrand M, Hogberg J, Stenius U. Sphingolipids suppress preneoplastic rat hepatocytes *in vitro* and *in vivo*. *Carcinogenesis* 2003; 24:1077–1083.

74. Polo A, Kirschner G, Guidotti A, Costa E. Brain content of glycosphingolipids after oral administration of monosialogangliosides GM1 and LIGA20 to rats. *Mol Chem Neuropathol* 1994; 21:41–53.

75. Sugawara T, Kinoshita M, Ohnishi M, Nagata J, Saito M. Digestion of maize sphingolipids in rats and uptake of sphingadienine by Caco-2 cells. *J Nutr* 2003; 133:2777–2782.

76. Schmelz EM, Bushnev AB, Dillehay DL, Liotta DC, Merrill AH Jr. Suppression of aberrant colonic crypt foci by synthetic sphingomyelins with saturated or unsaturated sphingoid base backbones. *Nutr Cancer* 1997; 28:81–85.

77. Bielawska A, Crane H, Liotta DC, Obeid LM, Hannun YA. Selectivity of ceramide-mediated biology. Lack of activity of erythro-dihydro-ceramide. *J Biol Chem* 1993; 268:26226–26232.

78. Schmelz EM, Bushnev AS, Dillehay DL, Sullards MC, Liotta DC, Merrill AH Jr. Ceramide-β-glucuronide:synthesis, digestion, and suppression of early markers of colon carcinogenesis. *Cancer Res* 1999; 59:5768–5772.

79. Jarvinen R, Knekt P, Hakulinen T, Aromaa A. Prospective study on milk products, calcium and cancers of the colon and rectum. *Eur J Clin Nutr* 2001; 55:1000–1007.

80. Negri E, La Vecchia C, D'Avanzo B, Francesci, S. Calcium, dairy products, and colorectal cancer. *Nutr Cancer* 1990; 10:255–262.

81. Terry P, Baron JA, Bergkvist L, Holmberg L, Wolk A. Dietary calcium and vitamin D intake and risk of colorectal cancer: a prospective cohort study in women. *Nutr Cancer* 2002; 43:39–46.

82. Jensen RG. *Handbook of Milk Composition.* New York: Academic Press; 1995.

83. Glinghammar B, Venturi M, Rowland IR, Rafter JJ. Shift from a dairy product-rich to a dairy product-free diet: influence on cytotoxicity and genotoxicity of fecal water — potential risk factors for colon cancer. *Am J Clin Nutr* 1997; 66:1277–1282.

84. Nichenametla SN, South EH, Exon JH. Interaction of conjugated linoleic acid, sphingomyelin, and butyrate on formation of colonic aberrant crypt foci and immune function in rats. *J Toxicol Environ Health* A 2004; 67:469–481.

85. Samsel L, Zaidel G, Drumgoole HM, Jelovac D, Drachenberg C, Rhee JG, Brodie AM, Bielawska A, Smyth MJ. The ceramide analog, B13, induces apoptosis in prostate cancer cell lines and inhibits tumor growth in prostate cancer xenografts. *Prostate* 2004; 58:382–393.

86. Modrak DE, Lew W, Goldenberg DM, Blumenthal R. Sphingomyelin potentiates chemotherapy of human cancer xenografts. *Biochem Biophys Res Commun* 2000; 268:603–606.

87. Veldman RJ, Zerp S, van Bitterswijk WJ, Verheij M. *N*-Hexanoyl-sphingomyelin potentiates *in vitro* doxorubicin cytotoxicity by enhancing its cellular influx. *Br J Cancer* 2004; 90:917–925.

88. Pfeifer M. Cell adhesion and signal transduction: the armadillo connection. *Trends Cell Biol* 1995; 5:224–229.

89. Orsulic S, Pfeifer M. An *in vitro* structure–function study of armadillo, the β-catenin homologue, reveals both separate and overlapping regions of the protein required for cell adhesion and for wingless signaling. *J Cell Biol* 1996; 134:1283–1300.

90. Shibamoto S, Hayakawa M, Takeuchi K, Hori T, Oku N, Miyazawa K, Kitamura N, Takeichi M, Ito F. Tyrosine phosphorylation of β-catenin and plakoglobin enhanced by hepatocyte growth factor and epidermal growth factor in human carcinoma cells. *Cell Adhes Commun* 1994; 1:295–305.

91. Jen J, Powell SM, Papdopoulos N, Smith KJ, Hamilton SR, Vogelstein B, Kinzler KW. Molecular determinants of dysplasia in colorectal lesions. *Cancer Res* 1994; 54:5523–5526.

92. Kim JS, Crooks H, Foxworth A, Waldman T. Proof-of-principle: oncogenic β-catenin is a valid molecular target for the development of pharmacological inhibitors. *Mol Cancer Ther* 2002; 1:1355–1359.

# Part IX

## Dietary Cancer Risk Factors

# 26 Obesity as a Cancer Risk Factor: Epidemiology

*Yang Mao, Sai Yi Pan, and Anne-Marie Ugnat*

## CONTENTS

26.1 Introduction ........................................................................................541
26.2 Prevalence of Overweight and Obesity ...........................................542
26.3 Health and Economic Impact of Obesity .........................................543
26.4 Obesity and Cancer ...........................................................................543
    26.4.1 Colorectal Cancer ...............................................................544
    26.4.2 Breast Cancer .......................................................................544
        26.4.2.1 Premenopausal Breast Cancer ...............................545
        26.4.2.2 Postmenopausal Breast Cancer ..............................545
        26.4.2.3 Stage of Breast Cancer at Diagnosis .....................546
        26.4.2.4 Breast Cancer Prognosis ........................................546
    26.4.3 Endometrial Cancer .............................................................547
    26.4.4 Kidney Cancer .....................................................................547
    26.4.5 Prostate Cancer ...................................................................548
    26.4.6 Adenocarcinoma of the Esophagus and Gastric Cardia .........548
    26.4.7 Ovarian Cancer ...................................................................549
    26.4.8 Pancreatic Cancer ...............................................................549
    26.4.9 Lung Cancer ........................................................................550
    26.4.10 Other Cancer Sites ..............................................................550
    26.4.11 All Cancers Combined ........................................................550
26.5 Conclusion .........................................................................................551
References ....................................................................................................551

## 26.1 INTRODUCTION

Obesity results from a chronic excess of energy intake over energy expenditure.[1] Several measurements are used to define obesity: body mass index (BMI) (weight in kilograms divided by height in meters squared), waist circumference (measured in centimeters at the midpoint between the lower border of the ribs and the upper border of the pelvis), skinfold thickness (measured in centimeters with callipers), bioimpedance (measurement of resistance to a weak current applied across extremities).[2] BMI is the most frequently used formula in epidemiological studies. The World Health Organization (WHO) has proposed a definition of overweight as BMI 25.0 to 29.9 kg/m[2] and obesity as BMI ≥30.0 kg/m[2], which apply to both sexes and to all adult age groups.[3]

## 26.2  PREVALENCE OF OVERWEIGHT AND OBESITY

The prevalence of obesity has increased rapidly over the past two decades, reaching epidemic levels in many parts of the world.[3] Currently worldwide, more than 1 billion adults are overweight and at least 300 million of them are obese.[3] Present levels of obesity vary from less than 5% in China, Japan, and certain African nations, to over 75% in urban Samoa.[3] Recent data from Europe found that the prevalence of obesity varied from 8 to 40% in men and from 5 to 53% in women, with high prevalence (>25%) in Spain, Greece, Ragusa and Naples (Italy), and the lowest prevalence (<10%) in France.[4] Obesity is more common in Eastern Europe than in other parts of Europe, especially among women.[5] Obesity prevalence remains at 1 to 5% in most populations in sub-Saharan Africa; however, it has risen to 8% in men and to 34% in women in some areas of South Africa and in neighboring countries.[6] Obesity is becoming a problem in some urban areas of developing countries, especially in those undergoing economic transition,[7] and the rates are almost 20% in some cities.[3]

The prevalence of obesity (BMI ≥30 kg/m[2]) in the U.S. adult population rose from 15% in 1976–1980 to 22.9% in 1988–1994 and 30.5% in 1999–2000, and excess weight (BMI ≥ 25 kg/m[2]) rose from 55.9% in 1988–1994 to 64.5% in 1999–2000; the increases occurred for both men and women in all age groups and for non-Hispanic whites, non-Hispanic blacks, and Mexican Americans.[8] A Canadian survey in 2000/2001, which used self-reported data, showed that about half of adult Canadians are overweight (56% in men and 39% in women) and 15% of them are obese (16% in men and 14% in women);[9] however, the true rate could be higher because of a tendency for individuals to underreport their weight.

Childhood obesity is epidemic in some areas of the world and increasing rapidly in others.[3,10] Worldwide, about 17.6 million children under 5 are estimated to be overweight.[3] The highest prevalences of overweight among children are in the U.S., Ireland, Greece, and Portugal.[11] The prevalence of overweight among U.S. children is increasing: in 1999–2000, 15.5% of 12- to 19-year-olds were overweight, 15.3% of 6- to 11-year-olds, and 10.4% of 2- to 5-year-olds, compared with 10.5, 11.3, and 7.2%, respectively, in 1988–1994.[12] In Canada, between 1981 and 1996–1997, the excess weight rate increased from 11 to 33% in 7- to 13-year-old boys and from 13 to 27% in girls, and the obesity rate rose from 2 to 10% in boys and from 2 to 9% in girls.[13] In a relatively short period of time

(1994–1995 to 1998–1999), the proportion of 2- to 11-year-olds who were overweight (including obese) rose from 34 to 37% and the obesity rate rose from 16 to 18%.[14]

## 26.3  HEALTH AND ECONOMIC IMPACT OF OBESITY

Obesity is now known to be a major contributor to the global burden of disease.[3] Obesity is associated not only with some nonfatal but debilitating health problems, such as respiratory difficulties, chronic musculoskeletal problems, skin problems, infertility, sleep apnea, and poor mental health, but also more life-threatening problems, including hypertension, type 2 diabetes, heart disease, stroke, some types of cancer.[3,15] Obese people have higher mortality from all causes;[16–19] more than 280,000 deaths annually have been attributed to obesity among U.S. adults.[20] In Europe, this number is at least 279,000 deaths, of which 175,000 are attributable to obesity and 104,000 to overweight.[21] Furthermore, a large decrease in life expectancy is observed among obese individuals, especially among younger adults.[22,23] Severely obese children and adolescents have lower health-related quality of life[24] and early-onset obesity has been suggested as a risk factor for morbidity and mortality later in life.[25,26]

Obesity is also associated significantly with excess medical costs.[3,27,28] It is estimated that obesity accounts for 2 to 6% of total health care costs in several industrialized countries[3] and for an even higher percentage in the U.S. where obesity-related health problems consume about 7 to 8% of the U.S. health care budget in direct medical costs.[29,30] The total cost (direct and indirect) for obesity-related health problems is around $117 billion annually in the U.S.[31] The total direct costs of obesity in Canada have been estimated at $1.8 billion, or 2.4% of total health care expenditures for all diseases in 1997.[32]

## 26.4  OBESITY AND CANCER

This chapter focuses on the epidemiological evidence of obesity as a risk factor for various cancers. Most studies used BMI as an indicator of overall obesity, and some had other measures as well, such as waist circumference or waist-to-hip ratio (WHR) (an indicator of body fat distribution) to examine whether central obesity is a risk factor for cancer. Different cut points for BMI, waist circumference, and WHR were used in various studies. We identified studies published between 1966 and 2004 via the MEDLINE database. Included in this chapter are published reviews and meta-analyses as well as individual studies published since the reviews. For individual studies, only those with at least 100 cases were included; however, all identified studies were included for less common cancers. When several articles were published from the same study, only the most recent is included.

### 26.4.1 COLORECTAL CANCER

Most of the cohort and case-control studies, included in three published reviews, as well as studies published subsequently[33–48] consistently demonstrated a positive association between the risk of colorectal cancer and body fatness, as indicated by BMI or WHR or waist circumference. Most studies found nearly a doubling of risk in those with BMI ≥30.0 kg/m$^2$ compared with those having BMI <23 kg/m$^2$.[33] A trend of increasing risk with increasing BMI across a wide range was also indicated in most investigations, with no clear evidence of a threshold effect.[33] Only three studies[49–51] showed no association of colorectal cancer and body fatness in both sexes.

The observed association between obesity and colorectal cancer is generally more consistent and stronger for men than for women and for colon cancer than for rectal cancer.[33] Some studies found that WHR is a strong predictor (of the same strength as BMI) of colorectal cancer risk, especially for women.[36,42,44,52–55] The association is also generally stronger and more consistent for cancer of the distal colon than the proximal colon.[36,39,40,52,54–58] A meta-analysis of 13 studies on BMI and colon cancer found that the observed associations were of similar strength for cohort and case-control studies, and that the pooled estimates were statistically significant for both male and female but larger for men than for women.[34] Excess weight early in life appears to be at least as important as recent excess weight in relation to colorectal cancer risk.[40,45,54,56,58] One large population-based case-control study found that estrogen modifies the association between BMI and colon cancer risk; i.e., obese women who were estrogen-positive (premenopausal women or women who used hormone replacement therapy) experienced a greater than twofold increase in risk, whereas obese women who were estrogen-negative (postmenopausal women not taking hormone replacement therapy) did not.[48]

A positive association of similar magnitude to the association with colorectal cancer was also observed between body fatness and colorectal adenomas,[50,53,59–66] which suggests that obesity may affect progression from adenoma to cancer. One study demonstrated the association in both sexes combined,[61] others found it for men only,[64,65] while another observed no association in either sex.[67] Studies also identified a stronger effect of BMI, WHR, or waist circumference on large adenomas than on small adenomas or an effect restricted to large adenomas.[53,50,62,64,65]

Although some studies suggest that weight gain between early adult ages and later adult ages increases the risks of developing colorectal cancer[56,57] and colorectal adenomas.[60,61] the findings have not been substantiated by other studies.[45,58,62]

### 26.4.2 BREAST CANCER

The relationship between breast cancer risk and various measures of body size at different periods of life and adult weight gain has been extensively explored in many epidemiological studies. Because the associations differ between pre-menopausal and postmenopausal women, we reviewed the literature separately for the two groups.

### 26.4.2.1 Premenopausal Breast Cancer

In general, obesity does not relate to or is inversely associated with premenopausal breast cancer risk, as demonstrated in four reviews and studies published after the reviews.[33-35,47,68-72] However, there were also studies that reported increased risk.[73-77] Two of these were studies of non-Caucasian women.[74,77]

Both race and the distribution of body fat, rather than obesity per se may be important factors. Increased risk with higher WHR but not with higher BMI has been reported,[78-80] as has decreased risk with higher BMI but not with higher WHR,[81-83] decreased risk with higher BMI and increased risk with higher WHR among white women, but increased risk with higher WHR and no change with BMI among black women,[84] and no change in risk with both higher BMI and higher WHR.[85]

Among the limited data on weight gain and premenopausal breast cancer risk, no association was observed in some case-control studies[78,82,86] and a decreased risk was reported in one cohort study[87] and several case-control studies.[76,88-90] One study found that adult weight gain was associated with increased risk among Hispanic white women but not among non-Hispanic white women.[77]

### 26.4.2.2 Postmenopausal Breast Cancer

Convincing evidence exists for an association between obesity and postmeno-pausal breast cancer.[33-35] The association remains after adjusting for various reproductive and lifestyle factors including physical activity. Most prospective cohort studies showed a significant increase in risk associated with recent obe-sity.[33-35,68-70,79,85,91-95] Various degrees of increased risk (from 10% to more than twofold) were reported in many case-control studies.[33-35,47,71,72,74,77,78,80,83,86,96-101] However, the increase is more modest in cohort studies than case-control studies. No increase in risk has also been found.[33,34]

Most studies suggested that obesity in young adulthood (at the age of 18 to 25 years) was either not associated with breast cancer risk[76,77,91,96,99,100,102] or was associated with a 10 to 30% decrease in risk.[69,84,86,90,93,95,103]

Adult weight gain appeared to be the strongest and most consistent predictor of increased postmenopausal breast cancer risk, in both cohort studies [69,87,92,103,104] and case-control studies.[33,74,77,78,86,90,96,98-100,102,105-108]

Family history of breast cancer, hormone replacement therapy (HRT) use, estrogen receptor status, tumor morphology, and age at diagnosis may modify the association between obesity/weight gain and postmenopausal breast cancer risk. Studies have found a stronger association with obesity for women with a family history of breast cancer than for those without.[75,95,96] Some studies also suggested that the association was restricted to non-HRT users[73,87,91,93,100,108] or stronger among women who had never used HRT;[72,92,106,109] however, one large case-control study observed a stronger association among women who had used estrogen replacement therapy.[76] Two studies have observed the association of breast cancer with weight gain among women who never used HRT but not among current HRT users.[91,93]

A study that examined breast cancer risk by estrogen receptor (ER) and progesterone receptor (PR) status[102] found that, among postmenopausal women, BMI-related risk was increased only among those with ER-/PR-positive tumors and not increased among those either with ER-/PR-negative tumors or among premenopausal women with any ER/PR subgroup. A Japanese study[71] demonstrated that among postmenopausal women, obesity-related risk increase was stronger for ER-positive than ER-negative tumors and for PR-positive than PR-negative tumors. Another study indicated an increased risk of breast cancer with weight gain among Hispanic and postmenopausal non-Hispanic white women with ER-/PR-positive tumors, but not those with ER-/PR-negative tumors.[77] However, one study suggested that the association between WHR and breast cancer is independent of ER status.[80] Furthermore, one case-control study found that obesity was more strongly associated with elevated risk of invasive ductal carcinoma than invasive lobular carcinoma.[97]

Age at diagnosis appears to modify obesity-related breast cancer risk. Among studies that examined the association stratified by age at diagnosis, the risk appeared to increase with age at diagnosis, from 1.1 to 1.3 for women younger than 60 years to 1.6 to 2.9 for women older than 65 years.[69,76,82,86,94,100,101] However, one cohort study of non-HRT users found that the effect of obesity was more pronounced among younger postmenopausal women (aged 50 to 69 years) than older women (aged 70 to 79 years).[93]

### 26.4.2.3 Stage of Breast Cancer at Diagnosis

Several studies have shown obesity to be associated with an increased risk of a more advanced stage of breast cancer at diagnosis.[110–114] However, obese women are less likely to be screened with mammography,[115] more likely to present late to a health-care professional,[116] and have lower socioeconomic status.[117,118] These factors are associated with delay in diagnosis of breast cancer and therefore may contribute to the more advanced stage at diagnosis for obese women.

### 26.4.2.4 Breast Cancer Prognosis

The literature suggests a modest negative effect of greater body size on breast cancer prognosis in both pre- and postmenopausal women even after adjustment for other prognostic factors.[94,119–121] However, some studies found no statistically significant difference in overall and disease-free survival between obese and non-obese women.[119,122,123] Some studies also found that the influence of obesity on prognosis was limited to or was stronger among women with negative nodes, ER- and PR-positive status, and early disease stages (I and II).[33]

### 26.4.3 ENDOMETRIAL CANCER

The evidence for a positive association between obesity and endometrial cancer risk is also convincing.[33–35] Obesity has been found consistently to be associated with a two- to fivefold increase in endometrial cancer risk in both pre- and postmenopausal women in a majority of cohort and case-control studies conducted in various countries.[33–35,37,41,44,69,124–131] Only two case-control studies observed no association.[132,133] Obesity has been estimated to account for 39% of endometrial cancer in European women.[35] Most studies observed a linear increase in risk with increasing BMI,[33] and the association was independent of other known risk factors in most studies. The association for older women was generally similar to[124,134,135] or somewhat stronger than for younger women.[70,129] However, one study observed an association only among older women (>60 years old).[136] One study identified a greater obesity-related risk increase among nonsmokers than among current smokers.[130] Several studies that assessed WHR, waist-to-thigh circumference ratio (WTR), and skinfold thickness also indicated a positive association.[129,137–140] Although some studies suggested that WHR or WTR influenced the risk independent of BMI,[129,138] other studies found that the association disappeared once the results were adjusted for BMI.[137,139,140] Large body weight among postmenopausal women was also found to increase the risk of hyperplasia of the endometrium.[126]

Body weight at early adulthood was not, or just weakly, associated with endometrial cancer risk.[129,134,136,138,139,141–143] However, one study found a similar magnitude of association as at late adulthood.[125] Weight gain during adult life substantially increased endometrial cancer risk in most studies that assessed adult weight gain[125,129,134,136,138,139,141,142] with a linear dose-dependent pattern.[33] However, studies that presented both crude and adjusted results showed that the association of risk with weight gain disappeared or became much weaker after adjusting for recent BMI or weight.[125,134] One study showed no increase in unadjusted risk.[143]

### 26.4.4 KIDNEY CANCER

Obesity has been consistently associated with an increased risk of renal cell cancer.[33–35] Of all the cohort and case-control studies[37,41,46,47] and reviews[33,34,144] examined, all but one study[145] demonstrated a more than twofold increase in renal-cell cancer risk among obese men and women compared with those of normal weight, with a dose–response effect. However, no association has been observed for cancer of the renal pelvis.[146,147] These studies were conducted on various populations in North America, northern and southern Europe, Asia, and Australia. The summary relative risk estimate from 14 studies on each sex in a meta-analysis was 1.07 (95% confidence interval 1.04 to 1.09) for men and 1.07 (95% confidence interval 1.05 to 1.09) for women per unit of increase of BMI.[144] It is estimated that 27% of the renal cell cancer cases among American men and 29% among women could be related to overweight and obesity.[144]

Some studies reported a stronger association among women than men;[148–153] however, the meta-analysis of 14 studies on each sex revealed no evidence of effect modification by sex, and BMI is equally strongly associated with the risk of renal cell cancer among men and women.[144] The meta-analyses also found comparable strengths of association of obesity with renal cell cancer between cohort studies and case-control studies, between small and large studies, between studies conducted in the U.S. and in other countries, and between studies adjusted and not adjusted for smoking.[144]

### 26.4.5 PROSTATE CANCER

The evidence of a link between prostate cancer incidence and obesity is insufficient: 13 cohort studies reported a small or modest positive association[37,43,44,154–163] and 12 other cohort studies, 6 of which were included in the three reviews, did not.[33–35,41,46,69,164–166] For case-control studies, only 4 studies observed a modest increase in prostate cancer risk associated with BMI[47,167–169] and others found no association with BMI;[33–35] one study found an inverse association with BMI.[170] Among the studies reporting a positive association with obesity, the association is stronger for, or restricted to, fatal or more aggressive tumors or is stronger with mortality than with incidence.[156–158,160,162] One meta-analysis of 6 studies of incident cases produced a modest relative risk of 1.01 (95% confidence interval 1.00 to 1.02) per unit of increase in BMI.[35] Two studies suggested that the larger effect found in men aged 50 to 59 years than in other age groups[154] and the increased risk only among those who never drank alcohol[47] might partly explain the inconsistent findings among studies.

Only a few studies examined the influence of abdominal obesity on prostate cancer risk. One case-control study conducted in China found no association with usual adult BMI, but an excess risk with high levels of WHR[171] and another study observed a nonsignificant increase in metastatic prostate cancer risk.[172]

Although epidemiological studies have not consistently shown that obesity is a risk factor for prostate cancer incidence, studies of mortality from prostate cancer have more clearly reported a positive association.[37,155,157,160,161] Some studies also suggested that a higher BMI has been associated with higher-grade prostate tumors, non-organ-confined disease, disease progression,[174] and poor prognosis.[173]

### 26.4.6 ADENOCARCINOMA OF THE ESOPHAGUS AND GASTRIC CARDIA

A limited number of cohort[44,175] and case-control studies[176–182] have consistently linked obesity with increased risk of adenocarcinoma of the esophagus and gastric cardia. Two case-control studies reported no association,[183,184] and one case-control study in Northern China suggested an inverse association between BMI and risk.[185]

The association between BMI and risk of adenocarcinoma of the esophagus and cardia is strong, as indicated by the 2.7 relative risk summary estimate of a meta-analysis[34] of seven studies.[175–181,184] The observed association seems not to be explained by bias and confounding.[33] The association also seems stronger for adenocarcinoma of the esophagus than of the cardia.[177,178,181] However, no association with BMI was reported for esophageal squamous cell carcinoma.[175,177,178,181]

## 26.4.7 OVARIAN CANCER

Results for the association between obesity and ovarian cancer risk are inconsistent.[33] However, a systematic review of 13 hospital case-control studies, 11 population case-control studies, and 5 cohort studies published through 2001 concluded that the evidence supports a small to moderate positive association between high BMI and ovarian cancer risk.[186] Seven cohort studies[37,69,187–191] and five case-control studies[47,192–195] were published later. Two cohort studies of mortality[37,187] and one cohort study of incidence[188] observed an increased risk with higher adult BMI. One cohort study identified a higher risk of ovarian cancer with higher WHR.[189]

The timing of overweight may be a risk modifier and may account for some of the inconsistent results. The Iowa Women's Health study found that higher BMI in early adulthood (but not current BMI) increased the risk of ovarian cancer.[189] An increased risk associated with higher BMI in adolescence and young adulthood but not in older women was also indicated in a large Norwegian cohort study.[190] A significantly increased risk associated with higher BMI at age 18 and for most of adult life, but not with change of weight between age 18 and adult life, was shown in one large case-control study with 1269 cases.[192] Two cohort studies found no association between recent BMI and ovarian cancer risk.[69,191] Although one case-control study indicated a positive association with recent BMI,[47] two others found no association with recent BMI for the overall group[193,194] but a significant positive association among premenopausal women[193] with BMI at age 30[194] and with higher WHR.[194]

High BMI was strongly related to risk of serous borderline ovarian cancer in three case-control studies,[186,193,195] especially among premenopausal women.[193] However, one nested case-control study suggested an inverse relation of risk with BMI.[196]

Among studies that examined BMI-related risk of ovarian cancer by menopause separately, a positive association was found among premenopausal women only in two studies[191,193] and among both groups in one study.[186] One study of mortality found that the increased risk with obesity was limited to women who had never used postmenopausal estrogen and was not seen among ever users.[187]

## 26.4.8 PANCREATIC CANCER

Although there have been limited studies published on this issue, a meta-analysis of six case-control studies and eight cohort studies provided evidence that obesity may be weakly associated with the risk of pancreatic cancer.[197] This meta-analysis observed a summary relative risk per unit increase in BMI of 1.02 (95% confidence interval 1.01 to 1.03). The estimates were slightly higher for studies that had adjusted for smoking and for case-control studies that had not used proxy respondents.[197] Of the four studies that were not included in the meta-analysis, both cohort studies[41,44] and one case-control study[47] suggested a positive association, whereas one case-control study conducted in China indicated a nonsignificant positive association.[198]

Although some studies found that the associations were of similar magnitude for men and women,[44,47,198–200] others suggested a larger effect of obesity on risk among men than among women.[41,201] One study observed a similar effect of obesity among white and black.[200]

### 26.4.9 LUNG CANCER

Most cohort[37,43,202–205] and case-control studies [47,206,207] have observed an inverse association between BMI and lung cancer risk. Three cohort studies[41,44,46] found no association and one case-control study[208] a positive relation. The inverse association may be explained by weight loss due to preclinical disease[43,202,204] or a residual confounding effect of smoking.[37,47,202,204,207] However, inconsistent results have been reported: the inverse relation with BMI was stronger among never-smokers in one cohort study[205] and among never-smoking women in another study,[207] and the positive association was found among both never-smokers and former-smokers.[208] The issue of whether BMI is related to lung cancer risk is still controversial.

### 26.4.10 OTHER CANCER SITES

One cohort study and seven case-control studies, including those studies reviewed by the *IARC Handbook*, suggested that overweight or obesity is not significantly associated with testicular cancer risk.[33,47,209,210] A significant positive association with obesity was observed for non-Hodgkin's lymphoma,[37,41,47] multiple myeloma,[37,47,211] and leukemia.[37,44,47] Very few studies have been published on other cancer sites. There are too few studies on these cancer sites to allow a firm conclusion to be drawn.

### 26.4.11 ALL CANCERS COMBINED

The results from several studies suggest that overweight and obesity are associated with the risk of incidence[41,46,47] and death[37,212] from all types of cancer combined. Overweight and obesity may account for 7.7% of all cancer in Canada[47] and 5% in Europe,[35] and in the U.S., for as high as 14% of all deaths from cancer in men and 20% in women.[37]

## 26.5 CONCLUSION

Epidemiological studies provide sufficient evidence that obesity is a risk factor for both cancer incidence and mortality. The evidence supports strong associations of obesity with the risk of cancers of the colon and rectum, breast (in postmenopausal women), endometrium, kidney, esophagus and gastric cardia, as well as weak associations with cancers of the pancreas, ovary, and prostate.

## ACKNOWLEDGMENTS

The authors would like to thank Dr. Shirley Huchcroft for her editing and insightful comments on the manuscript.

## REFERENCES

1. Bray GA. Obesity is a chronic, relapsing neurochemical disease. *Int J Obesity* 2004; 28:34–38.
2. Kopelman PG. Obesity as a medical problem. *Nature* 2000; 404:635–643.
3. World Health Organization. Global strategy on diet, physical activity and health — obesity and overweight. Geneva: World Health Organization; 2003.
4. Haftenberger M, Lahmann PH, Panico S, Gonzalez CA, Seidell JC, Boeing H, Giurdanella MC, Krogh V, Bueno-de-Mesquita HB, Peeters PH, Skeie G, Hjartaker A, Rodriguez M, Quiros JR, Berglund G, Janlert U, Khaw KT, Spencer EA, Overvad K, Tjonneland A, Clavel-Chapelon F, Tehard B, Miller AB, Klipstein-Grobusch K, Benetou V, Kiriazi G, Riboli E, Slimani N. Overweight, obesity and fat distribution in 50- to 64-year-old participants in the European Prospective Investigation into Cancer and Nutrition (EPIC). *Public Health Nutr* 2002; 5:1147–1162.
5. Visscher TLS, Seidell JC. The public health impact of obesity. *Annu Rev Public Health* 2001; 22:355–375.
6. Walker ARP, Adam F, Walker BF. World pandemic of obesity: the situation in Southern African populations. *Public Health* 2001; 115:368–372.
7. Hoffman DJ. Obesity in developing countries: causes and implications. *Food Nutr Agric* 2001; 28:35–44.
8. Flegal KM, Carroll MD, Ogden CL, Johnson CL. Prevalence and trends in obesity among U.S. adults, 1999–2000. *J Am Med Assoc* 2002; 288:1723–1727.
9. Statistics Canada. Canadian Community Health Survey: a first look. *The Daily*, May 8, 2002. Ottawa: Statistics Canada. Cat. No. 11-001E.
10. Wang Y, Monteiro C, Popkin BM. Trends of obesity and underweight in older children and adolescents in the United States, Brazil, China, and Russia. *Am J Clin Nutr* 2002; 75:971–977.
11. Lissau I, Overpaeck MD, Ruan WJ, Due P, Holstein BE, Hediger ML, the Health Behaviour in School-aged Children Obesity Working Group. Body mass index and overweight in adolescents in 13 European countries, Israel, and the United States. *Arch Pediatr Adolesc Med* 2004; 158:27–33.

12. Ogden CL, Flegal KM, Carroll MD, Johnson CL. Prevalence and trends in overweight among U.S. children and adolescents, 1999–2000. *J Am Med Assoc* 2002; 288:1728–1732.

13. Tremblay MS, Katzmarzyk PT, William JD. Temporal trends in overweight and obesity in Canada, 1981–1996. *Int J Obesity Relat Metab Disord* 2002; 26:538–543.

14. Statistics Canada. National Longitudinal Survey of Children and Youth: Childhood Obesity 1994–1999. *The Daily*, October 18, 2002.

15. Field AE, Coakley EH, Must A, Spadano JL, Laird N, Dietz WH, Rimm E, Colditz GA. Impact of overweight on the risk of developing common chronic diseases during a 10-year period. *Arch Intern Med* 2001; 161:1581–1586.

16. Engeland A, Bjorge T, Selmer RM, Tverdal A. Height and body mass index in relation to total mortality. *Epidemiology* 2003; 14:293–299.

17. Biggard J, Tjonneland A, Thomsen BL, Overvad K, Keitmann BL, Sorensen TI. Waist circumference, BMI, smoking, and mortality in middle-aged men and women. *Obesity Res* 2003; 11:895–903.

18. Lahmann PH, Lissner L, Gullberg B, Gerglund G. A prospective study of adiposity and all-cause mortality: the Malmo Diet and Cancer Study. *Obesity Res* 2002; 10:361–369.

19. Calle EE, Thun MJ, Petrelli JM, Rodriguez C, Heath CW Jr. Body mass index and mortality in a prospective cohort of U.S. adults. *N Engl J Med* 1999; 341:1097–1105.

20. Allison DB, Fontaine KR, Manson JE, Stevens J, VanItallie TB. Annual deaths attributable to obesity in the United States. *J Am Med Assoc* 1999; 282:1530–1538.

21. Banegas JR, Lopez-Garcia E, Gutierrez-Fisac JL, Guallar-Castillon P, Rodriguez-Artalejo F. A simple estimate of mortality attributable to excess weight in the European Union. *Eur J Clin Nutr* 2003; 57:201–208.

22. Fontaine KR, Redden DT, Wang C, Westfall AO, Allison DB. Years of life lost due to obesity. *J Am Med Assoc* 2003; 289:187–193.

23. Peeters A, Barendregt JJ, Willekens F, Mackenbach JP, Al Mamun A, Bonneux L, the Netherlands Epidemiology and Demography Compression of Morbidity Research Group. Obesity in adulthood and its consequences for life expectancy: a life-table analysis. *Ann Intern Med* 2003; 138:24–32.

24. Schwimmer JB, Burwinkle TM, Varni JW. Health-related quality of life of severely obese children and adolescents. *J Am Med Assoc* 2003; 289:1813–1819.

25. Engeland A, Bjorge T, Sogaard AJ, Tverdal A. Body mass index in adolescence in relation to total mortality: 32-year follow-up of 227,000 Norwegian boys and girls. *Am J Epidemiol* 2003; 157:517–523.

26. Jeffrey M, McCarron P, Gunnell D, McEwen J, Smith GD. Body mass index in early and mid-adulthood, and subsequent mortality: a historical cohort study. *Int J Obesity* 2003; 27:1391–1397.

27. Narbro K, Agren G, Jonsson E, Naslund I, Sjostrom L, Peltonen M. Pharmaceutical costs in obese individuals. Comparison with a randomly selected population sample and long-term changes after conventional and surgical treatment: the SOS Intervention Study. *Arch Intern Med* 2002; 162:2061–2069.

28. Kuriyama S, Tsuji I, Ohkubo T, Anzai Y, Takahashi K, Watanabe Y, Nishino Y, Hisamichi S. Medical care expenditure associated with body mass index in Japan: the Ohsaki study. *Int J Obesity* 2002; 26:1069–1074.

29. Colditz GA. Economic costs of obesity and inactivity. *Med Sci Sports Exerc* 1999; 31:S663–S667.
30. Josefson D. Obesity and inactivity fuel global cancer epidemic. *Br Med J* 2001; 322:945.
31. Centers for Disease Control, National Center for Chronic Disease Prevention and Health Promotion. Physical activity and good nutrition: essential elements to prevent chronic diseases and obesity 2003. *Nutr Clin Care* 2003; 6:135–138.
32. Birmingham CL, Muller JL, Palepu A, Spinelli JJ, Anis AH. The cost of obesity in Canada. *Can Med Assoc J* 1999; 160:483–488.
33. *IARC Handbooks of Cancer Prevention*. Vol 6. Weight control and physical activity. Lyons, France: International Agency for Research on Cancer; 2002.
34. Bianchini F, Kaaks R, Vainio H. Overweight, obesity, and cancer risk. *Lancet Oncol* 2002; 3:565–574.
35. Bergstrom A, Pisani P, Tenet V, Wolk A, Adami HO. Overweight as an avoidable cause of cancer in Europe. *Int J Cancer* 2001; 91:421–430.
36. MacInnis RJ, English DR, Hopper JL, Haydon AM, Gertig DM, Giles GG. Body size and composition and colon cancer risk in men. *Cancer Epidemiol Biomarkers Prev* 2004; 13:553–559.
37. Calle EE, Rodriguez C, Walker-Thurmond K, Thun MJ. Overweight, obesity, and mortality form cancer in a prospectively studied cohort of U.S. adults. *N Engl J Med* 2003; 348:1625–1638.
38. Shimizu N, Nagata C, Shimizu H, Kametani M, Takeyama N, Ohnuma T, Matsushita S. Height, weight, and alcohol consumption in relation to the risk of colorectal cancer in Japan: a prospective study. *Br J Cancer* 2003; 88:1038–1043.
39. Terry PD, Miller AB, Rohan TE. Obesity and colorectal cancer risk in women. *Gut* 2002; 51:191–194.
40. Terry P, Giovannucci E, Bergkvist L, Holmerg, Wolk A. Body weight and colorectal cancer risk in a cohort of Swedish women: relation varies by age and cancer site. *Br J Cancer* 2001; 85:346–349.
41. Wolk A, Gridley G, Svensson M, Nyren O, McLaughlin JK, Fraumeni JF, Adami HO. A prospective study of obesity and cancer risk (Sweden). *Cancer Causes Control* 2001; 12:13–21.
42. Schoen RE, Tangen CM, Kuller LH, Burke GL, Cushman M, Tracy RP, Dobs A, Savage PJ. Increased blood glucose and insulin, body size, and incident colorectal cancer. *J Natl Cancer Inst* 1999; 91:1147–1154.
43. Chyou PH, Nomura AM, Stemmermann GN. A prospective study of weight, body mass index and other anthropometric measurements in relation to site-specific cancers. *Int J Cancer* 1994; 57:313–317.
44. Moller H, Mellemgaard A, Lindvig K, Olsen JH. Obesity and cancer risk: a Danish record-linkage study. *Eur J Cancer* 1994; 30A:344–350.
45. Lee IM, Paffenbarger RS Jr. Quetelet's index and risk of colon cancer in college alumni. *J Natl Cancer Inst* 1992; 84:1326–1331.
46. Nomura A, Heilbrun LK, Stemmermann GN. Body mass index as a predictor of cancer in men. *J Natl Cancer Inst* 1985; 74:319–323.
47. Pan SY, Johnson KC, Ugnat AM, Wen SW, Mao Y, the Canadian Cancer Registries Epidemiology Research Group. Association of obesity and cancer risk in Canada. *Am J Epidemiol* 2004; 159:259–268.

48. Slattery ML, Ballard-Barbash R, Edwards S, Cann BJ, Potter JD. Body mass index and colon cancer: an evaluation of modifying effects of estrogen (United States). *Cancer Causes Control* 2003; 14:75–84.

49. Lund Nilsen TI, Vatten LJ. Prospective study of colorectal cancer risk and physical activity, diabetes, blood glucose and BMI: exploring the hyperinsulinaemia hypothesis. *Br J Cancer* 2001; 84:417–422.

50. Boutron-Ruault MC, Senesse P, Meance S, Belghiti C, Faivre J. Energy intake, body mass index, physical activity, and the colorectal adenoma-carcinoma sequence. *Nutr Cancer* 2001; 39:50–57.

51. Munoz SE, Navarro A, Lantieri MJ, Fabro ME, Peyrano MG, Ferraron M, Decarli A, La Vecchia C, Eynard AR. Alcohol, methylxanthine-containing beverages, and colorectal cancer in Cordoba, Argentina. *Eur J Cancer Prev* 1998; 7:207–213.

52. Martinez ME, Giovannucci E, Spiegelman D, Hunter DJ, Willett WC, Colditz GA. Leisure-time physical activity, body size, and colon cancer in women. *J Natl Cancer Inst* 1997; 89:948–955.

53. Giovannucci E, Ascherio A, Rimm EB, Colditz GA, Stampfer MJ, Willett WC. Physical activity, obesity, and risk for colon cancer and adenoma in men. *Ann Intern Med* 1995; 122:327–334.

54. Russo A, Franceschi S, La Vecchia C, Dal Maso L, Montella M, Conti E, Giacosa A, Falcini F, Negri E. Body size and colorectal-cancer risk. *Int J Cancer* 1998; 78:161–165.

55. Caan BJ, Coates AO, Slattery ML, Potter JD, Quesenberry CP Jr, Edwards SM. Body size and the risk of colon cancer in a large case-control study. *Int J Obesity* 1998; 22:178–184.

56. Le Marchand L, Wilkens LR, Kolonel LN, Hankin JH, Lyu LC. Associations of sedentary lifestyle, obesity, smoking, alcohol use, and diabetes with the risk of colorectal cancer. *Cancer Res* 1997; 57:4787–4797.

57. Dietz AT, Newcomb PA, Marcus PM, Storer BE. The association of body size and large bowel cancer risk in Wisconsin (United States) women. *Cancer Causes Control* 1995; 6:30–36.

58. Le Marchand L, Wilkens LR, Mi MP. Obesity in youth and middle age and risk of colorectal cancer in men. *Cancer Causes Control* 1992; 3:349–354.

59. Terry MB, Neugut AI, Bostick RM, Sandler RS, Haile RW, Jacobson JS, Fenoglio-Preiser CM, Potter JD. Risk factors for advanced colorectal adenomas: a pooled analysis. *Cancer Epidemiol Biomarkers Prev* 2002; 11:622–629.

60. Kono S, Handa K, Hayabuchi H, Kiyohara C, Inoue H, Narugame T, Shinomiya S, Hamada H, Onuma K, Koga H. Obesity, weight gain and risk of colon adenomas in Japanese men. *Jpn J Cancer Res* 1999; 90:805–811.

61. Bird CL, Frankl HD, Lee ER, Haile RW. Obesity, weight gain, large weight changes, and adenomatous polyps of the left colon and rectum. *Am J Epidemiol* 1998; 147:670–680.

62. Giovannucci E, Colditz GA, Stampfer MJ, Willett WC. Physical activity, obesity, and risk of colorectal adenoma in women (United States). *Cancer Causes Control* 1996; 7:253–263.

63. Davidow AL, Neugut AI, Jacobson JS, Ahsan H, Garbowski GC, Forde KA, Treat MR, Waye JD. Recurrent adenomatous polyps and body mass index. *Cancer Epidemiol Biomarkers Prev* 1996; 5:313–315.

64. Honjo S, Kono S, Shinchi K, Wakabayashi K, Todoroki I, Sakurai Y, Imanishi K, Nishikawa H, Ogawa S, Katsurada M. The relation of smoking, alcohol use and obesity to risk of sigmoid colon and rectal adenomas. *Jpn J Cancer Res* 1995; 86:1019–1026.

65. Shinchi K, Kono S, Honjo S, Todoroki I, Sakurai Y, Imanishi K, Nishikawa H, Ogawa S, Katsurada M, Hirohata T. Obesity and adenomatous polyps of the sigmoid colon. *Jpn J Cancer Res* 1994; 85:479–484.

66. Neugut AI, Lee WC, Gardowski GC, Waye JD, Forde KA, Treat MR, Fenoglio-Preiser C. Obesity and colorectal adenomatous polyps. *J Natl Cancer Inst* 1991; 83:359–361.

67. Little J, Logan RF, Hawtin PG, Hardcastle JD, Turner ID. Colorectal adenomas and energy intake, body size and physical activity: a case-control study of subjects participating in the Nottingham faecal occult blood screening programme. *Br J Cancer* 1993; 67:172–176.

68. Day Stephenson G, Rose DP. Breast cancer and obesity: an update. *Nutr Cancer* 2003; 45:1–16.

69. Jonsson F, Wolk A, Pedersen NL, Lichtenstein P, Terry P, Ahlbom A, Feychting M. Obesity and hormone-dependent tumors: cohort and co-twin control studies based on the Swedish twin registry. *Int J Cancer* 2003; 106:594–599.

70. Tornberg SA, Carstensen JM. Relationship between Quetelet's index and cancer of breast and female genital tract in 47,000 women followed for 25 years. *Br J Cancer* 1994; 69:358–361.

71. Yoo KY, Tajima K, Park SK, Kang D, Kim SU, Hirose K, Takeuchi T, Miura S. Postmenopausal obesity as a breast cancer risk factor according to estrogen and progesterone receptor status (Japan). *Cancer Lett* 2001; 167:57–63.

72. Lam PB, Vacek PM, Geller BM, Muss HB. The association of increased weight, body mass index and tissue density with the risk of breast carcinoma in Vermont. *Cancer* 2000; 89:369–375.

73. Huang Z, Willett WC, Colditz GA, Hunter DJ, Manson JE, Rosner B, Speizer FE, Hankinson SE. Waist circumference, waist:hip ratio, and risk of breast cancer in the Nurses' Health Study. *Am J Epidemiol* 1999; 150:1316–1324.

74. Ziegler RG, Hoover RN, Nomura AMY, West DW, Wu AH, Pike MC, Lake AJ, Horn-Ross PL, Kolonel LN, Siiteri PK, Fraumeni JF Jr. Relative weight, weight change, height, and breast cancer risk in Asian-American women. *J Natl Cancer Inst* 1996; 88:650–660.

75. Mayberry RM. Age-specific patterns of association between breast cancer and risk factors in black women, ages 20 to 39 and 40 to 54. *Ann Epidemiol* 1994; 4:205–213.

76. Chu SY, Lee NC, Wingo PA, Senie RT, Greenberg RS, Peterson HB. The relationship between body mass and breast cancer among women enrolled in the Cancer and Steroid Hormone Study. *J Clin Epidemiol* 1991; 44:1197–1206.

77. Wenten M, Gilliland FD, Baumgartner K, Samet JM. Associations of weight, weight change, and body mass with breast cancer risk in Hispanic and non-Hispanic white women. *Ann Epidemiol* 2002; 12:435–444.

78. Shu XO, Jin F, Shi JR, Potter JD, Brinton LA, Hebert JR, Ruan Z, Gao YT, Zheng W. Association of body size and fat distribution with risk of breast cancer among Chinese women. *Int J Cancer* 2001; 94:449–455.

79. Sonnenschein E, Toniolo P, Terry MB, Bruning PF, Kato I, Koenig KL, Shore RE. Body fat distribution and obesity in pre- and postmenopausal breast cancer. *Int J Epidemiol* 1999; 28:1026–1031.

80. Mannisto S, Pietinen P, Pyy M, Palmgren J, Eskelinen M, Uusitupa M. Body-size indicators and risk of breast cancer according to menopause and estrogen-receptor status. *Int J Cancer* 1996; 68:8–13.

81. Swanson CA, Coates RJ, Schoenberg JB, Malone KE, Gammon MD, Stanford JL, Shorr IJ, Potischman NA, Brinton LA. Body size and breast cancer risk among women under age 45 years. *Am J Epidemiol* 1996; 143:698–706.

82. Franceschi S, Favero A, La Vecchia C, Baron AE, Negri E, Dal Maso L, Giacosa A, Montella M, Conti E, Amadori D. Body size indices and breast cancer risk before and after menopause. *Int J Cancer* 1996; 67:181–186.

83. Bruning PF, Bonfrer JM, Hart AA, van Noord PA, van der Hoeven H, Collette HJ, Battermann JJ, de Jong-Bakker M, Nooijen WJ, de Waard F. Body measurements, estrogen availability and the risk of human breast cancer: a case-control study. *Int J Cancer* 1992; 51:14–19.

84. Vatten LJ, Kvinnsland S. Prospective study of height, body mass index and risk of breast cancer. *Acta Oncol* 1992; 31:195–200.

85. Kaaks R, Van Noord PAH, Den Tonkelaar ID, Peeters PHM, Riboli E, Grobbee DE. Breast-cancer incidence in relation to height, weight and body-fat distribution in the Dutch "DOM" cohort. *Int J Cancer* 1998; 76:647–651.

86. Hirose K, Tajima K, Hamajima N, Takezaki T, Inoue M, Kuroishi T, Miura S, Tokudome S. Effect of body size on breast-cancer among Japanese women. *Int J Cancer* 1999; 80:349–355.

87. Huang Z, Hankinson SE, Colditz GA, Stampfer MJ, Hunter DJ, Manson JE, Hennekens CH, Rosner B, Speizer FE, Willett WC. Dual effects of weight and weight gain on breast cancer risk. *J Am Med Assoc* 1997; 278:1407–1411.

88. Coates RJ, Uhler RJ, Hall HI, Potischman N, Brinton LA, Ballard-Barbash R, Gammon MD, Brogan DR, Daling JR, Malone KE, Schoenberg JB, Swanson CA. Risk of breast cancer in young women in relation to body size and weight gain in adolescence and early adulthood. *Br J Cancer* 1999; 81:167–174.

89. Peacock SL, White E, Daling JR, Voigt LF, Malone KE. Relation between obesity and breast cancer in young women. *Am J Epidemiol* 1999; 149:339–346.

90. Brinton LA, Swanson CA. Height and weight at various age and risk of breast cancer. *Ann Epidemiol* 1992; 2:597–609.

91. Feigelson HS, Jonas CR, Teras LR, Thun MJ, Calle EE. Weight gain, body mass index, hormone replacement therapy, and postmenopausal breast cancer in a large prospective study. *Cancer Epidemiol Biomarkers Prev* 2004; 13:220–224.

92. Lahmann PH, Lissner L, Gullberg B, Olsson H, Berglund G. A prospective study of adiposity and postmenopausal breast cancer risk: the Malmo Diet and Cancer Study. *Int J Cancer* 2003; 103:246–252.

93. Morimoto LM, White E, Chen Z, Chlebowski RT, Hays J, Kuller L, Lopez AM, Manson J, Margolis KL, Muti PC, Stefanick ML, McTiernan A. Obesity, body size, and risk of postmenopausal breast cancer: the Women's Health Initiative (United States). *Cancer Causes Control* 2002; 13:741–751.

94. Galanis DJ, Kolonel LN, Lee J, Le Marchand L. Anthropometric predictors of breast cancer incidence and survival in multi-ethnic cohort of female residents of Hawaii United States. *Cancer Causes Control* 1998; 9:217–224.

95. Sellers TA, Kushi LH, Potter JD, Kaye SA, Nelson CL, McGovern PG, Folsom AR. Effect of family history, body-fat distribution, and reproductive factors on the risk of postmenopausal breast cancer. *N Engl J Med* 1992; 326:1323–1329.

96. Carpenter CL, Ross RK, Paganini-Hill A, Bernstein L. Effect of family history, obesity and exercise on breast cancer risk among postmenopausal women. *Int J Cancer* 2003; 106:96–102.

97. Li CI, Malone KE, Porter PL, Weiss NS, Tang MT, Daling JR. Reproductive and anthropometric factors in relation to the risk of lobular and ductal breast carcinoma among women 65–79 years of age. *Int J Cancer* 2003; 107:647–651.

98. Li CI, Stanford JL, Daling JR. Anthropometric variables in relation to risk of breast cancer in middle-aged women. *Int J Epidemiol* 2000; 29:208–213.

99. Shoff SM, Newcomb PA, Trentham-Dietz A, Remington PL, Mittendorf R, Greenberg R, Willett WC. Early-life physical activity and postmenopausal breast cancer: effect of body size and weight change. *Cancer Epidemiol Biomarkers Prev* 2000; 9:591–595.

100. Magnusson C, Baron J, Persson I, Wolk A, Bergstrom R, Trichopoulso D, Adami HO. Body size in different periods of life and breast cancer risk in postmenopausal women. *Int J Cancer* 1998; 76:29–34.

101. La Vecchia C, Negri E, Franceschi S, Talamini R, Bruzzi P, Palli D, Decarli A. Body mass index and post-menopausal breast cancer: an age-specific analysis. *Br J Cancer* 1997; 75:441–444.

102. Enger SM, Ross RK, Paganini-Hill A, Carpenter CL, Bernstein L. Body size, physical activity, and breast cancer hormone receptor status: results from two case-control studies. *Cancer Epidemiol Biomarkers Prev* 2000; 9:681–687.

103. Barnes-Josiah D, Potter J, Sellers T, Himes J. Early body size and subsequent weight gain as predictors of breast cancer incidence (Iowa, United States). *Cancer Causes Control* 1995; 6:112–118.

104. Folsom AR, Kaye SA, Prineas RJ, Potter JD, Gapshur SM, Wallace RB. Increased incidence of carcinoma of the breast associated with abdominal adiposity in postmenopausal women. *Am J Epidemiol* 1990; 131:794–803.

105. Trentham-Dietz A, Newcomb P, Egan K, Tirus-Ernstoff L, Baron J, Storer B, Stampfer M, Willett W. Weight change and risk of postmenopausal breast cancer (United States). *Cancer Causes Control* 2000; 11:533–542.

106. Harris RE, Namboodiri KK, Wynder EL. Breast cancer risk: effects of estrogen replacement therapy and body mass. *J Natl Cancer Inst* 1992; 84:1575–1582.

107. Lubin F, Ruder AM, Wax Y, Modan B. Overweight and changes in weight throughout adult life in breast cancer etiology. A case-control study. *Am J Epidemiol* 1985; 122:579–588.

108. Friedenreich C, Courneya K, Bryant H. Case-control study of anthropometric measures and breast cancer risk. *Int J Cancer* 2002; 99:445–452.

109. van den Brandt PA, Spiegelman D, Yaun SS, Adami HO, Beeson L, Folsom AR, Goldbohm RA, Graham S, Kushi L, Marshall JR, Miller AB, Rohan T, Smith-Warner SA, Speizer FE, Willett WC, Wolk A, Hunter DJ. Pooled analysis of prospective cohort studies on height, weight and breast cancer risk. *Am J Epidemiol* 2000; 152:514–527.

110. Cui Y, Whiteman MK, Flaws JA, Langenberg P, Tkaczuk KH, Bush TL. Body mass and stage of breast cancer at diagnosis. *Int J Cancer* 2002; 98:279–283.

111. Moorman PG, Jones BA, Millikan RC, Hall IJ, Newman B. Race, anthropometric factors, and stage at diagnosis of breast cancer. *Am J Epidemiol* 2001; 153:284–291.

112. Hall HI, Coates RJ, Uhler RJ, et al. Stage of breast cancer in relation to body mass index and bra cup size. *Int J Cancer* 1999; 82:23–27.

113. Jones BA, Kasi SV, Curnen MG, Owens PH, Dubrow R. Severe obesity as an explanatory factor for the black/white difference in stage at diagnosis of breast cancer. *Am J Epidemiol* 1997; 146:394–404.

114. Reeves MJ, Newcomb PA, Remington PL, Marcus PM, MacKenzie WR. Body mass and breast cancer — relationship between method of detection and stage of disease. *Cancer* 1996; 77:301–307.

115. Wee CC, McCarthy EP, Davis RB, Phillips RS. Screening for cervical and breast cancer: is obesity an unrecognized barrier to preventive care? *Ann Intern Med* 2000; 132:697–704.

116. Arndt V, Sturmer T, Stegmaier C, et al. Patient delay and stage of diagnosis among breast cancer patients in Germany — a population-based study. *Br J Cancer* 2002; 86:1034–1040.

117. Richardson JL, Langholz B, Bernstein L, et al. Stage and delay in breast cancer diagnosis by race, socioeconomic status, age and year. *Br J Cancer* 1992; 65:922–926.

118. Schrijvers CT, Mackenbach JP, Lutz JM, Quinn MJ, Coleman MP. Deprivation and survival from breast cancer. *Br J Cancer* 1995; 72:738–743.

119. Chlebowski RT, Aiello E, McTiernan A. Weight loss in breast cancer patient management. *J Clin Oncol* 2002; 20:1128–1143.

120. Berclaz G, Li S, Price KN, Coates AS, Castiglione-Gertsch M, Rudenstam CM, Holmberg SB, Lindtner J, Erien D, Collins J, Snyder R, Thurlimann B, Fey MF, Mendiola C, Dudley Werner I, Simoncini E, Crivellari D, Gelber RD, Goldhirsch A. Body mass index as a prognostic feature in operable breast cancer: the International Breast Cancer Study Group experience. *Ann Oncol* 2004; 15:875–884.

121. Daling JR, Malone KE, Doody DR, Johnson LG, Gralow JR, Porter PL. Relation of body mass index to tumor markers and survival among young women with invasive ductal breast carcinoma. *Cancer* 2001; 92:720–729.

122. Carmichael AR, Bendall S, Lockerbie L, Prescott RJ, Bates T. Does obesity compromise survival in women with breast cancer? *Breast* 2004; 13:93–96.

123. Dignam JJ, Wieand K, Johnson KA, Fisher B, Xu L, Mamounas EP. Obesity, tamoxifen use, and outcomes in women with estrogen receptor-positive early-stage breast cancer. *J Natl Cancer Inst* 2003; 95:1467–1476.

124. Furberg AS, Thune I. Metabolic abnormalities (hypertension, hyperglycemia and overweight), lifestyles (high energy intake and physical inactivity) and endometrial cancer risk in a Norwegian cohort. *Int J Cancer* 2003; 104:669–676.

125. Terry P, Baron JA, Weiderpass E, Yuen J, Lichtenstein P, Nyren O. Lifestyle and endometrial cancer risk: a cohort study from the Swedish twin registry. *Int J Cancer* 1999; 82:38–42.

126. Baanders-van Halewyn EA, Blankenstein MA, Thijssen JHH, de Ridder CM, de Waard F. A comparative study of risk factors for hyperplasia and cancer of the endometrium. *Eur J Cancer Prev* 1996; 5:105–112.

127. Horn-Ross PL, John EM, Canchola AJ, Stewart SL, Lee MM. Phytoestrogen intake and endometrial cancer risk. *J Natl Cancer Inst* 2003; 95:1158–1164.

128. Augustin LSA, Gallus S, Bosetti C, Levi F, Negri E, Franceschi S, Dal Maso L, Jenkins DJA, Kendall CWC, La Vecchia C. Glycemic index and glycemic load in endometrial cancer. *Int J Cancer* 2003; 105:404–407.

129. Xu W, Dai Q, Ruan Z, Cheng J, Jin F, Shu X. Obesity at different ages and endometrial cancer risk factors in urban Shanghai, China. *Zhonghua Liu Xing Bing Xue Za Zhi* 2002; 23:347–351.

130. Newcomer LM, Newcomb PA, Trentham-Dietz A, Storer BE. Hormonal risk factors for endometrial cancer: modification by cigarette smoking (United States). *Cancer Causes Control* 2001; 12:829–835.

131. Niwa K, Imai A, Hashimoto M, Yokoyama Y, Mori H, Matsuda Y, Tamaya T. A case-control study of uterine endometrial cancer of pre- and post-menopausal women. *Oncol Rep* 2000; 7:89–93.

132. Parslov M, Lidegaard O, Klintorp S, Pedersen B, Jonsson L, Eriksen PS, Ottesen B. Risk factors among young women with endometrial cancer: a Danish case-control study. *Am J Obstet Gynecol* 2000; 182(1 Pt 1):23–29.

133. Koumantaki Y, Tzonou A, Koumantakis E, Kaklamani E, Aravantinos D, Trichopoulos D. A case-control study of cancer of endometrium in Athens. *Int J Cancer* 1989; 43:795–799.

134. La Vecchia C, Franceschi S, Decarli A, Gallus G, Tognoni G. Risk factors for endometrial cancer at different ages. *J Natl Cancer Inst* 1984; 73:667–671.

135. Le Marchand L, Wilkens LR, Mi MP. Early-age body size, adult weight gain and endometrial cancer risk. *Int J Cancer* 1991; 48:807–811.

136. Goodman MT, Hankin JH, Wilkens LR, Lyu LC, McDuffie K, Liu LQ, Kolonel LN. Diet, body size, physical activity, and the risk of endometrial cancer. *Cancer Res* 1997; 57:5077–5085.

137. Swanson CA, Potischman N, Wilbanks GD, Twiggs LB, Mortel R, Berman ML, Barrett RJ, Baumgartner RN, Brinton LA. Relation of endometrial cancer risk to past and contemporary body size and body fat distribution. *Cancer Epidemiol Biomarkers Prev* 1993; 2:321–327.

138. Shu XO, Brinton LA, Zheng W, Swanson CA, Hatch MC, Gao YT, Fraumeni JF Jr. Relation of obesity and body fat distribution to endometrial cancer in Shanghai, China. *Cancer Res* 1992; 52:3865–3870.

139. Austin H, Austin JM Jr, Partridge EE, Hatch KD, Shingleton HM. Endometrial cancer, obesity, and body fat distribution. *Cancer Res* 1991; 51:568–572.

140. Olson SH, Trevisan M, Marshall JR, Graham S, Zielezny M, Vena JE, Hellmann R, Freudenheim JL. Body mass index, weight gain, and risk of endometrial cancer. *Nutr Cancer* 1995; 23:141–149.

141. Weiderpass E, Persson I, Adami HO, Magnusson C, Lindgren A, Baron JA. Body size in different periods of life, diabetes mellitus, hypertension, and risk of post-menopausal endometrial cancer (Sweden). *Cancer Causes Control* 2000; 11:185–192.

142. Hirose K, Tajima K, Hamajima N, Kuroishi T, Kuzuya K, Miura S, Tokudome S. Comparative case-referent study of risk factors among hormone-related female cancers in Japan. *Jpn J Cancer Res* 1999; 90:255–261.

143. Levi F, La Vecchia C, Negri E, Parazzini F, Franceschi S. Body mass at different ages and subsequent endometrial cancer risk. *Int J Cancer* 1992; 50:567–571.

144. Bergstrom A, Hsieh CC, Lindblad P, Lu CM, Cook NR, Wolk A. Obesity and renal cell cancer — a quantitative review. *Br J Cancer* 2001; 85:984–990.

145. Talamini R, Baron AE, Barra S, Bidoli E, La Vecchia C, Negri E, Serraino D, Franceschi S. A case-control study of risk factor for renal cell cancer in northern Italy. *Cancer Causes Control* 1990; 1:125–131.

146. Chow WH, Gridley G, Fraumeni JF, Jarvholm B. Obesity, hypertension, and the risk of kidney cancer in men. *N Engl J Med* 2000; 343:1305–1311.

147. McCredie M, Stewart JH. Risk factors for kidney cancer in New South Wales, Australia. II. Urologic disease, hypertension, obesity, and hormonal factors. *Cancer Causes Control* 1992; 3:323–331.

148. Heath CW Jr, Lally CA, Calle EE, McLaughlin JK, Thun MJ. Hypertension, diuretics, and antihypertensive medications as possible risk factors for renal cell cancer. *Am J Epidemiol* 1997; 145:607–613.

149. Chow WH, McLaughlin JK, Mandel JS, Wacholder S, Niwa S, Fraumeni JF Jr. Obesity and risk of renal cell cancer. *Cancer Epidemiol Biomarkers Prev* 1996; 5:17–21.

150. Mellemgaard A, Lindblad P, Schlehofer B, Bergstrom R, Mandel JS, McCredie M, McLaughlin JK, Niwa S, Odaka N, Pommer W, et al. International renal-cell cancer study. III. Role of weight, height, physical activity, and use of amphetamines. *Int J Cancer* 1995; 60:350–354.

151. Kreiger N, Marrett LD, Dodds L, Hilditch S, Darlington GA. Risk factors for renal cell carcinoma: results of a population-based case-control study. *Cancer Causes Control* 1993; 4:101–110.

152. Benhamou S, Lenfant MH, Ory-Paoletti C, Flamant R. Risk factors for renal cell carcinoma in a French case-control study. *Int J Cancer* 1993; 55:32–36.

153. McLaughlin JK, Gao YT, Gao RN, Zheng W, Ji BT, Blot WJ, Fraumeni JF Jr. Risk factors for renal cell cancer in Shanghai, China. *Int J Cancer* 1992; 52:562–565.

154. Engeland A, Tretli S, Bjorge T. Height, body mass index, and prostate cancer: a follow-up of 950,000 Norwegian men. *Br J Cancer* 2003; 89:1237–1242.

155. Rodriguez C, Patel AV, Calle EE, Jacobs EJ, Thun MJ. Body mass index, height and prostate cancer mortality in two large cohorts of adult men in the United States. *Cancer Epidemiol Biomarkers Prev* 2001; 10:345–353.

156. Putnam SD, Cerhan JR, Parker AS, Bianchi GD, Wallace RB, Cantor KP, Lynch CF. Lifestyle and anthropometric risk factors for prostate cancer in a cohort of Iowa men. *Ann Epidemiol* 2000; 10:361–369.

157. Andersson SO, Wolk A, Bergstrom R, Adami HO, Engholm G, Englund A, Nyren O. Body size and prostate cancer: a 20-year follow-up study among 135,006 Swedish construction workers. *J Natl Cancer Inst* 1997; 89:385–389.

158. Cerhan JR, Torner JC, Lynch CF, Rubenstein LM, Lemke JH, Cohen MB, Lubaroff DM, Wallace RB. Association of smoking, body mass, and physical activity with risk of prostate cancer in the Iowa 65+ Rural Health Study (United States). *Cancer Causes Control* 1997; 8:229–238.

159. Thompson MM, Garland C, Barrett-Connor E, Khaw KT, Friedlander NJ, Wingard DL. Heart disease risk factors, diabetes, and prostate cancer in an adult community. *Am J Epidemiol* 1989; 129:511–517.

160. Snowdon DA, Phillips RL, Choi W. Diet, obesity, and risk of fatal prostate cancer. *Am J Epidemiol* 1984; 120:244–250.

161. Lew EA, Garfinkel L. Variations in mortality by weight among 750,000 men and women. *J Chronic Dis* 1979; 32:563–576.

162. MacInnis RJ, English DR, Gertig DM, Hopper JL, Giles GG. Body size and composition and prostate cancer risk. *Cancer Epidemiol Biomarkers Prev* 2003; 12:1417–1421.

163. Thune I, Lund E. Physical activity and the risk of prostate and testicular cancer: a cohort study of 53,000 Norwegian men. *Cancer Causes Control* 1994; 5:549–556.

164. Giovannucci E, Rimm EB, Liu Y, Leitzmann M, Wu K, Stampfer MJ, Willett WC. Body mass index and risk of prostate cancer in U.S. health professionals. *J Natl Cancer Inst* 2003; 95:1240–1244.

165. Lee IM, Sesso HD, Paffenbarger RS Jr. A prospective cohort study of physical activity and body size in relation to prostate cancer risk (United States). *Cancer Causes Control* 2001; 12:187–193.

166. Habel LA, Van Den Eeden SK, Friedman GD. Body size, age at shaving initiation, and prostate cancer in a large, multiracial cohort. *Prostate* 2000; 43:136–143.

167. Gronberg H, Damber L, Damber JE. Total food consumption and body mass index in relation to prostate cancer risk: a case-control study in Sweden with prospectively collected exposure data. *J Urol* 1996; 155:969–974.

168. Talamini R, La Vecchia C, Decarli A, Negri E, Franceschi S. Nutrition, social factors and prostatic cancer in a Northern Italian population. *Br J Cancer* 1986; 53:817–821.

169. Key TJ, Silcocks PB, Davey GK, Appleby PN, Bishop DT. A case-control study of diet and prostate cancer. *Br J Cancer* 1997; 76:678–687.

170. Sung JFC, Lin RS, Pu YS, Chen YC, Chang HC, Lai MK. Risk factors for prostate carcinoma in Taiwan. A case-control study in a Chinese population. *Cancer* 1999; 86:484–491.

171. Hsing AW, Deng J, Sesterhenn IA, Mostofi FK, Stanczyk FZ, Benichou J, Xie T, Gao YT. Body size and prostate cancer: a population-based case-control study in China. *Cancer Epidemiol Biomarkers Prev* 2000; 9:1335–1341.

172. Giovannucci E, Rimm EB, Stampfer MJ, Colditz GA, Willett WC. Height, body weight, and risk of prostate cancer. *Cancer Epidemiol Biomarkers Prev* 1997; 6:557–563.

173. Neugut AI, Chen AC, Petrylak DP. The "skinny" on obesity and prostate cancer prognosis. *J Clin Oncol* 2004; 22:395–398.

174. Furuya Y, Akimoto S, Akakura K, Ito H. Smoking and obesity in relation to the etiology and disease progression of prostate cancer in Japan. *Int J Urol* 1998; 5:134–137.

175. Tretli S, Robsahm TE. Height, weight and cancer of the oesophagus and stomach: a follow-up study in Norway. *Eur J Cancer Prev* 1999; 8:115–122.

176. Cheng KK, Sharp L, McKinney PA, Logan RFA, Chilvers CED, Cook-Mozaffari P, Ahmed A, Day NE. A case-control study of oesophageal adenocarcinoma in women: a preventable disease. *Br J Cancer* 2000; 83:127–132.

177. Lagergren J, Bergstrom R, Nyren O. Association between body mass and adenocarcinoma of the esophagus and gastric cardia. *Ann Intern Med* 1999; 130:883–890.

178. Chow WH, Blot WJ, Vaughan TL, Risch HA, Gammon MD, Stanford JL, Dubrow R, Schoenberg JB, Mayne ST, Farrow DC, Ahsan H, West AB, Rotterdam H, Niwa S, Fraumeni JF Jr. Body mass index and risk of adenocarcinomas of the esophagus and gastric cardia. *J Natl Cancer Inst* 1998; 90:150–155.

179. Ji BT, Chow WH, Yang G, McLaughlin JK, Gao RN, Zheng W, Shu XO, Jin F, Fraumeni JF Jr, Gao YT. Body mass index and the risk of cancers of the gastric cardia and distal stomach in Shanghai, China. *Cancer Epidemiol Biomarkers Prev* 1997; 6:481–485.

180. Brown LM, Swanson CA, Gridely G, Swanson GM, Schoenberg JB, Greenberg RS, Silverman DT, Pottern LM, Hayes RB, Scheartz AG, et al. Adenocarcinoma of the esophagus: role of obesity and diet. *J Natl Cancer Inst* 1995; 87:104–109.

181. Vaughan TL, Davis S, Kristal A, Thomas DB. Obesity, alcohol, and tobacco as risk factors for cancers of the esophagus and gastric cardia: adenocarcinoma versus squamous cell carcinoma. *Cancer Epidemiol Biomarkers Prev* 1995; 4:85–92.

182. Wu AH, Wan P, Bernstein L. A multiethnic population-based study of smoking, alcohol and body size and risk of adenocarcinomas of the stomach and esophagus (United States). *Cancer Causes Control* 2001; 12:721–732.

183. Zhang ZF, Kurtz RC, Sun M, Karpeh M Jr, Yu GP, Gargon N, Fein JS, Georgopoulos SK, Harlap S. Adenocarcinomas of the esophagus and gastric cardia: medical conditions, tobacco, alcohol, and socioeconomic factors. *Cancer Epidemiol Biomarkers Prev* 1996; 5:761–768.

184. Kabat GC, Ng SK, Wynder EL. Tobacco, alcohol intake, and diet in relation to adenocarcinoma of the esophagus and gastric cardia. *Cancer Causes Control* 1993; 4:123–132.

185. Zhang J, Su SQ, Wu XJ, Liu YH, Wang H, Zong XN, Wang Y, Ji JF. Effect of body mass index on adenocarcinoma of gastric cardia. *World J Gastroenterol* 2003; 9:2658–2661.

186. Purdie DM, Bain CJ, Webb PM, Whiteman DC, Pirozzo S, Green AC. Body size and ovarian cancer: case-control study and systematic review (Australia). *Cancer Causes Control* 2001; 12:855–863.

187. Rodriguez C, Calle EE, Fakhrabadi-Shokoohi D, Jacobs EJ, Thun MJ. Body mass index, height, and the risk of ovarian cancer mortality in a prospective cohort of postmenopausal women. *Cancer Epidemiol Biomarkers Prev* 2002; 11:822–828.

188. Schouten LJ, Goldbouhm RA, van den Brandt PA. Height, weight, weight change, and ovarian cancer risk in the Netherlands cohort study on Diet and Cancer. *Am J Epidemiol* 2003; 157:424–433.

189. Anderson JP, Ross JA, Folsom AR. Anthropometric variables, physical activity, and incidence of ovarian cancer. *Cancer* 2004; 100:1515–1521.

190. Engeland A, Tretli S, Bjorge T. Height, body mass index, and ovarian cancer: a follow-up of 1.1 million Norwegian women. *J Natl Cancer Inst* 2003; 95:1244–1248.

191. Fairfield KM, Willett WC, Rosner BA, Manson JE, Speizer FE, Hankinson SE. Obesity, weight gain, and ovarian cancer. *Obstet Gynecol* 2002; 100:288–296.

192. Lubin F, Chetrit A, Freedman LS, Alfandary E, Fishler Y, Nitzan H, Zultan A, Modan B. Body mass index at age 18 years and during adult life and ovarian cancer risk. *Am J Epidemiol* 2003; 157:113–120.

193. Kuper H, Cramer DW, Tirus-Ernstoff L. Risk of ovarian cancer in the United States in relation to anthropometric measures: does the association depend on menopausal status? *Cancer Causes Control* 2002; 13:455–463.

194. Dal Maso L, Franceschi S, Negri E, Conti E, Montella M, Vaccarella S, Canzonieri V, Parazzini F, La Vecchia C. Body size indices at different ages and epithelial ovarian cancer risk. *Eur J Cancer* 2002; 38:1769–1774.

195. Riman T, Dichman PW, Nilsson S, Correia N, Nordlinder H, Magnusson CM, Persson IR. Risk factors for epithelial borderline ovarian tumors: results of Swedish case-control study. *Gynecol Oncol* 2001; 83:575–585.

196. Lukanova A, Toniolo P, Lundin E, et al. Body mass index in relation to ovarian cancer: a multi-centre nested case-control study. *Int J Cancer* 2002; 99:603–608.

197. Berrington de Gonzalez A, Sweetland S, Spencer E. A meta-analysis of obesity and the risk of pancreatic cancer. *Br J Cancer* 2003; 89:519–523.

198. Ji BT, Hatch MC, Chow WH, McLaughlin JK, Dai Q, Howe GR. Anthropometric and reproductive factors and the risk of pancreatic cancer: a case-control study in Shanghai, China. *Int J Cancer* 1996; 66:432–437.

199. Michaud DS, Giovannucci E, Willett WC, Colditz GA, Stampfer MJ, Fuchs CS. Physical activity, obesity, height, and the risk of pancreatic cancer. *J Am Med Assoc* 2001; 286:921–929.

200. Silverman DT, Swanson CA, Gridley G, Wacholder S, Greenberg RS, Brown LM, Hayes RB, Swanson GM, Schoenberg RS, Pottern LM, Schwartz AG, Fraumeni JF Jr, Hoover RN. Dietary and nutritional factors and pancreatic cancer: a case-control study on direct interviews. *J Natl Cancer Inst* 1998; 90:1710–1719.

201. Gapstur SM, Gann PH, Lowe W, Liu K, Colangelo L, Dyer A. Abnormal glucose metabolism and pancreatic cancer mortality. *J Am Med Assoc* 2000; 283:2552–2558.

202. Henley SJ, Flanders WD, Manatunga A, Thun MJ. Leanness and lung cancer risk: fact or artifact? *Epidemiology* 2002; 13:268–276.

203. Kark JD, Yaari S, Rasooly I, Goldbourt U. Are lean smokers at increased risk of lung cancer? The Israel Civil Servant Cancer Study. *Arch Intern Med* 1995; 155:2409–2416.

204. Drinkard CR, Sellers TA, Potter JD, Zheng W, Bostick RM, Nelson CL, Folsom AR. Association of body mass index and body fat distribution with risk of lung cancer in older women. *Am J Epidemiol* 1995; 142:600–607.

205. Knekt P, Heliovaara M, Rissanen A, Aromaa A, Seppanen R, Teppo L, Pukkala E. *Int J Cancer* 1991; 49:208–213.

206. Goodman MT, Wilkens LR. Relation of body size and the risk of lung cancer. *Nutr Cancer* 1993; 20:179–186.

207. Kabat GC, Wynder EL. Body mass index and lung cancer risk. *Am J Epidemiol* 1992; 135:769–774.

208. Rauscher GH, Mayne ST, Janerich DT. Relation between body mass index and lung cancer risk in men and women never and former smokers. *Am J Epidemiol* 2000; 152:506–513.

209. Richiardi L, Askling J, Granath F, Akre O. Body size at birth and adulthood and the risk for germ-cell testicular cancer. *Cancer Epidemiol Biomarkers Prev* 2003; 12:669–673.

210. Davies TW, Prener A, Engholm G. Body size and cancer of the testis. *Acta Oncol* 1990; 29:287–290.

211. Friedman GD, Herrinton LK, Stemmermann GN. Obesity and multiple myeloma. *Cancer Causes Control* 1994; 5:479–483.

212. Okasha M, McCarron P, McEwen P, Davey Smith G. Body mass index in young adulthood and cancer mortality: a retrospective cohort study. *J Epidemiol Community Health* 2002; 56:780–784.

# 27 Obesity as a Cancer Risk Factor: Potential Mechanisms of Action

*Henry J. Thompson, Weiqin Jiang, and Zongjian Zhu*

## CONTENTS

27.1 Introduction ..................................................................................565
27.2 Obesity: A Misdirected Focus of Attention? ...................................567
27.3 Revisiting a Misunderstood Paradigm and a New Working
Hypothesis ...................................................................................567
27.4 A Specific Model for Energy Balance, Weight Gain, and
Cancer Risk ..................................................................................568
27.5 Cellular Processes and Carcinogenesis ..........................................569
27.6 Cell Proliferation .........................................................................570
27.7 Apoptosis ....................................................................................571
27.8 Vascularization ............................................................................571
27.9 Candidate Chemical Mediators .....................................................572
    27.9.1 Adrenal Cortical Steroids ..................................................572
    27.9.2 Insulin and Insulin-Like Growth Factors ............................573
27.10 Summary .....................................................................................574
Acknowledgments ..................................................................................574
References .............................................................................................575

## 27.1 INTRODUCTION

Obesity is an operationally defined stage in a disease process characterized by the accumulation of body fat due to an excess of energy intake relative to energy expenditure (Figure 27.1A).[1] Accumulation of energy in the body is referred to as positive energy balance (PEB). In the adult, a lifestyle characterized by chronic PEB leads to the development of obesity.

The prevalence of obesity is increasing at an unprecedented rate,[2,3] and the occurrence of this disorder in humans is reported to be associated with an increased risk for a number of chronic diseases including several types of cancer.[4]

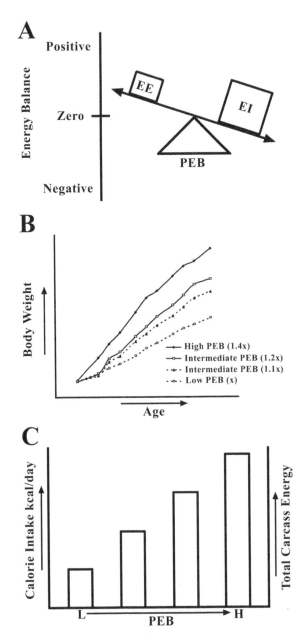

**FIGURE 27.1** (A) When energy intake (EI) is greater than energy expenditure (EE), a condition of positive energy balance (PEB) exists. (B) Animals in PEB grow at rates proportional to the magnitude of PEB. (C) EE is held relatively constant in most preclinical experiments using rodents. When this is the case, the magnitude of PEB (low, L, to high, H) is proportional to the level of caloric intake. During the course of an experiment, the levels of caloric intake and PEB are proportional to total carcass energy.

This chapter reviews mechanisms that may account for the perceived risk for cancer associated with obesity based on data drawn from preclinical models for cancer.

## 27.2 OBESITY: A MISDIRECTED FOCUS OF ATTENTION?

Although there is a natural tendency to focus on the relationship between obesity per se and the development of cancer, the designation of the obese state is arbitrary, i.e., an operational definition, and indicates only that a particular magnitude of excess energy accumulation, frequently measured as body weight relative to height, has been attained in a disease process that in most cases has been ongoing for many years. The thesis presented in this chapter is that the cause-and-effect relationship between energy accumulation in the body and cancer risk is initiated at an early stage in the misregulation of energy balance resulting in obesity. Moreover, while there may be effects of the obese state on the manifestations of clinically detectable cancer or cancer treatment outcomes,[4] the extrapolation of such effects to understanding how chronic PEB affects cancer risk may obscure critical relationships and/or generate false leads about candidate mechanisms that relate to cancer risk. Consistent with this viewpoint is the report of an expert panel on the role of weight control and physical activity in cancer prevention; it was concluded that adult weight gain in excess of 5 kg is associated with an increased risk for cancer.[4] For individuals that have maintained a body mass index below 25 as they enter adulthood, this margin of excess weight gain would not be sufficient to qualify an individual as obese. Moreover, while the number of preclinical studies in which experimental models for obesity and cancer have been combined to investigate the obesity–cancer risk hypothesis is limited, the results of those studies designed to investigate the role of body fat, i.e., obesity per se, failed to support a direct relationship between body fatness and the occurrence of cancer in the model systems investigated.[5–8] Thus, rather than proposing that a relationship exists between obesity per se and cancer risk, both the preclinical and clinical data argue that a more appropriate statement of the relationship is that cancer risk is associated with PEB.

## 27.3 REVISITING A MISUNDERSTOOD PARADIGM AND A NEW WORKING HYPOTHESIS

There is a substantial body of preclinical literature that has a direct bearing on the PEB–cancer risk hypothesis, but the existence of this evidence is obscured by misconception. As noted in two recent reviews,[9,10] dietary energy restriction (DER) is a powerful physiological approach to the prevention of cancer and DER also reduces the risk for other chronic diseases and is associated with increased longevity and de-acceleration of the process of aging. However, there is an understandable perception that DER is a model for starvation, famine, and/or profound undernutrition. While the scientific literature, particularly prior to 1980, is replete with examples of experiments in which it can legitimately be argued that this was the case, there also is a body of preclinical data on DER in which experiments have been carefully designed so that the magnitude of PEB is altered by regulating the amount of energy ingested while providing animals the same amounts of all other dietary components.[11] Moreover, in some experiments this approach has been refined by introducing the concept of meal feeding all animals in an experiment.[12] While experimental approaches in which meal feeding is used are not novel, the application of this approach in cancer research is limited. Most investigators conducting DER–cancer studies provide food to restricted animals once per day whereas *ad libitum* fed animals that serve as the control group are given unlimited access to food. Using this traditional approach, *ad libitum* fed animals will eat throughout a 24-hour period, the so-called nibbling pattern of food intake, whereas energy-restricted animals consume most of their diet soon after it is delivered to the food cup. The time in which the food provided is eaten varies, depending on the magnitude of energy restriction, but for an animal given 60% of *ad libitum* intake, which is the most common level of restriction investigated, the food is consumed within 2 hours. After the day's allotment of food is eaten, the animals then remain fasted until the next daily feeding. On the other hand, by meal feeding both *ad libitum* and restricted-fed animals the same number of meals per day for the same duration, the potential effects of differential patterns of eating are minimized and the pattern of food intake better reflects the meal feeding behavior typical in human populations.

Given the observations put forward in the preceding paragraph, the working hypothesis formulated for this discussion of mechanisms is that studies of DER, when they use dietary formulations as defined in Reference 12, and particularly when patterns of meal feeding are standardized among experimental groups, actually provide a model for identifying the consequences of PEB that, if left unchecked, will result in overweight and obesity. As with most concepts, a variant of this idea was actually advanced in 1987.[13,14] However, this idea is not reflected in current reports on DER or obesity and cancer risk; it is hoped that this restatement of the concept will promote a new analysis and consideration of its tenets.

## 27.4  A SPECIFIC MODEL FOR ENERGY BALANCE, WEIGHT GAIN, AND CANCER RISK

Given that the risk for breast cancer in women has been reported to have a significant association with obesity,[4] and that the majority of preclinical studies of the PEB–cancer risk hypothesis have been conducted using experimental models for breast cancer,[10] the review of mechanisms presented in this chapter is based on studies of experimentally induced breast cancer. Nonetheless, the mechanisms discussed are likely to be applicable to cancer at organ sites other than the breast because the underlying mechanism or mechanisms responsible for the energy balance–cancer linkage appear unlikely to be driven by effects on the metabolism of sex steroid hormones.[15–17] Rather, available data indicate that such effects are secondary and may serve to amplify the primary effects of different states of energy balance on chemical mediators that modulate cancer risk depending on the responsiveness to these hormones of the target tissue of interest.

As reported in References 11 and 12, female rats fed 60 to 90% of the number of calories consumed by their counterparts allowed to eat *ad libitum* for the same number of meals and same duration of time each day do not lose weight (Figure 27.1B). Rather, they are in PEB and grow at a constant, albeit slower, rate depending on the number of calories consumed per day. Animals with slower rates of growth also experience a lower rate of other chronic diseases and live markedly longer. Animals in these different states are being maintained on different planes of PEB. For this discussion, animals that consume 40% fewer calories than animals fed *ad libitum* are referred to as having a low PEB (LPEB) and provide a model to identify and study mechanisms that may be operative in individuals that limit weight gain resulting in the accumulation of body fat by monitoring their caloric intake and balancing it with energy expenditure. On the other hand, animals eating *ad libitum* experience a high PEB (HPEB) providing a model to identify and study mechanisms relevant to the effects of increased energy availability on the carcinogenic process. In subsequent paragraphs, the candidate mechanisms being reported to account for the effects of different levels of PEB on carcinogenesis are presented with the goal of identifying how PEB affects the process of tissue size homeostasis, the failure of which is a prerequisite for the development of cancer.

## 27.5 CELLULAR PROCESSES AND CARCINOGENESIS

Carcinogenesis is characterized by a failure in the regulation of tissue size homeostasis in which a clone of transformed cells achieves growth advantage due to an increased rate of cell proliferation and/or a decreased rate of cell death in comparison to neighboring populations of cells.[18,19] The development of a carcinoma can be considered a failure of tissue size regulation attributed to the formation, selection, expansion, and progression of clones of transformed cells.[18] In addition, it appears that a co-requisite event in the progression of premalignant clones of cells to those diagnosed as malignant is the induction of vascularization.[19] Evidence is now presented that excessive caloric intake (HPEB) creates a permissive environment in which normal controls to cellular proliferation are abrogated, the checks on cell number accumulation by apoptosis are diminished, and restraints on the vascular system to increase blood supply are relaxed (Figure 27.2). Candidate molecular mechanisms and chemical mediators of these cellular conditions also are discussed.

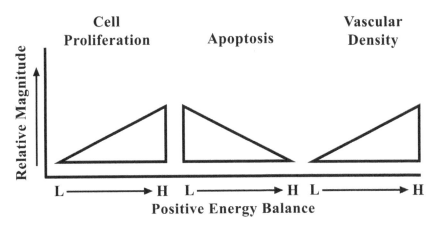

**FIGURE 27.2** The level of positive energy balance has differential effects on three cellular processes, the misregulation of which are involved in the carcinogenic process. The relative effects of level of positive energy balance, low (L) to high (H) on these processes, are shown.

## 27.6  CELL PROLIFERATION

Rates of cell proliferation are generally low in populations of mammary epithelial cells at low risk for the development of cancer, but during premalignant and malignant stages of this disease process, cell proliferation is markedly increased.[20] In animals maintained on LPEB, rates of cell proliferation remain low despite that cells harbor the genetic defects requisite for the development of cancer. On the other hand, HPEB is associated with increased rates of cell proliferation.[20,21] Emerging evidence indicates that LPEB results in the arrest of the cycle cell at the $G_1$/S transition.[22] Mammary carcinomas that emerge in LPEB-treated rats are only 15% the size of age-matched carcinomas that occur in animals receiving HPEB. By using these carcinomas to mirror the effects of LPEB on the carcinogenic process, levels of phosphorylated Rb and E2F-1 were observed to be significantly reduced by LPEB.[23] Reductions in CDK2 and CDK4 kinase activity in LPEB carcinomas were likely to account for the observed effects on Rb and E2F-1. Both Cip1/p21 and Kip1/p27 and levels of these proteins complexed with CDK2 were significantly elevated in LPEB carcinomas, and levels of cyclin E were reduced. On the other hand, regulation of CDK4 kinase activity by LPEB was likely due to a reduction in cyclin D1 protein as well as increased binding of P16 and P19 to CDK4. The majority of changes induced were reported to be reversed when animals were changed to HPEB. Thus, it appears that HPEB is permissive to increases in levels of cyclin D and E and to lower levels of proteins in the Kip/Cip and p16 families of CKIs; these effects work in concert to promote higher levels of activity of the cyclin D–CDK4 and cyclin E–CDK2 complexes. Such changes result in the phosphorylation of the Rb protein and the release of E2F and related transcription factors, all of which support the sustained increase in cell proliferation that is considered a prerequisite for the development of cancer.

These observations are consistent with the hypothesis that HPEB, which unchecked will lead to overweight and obesity, increases cancer risk by perpetuating an environment permissive to the deregulation of the cell cycle that is characteristic of carcinogenesis.

## 27.7 APOPTOSIS

Apoptosis is a critical process in the regulation of tissue size, and defects in this cell death pathway are a prerequisite for the clinical manifestation of cancer.[19] Available data indicate that LPEB favors the maintenance of constraints on the expansion of cell populations through the upregulation of cellular machinery that facilitates the activation of caspases and the suppression of caspase inhibitors. LPEB has been reported to induce apoptosis in both premalignant and malignant mammary gland pathologies,[20] and the pathway by which cell death was induced has been investigated[24] using the experimental approach reported in Reference 25. By using caspase activity assays, it was shown that the activities of caspases 9 and 3 were elevated approximately twofold in carcinomas from LPEB rats compared to carcinomas from animals receiving HPEB, whereas caspase 8 activity was similar in carcinomas from both groups. This finding implies that LPEB induces the mitochondrial pathway of apoptosis activation, and is consistent with the finding that levels of Bcl-2 and Bcl-XL protein were significantly lower and levels of Bax and Apaf-1 were elevated in carcinomas from LPEB vs. HPEB treated animals. Expression levels of transcripts for IAP1, IAP2, X-linked IAP, and survivin, proteins that can block the activity of activated caspases, were also found to be significantly lower in mammary carcinomas from LPEB vs. HPEB animals. Thus, HPEB favors a growth environment that is permissive to the expansion of both nontransformed and transformed cell populations within a tissue. Given that HPEB is permissive to suppression of apoptotic pathways and the relaxation of cell cycle restraints observed in transformed cell populations, it is not surprising that the magnitude of the PEB has been reported to be proportional to the magnitude of the carcinogenic response.[12]

## 27.8 VASCULARIZATION

Spatial limitations on the diffusion of nutrients and metabolic wastes between the vascular system and the cells that it supplies impose restraints on the growth of both nontransformed and transformed cell populations.[19] Vascular supply to a tissue and its component cells can be induced via the expansion in size of existing blood vessels and/or the formation of new vessels. As reported in Reference 26, premalignant mammary pathologies (PMMP) and mammary adenocarcinomas (AC) from LPEB vs. HPEB maintained animals were assessed for pathology associated differences in vascularity. The density of blood vessels associated with premalignant mammary pathologies, as well as the density of blood vessels in immediate proximity to mammary carcinomas, was lower in animals maintained on LPEB vs. HPEB, although PEB had no effect on intratumoral vascular density. However, it remains unclear whether these differences in vascular density were due to differences in concentrations of growth factors required for maintenance or growth of blood vessels or to the inability of endothelial cells to respond to growth factors when LPEB is maintained. Efforts to identify effects of PEB on the expression of an array of genes involved in vascularization were inconclusive, although the evidence suggested involvement of signaling pathways of which vascular endothelial growth factor (VEGF) is a component.[26] Based on the effects of PEB on vascular density, it can be inferred that LPEB imposes limitations on the supply of nutrients to and elimination of wastes from developing pathologies; these limitations could exert direct effects on cell proliferation and apoptosis in transformed epithelial cell populations undergoing clonal selection and expansion. HPEB appears to relax restraints to vascularization thereby maintaining an environment conducive to the expansion of cell populations. This effect is consistent with a positive association between energy balance and the risk for cancer.

## 27.9  CANDIDATE CHEMICAL MEDIATORS

For a comprehensive review of potential chemical mediators of the effects of energy balance on carcinogenesis, the reader is referred to References 4 and 27. In this section, discussion is limited to one prominent mechanism that could account, at least in part, for the effects of PEB on cell proliferation, apoptosis, and vascularization that were summarized in preceding sections.

Available energy in the form of high-energy phosphate bonds is essential for life and a primary source of energy-rich compounds formed during metabolism is glucose. There are well established but frequently overlooked effects of PEB on glucose homeostasis. In general, LPEB reduces dietary carbohydrate availability, whereas HPEB is associated with dietary carbohydrate available in amounts in excess of that needed to support basal metabolic rate. For glucose homeostasis to be maintained under different PEBs, there are marked differences in circulating levels of insulin, insulin-like growth factors (IGFs), and adrenal cortical steroids in LPEB vs. HPEB. The following evidence indicates that these differences in part may account for the effects of PEB on cancer risk.

### 27.9.1  ADRENAL CORTICAL STEROIDS

As early as 1949, a role was hypothesized for the adrenal gland in accounting for the effects of LPEB in preventing tumor development,[28] and as reported in Reference 12 in comparison to HPEB, LPEB has been shown to increase urinary excretion of immunoreactive adrenal cortical steroids and levels of urinary corticosteroids were reported to be inversely associated with mammary carcinoma multiplicity. These observations were followed by a series of reports by the same laboratory.[22,29,30] Briefly, it was shown both *in vivo*[22,29] and *in vitro*[30] that provision of supplemental corticosterone has effects on cell proliferation but not apoptosis that are similar to those observed in response to LPEB. In particular, corticosterone induced higher levels of the CKI p27 and lower levels of cyclin D1, effects that would be expected to occur when cell cycle progression is arrested at the $G_1/S$ transition. However, two recently published observations from this laboratory raise questions about the degree to which increased adrenal cortical steroid activity alone accounts for the protective effects of LPEB against mammary carcinogenesis.[31,32] They are (1) in an animal study in which dietary corticosterone was fed to rats at a concentration that increased plasma corticosterone to levels comparable to those observed in animals that were LPEB, mammary carcinogenesis was inhibited, but the degree of inhibition was markedly less than observed in response to LPEB; and (2) unlike observations reported in Reference 33, adrenalectomy failed to negate the inhibitory activity of LPEB against mammary carcinogenesis.

### 27.9.2 INSULIN AND INSULIN-LIKE GROWTH FACTORS

Studies in rodents have shown that HPEB accelerates DMBA-induced mammary tumorigenesis in proportion to the magnitude of PEB. In those studies, HPEB was associated with higher plasma insulin levels again in proportion to the magnitude of PEB maintained.[34,35] The relevance of these observations is based in part on reports that the development of DMBA-induced mammary tumors was inhibited by alloxan-induced diabetes and that alloxan- or streptozotocin-induced diabetes in rats caused a regression of 60 to 90% of DMBA-induced mammary tumors.[36–39] Tumor growth was restored and tumor latency reduced upon insulin administration to diabetic rats.

The effects of different PEB that modulate mammary carcinoma development on IGF metabolism have been investigated. In a number of model systems, LPEB is associated with a decrease in circulating levels of IGF-1. For example, Ruggeri and co-workers[34] reported that PEBs that inhibited DMBA-induced mammary tumorigenesis were associated with reduced circulating levels of insulin and IGF-1, but not IGF-II. A causal role of IGF-1 in mediating the protective effects of LPEB was hypothesized; in that paradigm, the effects of PEB were hypothesized to be mediated via a change in the availability of IGF-1, which in turn modulated tissue size homeostasis by decreasing cell proliferation and increasing the rate of apoptosis.[40] Zhu and co-workers have recently reported that protection against cancer is lost, and plasma IGF-1 levels are restored to control values when animals are switched from LPEB to HPEB also supporting a causal role of IGF-1 in accounting for the effects of PEB on the carcinogenic response. However, in a recent work, those investigators found that infusion of recombinant human IGF-1 to LPEB treated animals failed to mimic the effects on the carcinogenic response of switching animals from LPEB to HPEB. Collectively, these data imply a permissive but not obligatory role of insulin and its related growth factors in accounting for the effects of PEB on the carcinogenic response.

## 27.10 SUMMARY

The thesis presented in this chapter is that chronic PEB results in the accumulation of body energy and over time to the development of overweight and obesity. Consequently, efforts to elucidate the linkage between obesity and cancer risk should actually be focused on how energy balance influences the carcinogenic process. The following working hypotheses summarize what is currently known about the mechanisms underlying the role of PEB in the modulation of cancer risk. It is hoped that this will provide a coherent framework upon which to formulate new research initiatives.

HPEB promotes the development of the cancer phenotype by fostering conditions favorable to the clonal expansion of transformed cell populations. It does this by promoting cells to leave the $G_0$ (quiescent) phase of the cell cycle. For cells that enter the cell cycle, HPEB favors cell cycle progression due to its effects on the phosphorylation of Rb and the release of E2F1 from its binding to Rb. Increased phosphorylation of Rb is a consequence of the effects of HPEB on the activity of CDK-4 and CDK-2 per the mechanisms described earlier. In addition, HPEB promotes the maintenance of the cellular anti-apoptotic machinery by inducing changes in the metabolism of the Bcl-2 and IAP families of proteins. It is speculated that the effects of HPEB on cell proliferation and apoptosis affect not only the expansion of transformed clones of mammary epithelial cells, but also the ability of endothelial cells to respond to growth factors that induce vascular expansion. The coordinated regulation of proliferation, apoptosis, and vascularization are responsible for the promotional activity of HPEB on the carcinogenic process.

That the activity of three cellular processes is coordinately regulated suggests that a common molecular mechanism is at work. Again, the hypothesis advanced is that a primary consequence of PEB is its effect on glucose homeostasis. In response to reduced glucose availability, levels of insulin and IGF-1 are reduced and levels of glucocorticoids are increased. One outcome of these changes is the limitation within a tissue of intracellular growth and survival factors. Thus, it is hypothesized that the ultimate regulation of carcinogenesis by PEB can be linked directly to glucose availability. The effects of glucose homeostasis on cancer risk have received only limited attention but clearly merit in-depth investigation.

## ACKNOWLEDGMENTS

The excellent technical assistance of John McGinley in the preparation of this manuscript is greatly appreciated. This work was supported by PHS Grants CA52626 and CA100693 from the National Cancer Institute.

# REFERENCES

1. Clinical Guidelines on the Identification, Evaluation, and Treatment of Overweight and Obesity in Adults. NIH Publication 98-4083; 1998.
2. Mokdad AH, Bowman BA, Ford ES, Vinicor F, Marks JS, Koplan JP. The continuing epidemics of obesity and diabetes in the United States. *J Am Med Assoc* 2001; 286:1195–1200.
3. Statistics Related to Overweight and Obesity. NIH Publication 03-4158, http://www.niddk.nih.gov/health/nutrit/pubs/statobes.htm; 2003.
4. IARC. *Weight Control and Physical Activity.* Lyon: IARC Press; 2002.
5. Klurfeld DM, Lloyd LM, Welch CB, Davis MJ, Tulp OL, Kritchevsky D. Reduction of enhanced mammary carcinogenesis in LA/N-cp (corpulent) rats by energy restriction. *Proc Soc Exp Biol Med* 1991; 196:381–384.
6. Lee WM, Lu S, Medline A, Archer MC. Susceptibility of lean and obese Zucker rats to tumorigenesis induced by *N*-methyl-*N*-nitrosourea. *Cancer Lett* 2001; 162:155–160.
7. Cleary MP, Phillips FC, Getzin SC, Jacobson TL, Jacobson MK, Christensen TA, Juneja SC, Grande JP, Maihle NJ. Genetically obese MMTV-TGF-alpha/Lep(ob)Lep(ob) female mice do not develop mammary tumors. *Breast Cancer Res Treat* 2003; 77:205–215.
8. Cleary MP, Juneja SC, Phillips FC, Hu X, Grande JP, Maihle NJ. Leptin receptor-deficient MMTV-TGF-alpha/Lepr(db)Lepr(db) female mice do not develop oncogene-induced mammary tumors. *Exp Biol Med (Maywood)* 2004; 229:182–193.
9. Hursting SD, Lavigne JA, Berrigan D, Perkins SN, Barrett JC. Calorie restriction, aging, and cancer prevention: mechanisms of action and applicability to humans. *Annu Rev Med* 2003; 54:131–152.
10. Thompson HJ, Zhu Z, Jiang W. Dietary energy restriction in breast cancer prevention. *J Mammary Gland Biol Neoplasia* 2003; 8:133–142.
11. Thompson HJ, Zhu Z, Jiang W. Protection against cancer by energy restriction: all experimental approaches are not equal. *J Nutr* 2002; 132:1047–1049.
12. Zhu Z, Haegele AD, Thompson HJ. Effect of caloric restriction on pre-malignant and malignant stages of mammary carcinogenesis. *Carcinogenesis* 1997; 18:1007–1012.
13. Pariza MW, Boutwell RK. Historical perspective: calories and energy expenditure in carcinogenesis. *Am J Clin Nutr* 1987; 45:151–156.
14. Pariza MW. Dietary fat, calorie restriction, ad libitum feeding, and cancer risk. *Nutr Rev* 1987; 45:1–7.
15. Sylvester PW, Aylsworth CF, Meites J. Relationship of hormones to inhibition of mammary tumor development by underfeeding during the "critical period" after carcinogen administration. *Cancer Res* 1981; 41:1384–1388.
16. Sarkar NH, Fernandes G, Telang NT, Kourides IA, Good RA. Low-calorie diet prevents the development of mammary tumors in C3H mice and reduces circulating prolactin level, murine mammary tumor virus expression, and proliferation of mammary alveolar cells. *Proc Natl Acad Sci USA* 1982; 79:7758–7762.
17. Sinha DK, Gebhard RL, Pazik JE. Inhibition of mammary carcinogenesis in rats by dietary restriction. *Cancer Lett* 1988; 40:133–141.
18. Thompson HJ, Strange R, Schedin PJ. Apoptosis in the genesis and prevention of cancer. *Cancer Epidemiol Biomarkers Prev* 1992; 1:597–602.

19. Hanahan D, Weinberg RA. The hallmarks of cancer. *Cell* 2000; 100:57–70.
20. Zhu Z, Jiang W, Thompson HJ. Effect of energy restriction on tissue size regulation during chemically induced mammary carcinogenesis. *Carcinogenesis* 1999; 20:1721–1726.
21. Lok E, Scott FW, Mongeau R, Nera EA, Malcolm S, Clayson DB. Calorie restriction and cellular proliferation in various tissues of the female Swiss Webster mouse. *Cancer Lett* 1990; 51:67–73.
22. Zhu Z, Jiang W, Thompson HJ. Effect of energy restriction on the expression of cyclin D1 and p27 during premalignant and malignant stages of chemically induced mammary carcinogenesis. *Mol Carcinog* 1999; 24:241–245.
23. Jiang W, Zhu Z, Thompson HJ. Effect of energy restriction on cell cycle machinery in 1-methyl-1-nitrosourea-induced mammary carcinomas in rats. *Cancer Res* 2003; 63:1228–1234.
24. Thompson HJ, Zhu Z, Jiang W. Identification of the apoptosis activation cascade induced in mammary carcinomas by energy restriction. *Cancer Res* 2004; 64:1541–1545.
25. Zhu Z, Jiang W, Thompson HJ. An experimental paradigm for studying the cellular and molecular mechanisms of cancer inhibition by energy restriction. *Mol Carcinog* 2002; 35:51–56.
26. Thompson HJ, McGinley JN, Spoelstra NS, Jiang W, Zhu Z, Wolfe P. Effect of dietary energy restriction on vascular density during mammary carcinogenesis. *Cancer Res* 2004; 64:5643–5650.
27. Hursting SD, Kari FW. The anti-carcinogenic effects of dietary restriction: mechanisms and future directions. *Mutat Res* 1999; 443:235–249.
28. Boutwell RK, Brush MK, Rusch HP. The stimulating effect of dietary fat on carcinogenesis. *Cancer Res* 1949; 9:741–746.
29. Zhu Z, Jiang W, Thompson HJ. Effect of corticosterone administration on mammary gland development and p27 expression and their relationship to the effects of energy restriction on mammary carcinogenesis. *Carcinogenesis* 1998; 19:2101–2106.
30. Jiang W, Zhu Z, Bhatia N, Agarwal R, Thompson HJ. Mechanisms of energy restriction: effects of corticosterone on cell growth, cell cycle machinery, and apoptosis. *Cancer Res* 2002; 62:5280–5287.
31. Jiang W, Zhu Z, McGinley JN, Thompson HJ. Adrenalectomy does not block the inhibition of mammary carcinogenesis by dietary energy restriction in rats. *J Nutr* 2004; 134:1152–1156.
32. Zhu Z, Jiang W, Thompson HJ. Mechanisms by which energy restriction inhibits rat mammary carcinogenesis: *in vivo* effects of corticosterone on cell cycle machinery in mammary carcinomas. *Carcinogenesis* 2003; 24:1225–1231.
33. Pashko LL, Schwartz AG. Reversal of food restriction-induced inhibition of mouse skin tumor promotion by adrenalectomy. *Carcinogenesis* 1992; 13:1925–1928.
34. Ruggeri BA, Klurfeld DM, Kritchevsky D, Furlanetto RW. Caloric restriction and 7,12-dimethylbenz(a)anthracene-induced mammary tumor growth in rats: alterations in circulating insulin, insulin-like growth factors I and II, and epidermal growth factor. *Cancer Res* 1989; 49:4130–4134.
35. Klurfeld DM, Welch CB, Davis MJ, Kritchevsky D. Determination of degree of energy restriction necessary to reduce DMBA-induced mammary tumorigenesis in rats during the promotion phase. *J Nutr* 1989; 119:286–291.

36. Heuson JC, Legros N. Influence of insulin deprivation on growth of the 7,12-dimethylbenz(a)anthracene-induced mammary carcinoma in rats subjected to alloxan diabetes and food restriction. *Cancer Res* 1972; 32:226–232.

37. Cohen ND, Hilf R. Influence of insulin on growth and metabolism of 7,12-dimethylbenz(alpha)anthracene-induced mammary tumors. *Cancer Res* 1974; 34:3245–3252.

38. Hilf R, Hissin PJ, Shafie SM. Regulatory interrelationships for insulin and estrogen action in mammary tumors. *Cancer Res* 1978; 38:4076–4085.

39. Gibson SL, Hilf R. Regulation of estrogen-binding capacity by insulin in 7,12-dimethylbenz(a)anthracene-induced mammary tumors in rats. *Cancer Res* 1980; 40:2343–2348.

40. Kari FW, Dunn SE, French JE, Barrett JC. Roles for insulin-like growth factor-1 in mediating the anti-carcinogenic effects of caloric restriction. *J Nutr Health Aging* 1999; 3:92–101.

# 28 Alcohol and Cancer: Cellular Mechanisms of Action

*Xiang-Dong Wang and Hiroko Inoue-Fruehauf*

## CONTENTS

28.1 Introduction ........................................................................................579
28.2 Multiple Mechanisms Involved in Alcohol-Associated
Carcinogenesis ..................................................................................580
    28.2.1 Increased Generation of Acetaldehyde .................................580
    28.2.2 Induction of Cytochrome P4502E1 and Activation of
    Chemical Procarcinogens ......................................................582
    28.2.3 Generation of Reactive Free Radicals That Cause DNA
    Damage ..................................................................................584
    28.2.4 Impairment of Immune Function .........................................585
    28.2.5 Induction of Cell Hyperproliferation That Promotes
    Genomic Instability ..............................................................586
    28.2.6 Deregulation of Apoptosis and Promotion of
    Tumorigenesis .......................................................................587
    28.2.7 Impaired Nutritional Status ..................................................588
        28.2.7.1 Folate and Vitamin $B_6$ (pyridoxal-5′-phosphate).....588
        28.2.7.2 Selenium and Zinc ..................................................589
        28.2.7.3 Vitamin A ................................................................589
28.3 Summary ............................................................................................590
Acknowledgment ......................................................................................590
References ................................................................................................590

## 28.1 INTRODUCTION

A number of epidemiological studies have indicated that long-term and excessive alcohol consumption is a significant risk factor for upper aerodigestive tract cancers (oropharynx, larynx, esophagus, stomach) and liver cancer.[1,2] High alcohol consumption also increases the risk for other types of cancer, such as colorectal, lung, and breast.[1] In examining the role of alcohol in cancer development, effects of both alcohol and its metabolites have to be considered, as well as other nutritional and lifestyle factors associated with alcoholism.[3] Several mechanisms have been proposed to explain the contribution of chronic alcohol consumption to the alcohol-associated carcinogenesis (Figure 28.1), but these mechanisms need to be further defined at cellular and molecular levels. While alcohol is not considered to be a direct carcinogen, the metabolite acetaldehyde is mutagenic and carcinogenic.[4] More importantly, chronic alcohol intake can induce a number of biochemical and molecular alterations, thereby providing a promoting environment for carcinogenesis. The purpose of this chapter is to summarize the available evidence and hypotheses that address the carcinogenic effects of alcohol and its mechanisms (Figure 28.1).

## 28.2  MULTIPLE MECHANISMS INVOLVED IN ALCOHOL-ASSOCIATED CARCINOGENESIS

### 28.2.1  Increased Generation of Acetaldehyde

Acetaldehyde is probably the most important single mechanism through which alcohol contributes to increased cancer risk.[4] Acetaldehyde is produced as a metabolite from ethanol by the action of cellular alcohol dehydrogenase (ADH), mainly in the liver, but also in peripheral tissues and through the action of bacterial ADH in the colon and saliva.[5] Acetaldehyde is highly reactive and binds rapidly to cellular proteins as well as to DNA, resulting in protein malfunction and formation of stable DNA adducts.[6] It can induce cross-links between DNA molecules and between DNA and proteins. Alterations to DNA by acetaldehyde increase the risk of replication errors and mutations, and trigger replication errors and/or mutations of oncogenes and tumor suppressor genes.[6] Acetaldehyde also exerts direct mutagenic effects on mammalian DNA by causing point mutations, sister chromatid exchanges, and chromosomal aberrations, as demonstrated by *in vitro* experiments.[7,8] Furthermore, acetaldehyde interferes with DNA repair machinery by inhibiting *O*6-methyl-guanyltransferase, an enzyme responsible for the removal of DNA adducts.[9]

High levels of acetaldehyde in saliva have been proposed to contribute to carcinogenesis.[10–12] Even in volunteers who consumed moderate amounts of alcohol, a substantial production of acetaldehyde was detected in their saliva at concentrations (19 to 143 $\mu M$) which could cause mutagenic damage.[10–12] In addition, acetaldehyde contributes significantly to the development of autoimmunity in alcoholic patients through the formation of protein adducts to enzymes, collagen, albumin, hemoglobin, and microtubules.[13] These acetaldehyde-protein adducts can act as autoantigens and mediate inflammatory responses with increases immunoglobulin levels and cellular cytotoxicity, resulting in tissue damage.

The important role for acetaldehyde as a mediator of increased cancer risk in alcoholic individuals is further highlighted by the fact that patients with deficient acetaldehyde metabolism (e.g., through mutations in acetaldehyde

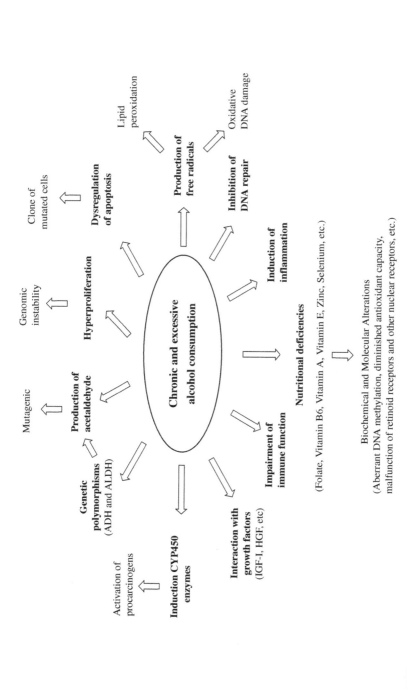

**FIGURE 28.1** Simplified schematic illustration of possible mechanisms for excessive ethanol effects on carcinogenesis. (See the text for more detail.)

dehydrogenase 2, ALDH2, gene) have significantly elevated acetaldehyde levels and increased risk of cancer.[14–16] Inactivating polymorphisms of ALDH2 lead to significantly slowed acetaldehyde metabolism and are strongly associated with esophageal squamous cell carcinoma in Asian drinkers.[14] Patients with ALDH2 polymorphisms also have a higher risk for multiple cancers, especially of the oropharynx and stomach. When the ALDH2 polymorphism occurs in combination with a less active form of ADH2, this risk is further increased.[17] For Caucasians, ADH1 polymorphisms (ADH1C*1) resulting in increased enzyme activity and increased acetaldehyde production lead to higher risk of upper aerodigestive tract and liver cancer in heavy alcohol drinkers.[18] It should be mentioned that ADH plays a role in the oxidation of vitamin A (retinol) to retinoic acid.[19] In the presence of alcohol, the reaction velocity for retinal formation from retinol, the rate-limiting step in the synthesis of retinoic acid, is dramatically reduced through competitive inhibition.[20] Han et al.[21] showed that the retinol-oxidizing activity of ADH1 was 90% inhibited by 5 m$M$ ethanol (blood ethanol levels of 5 to 20 m$M$ are usually reached after social drinking), and the retinol-oxidizing activity of some forms of ADH2 and ADH3 was 60 to 80% inhibited by 20 or 50 m$M$ ethanol (only seen in heavy drinking). Kedishvili et al.[22] showed that the contribution of ADH isozymes to retinoic acid biosynthesis depends on the amount of free retinol in cells, and that physiological levels of ethanol can substantially inhibit the oxidation of retinol by human ADHs. These earlier observations have been substantiated by the demonstration that biosynthesis of retinoic acid following a dose of retinol was reduced by 82% in ADH null mutant mice ($ADH1^{-/-}$).[23] This reduction was similar in magnitude to the inhibition in retinoic acid biosynthesis seen in wild-type mice treated with ethanol (87% decrease). In addition, it has been reported that ethanol inhibits the oxidation of retinol into retinoic acid in the human gastric and esophageal mucosa and rat colon mucosa[24] and the acetaldehyde inhibits the generation of retinoic acid in human prenatal tissue.[25] The importance of the ADH system for the oxidation of retinol to retinoic acid is supported by the observation that retinol oxidation is inhibited to a similar degree in ADH$^{-/-}$ mice as it is after ethanol pretreatment.[20] These studies clearly demonstrate that retinoic acid biosynthesis can be impaired by ethanol via competition for ADH and ALDH, which may contribute to the increased risk of developing certain alcohol-related cancers. This has been shown for the liver and colon, two primary organs affected by cancer in alcoholic patients.[26–28] It has been reported that the presence of an inactivating ADH2 polymorphism leads to slower metabolism of alcohol to acetaldehyde;[16] however, whether the presence of inactivating ADH and ALDH polymorphisms lead to slower conversion of retinol to retinal and, further, to retinoic acid is currently unknown.

### 28.2.2 INDUCTION OF CYTOCHROME P4502E1 AND ACTIVATION OF CHEMICAL PROCARCINOGENS

Chronic alcohol consumption induces cytochrome P450 isoform 2E1 (CYP2E1) in the liver and, to a lesser degree, in other target organs such as the lungs and the mucosal layers of the esophagus and lower gastrointestinal tract.[1] This enzyme, a microsomal cytochrome oxidase, catalyses the conversion of ethanol into acetaldehyde, and is able to metabolize a wide variety of xenobiotics.[29,30] After ethanol consumption, the activity of CYP2E1 is increased to four- to tenfold levels in the liver, with a high rate of individual variation.[31] Activation of CYP2E1 activity can be observed after 1 week at relatively low levels of alcohol intake (40 g/day).[31] It is assumed that CYP2E1 induction after ethanol consumption occurs through two distinct pathways, post-translational mechanisms at low ethanol concentrations, and increased mRNA transcription at high ethanol concentrations.[32] The activation of CYP2E1 may be modulated by hormones and growth factors, but the details regarding this regulation are not yet understood.

The important role for CYP2E1 induction as a link between alcohol abuse and cancer is highlighted by the fact that high CYP2E1 expression has been found in the liver and in peripheral tissues (oral cavity, esophagus, colon, and rectum), which are known from epidemiological studies to have increased risk of cancer formation associated with chronic alcohol consumption.[1,30] In the presence of alcohol, the hepatic first-pass metabolism is reduced for many carcinogens, including nitrosamines. This leads to higher peripheral tissue levels of nitrosamines, which are then activated by mucosal CYP2E1. Inducible expression of CYP2E1 exposes the liver and peripheral tissues to a range of pathogenic and potentially carcinogenic substances due to this enzyme's low substrate specificity.[29] Inducible expression of CYP2E1 leads to generation of reactive and harmful acetaldehyde in peripheral tissues, along with increased oxidative stress.[1] It also exposes the peripheral epithelium to activated carcinogenic metabolites from procarcinogens such as nitrosamines, alkanes, aflatoxin, vinylchloride, and aromatic hydrocarbons, which would otherwise be metabolized in the liver. CYP2E1 induction by alcohol leads to accelerated metabolism of a multitude of therapeutic drugs, thereby leading to increased toxicity in some (e.g., acetaminophen) and decreased therapeutic effect in others (e.g., inhalation anesthetics), a fact that should be considered when drugs are prescribed.[31] For example, chronic ethanol intake increases catabolism of vitamin A (retinol and retinoic acid) into more polar metabolites in the liver.[33–35] Recent studies have shown that the enhanced catabolism of retinol and retinoic acid in ethanol-fed rats can be inhibited by chlormethiazole (an inhibitor of CYP2E1) *in vitro* and *in vivo*,[34,35] indicating that CYP2E1 is the major enzyme responsible for the ethanol-enhanced catabolism of retinoic acid in hepatic tissue after exposure to alcohol. It is possible that CYP2E1 enzyme induction in chronic intermittent drinking could continue to be a factor mediating oxidative stress and destroying retinol and retinoic acid, even after alcohol is cleared. This may provide one explanation for why chronic and excessive alcohol intake is a risk not only for hepatic, but also for extra-hepatic cell proliferation and carcinogenesis, as it has been reported that CYP2E1 is also present and inducible by alcohol in the esophagus, forestomach, and surface epithelium of the proximal colon.[36] It has been shown that treatment with CYP2E1 inhibitors (e.g., chlormethiazole) protects against ethanol-induced liver injury.[37–39] The restoration of hepatic vitamin A status in ethanol-fed rats by chlormethiazole may provide a possible mechanism for the protective effect of chlormethiazole on ethanol-induced liver injury.[35]

### 28.2.3 GENERATION OF REACTIVE FREE RADICALS THAT CAUSE DNA DAMAGE

Oxidative stress is caused by an imbalance in protective cellular antioxidant systems and generation of free radicals and their metabolites. Reactive oxygen species can interact with membrane lipids to form lipid peroxides and reactive aldehydes, such as hydroxynonenal and malondialdehyde, and form DNA adducts, which increase the risk of mutations during mitosis. The formation of DNA adducts is one of the earliest events in the multistage development of cancer. Chronic alcohol consumption has been shown to increase oxidative stress on cellular and systemic levels.[40] Markers of oxidative stress are increased in heavy drinkers and experimental animals, and reduced levels of plasma and tissue antioxidants have been reported.[40]

Several cellular mechanisms contribute to the increased generation of free radicals after acute or chronic alcohol intake. Cellular induction of the microsomal cytochrome P450 enzymes, especially the inducible isoform CYP2E1, results in a surplus formation of oxygen-derived free radicals and hydrogen peroxide ($H_2O_2$) within the microsomes. This enzyme has a high redox potential and was found to produce $H_2O_2$ even in the absence of hydroxylable substrates. Under *in vitro* conditions, cells overexpressing CYP2E1 can only survive when adequate levels of antioxidant substances (e.g., glutathione) are provided, highlighting the potential of this enzyme to increase oxidative stress.[41] Independent of CYP2E1 induction, other alcohol-induced changes can result in a net increase in oxidative stress. For example, in the presence of ethanol, hydroxyethyl radicals can be formed, which have a more toxic potential than hydroxyl radicals. They interact freely with lipids and proteins, have a longer lifespan compared to hydroxyl radicals, and are able to diffuse through membrane barriers more easily based on their more hydrophobic structure. Chronic alcohol consumption also leads to alterations in mitochondrial respiratory chain enzymes, with resulting disturbances in the electron transfer from flavinmononucleotide of complex I to complex III.[42] The subsequent accumulation of semiquinones is thought to contribute to increased formation of reactive oxygen species.[42]

In the early stages of alcohol-induced liver damage, proinflammatory cytokines such as tumor necrosis factor-alpha (TNF-$\alpha$), interleukin 1 beta (IL-1$\beta$), and IL-6 are released by neutrophils and macrophages and mediate a pronounced inflammatory reaction within the hepatic parenchyma. Hepatocytes react to these inflammatory signals by increased intracellular formation of reactive oxygen species and reactive nitrogen species. On the other hand, chronic alcohol treatment decreases glutathione peroxidase-1 levels and leads to a disturbance of the glutathione-based intracellular antioxidative system. This results in decreased clearance of free radicals and increased oxidative stress. Further mechanisms include vitamin E (tocopherol) depletion and alterations in the mitochondrial respiratory chain enzymes. Vitamin E is one of the most important intracellular antioxidants within the lipophilic compartment of the cell. Chronic alcohol consumption leads to lower tocopherol levels in experimental animals, independent of the level of dietary vitamin E, and increases oxidative stress. Eskelson[43] has demonstrated that free radicals produced during ethanol metabolism promote tumor formation in the esophagus, whereas diets supplemented with high levels of vitamin E inhibit ethanol-induced free radical activity and suppress the promotion of cancer by ethanol. A recent study also showed that alcohol-associated colorectal hyperproliferation can be prevented by supplementation with α-tocopherol.[44]

## 28.2.4 IMPAIRMENT OF IMMUNE FUNCTION

Both chronic and acute alcohol consumption lead to a change in the overall immune system function, thereby reducing the individual's defenses against pathogenic stimuli.[45] Clinically, this compromised immune system is reflected in higher rates of pneumonia and other bacterial infections. It is plausible that a compromised immune defense also leaves the organism more susceptible to cancer development. Several mechanisms contribute to the reduction of the individual's immune function, indicating direct effects of ethanol and its metabolites and indirect effects through deficient nutrient supply in alcoholic individuals.[46]

General changes to the immune system that can be observed in alcoholic individuals and experimental animals include atrophy of lymphoid organs, loss or redistribution of peripheral blood leukocytes, diminished hormonal and cell-mediated immune response, and impaired epithelial barrier function, especially in the gastrointestinal tract.[47] Alcohol displays an inhibitory effect on the function of natural killer (NK) cells in alcohol-fed animals as well as in alcohol consuming patients.[48–52] It is assumed that ethanol or its metabolites has an inhibiting effect on NK cell calcium-dependent programming and signal transduction. After long-term alcohol exposure, numerical reduction in NK cells and circulating lymphocytes also contributes to a loss in NK cell function.[53] Neutrophils, circulating blood cells with a key function in the defense against bacteria, show functional changes in the presence of alcohol, such as impaired migration to inflammatory foci and reduced capability to kill bacteria. Alcohol interferes with the cell–cell interactions of different immune cells, including interactions between monocytes and T lymphocytes.[45] After pretreatment with alcohol, human monocytes are less able to present a pathogenic antigen to T lymphocytes, leading to reduced antigen-specific T-cell response and proliferation.[54]

Chronic alcoholism leads to a shift in immune cytokine signaling resulting in a reduction of cellular and increase of hormonal responses. Frequently, increases in proinflammatory cytokines IL-1, IL-6, IL-8, and TNF-α have been observed and are attributed to oversecretion by monocytes. These changes are also likely to contribute to the inflammatory response within the liver, resulting in the formation of fibrosis. Frequently an increased level of immunoglobulins can be found in alcoholic individuals, even in a situation of immunodeficiency. Some of this immunoglobulin increase is attributable to autoimmunity arising from antibody formation against protein adducts formed under the influence of highly reactive acetaldehyde.

## 28.2.5 Induction of Cell Hyperproliferation That Promotes Genomic Instability

Chronic alcohol intake leads to increased cellular proliferation in various tissues, such as liver, colon, and rectum.[26,27,55] Such hyperproliferation predisposes development of genetic instability and cancer development by increasing the number of cellular divisions. Several mechanisms contribute to increased cellular turnover after acute and chronic ethanol intake.[56] One of the effects of ethanol on proliferative signaling pathways within the cells includes alteration of the mitogen-activated protein kinase (MAPK including Jun N-terminal kinase, JNK, extracellular signal-regulated kinase, ERK, and p38 kinase) pathway and its downstream cascades (e.g., C-jun is phosphorylated by JNKs, resulting in increased AP-1 transcriptional activity; Figure 28.2). Products of the two proto-oncogenes, c-Jun and c-Fos, form a complex in the nucleus, termed AP-1, that binds to a DNA sequence motif referred to as the AP-1 response element (AP-1 RE). Recent evidence has accumulated supporting a role for ethanol in the regulation of AP-1 gene expression. It has been shown that components of AP-1 are important in modulating carcinogenesis, and transactivation of AP-1-dependent genes is required for tumor promotion.[57]

We have observed that chronic ethanol intake in rats significantly increases hepatic c-Jun and c-Fos protein levels, as compared with control animals.[58] AP-1 plays a key role in regulating proliferative target gene expression. It mediates signals from a variety of sources of proliferative stimuli, including growth factors, cytokines, oxidative stress, and others. One of its key target genes is the cell cycle regulating gene, cyclin D1, which controls progression from $G_1$ to S phase during mitosis. In the livers of chronically ethanol fed rats, phosphorylation of c-jun and also of JNKs is significantly increased, resulting in increased AP-1-mediated transcription and cellular proliferation.[27,59] In transformed hepatocytes, alcohol administration leads to activation of ERK and increased DNA synthesis, and enhances the MAPK activation after G protein signaling.[60] Increased ERK activation is also found in human cancers related to alcohol, such as hepatocellular carcinoma and breast cancer.

Antiproliferative and antioncogenic effects of retinoids may be mediated by inhibiting AP-1 activity.[61] We have shown that the retinoic acid treatment in ethanol-fed rats dramatically inhibited the ethanol-induced overexpression of c-Jun and cyclin D1, AP-1 DNA binding activities, as well as the ethanol-induced proliferating cellular nuclear antigen-positive hepatocytes.[27] Because transactivation of AP-1-dependent genes is required for tumor promotion[57] and cyclin D1 plays an important role in tumorigenesis and tumor progression in hepatocellular carcinoma,[62] the identification of c-Jun and cyclin D1 as two potential targets of retinoic acid action in ethanol-fed rats indicates that retinoids play an important role in preventing certain types of ethanol-promoted cancer. Furthermore, we have

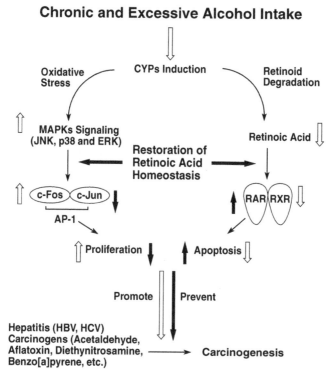

**FIGURE 28.2** Simplified schematic illustration of possible interactions of ethanol (open arrows) with retinoic acid (closed arrows) MAPK (including JNK, ERK, and p38 kinase) pathway and AP-1 (c-Jun and c-Fos) nuclear complex in ethanol-promoted carcinogenesis; see text for more detail. (Adapted from Wang XD. *J Nutr* 2003; 133:287S–290S.)

observed that all-*trans*-retinoic acid supplementation in ethanol-fed rats greatly attenuated the ethanol-induced phosphorylation of JNK and increased the levels of mitogen-activated kinase phosphatase-1 (MKP-1) in liver tissue.[59] It has been shown that JNK is required for tumorigenesis using a multistep carcinogenesis model in mice lacking the JNK2 gene.[63] These studies support our notion that JNK signaling may mediate ethanol-promoted hepatocyte proliferation and oncogenic transformation, due to alcohol-impaired retinoic acid action, and "cross talk" with the JNK signaling pathway. Retinoic acid is involved in the checkpoint function at the $G_1$/S phase transition and helps delay the progress of damaged cells into S phase during mitosis. This leaves more time for repair of damaged DNA or the initiation of apoptosis, thereby reducing the risk of malignant development.

## 28.2.6 DEREGULATION OF APOPTOSIS AND PROMOTION OF TUMORIGENESIS

Apoptosis is an important regulating mechanism in an organism's defense against cancer. Especially in a setting of increased tissue proliferation and frequent mitosis, the risk of genetic instability is increased, making more important the self-regulating function of apoptosis, which eliminates malfunctioning or mutated cells to prevent harm to the organism. Chronic alcohol intake can lead to a reduction in apoptosis, as demonstrated in the liver of alcohol-fed rats where decreased apoptosis coincides with increased proliferation.[27,59] Retinoids have been implicated in the induction of cell death in many tumor-derived cultured cell systems in retinoid receptor-dependent or receptor-independent manners.[64] It is possible that under certain risk conditions, such as diminished hepatic retinoid signaling due to prolonged alcohol intake, apoptosis may become deregulated, thereby promoting genomic instability and neoplasia. Recently, we investigated whether hepatocellular apoptosis can be regulated by either ethanol feeding or retinoic acid supplementation. We showed that ethanol feeding in rats for a 1-month period (subacute phase) significantly increased apoptosis; however, after 6 months of ethanol feeding, hepatic apoptosis decreased significantly relative to controls.[27,59] Interestingly, retinoic acid supplementation increased apoptosis four-fold in ethanol-fed rats, as compared with ethanol treatment alone.[27,59] Although the mechanism is not well defined, these data indicate that retinoic acid plays an important role in preventing ethanol-promoted carcinogenesis by inducing apoptosis.

### 28.2.7 IMPAIRED NUTRITIONAL STATUS

### 28.2.7.1 Folate and Vitamin $B_6$ (pyridoxal-5′-phosphate)

Folate and vitamin $B_6$ are important nutrients required for methylation reactions. Chronic alcohol intake interferes with one carbon metabolism, in which folate functions as a methyl donor for DNA methylation and nucleotide synthesis.[65] Folate deficiency leads to hypomethylation of DNA, which might contribute to increased cancer risk.[66] Alcoholic patients are at increased risk of folate deficiency due to a general pattern of micronutrient deficiency in chronic alcoholism. High acetaldehyde levels have been shown to lead to destruction of folic acid *in vitro*,[67] suggesting acetaldehyde can further contribute to the deterioration of folate levels in specific tissues. While systemic acetaldehyde levels are kept usually very low, bacterial degradation of ethanol within the lumen of the colon leads to very high local levels of acetaldehyde. This in turn leads to a significant reduction in tissue folic acid levels in the colonic mucosa and might contribute to the increased risk of colon cancer in alcoholic individuals.[12] Epidemiologic studies show an increased risk of colon cancer in alcoholic patients with a low folate diet, but high folic acid intake seems to alleviate this risk, giving further support for the hypothesis that local depletion of folic acid is a contributing factor in colon carcinogenesis in chronic alcohol users.[12] Chronic alcohol intake also affects both absorption and metabolism of vitamin $B_6$, resulting in impaired methyl group synthesis and transfer.[68–70]

### 28.2.7.2 Selenium and Zinc

The deficiency of selenium and zinc may contribute to cancer development.[1] Selenium is an important nutrient for the cellular antioxidant defense based on its essential role in the enzyme glutathione-peroxidase. Selenium deficiency is associated with increased oxidative stress and epidemiologic studies suggest that low selenium intake is related to an increased risk of cancer. Selenium supplementation is able to reduce cancer incidence and cancer mortality for many types of cancer, including colon cancer.[71] Selenium was shown to prevent experimental colon carcinogenesis induced by aromatic amines in a rat model.[72] Alcohol consumption does not seem to interfere with selenium uptake or utilization, but intake studies demonstrate that insufficient selenium intake is present in nearly all alcoholic patients,[73] and this nutritional deficiency might significantly contribute to the increased cancer risk in such patients. Zinc levels are also frequently decreased in chronic alcohol users through a combination of low absorption and increased excretion. Zinc deficiency and environmental exposure to nitrosamines are associated with esophageal carcinoma.[74] Zinc treatment at the time of ethanol exposure reduced the incidence of fetal abnormalities to basal levels.[75]

### 28.2.7.3 Vitamin A

Retinoids (vitamin A and its derivatives) are known to exert profound effects on cellular growth, differentiation, and apoptosis, thereby controlling carcinogenesis.[76] Retinoic acid receptors (RARs) and retinoid X receptors (RXRs) function as ligand-dependent transcription factors, thereby transcriptionally activating a series of genes with distinct antiproliferative activity and tumor suppressor function. Lower hepatic vitamin A levels have been well documented in chronic alcohol users.[77] Our previous animal studies have shown that long-term and excessive alcohol intake results in decreased hepatic retinoic acid,[58] the most active derivative of vitamin A and a ligand for both RARs and RXRs. It has been reported that the expression of the RARβ gene, a tumor suppressor, was downregulated by ethanol, even in the presence of retinol[78] as well as in tumorigenic hepatoma cell lines.[79,80] Substantial research has recently been done regarding the mechanisms by which excessive alcohol interferes with retinoid metabolism.[56,81] Specifically, alcohol (1) acts as a competitive inhibitor of vitamin A oxidation to retinoic acid involving ADHs and ALDHs; (2) enhances catabolism of vitamin A and retinoic acid by inducing cytochrome P450 enzymes, particularly CYP2E1, which contributes greatly to alcohol-related disease; and (3) alters retinoid homeostasis by increasing vitamin A mobilization from liver to extrahepatic tissues. This alcohol-impaired retinoic acid homeostasis (Figure 28.2) interferes with retinoic acid signaling (e.g., diminishes RARs binding activity to retinoic acid responsive elements (RAREs) and downstream target gene expression); and retinoic acid "cross talk" with the MAPK signaling cascade, which plays an essential role in cellular proliferation, apoptosis, stress, inflammatory response, and carcinogenesis. Furthermore, we have shown that restoration of retinoic acid homeostasis by retinoic acid supplementation restored the normal status of both JNK and IGF-I signal transduction pathways and maintained normal cell proliferation and apoptosis in the liver of ethanol-fed rats.[59,82] The implications for the prevention of ethanol-promoted liver (and peripheral tissue) carcinogenesis are clear. However, a better understanding of the retinoid–alcohol interaction and the molecular mechanism or mechanisms involved are needed before pursuing retinoids in the prevention of alcohol-related carcinogenesis in humans. This is particularly important in terms of the toxicity of retinoids in alcoholic individuals.[24,83]

## 28.3 SUMMARY

Carcinogenesis is a multistage process consisting of initiation, promotion, and progression. Initiation is rapid and occurs with high frequency (e.g., with exposure to a carcinogen, such as high levels of acetaldehyde from excessive alcohol intake), whereas promotion is a long-term process that requires chronic exposure to a tumor promoter (e.g., both biochemical and molecular alterations and nutritional deficiencies induced by chronic alcohol consumption). Although the exact process by which chronic alcohol intake promotes carcinogenesis needs further investigation, current evidence supports the following general mechanisms: (1) Increased generation of mutagenic acetaldehyde from alcohol, particularly related with ALDH/ADH genetic polymorphisms; (2) induction of cytochrome P450 enzymes that activate chemical procarcinogens and enhance degradation of retinoids; (3) generation of reactive free radicals that cause DNA damage and lipid peroxidation; (4) altered and deficient immune responses; (5) interaction with cell growth signaling and induction of cell hyperproliferation that promotes genomic instability; (6) dysregulation of apoptosis that allows cloning of transformed cells; and (7) impaired nutritional status. These multiple mechanisms may act together to play a role in carcinogenesis at both the initiation and promotion stages. A greater understanding of these molecular mechanisms is needed for the prevention and treatment of alcohol-related carcinogenesis.

## ACKNOWLEDGMENT

This work was supported by NIH/NIAAA Grant R01AA12628. The authors thank Heather Mernitz for her assistance in the preparation of the manuscript.

## REFERENCES

1. Seitz HK, Poschl G, Simanowski UA. Alcohol and cancer. *Recent Dev Alcohol* 1998; 14:67–95.
2. Poschl G, Seitz HK. Alcohol and cancer. *Alcohol Alcohol* 2004; 39:155–165.

3. Poschl G, Stickel F, Wang XD, Seitz HK. Alcohol and cancer: genetic and nutritional aspects. *Proc Nutr Soc* 2004; 63:65–71.

4. Seitz HK, Matsuzaki S, Yokoyama A, Homann N, Vakevainen S, Wang XD. Alcohol and cancer. *Alcohol Clin Exp Res* 2001; 25:137S–143S.

5. Seitz HK, Oneta CM. Gastrointestinal alcohol dehydrogenase. *Nutr Rev* 1998; 56:52–60.

6. Fang JL, Vaca CE. Detection of DNA adducts of acetaldehyde in peripheral white blood cells of alcohol abusers. *Carcinogenesis* 1997; 18:627–632.

7. Obe G, Jonas R, Schmidt S. Metabolism of ethanol *in vitro* produces a compound which induces sister-chromatid exchanges in human peripheral lymphocytes *in vitro*: acetaldehyde not ethanol is mutagenic. *Mutat Res* 1986; 174:47–51.

8. Helander A, Lindahl-Kiessling K. Increased frequency of acetaldehyde-induced sister-chromatid exchanges in human lymphocytes treated with an aldehyde dehydrogenase inhibitor. *Mutat Res* 1991; 264:103–107.

9. Espina N, Lima V, Lieber CS, Garro AJ. *In vitro* and *in vivo* inhibitory effect of ethanol and acetaldehyde on O6-methylguanine transferase. *Carcinogenesis* 1988; 9:761–766.

10. Homann N, Jousimies-Somer H, Jokelainen K, Heine R, Salaspuro M. High acetaldehyde levels in saliva after ethanol consumption: methodological aspects and pathogenetic implications. *Carcinogenesis* 1997; 18:1739–1743.

11. Homann N, Tillonen J, Rintamaki H, Salaspuro M, Lindqvist C, Meurman JH. Poor dental status increases acetaldehyde production from ethanol in saliva: a possible link to increased oral cancer risk among heavy drinkers. *Oral Oncol* 2001; 37:153–158.

12. Homann N, Tillonen J, Salaspuro M. Microbially produced acetaldehyde from ethanol may increase the risk of colon cancer via folate deficiency. *Int J Cancer* 2000; 86:169–173.

13. Nakamura Y, Yokoyama H, Higuchi S, Hara S, Kato S, Ishii H. Acetaldehyde accumulation suppresses Kupffer cell release of TNF-Alpha and modifies acute hepatic inflammation in rats. *J Gastroenterol* 2004; 39:140–147.

14. Yokoyama A, Muramatsu T, Ohmori T, Higuchi S, Hayashida M, Ishii H. Esophageal cancer and aldehyde dehydrogenase-2 genotypes in Japanese males. *Cancer Epidemiol Biomarkers Prev* 1996; 5:99–102.

15. Yokoyama T, Yokoyama A, Kato H, et al. Alcohol flushing, alcohol and aldehyde dehydrogenase genotypes, and risk for esophageal squamous cell carcinoma in Japanese men. *Cancer Epidemiol Biomarkers Prev* 2003; 12:1227–1233.

16. Yokoyama A, Muramatsu T, Ohmori T, et al. Alcohol-related cancers and aldehyde dehydrogenase-2 in Japanese alcoholics. *Carcinogenesis* 1998; 19:1383–1387.

17. Yokoyama A, Kato H, Yokoyama T, et al. Genetic polymorphisms of alcohol and aldehyde dehydrogenases and glutathione S-transferase M1 and drinking, smoking, and diet in Japanese men with esophageal squamous cell carcinoma. *Carcinogenesis* 2002; 23:1851–1859.

18. Visapaa JP, Gotte K, Benesova M, et al. Increased cancer risk in heavy drinkers with the alcohol dehydrogenase 1C*1 allele, possibly due to salivary acetaldehyde. *Gut* 2004; 53:871–876.

19. Wang XD. Retinoids and alcoholic liver disease. In: Agarwal DP, Seitz HK, eds. *Alcohol in Health and Disease.* New York: Marcel Dekker; 2001:427–452.

20. Duester G. Genetic dissection of retinoid dehydrogenases. *Chem Biol Interact* 2001; 130–132:469–480.

21. Han CL, Liao CS, Wu CW, Hwong CL, Lee AR, Yin SJ. Contribution to first-pass metabolism of ethanol and inhibition by ethanol for retinol oxidation in human alcohol dehydrogenase family — implications for etiology of fetal alcohol syndrome and alcohol-related diseases. *Eur J Biochem* 1998; 254:25–31.

22. Kedishvili NY, Gough WH, Davis WI, Parsons S, Li TK, Bosron WF. Effect of cellular retinol-binding protein on retinol oxidation by human class IV retinol/alcohol dehydrogenase and inhibition by ethanol. *Biochem Biophys Res Commun* 1998; 249:191–196.

23. Molotkov A, Duester G. Retinol/ethanol drug interaction during acute alcohol intoxication in mice involves inhibition of retinol metabolism to retinoic acid by alcohol dehydrogenase. *J Biol Chem* 2002; 277:22553–22557.

24. Crabb DW, Pinairs J, Hasanadka R, et al. Alcohol and retinoids. *Alcohol Clin Exp Res* 2001; 25:207S–217S.

25. Khalighi M, Brzezinski MR, Chen H, Juchau MR. Inhibition of human prenatal biosynthesis of all-*trans*-retinoic acid by ethanol, ethanol metabolites, and products of lipid peroxidation reactions: a possible role for CYP2E1. *Biochem Pharmacol* 1999; 57:811–821.

26. Halsted CH, Villanueva J, Chandler CJ, et al. Ethanol feeding of micropigs alters methionine metabolism and increases hepatocellular apoptosis and proliferation. *Hepatology* 1996; 23:497–505.

27. Chung J, Liu C, Smith DE, Seitz HK, Russell RM, Wang XD. Restoration of retinoic acid concentration suppresses ethanol-enhanced c-Jun expression and hepatocyte proliferation in rat liver. *Carcinogenesis* 2001; 22:1213–1219.

28. Parlesak A, Menzl I, Feuchter A, Bode JC, Bode C. Inhibition of retinol oxidation by ethanol in the rat liver and colon. *Gut* 2000; 47:825–831.

29. Lieber CS. The discovery of the microsomal ethanol oxidizing system and its physiologic and pathologic role. *Drug Metab Rev* 2004; 36:511–529.

30. Lieber CS. Cytochrome P-4502E1: its physiological and pathological role. *Physiol Rev* 1997; 77:517–544.

31. Oneta CM, Lieber CS, Li J, et al. Dynamics of cytochrome P4502E1 activity in man: induction by ethanol and disappearance during withdrawal phase. *J Hepatol* 2002; 36:47–52.

32. Lieber CS. Alcohol: its metabolism and interaction with nutrients. *Annu Rev Nutr* 2000; 20:395–430.

33. Sato M, Lieber CS. Increased metabolism of retinoic acid after chronic ethanol consumption in rat liver microsomes. *Arch Biochem Biophys* 1982; 213:557–564.

34. Liu C, Russell RM, Seitz HK, Wang XD. Ethanol enhances retinoic acid metabolism into polar metabolites in rat liver via induction of cytochrome P4502E1. *Gastroenterology* 2001; 120:179–189.

35. Liu C, Chung J, Seitz HK, Russell RM, Wang XD. Chlormethiazole treatment prevents reduced hepatic vitamin A levels in ethanol-fed rats. *Alcohol Clin Exp Res* 2002; 26:1703–1709.

36. Shimizu M, Lasker JM, Tsutsumi M, Lieber CS. Immunohistochemical localization of ethanol-inducible P450IIE1 in the rat alimentary tract. *Gastroenterology* 1990; 99:1044–1053.

37. Gouillon Z, Lucas D, Li J, et al. Inhibition of ethanol-induced liver disease in the intragastric feeding rat model by chlormethiazole. *Proc Soc Exp Biol Med* 2000; 224:302–308.

38. Morimoto M, Reitz RC, Morin RJ, Nguyen K, Ingelman-Sundberg M, French SW. CYP-2E1 inhibitors partially ameliorate the changes in hepatic fatty acid composition induced in rats by chronic administration of ethanol and a high fat diet. *J Nutr* 1995; 125:2953–2964.

39. Morimoto M, Hagbjork AL, Wan YJ, et al. Modulation of experimental alcohol-induced liver disease by cytochrome P450 2E1 inhibitors. *Hepatology* 1995; 21:1610–1617.

40. Sun AY, Ingelman-Sundberg M, Neve E, et al. Ethanol and oxidative stress. *Alcohol Clin Exp Res* 2001; 25:237S–243S.

41. Mari M, Wu D, Nieto N, Cederbaum AI. CYP2E1-dependent toxicity and up-regulation of antioxidant genes. *J Biomed Sci* 2001; 8:52–58.

42. Cunningham CC, Bailey SM. Ethanol consumption and liver mitochondria function. *Biol Signals Recept* 2001; 10:271–282.

43. Eskelson CD, Odeleye OE, Watson RR, Earnest DL, Mufti SI. Modulation of cancer growth by vitamin E and alcohol. *Alcohol Alcohol* 1993; 28:117–125.

44. Vincon P, Wunderer J, Simanowski UA, et al. Inhibition of alcohol-associated colonic hyperregeneration by alpha-tocopherol in the rat. *Alcohol Clin Exp Res* 2003; 27:100–106.

45. Szabo G. Consequences of alcohol consumption on host defence. *Alcohol Alcohol* 1999; 34:830–841.

46. Cook RT. Alcohol abuse, alcoholism, and damage to the immune system — a review. *Alcohol Clin Exp Res* 1998; 22:1927–1942.

47. Saada HN, Azab KS. Role of lycopene in recovery of radiation induced injury to mammalian cellular organelles. *Pharmazie* 2001; 56:239–241.

48. Abdallah RM, Starkey JR, Meadows GG. Toxicity of chronic high alcohol intake on mouse natural killer cell activity. *Res Commun Chem Pathol Pharmacol* 1988; 59:245–258.

49. Chadha KC, Stadler I, Albini B, Nakeeb SM, Thacore HR. Effect of alcohol on spleen cells and their functions in C57BL/6 mice. *Alcohol* 1991; 8:481–485.

50. Blank SE, Duncan DA, Meadows GG. Suppression of natural killer cell activity by ethanol consumption and food restriction. *Alcohol Clin Exp Res* 1991; 15:16–22.

51. Meadows GG, Blank SE, Duncan DD. Influence of ethanol consumption on natural killer cell activity in mice. *Alcohol Clin Exp Res* 1989; 13:476–479.

52. Laso FJ, Madruga JI, Giron JA, et al. Decreased natural killer cytotoxic activity in chronic alcoholism is associated with alcohol liver disease but not active ethanol consumption. *Hepatology* 1997; 25:1096–1100.

53. Blank SE, Gallucci RM, Wang JH, Meadows GG. Factors involved in modulation of NK cell activity by ethanol consumption. *Alcohol Alcohol Suppl* 1994; 2:439–445.

54. Szabo G, Verma B, Catalano D. Selective inhibition of antigen-specific T lymphocyte proliferation by acute ethanol exposure: the role of impaired monocyte antigen presentation capacity and mediator production. *J Leukoc Biol* 1993; 54:534–544.

55. Simanowski UA, Homann N, Knuhl M, et al. Increased rectal cell proliferation following alcohol abuse. *Gut* 2001; 49:418–422.

56. Wang XD. Retinoids and alcohol-related carcinogenesis. *J Nutr* 2003; 133:287S–290S.

57. Young MR, Li JJ, Rincon M, et al. Transgenic mice demonstrate AP-1 (activator protein-1) transactivation is required for tumor promotion. *Proc Natl Acad Sci USA* 1999; 96:9827–9832.

58. Wang XD, Liu C, Chung J, Stickel F, Seitz HK, Russell RM. Chronic alcohol intake reduces retinoic acid concentration and enhances AP-1 (c-Jun and c-Fos) expression in rat liver. *Hepatology* 1998; 28:744–750.

59. Chung J, Chavez PR, Russell RM, Wang XD. Retinoic acid inhibits hepatic Jun N-terminal kinase-dependent signaling pathway in ethanol-fed rats. *Oncogene* 2002; 21:1539–1547.

60. Aroor AR, Shukla SD. MAP kinase signaling in diverse effects of ethanol. *Life Sci* 2004; 74:2339–2364.

61. Altucci L, Gronemeyer H. The promise of retinoids to fight against cancer. *Nat Rev Cancer* 2001; 1:181–193.

62. Uto H, Ido A, Moriuchi A, et al. Transduction of antisense cyclin D1 using two-step gene transfer inhibits the growth of rat hepatoma cells. *Cancer Res* 2001; 61:4779–4783.

63. Chen N, Nomura M, She QB, et al. Suppression of skin tumorigenesis in c-Jun NH(2)-terminal kinase-2-deficient mice. *Cancer Res* 2001; 61:3908–3912.

64. Simoni D, Tolomeo M. Retinoids, apoptosis and cancer. *Curr Pharm Des* 2001; 7:1823–1837.

65. Davis CD, Uthus EO. DNA methylation, cancer susceptibility, and nutrient interactions. *Exp Biol Med (Maywood)* 2004; 229:988–995.

66. Choi SW, Stickel F, Baik HW, Kim YI, Seitz HK, Mason JB. Chronic alcohol consumption induces genomic but not p53-specific DNA hypomethylation in rat colon. *J Nutr* 1999; 129:1945–1950.

67. Shaw S, Jayatilleke E, Herbert V, Colman N. Cleavage of folates during ethanol metabolism: role of acetaldehyde/xanthine oxidase-generated superoxide. *Biochem J* 1989; 257:277–280.

68. Lumeng L, Li TK. Vitamin $B_6$ metabolism in chronic alcohol abuse. Pyridoxal phosphate levels in plasma and the effects of acetaldehyde on pyridoxal phosphate synthesis and degradation in human erythrocytes. *J Clin Invest* 1974; 53:693–704.

69. Labadarios D, Rossouw JE, McConnell JB, Davis M, Williams R. Vitamin $B_6$ deficiency in chronic liver disease — evidence for increased degradation of pyridoxal-5'-phosphate. *Gut* 1977; 18:23–27.

70. Stickel F, Choi SW, Kim YI, et al. Effect of chronic alcohol consumption on total plasma homocysteine level in rats. *Alcohol Clin Exp Res* 2000; 24:259–264.

71. Clark LC, Combs GF Jr, Turnbull BW, et al. Effects of selenium supplementation for cancer prevention in patients with carcinoma of the skin. A randomized controlled trial. Nutritional Prevention of Cancer Study Group. *J Am Med Assoc* 1996; 276:1957–1963.

72. Finley JW, Davis CD, Feng Y. Selenium from high selenium broccoli protects rats from colon cancer. *J Nutr* 2000; 130:2384–2389.

73. Manari AP, Preedy VR, Peters TJ. Nutritional intake of hazardous drinkers and dependent alcoholics in the UK. *Addict Biol* 2003; 8:201–210.

74. Barch DH, Kuemmerle SC, Hollenberg PF, Iannaccone PM. Esophageal microsomal metabolism of N-nitrosomethylbenzylamine in the zinc-deficient rat. *Cancer Res* 1984; 44:5629–5633.

75. Carey LC, Coyle P, Philcox JC, Rofe AM. Zinc supplementation at the time of ethanol exposure ameliorates teratogenicity in mice. *Alcohol Clin Exp Res* 2003; 27:107–110.

76. Lippman SM, Lotan R. Advances in the development of retinoids as chemopreventive agents. *J Nutr* 2000; 130:479S–482S.

77. Leo MA, Lieber CS. Hepatic vitamin A depletion in alcoholic liver injury. *N Engl J Med* 1982; 307:597–601.

78. Grummer MA, Zachman RD. Interaction of ethanol with retinol and retinoic acid in RAR beta and GAP-43 expression. *Neurotoxicol Teratol* 2000; 22:829–836.

79. Li C, Wan YJ. Differentiation and antiproliferation effects of retinoic acid receptor beta in hepatoma cells. *Cancer Lett* 1998; 124:205–211.

80. Wan YJ, Cai Y, Magee TR. Retinoic acid differentially regulates retinoic acid receptor-mediated pathways in the Hep3B cell line. *Exp Cell Res* 1998; 238:241–247.

81. Wang XD. Chronic alcohol intake interferes with retinoid metabolism and signaling. *Nutr Rev* 1999; 57:51–59.

82. Lian F, Chung J, Russell RM, Wang XD. Alcohol-reduced plasma IGF-I levels and hepatic IGF-I expression can be partially restored by retinoic acid supplementation in rats. *J Nutr* 2004; 134:2953–2956.

83. Leo MA, Lieber CS. Alcohol, vitamin A, and beta-carotene: adverse interactions, including hepatotoxicity and carcinogenicity. *Am J Clin Nutr* 1999; 69:1071–1085.

# Index

## A

ABCG5, 252
ABCG8, 252
ABC transporter proteins, and phytosterol
    absorption, 235–236
Aberrant crypt foci (ACF)
    effect of MNU on, 79, 81
    and sphingolipids, 525–527
    and synthetic sphingolipids, 527–528
Absorption
    and antioxidant activity, 417–418
    of flavonoids, 280
Acetaldehyde, in alcohol-associated
    carcinogenesis, 580
Acitretin, and cutaneous T-cell lymphomas, 69
Activator protein-1 (AP-1), 352, 356, 359
Acute lymphoblastic leukemia (ALL)
    in children, 161, 165, 167
    and resveratrol analogues, 379
Acute myeloid (AML) cells, and resveratrol,
    374
Acute promyelocytic leukemia (APL), retinoid
    treatment in, 69
Adenocarcinoma
    breast, 264
    of esophagus and gastric cardia, 548–549
Adenomas
    malignant potential of, 16
    and obesity, 544
Adenomatous polyps, and selenium, 195
Adequate Intake, 92, 93
Adhesion of cancer cells, and flavonoids,
    341–342
Adhesions, integrin-mediated, 178. See also
    Cell adhesions
Adrenal cortical steroids, and energy balance,
    572–573
African Americans, prostate cancer in, 13
Age
    and cancer, 371
    and cancer diagnosis, 50
    and DER, 567
    and incidence of cancer, 321
    and postmenopausal breast cancer, 545, 546
Aglycones, 296

AICR, 29, 32
AITC, and caspase activity, 448
Akt pathway, effects of genistein on, 302
Alcohol consumption, 46
    and breast cancer risk, 7
    and cancer risk, 28
    and cancers, 579–580, 581, 590
    and cellular proliferation, 586
    and DNA methylation, 47
    and oxidative stress, 584–585
Alcohol dehydrogenase (ADH), genetics of,
    580, 582
All-*trans*-retinol. *See* Vitamin A
Alpha-Tocopherol, Beta-Carotene Cancer
    Prevention (ATBC) trial, 114
American Cancer Society, 32
American Institute for Cancer Research
    (AICR), 28
Androgen receptor (AR) signaling pathway,
    effects of genistein on, 302
Androgens
    and breast cancer risk, 8, 9
    in prostatic carcinogenesis, 13
Angiogenesis
    effect of genistein on, 303–304
    effect of selenium on, 204
    effects of tea polyphenols on, 338
    flavonoids and, 337–338
    inhibited by VE analogs, 126–127
    inhibition of, 43, 142
    and selenium levels, 196
    and soy isoflavones, 338–339
    VE analog inhibition of, 126
    and VEGF, 319
Animal models. *See also* Rat models; Rodent
    models
    antimetastatic effects of flavonoids in,
        329–331
    catechin inhibition of carcinogenesis in, 355
    of colon cancer, 489
    effects of ITCs on cancer in, 443
    ginseng studies in, 470–471
    for growth and metastasis, 343
    ITC anticarcinogenic activities in, 441–442,
        443
    lycopene in, 81

testing in, 32
vitamin A deficiency in, 65–66
vitamin E analogs in, 120–121
Anthocyanidins, 30, 413
chemical structure of, 275, 276, 327
common, 414
Anthocyanins
anticancer properties of, 426
anticarcinogenic mechanisms of, 415
antioxidant activity of, 416–419
antioxidant characteristics of, 414, 425
in berries, 415
biological activity of, 426
and cancer, 414–415
and DNA damage, 419
enzymatic antioxidant defense of, 419–420
in foods, 277
properties of, 413–414
sources of, 274
and tumor development, 420–421
Anticancer agents. *See also specific anticancer
agents*
vitamin E analogs as, 120–122
vitamin E as, 113–116
Antigrowth signals, increased response to,
40–41
Antimetastasis
role of flavonoids in, 344
tea polyphenols and, 328, 332
Antimutagenesis, mechanisms for, 36
Antioxidants
anthocyanins as, 414, 416–419
and cancer risk, 44
catechins as, 352, 356–357
and disease, 139
flavonoids as, 273, 276, 277, 278
ginseng, 460–461
isoflavones as, 304
phytosterols as, 232
resveratrol as, 371
and ROS, 44
soyasaponins, 472
vitamin C, 134–144, 146–147
vitamin E analogs as, 117
Antiprogression, mechanisms for, 36–37
Antiproliferation, mechanisms for, 36–37
Antitumor agents, vitamin E analogs as,
126–127
*Apc* gene, in colorectal cancer, 33
Apigenin
antimetastatic activity of, 326, 328, 336–337
and tumor metastasis, 331
tumor metastasis prevented by, 343

Apoptosis
beta-sitosterol-mediated, 260
and beta-sitosterol supplementation, 262
in chronic alcohol consumption, 587–589
CLA induced, 508
effects of phytosterols on, 258–261
enhancement of, 41–42
induced by ginsenosides, 463
induction of, 42, 123
occurrence of, 41
and PEB, 571, 574
for protein kinase pathways, 126
selenium and, 201–203
by tea metabolites, 358
α-TOS induction of, 125
Arachidonic acid, eicosanoid synthesis from,
509–510
Arachidonic acid metabolism, inflammation
and, 422–423
Aromatase, in estrogen synthesis, 401
Ascorbic acid, beneficial effects of, 412
Asian populations, effects of tea on cancer in,
355
Aspirin, and colorectal cancer, 16
Astaxanthin, 82
Atherosclerosis, effect of phytosterols on,
231–232
Athymic mice, ginseng studies in, 470–471
ATP binding cassette cotransporters, 252
Australia, breast cancer study in, 388–389, 393
Azoxymethane (AOM), 489
AZT (zidovudine), 462


**B**


Bavachinin, and colon cancer, 317
β-Carotene
anticarcinogenic activity of, 78–79
and cancer, 68
β-catenin, in colon carcinogenesis, 530–531
β-Cryptoxanthin, anticarcinogenic activity of,
82
Benign prostatic hypertrophy (BPH)
and β-sitosterol, 253–254
effects of phytosterols on, 232–233
Benzyl ITC (BITC), 439
effects on cancer of, 443
phase II enzyme induction by, 446
*in vitro* cytotoxic effects of, 439
Berry fruits, anthocyanins in, 415
Biacalein, and colon cancer, 317
Bile acids
and colon cancer, 492

and phytosterols, 239
Biliary carcinoma cells, and polyphenols, 333
Bio-chemoprevention, 85
Bioimpedance, 542
Biological activity, and antioxidant activity,
    417–418
Biomarkers, of chemopreventive effects,
    141–142
Biosynthesis, folate-dependent, 154, 155
Birth defects, and folate supplementation, 167
Bisbenzamide spectrofluorometric assays, 102
Blackberries, as anti-inflammatory agent, 422
Bladder cancer
    and cruciferous intake, 444
    and isotretinoin, 70
Body mass index (BMI)
    and breast cancer risk, 316
    and cancer risk, 545
    as indicator of obesity, 543
    as obesity measure, 541
    and ovarian cancer risk, 549
    and prostate cancer, 548
    and renal cell cancer, 547
Boswellia, and carcinogenesis, 45
Bovine brain-derived capillary endothelial cells
    (BBCE), genistein inhibition of,
    338
Boyarsky scores, in BPH studies, 254
*Brassica,* 435
*Brassica oleracea* species, 46
Brassicasterol, 227, 240
BRCA-1, 11
BRCA-2, 11
Breads
    phytosterols from, 252
    plant sterols in, 230
Breast adenocarcinoma, and phytosterols, 264
Breast cancer
    and cruciferous intake, 444
    cytotoxicity in, 440–441
    delay in diagnosis of, 546
    effect of soy isoflavones on, 334
    ER-negative, 397–398
    ER-positive, 398–400
    flaxseed in, 394
    incidence of, 297, 320, 321
    isoflavones and, 297–298
    and lignans, 387–391
    and obesity, 544–546, 568
    and phytoestrogens, 315–317
    and phytosterol diet, 257–258
    and phytosterol supplementation, 261
    postmenopausal, 545–546

premenopausal, 545
prognosis for, 546
protective effects of lignans on, 400–405
and vitamin D, 97–99
and vitamin $D_3$ status, 103
Breast cancer, female
    and early life exposures, 8
    and endogenous hormones, 8–10
    epidemiology of, 6
    and exogenous hormones, 10–11
    and lifestyle factors, 7–8
    mammographic density and, 12
    markers of risk for, 11–12
    reproductive factors and, 6–7
Breast cancer risk, 6. *See also* Cancer risk
    ENL concentrations and, 393
    and lignans, 387–391, 392, 405
Breast cancer studies
    in athymic nude mice model, 397–400
    with ITCs, 442, 444
Breastfeeding, and breast cancer risk, 8, 9
Breast milk, selenium in, 207
Breast tumor models, and deltanoids, 101
Broccoli
    and carcinogenesis, 47
    and colon cancer risk, 51
    selenium enriched, 206–207
Bromelain, and carcinogenesis, 45

**C**

Cadherin, loss of, 43–44
Caffeic acid phenethyl ester, apoptosis induced
    by, 42
Calciferol, 89. *See also* Vitamin D
Calcium, 30
    and CaSR function in colon, 181
    and chemoprevention, 36, 178
    and E-Cadherin molecules, 179
    extracellular, 180
    intracellular, 180
    protective effects of, 50
Calcium-sensing receptor (CaSR), 178, 180
    cell-ECM adhesion regulated by, 182
    and function in colon, 181
Campesterol, 227
    chemical structure of, 251, 252
    and colon cancer, 257
    in dietary intake, 234
    in human studies, 252, 254
    metabolism of, 240
    and metastasis, 263

Cancer. *See also* Breast cancer; Colon cancer;
    Prostate cancer; *specific cancers*
  anthocyanins and, 414–415
  and 1α,25-(OH)₂D₃ analogs, 100–103
  chemopreventive agents for, 496
  CLA intake and, 511
  conceptual framework for, 38, 50
  in developing *vs.* developed world, 28
  diet, 412
  and dietary phytosterols, 256–257
  effects of selenium on, 194–195
  epidemiology of, 3–5, 192 (*see also*
      Epidemiology)
  epithelial, 32
  female breast, 6–12
  and flavonoids, 412–413
  genetic predisposition for, 5
  and ginsenosides, 469
  and hormone activity, 421–422
  hormone-dependent, 421–422
  incidence of, 5, 295–296, 320
  and nutritional factors, 28
  and obesity, 543–550, 567
  pathogenesis of, 32–35
  and phytoestrogens, 315–318
  role of alcohol in, 579–580, 581, 590
  and selenium supplementation, 195
  and vitamin A, 65–68
  and vitamin A deficiency, 76
  and vitamin D, 95–97
Cancer cell apoptosis, resveratrol-induced,
    373–374. *See also* Apoptosis
Cancer cells, sphingolipids in, 521–523
Cancer predisposition syndromes, 16
Cancer prevention, 147. *See also*
    Chemoprevention
  and dietary phytosterols, 255
  by exogenous sphingolipids, 530–531
  isoflavones in, 297
  by resveratrol, 377–379
  role of food in, 51–52
Cancer risk
  age and obesity-related, 546
  in alcoholic individuals, 580–581
  and chronic PEB, 567
  colon cancer in, 487–488
  colorectal, 544
  and ginseng intake, 471
  and glucose homeostasis, 574
  and obesity, 546, 547, 550–551, 568
  and saponins, 476
Cancer treatment
  combinatorial, 528–530
  efficacy of sphingolipids in, 531

Capsanthin, 82
Carcinogenesis. *See also* Tumorigenesis
  alcohol-associated, 580–590
  biomarkers related to, 141–142
  characteristics of, 492
  chemical-induced, 424–425
  chemoprevention of, 352
  CLA inhibition of, 505–506, 506–509, 511
  diet in, 28
  experimentally induced models of, 140
  through folate deficiency, 162–134
  and HPEB, 569, 570
  inhibition of catechin in, 355
  and isoflavones, 304–305
  ITCs blocked by, 437
  oxidative stress in, 142–143
  role of inflammation in, 16
  and VE, 114
Carcinogenicity
  effects of selenium on, 199
  and inhibition of cell-to-cell
      communication, 145
  inhibition of GJIC and, 145–146
  of oxidative stress, 140
Carcinogens. *See also specific carcinogens*
  dietary, 46
  and vitamin A, 66
CARET study, 78
α-Carotene
  anticarcinogenic activity of, 78–79
ß-Carotene, 30
  apoptosis induced by, 42
  protective effects of, 76–77
  provitamin A activity of, 76
Carotenoids, 30
  anticarcinogenic activity of, 76, 77–78
  beneficial effects of, 412
  and cancer, 68
  and chemoprevention, 36
  multicarotenoids, 82–83
  and plant sterols, 234
  protective effects of, 76–77
  provitamin A activity of, 76
Catabolic reactions, folate-dependent, 154, 155
Catechins, 351
  action mechanisms of, 361–362
  antioxidant effects of, 356–357
  biological activities of, 354
  carcinogenesis inhibition by, 355
  chemical structure of, 352, 353
  chemoprevention by, 356–361
  FAS expression suppressed by, 360
  green tea, 328, 357
  occurrence of, 354

pro-oxidant effects of, 357–358
source of, 352
suppression of fatty acid synthase
expression by, 360
ubiquitin-proteasome pathway inhibited by,
361
Cathepsin D, ceramide regulation of, 260
CDK4 kinase activity, and PEB, 570
Cell adhesion molecules (CAMS), in metastasis,
43
Cell adhesions, types of, 178
Cell-cell adhesion, E-Cadherin mediated, 179
Cell cycle, 35, 37
and differentiation, 180
effects of phytosterols on, 261–262
effects of resveratrol on, 372
inhibitory effects of α-TOS on, 126
ITC inhibition of, 439
and tumor development, 420–421
Cell cycle arrest, by tea metabolites, 358
Cellular replication, inhibition of, 35, 37–40
Ceramides
and ACF suppression, 527–528
apoptosis induced by, 259
and beta-sitosterol supplementation, 261
in cancer cells, 521, 522
in intestinal cells, 524–525
phytosterol generation of, 265
in sphingolipid metabolism, 520
Cereals
antioxidant capacities of, 45
phytosterols in, 229, 252
Cerebrosides, in plants, 524
Cervical cancer, and folate deficiency, 162
CF1 mice, 525, 530. *See also* Rodent models
Chalcone, chemical structure of, 327
Chalcone synthase, 274
CHD risk, and sitosterolemia, 233–234
Chemoprevention
by catechins, 356–361
concepts of, 140–141
defined, 177
of tea, 355–356
Chemopreventive agents
EGCG, 360
ideal, 520
Chemotherapy
in combination with sphingolipids, 529–530
expression of *MDR1* after, 469
Childhood
cancer in, 161 (*See also* Leukemia)
obesity in, 542–543
Chlormethiazole, protective effect of, 583–584
Cholecalciferol, 89, 90 *See also* Vitamin D, 91

Cholesterol, 223, 227
effect of phytosterols on, 230–231,
237–238, 261
HDL, 238
LDL, 232, 238
metabolism of, 240
Choline, and DNA methylation, 47
Chromosomal fragile sites, and folate
deficiency, 158. *See also*
Genomics
Cigarette smoking, and breast cancer risk, 7–8.
*See also* Smoking
Cisplatin, 301
Collaborative Group on Hormonal Factors in
Breast Cancer, 8, 10
Colon
and CaSR function in, 181
and protective effects of flavonoids, 317
Colon cancer
and calcium's chemoprevention, 181
chemoprevention of, 177–178
and dietary fat, 495
early stages of, 525
effect of ß-Cryptoxanthin on, 82
and folate status, 160–161
high-risk patients for, 496
incidence of, 487
in Japan, 488
and phytosterol animal studies, 255–257
prevention of, 496
resveratrol-induced apoptosis in, 373–374
in rodent models, 525–526
soysaponins and, 476
sphingolipid treatment of, 528–530
and α-TOS, 120, 122
and VE analogs, 124
and vitamin D, 96
and vitamin $D_3$ status, 103
Colorectal cancer
and adenomatous polyps, 16
epidemiology of, 15–16, 17
incidence of, 15, 320, 321
and inflammation, 16
and obesity, 544
and plant sterol intake, 254
prevention of, 489, 495–496
progression of, 14–15
risk of, 15
and selenium supplementation, 195, 196
Vitamin D in, 48–50
Compartmentalization, and antioxidant activity,
418–419
Conjugated linoleic acid (CLA)
anticancer activity of

*in vitro* cell culture model, 504, 505
*in vivo* animal model, 505–506
and cancer risk, 511
chemical structure of, 503, 504
properties of, 503
Continuing Survey of Food Intakes by
    Individuals, 92
Corn oil, and colon cancer, 490
Coronary heart disease (CHD), effect of
    phytosterols on, 231–232
Cortical steroids, and energy balance, 572–573
Crocetin, 82
Cruciferae, 435
Cruciferous intake, clinical studies of, 444
Cruciferous vegetables, 46
Curcumin
    apoptosis induced by, 42
    and carcinogenesis, 45
    and chemoprevention, 36, 37
    and telomerase activity, 42
Curcuminoids, 31
Cyanidin
    antitumor promoting effects of, 420–421
    estrogenic activity of, 421
Cyclin, formation of, 35
Cyclin-dependent kinase (CDK), regulation of,
    35, 37
Cyclin dependent kinase inhibitors (CDKIs),
    300, 372
Cyclooxygenase-1 (COX-1), 371
    CLA modulation of, 509–510
    and inflammation, 423
    and resveratrol, 375
Cyclooxygenase-2 (COX-2), 371, 492
    as biomarker, 141
    CLA modulation of, 509–510
    in colon carcinogenesis, 494
    in colon tumors, 489–490
    and inflammation, 423
    and resveratrol, 375
Cyclooxygenase-2 (COX-2) inhibitors
    and colorectal cancer, 16
    long-term safety of, 45
Cyclooxygenases, CLA modulation of,
    509–510
CYP2E1, induced after ethanol consumption,
    583
Cytochrome P-450 (CYP), ITC inhibition of,
    444–445
Cytochrome P450 isoform 2E1 (CYP2E1), in
    chronic alcohol consumption,
    582–584

# D

Daidzein, 296
Dallas Heart Study, 234
Daunomycin (DNM), 439
Death-receptor apoptosis pathway, 373–374
Delphinidin
    antitumor promoting effects of, 420–421
    estrogenic activity of, 421
Deltanoids
    as anticancer agents, 101, 103
    combined with anticancer agents, 102
Deoxynucleotide (dNTP), in folate deficiency,
    163
DHEA, and chemoprevention, 37
Diabetes, and colorectal cancer risk, 17
*Sn*-1,2-diacylglycerol (DAG), 376, 377

Dietary components
    bioactive, 29–32
    chemopreventive action of, 35–48
Dietary energy restriction (DER), 567–568
Dietary supplements, antineoplastic, 111, 112
Diets
    cancer, 412
    and cancer, 28–29
    and carcinogenesis, 38
    with CLA, 509
    and colorectal cancer, 16
    fatty acids in, 493
    HFML, 494
    high-fat fish oil, 494
    interaction with environment of, 51
    ITCs in, 437
    molecular analysis of, 51
    and prostate cancer risk, 14
    soy products in, 296
    Western, 490, 492
Differentiation
    abnormal pathway in, 181, 182
    cell adhesions and, 178–179
    induction of, 40–41, 178, 180
    reduced, 520
Differentiation-inducing agents, 177
Dihydrobrassicasterol, and colon cancer, 257
$1\alpha,25$-dihydroxyvitamin $D_3$ $(1\alpha,25(OH)_2D_3)$.
    *See also* Vitamin D
    anticarcinogenic activity of, 48
    antiproliferative properties of, 48
1,2-dimethylhydrazine (DMH), 50
4,4-dimethylsterol, 225, 226
Disease, flavonoid intake and, 413
DNA damage
    in cell cycle, 37

oxidative, 44
DNA methylation, alterations in patterns of, 47
DNA radicals, and catechins in, 357
DNA repair, selenium and, 203
DNA synthesis
  in folate deficiency, 165–166
  folates in, 156
Docetaxel, 301
Docosahexaenoic acid (DHA), 488, 491
  and carcinogenesis, 45
  and cell proliferation, 493
  colon cancer inhibited by, 495
  and differentiation promotion, 41
  inhibition of colon carcinogenesis by, 493
Doxorubicin, 522, 529
Drug metabolizing enzymes (DMEs), 46

**E**

EB 1089 (deltanoid)
  and breast tumor cells, 101–102
  treatment with, 102
E-Cadherin, 179
Eggs, sphingolipids in, 524
Eicosanoid synthesis, from arachidonic acid,
  509–510
Eicosapentaenoic acid (EPA), 491–492
  and carcinogenesis, 45
  and cell proliferation, 493
  and differentiation promotion, 41
Endometrial cancer
  and consumption of soy foods, 318
  and obesity, 547
Energy balance, chemical mediators of effects
  of, 572–574. See also Positive
  energy balance
Enterocyte membrane proteins, and sterol
  absorption, 236
Enterodiol (END)
  structure of, 386
  transcriptional activation potential of, 403
Enterolactone (ENL)
  structure of, 386
  transcriptional activation potential of, 403
Environment, and breast cancer risk, 6
Enzymes, and carcinogens, 46
Epicatechin (EC), 328
Epicatechin gallate (ECG), 328
Epidemiology
  of alcohol and cancer, 579–580, 590
  of cancer, 3–5, 296
  of colorectal cancer, 15–16, 17, 488–489
  of female breast cancer, 6

of folate deficiency, 159–160
of folate status and cancer, 161–162
of isoflavones, 304
of lignans and breast cancer, 387
of lycopene, 80–81
of obesity and cancer risk, 551
of phytosterol and cancer, 253–255
of phytosterol concentrations, 233
of prostate cancer, 12–13, 298
of selenium and cancer, 192–193
of selenium intake, 189–190
of tea drinking with cancer incidence, 355
usefulness of, 5
of vitamin E and cancer risk, 115, 116
Epidermal growth factor (EGF)
  and breast cancer risk, 404
  and cell proliferation, 39
Epidermal growth factor (EGF)-receptor,
  EGCG inhibition of, 359
Epigallocatechin (EGC), 328
Epigallocatechin gallate (EGCG), 44, 328, 329
  antiangiogenic activity of, 338
  anticancer-promoting effects of, 359
  apoptotic inducing effects of, 358
  and carcinogenesis, 45
  and chemoprevention, 36, 37
  growth inhibitory effect of, 358
  pro-oxidant effects of, 357
  and telomerase activity, 42
  TPA-induced transformation inhibited by,
  358
Epstein-Barr virus, 82
Equol, chemical structure of, 314
Ergocalciferol, 89, 90 See also Vitamin D
Ergosterol, 227
ER signaling pathway, 303
Esophageal dysplasia, in selenium studies, 194
Esophagus, adenocarcinoma of, 548–549
17 β-Estradiol, chemical structure of, 314
Estrogenic actions, of phytosterols, 263–264
Estrogen-receptor (ER), and resveratrol, 376
Estrogen receptor status, and postmenopausal
  breast cancer, 545, 546
Estrogen response elements (EREs), and
  resveratrol, 376
Estrogens
  bioavailability of, 400–401
  and breast cancer risk, 8–9
  chemical structure of, 313, 314
  effect of lignans on metabolism of, 400,
  402–403
  and prostate cancer risk, 13–14
  synthesis of altered by lignans, 401–402
Etretinate, and cutaneous T-cell lymphomas, 69

European Prospective Investigation into Cancer
and Nutrition (EPIC) study, 392
Extracellular matrix (ECM), 146, 178
Ezetimibe (Zetia), 251

**F**

Familial adenomatous polyposis (FAP), 16
Familial factors, in colorectal cancer, 16
Fas-associated death domain (FADD), 259
Fats, dietary
animal, 489
and cancer risk, 28
in colon cancer, 487–488
and colon tumor development, 490
phytosterols in, 229
plant sterols in, 230
Fatty acids, 31
and carcinogenesis, 45
and cell proliferation, 493
and differentiation promotion, 41
omega (*see* Omega fatty acids)
tumor-promoting effects of saturated, 490
Fatty acid synthase, EGCG inhibition of, 360
Fenretinide
as chemopreventive agent, 69–70
and prostate cancer, 67
Fiber, and cancer risk, 28
Fibroblast growth factor (FGF), and cell
proliferation, 39
Fibroblast growth factor (FGF)-receptor,
EGCG inhibition of, 359
Fibrosarcoma
and polyphenols, 333
and soy isoflavones, 335
Fibrous foods, and colorectal cancer, 496
Finland, breast cancer study in, 389, 391, 393
Fish oils, 488, 490, 491
and colon tumors, 490
high-fat diet with, 494
5-a-Day Program, 32
5FU, for colon cancer, 529
Flavanols
chemical structure of, 276
colonic-derived metabolites of, 283
in foods, 277
formation of hippuric acid from, 284
Flavan-3-ols, 283
Flavanones
chemical structure of, 275, 276, 327
in foods, 277
sources of, 274
Flavans, chemical structure of, 327

Flavones, 30
chemical structure of, 327
in foods, 277
Flavonoids
absorption of, 277–280
and angiogenesis, 337–338
antimetastatic effects of, 328, 329–331
antioxidant potential of, 278
apoptosis induced by, 42
beneficial properties of, 273
bioavailable metabolites of, 286
biosynthesis of, 275
and cancer, 412–413
and cancer cell adhesion, 341–342
cellular uptake of, 286
chemical structure of, 274, 275, 282, 326,
327, 413
circulating metabolites of, 282
as classical antioxidants, 276, 277
classification of, 274, 326, 327
and colon cancer, 317
conjugation of, 284
and differentiation promotion, 41
in foods, 277
formation of metabolites and conjugates of,
285
and infant leukemia, 318
interactive effects of, 344
metabolism of, 280–284
and MMPs, 339
*O*-methylation of, 281
properties of, 413
sources of, 274, 326, 327
and tumor metastasis, 342–344
Flavonols, 30
chemical structure of, 275, 276
in foods, 277
sources of, 274
Flavonones, 30
Flaxseed (FS)
anticancer effects of, 313
beneficial effects of, 405
and breast cancer treatment, 397
and carcinogenesis, 319
in carcinogen-treated rat model, 397
disease risk-reducing capabilities of, 385,
386
experimental studies with, 394–400
lignans of, 313–314
and tumor initiation and promotion, 396
and tumor proliferation, 400
Folate
beneficial effects of, 412
in chronic alcohol intake, 588

and DNA methylation, 47
protective effect of, 161
Folate antagonists, in cancer chemotherapy, 156
Folate deficiency
and cancer, 159–160
in cancer treatment, 156
and childhood leukemia, 161
and colorectal cancer, 160
defining, 157
and DNA damage, 158
functional, 157
genomic instability in, 164
mechanisms of carcinogenesis through,
162–164
Folates
and cancer prevention, 156–167
in cancer therapy, 156
intracellular, 154
metabolism of, 153
supplementation with, 166
Folate status, determining, 159
Folic acid, 30
chemical structure of, 153, 154
and chemoprevention, 37
supplementation with, 166, 167
Food frequency questionnaires (FFQs), 392
Food intake, nibbling pattern of, 568
Foods. *See also* Diets
flavonoid-containing, 277
functional, 76
infant, 45
Free radicals, cellular injuries induced by, 139.
*See also* Oxidative stress
Fruits
antioxidant capacities of, 31, 45
and cancer incidence, 412, 435
and cancer risk, 28
and colorectal cancer, 496
DOA recommendations for, 139
evaluation of, 344
flavonoids in, 274
phytosterols in, 229
Fucoxanthin, 82
Functional foods, 76

**G**

Gap-junction intercellular communication
(GJIC), 140
and carcinogenicity, 145
homeostatic balance maintained by, 141
Garlic
apoptosis induced by, 42

selenium-enriched, 206
Garlic/onion, and chemoprevention, 36
Gastric cancer
and polyphenols, 333
protective effect of soy intake on, 318
Gastric cardia, adenocarcinoma of, 548–549
Gastrointestinal (GI) tract
flavonoid absorption in, 278–279
flavonoid metabolism in, 281
saponins in, 462
GEN, and tumor growth, 399
Gene-environment interaction, 5
Gene-nutrient interactions, 51
Generally recognized as safe (GRAS),
phytosterol esters as, 233
Genes
associated with breast cancer, 11
oncogenes, 32
p53, 33, 48
Genetic defects, and cancer cell production,
32–33, 34. *See also* Mutations
Genetics, of prostate cancer, 14
Genistein, 296, 298, 330
and Akt pathway, 302
antiangiogenic activity of, 338, 339
anti-angiogenic effects of, 303–304
anti-metastatic effects of, 303–304
and AR signaling pathway, 302–303
cell cycle arrest induced by, 300
cellular growth inhibited by, 39–40
and colon cancer, 317
and ER pathway, 303
and estrogen receptors, 39, 40
metastasis inhibited by, 335
and MMP activities, 341
Genomics
in clinically relevant animal models, 344
of ginsenosides, 463–464
increased stability in, 44
nutritional, 51
Germany, breast cancer study in, 389, 392
Ginseng, 458
anticancer activity of, 462–463
antioxidant properties of, 460–461
cancer preventative properties of, 459–471
and cancer risk, 471
effect on cultured cancer cells of, 463–466
effect on membrane homolysis of, 467–468
immune-stimulating properties of, 461–462
types of, 460
Ginseng extracts
and cellular immunity, 461–462
and cultured cancer cells, 463
standardized, 461

Ginsenosides
  anticancer activity of, 462–463
  cancer preventative properties of, 459–471
  chemical structure of, 458, 459
  cytotoxic effects of, 469
  effect on cultured cancer cells of, 463–466
  effect on membrane homolysis of, 467–468
  genomic effects of, 463–464
  and membrane function, 467
  in plants, 459
Glioblastoma, and soy isoflavones, 335
Glioma cell lines, sphingolipid composition in,
    523
Glucose homeostasis, and cancer risk, 574
Glucose metabolism, and breast cancer risk, 9
Glucosinolates, 46
Glutathione peroxidase (GPX), 191, 198–199
Glutathione-*S*-transferases (GSTs)
  detoxification with, 46, 47
  ITCs catalyzed by, 438
Glycoside processing, flavonoid, 279
Glycosylation, and antioxidant capacity,
    416–417
Golden hamsters, vitamin A depletion in, 66.
    *See also* Rodent models
Grains, 320
  and cancer risk, 28
  phytosterols in, 229
Grapes, 369, 370
Green tea, 44, 329
  benefits of, 352
  cancer-prevention effect of, 328
  and onset of cancer, 356
Green tea catechins, 328, 357
Green tea polyphenols (GTPs), 333
Growth factors
  effects of lignans on, 404–405
  fibroblast, 39, 359
  insulin-like, 9–10, 14, 404, 573
  platelet derived, 39, 359
Growth hormone (GH), and prostate cancer, 14

**H**

Head and neck cancer, and soy isoflavones, 335
Health, and obesity, 543
*Helicobacter pylori,* 28
Hemolysis, protective effect of ginsenosides on,
    467
Hepatitis, viral, 28
Hepatocarcinoma, and isotretinoin, 71. *See also*
    Liver carcinogenesis
Hepatocytes, effects of soyasaponins on, 476

Hepatomas
  and methyl-deficient diet, 47
  and polyphenols, 333
Herbal medicines, traditional, 29
Herbal supplements, 437
Hereditary factors, in colorectal cancer, 16
Hereditary nonpolyposis colorectal cancer
    (HNPCC) syndrome, 16
Heterocyclic amines, 46
High-fat fish oil (HFO) diet, 494
High-fat mixed lipid (HFML) diet, 494
High PEB (HPEB), 569
Hippuric acid, 284
Histopathology, of neoplastic progression, 33
HIV patients, ginseng for, 462
Honeybee propolis, apoptosis induced by, 42
Hormone-independent cancers, and isoflavones,
    299
Hormone-related cancers, and isoflavones, 299.
    *See also* Breast cancer; Prostate
    cancer
Hormone replacement therapy (HRT), 6
  and breast cancer risk, 11
  and postmenopausal breast cancer, 545–546
Hormones
  and breast cancer risk, 8–10, 10–11
  and cancer development, 421
H-*ras* oncogene, in phytoene-producing cells,
    85
17-hydroxysteroid dehydrogenase (HSD), in
    estrogen synthesis, 401
25-hydroxyvitamin D$_3$ (25-(OH)$_2$D$_3$), 90, 91
  anticancer properties of, 103
  and cancer risk, 95
  and colon cancer, 96–97
  differentiation-promoting effect of, 49
  in treatment of cancer, 100–103
Hyperglycemia, and colorectal cancer, 16
Hyperinsulinemia, and colorectal cancer, 16
Hypermethylation, 47
Hyperoxia, and anthocyanins, 420
Hypomethylation, 47
Hypotheses, testing, 5

**I**

IGF-1 receptors, and colorectal cancer, 16
I$\kappa$B kinase (IKK), and cell signaling pathways,
    301
Ileum, and flavonoids, 285
Immune system
  in chronic alcohol consumption, 585–586
  effects of dietary phytosterols on, 232, 263

effects of ginseng on, 461
effects of selenium on, 200
and soyasaponins, 474
Incidence
    for colorectal cancer, 15
    defined, 4
    of female breast cancer, 6
    for prostate cancer, 12–13
Inducible nitric oxide synthase (iNOS)
    in colon tumors, 489–490, 492–493
    inflammatory processes mediated by, 141
    and tea polyphenols, 359
Infant food, antioxidant capacities of, 45
Inflammation, 141
    and arachidonic acid metabolism, 422–423
    and carcinogenesis, 45, 424
    and colorectal cancer, 16
    effect of phytosterols on, 232
    inhibition of, 141
    oxidative stress in, 143
    process of, 422
    ROS in, 145
    and vitamin C, 147
Initiation, 370, 506, 590
    flaxseed and lignans and, 396
    role of CLA in, 506–507
    role of NO in, 492–493
    sphingolipid suppression of, 528
Insulin
    and colorectal cancer, 16
    and energy balance, 573
Insulin-like growth factors (IGFs)
    and breast cancer risk, 9–10, 404
    and energy balance, 573
    and prostate cancer, 14
Insulin resistance, and breast cancer risk, 9
Integrins, 178
Intercellular adhesion molecule 1 (ICAM),
    231–232
Interferon γ (IFNγ), and dietary phytosterols,
    263
Interleukins
    in alcohol-induced liver damage, 584
    in chronic alcoholism, 585
    and dietary phytosterols, 263
International Prostate Symptoms scores, in BPH
    studies, 254
Invasion. See also Metastasis
    effects of apigenin on, 336–337
    effects of tea polyphenols on, 333
    and quercetin on, 336–337
    soy isoflavones and, 335
Iowa Women's Health Study, 29, 549
Isoflavones, 30, 320
    anticancer effects of, 313
    as antioxidants, 304
    bioavailability of, 297
    and cancer, 297–300, 304–305
    chemical structure of, 275, 276, 313, 327
    as estrogens, 314
    in foods, 277
    and hormone-independent cancers, 299–300
    and hormone-related cancers, 296, 299
    and melanoma, 335
    metabolism of, 296–297
    molecular mechanisms of action of,
        300–304
    sources of, 296
    and tumor metastasis, 330
Isoflavone supplements, lifelong intake of, 320
Isolariciresinol, 386
Isothiocyanates (ITCs), 31, 435
    absorption of, 437
    anticarcinogenic activities of
        clinical studies, 442, 444
        in vivo, 441–442, 443
    bioavailability of, 438
    chemical structures of, 436
    development of analogues of, 448
    in diet, 437
    excretion of, 438
    formation of, 436
    phase I enzymes inhibited by, 444–446
    phase II enzymes inducted by, 446–447
    in vitro cytotoxic effects of, 439
Isotretinoin
    chemopreventive properties of, 70, 71
    and cutaneous T-cell lymphomas, 69
Italy, breast cancer study in, 391

**J**

Jejunum, flavonoids in, 285
Jun N-terminal kinase (JNK), 586

**K**

Kaposi's sarcoma, and isotretinoin, 71
Kidney cancer, and obesity, 547–548
K-ras, in colorectal cancer, 33

**L**

Lactation, and breast cancer risk, 7
Legumes, 320. See also Vegetables

Leukemia, 161
   AML, 374
   and ginsenosides, 463
   infant, 318
   and obesity, 550
   and resveratrol-induced apoptosis, 373
Leukoplakia, oral, 71
Leukotrienes
   in inflammatory processes, 423
   as mediators of inflammation, 423
LGD1069 (Targretin®), 77
Lifespans, resveratrol extension of, 371
Life Span Study, in Hiroshima and Nagasaki,
   316
Lifestyle factors
   and breast cancer risk, 6, 7–8
   and carcinogenesis, 28
   diet nutrition, 265
Lignans, 30, 320
   absorption and metabolism of, 386
   anticancer effects of, 313
   in athymic nude mice model, 397–400
   and breast cancer
      prevention of, 394
      risk of, 387, 405
      treatment for, 397
   in carcinogen-treated rat model, 397
   estimating intake of, 392–393
   as estrogens, 314
   estrogen synthesis altered by, 400–403
   in flaxseed, 386
   and mammary gland development, 394–396
   non-ER-mediated mechanism of, 403–405
   serum, 393–394
   and tumor initiation and promotion, 396
Limonene, and chemoprevention, 36
Linoleic acid (LA). *See also* Conjugated linoleic
   acid
   chemical structure of, 488
   and colon carcinogenesis, 491–492
*Linum usitatissimum,* 385. *See also* Flaxseed
Linxian 1 study, 78
Lipid metabolism, CLA modulation of,
   509–511
Lipid peroxidation, and tumorigenesis, 84
Lipoproteins, ginseng protection of, 460
Lipoxygenases, in inflammatory processes, 423
Lithocholic acid (LCA), 50
Liver, flavonoid absorption in, 279
Liver cancer, and selenium, 193–194
Liver carcinogenesis
   and lycopene treatment, 81
   ß-Carotene in, 79
   and treatment with zeaxanthin, 80

Liver injury, ethanol-induced, 583–584
Lung cancer
   and cruciferous intake, 444
   and lycopene, 81
   obesity and, 550
   and retinoids, 70
   and selenium supplementation, 195, 196
   and soy isoflavones, 335
Lung cancer risk, and flavonoids, 412
Lung tumor, lutein treatment for, 80
Lutein, 30
   anticarcinogenic activity of, 79–80
   antitumor-promoting activity of, 80
Lycopene, 30, 76
   anticarcinogenic activity of, 80–82
   apoptosis induced by, 42
   and chemoprevention, 36
Lymphoma, and obesity, 550

**M**

Macronutrients, cancer-preventive properties of,
   29. *See also specific*
     *macronutrients*
Malignant cells, and differentiation-inducing
   agents, 177
Mammary carcinogenesis, CLA in, 506. *See*
     *also* Breast cancer
Mammary glands
   developing, 319
   and exposure to phytoestrogens, 394–396
Mammary tumors, efficacy of selenocompounds
   on, 204–205
Mammographic density
   interpretation of, 315–316
   as predictor of breast cancer, 12
Matairsinol (MAT), 386, 392–393
Matrix metalloproteinases (MMPs), 337
   effects of soy isoflavones on, 340–341
   effects of tea polyphenols on, 340
   inhibition of, 339
   in tumor promotion, 140, 142, 146
   upregulation of, 44
*MDR1,* 469
Meal feeding, experiments with, 568
Meat consumption, and colon adenomas in
   Japan, 488
Meat products, sphingolipids in, 524
Mediterranean diet, 489
Medulloblastoma cells, and polyphenols, 333
Melanoma
   effects of soy isoflavones on, 335
   effects of tea polyphenols on, 332

and α-TOS, 120, 122
Melatonin, and breast cancer risk, 10
Membrane-bound enzymes activities, effect of phytosterols on, 262
Membrane-bound folate binding proteins (FBPs), 154
Membranes, effects of phytosterols on, 235, 264
Menarche, and breast cancer incidence, 6–7
Menopause, and breast cancer incidence, 7
Mesotheliomas, and α-TOS, 120, 122, 126
Metabolism, and antioxidant activity, 417–418
Metals, carcinogenic properties of, 46
Metastasis. *See also* Carcinogenesis
    and apigenin, 336–337
    effect of genistein on, 303–304
    effect on soy isoflavones on, 334
    effects of flavonoids on, 329–331, 342–344
    effects of phytosterols on, 262–263
    effects of soy isoflavones on, 335
    effects of tea polyphenols on, 333
    flavonoid inhibition of, 337–342
    inhibition of, 43–44
    lignans and, 403–404
    protective effect of phytosterols against, 257–258
    quercetin and, 336–337
    treatment of, 326
Methionine
    biosynthesis, 157
    and DNA methylation, 47
    and folate deficiency, 165
Methotrexate (MTX)
    in chemotherapy protocols, 156
    and folate deficiency, 159
Methylation
    DNA, 47
    in folate deficiency, 164
Methyl group synthesis, in chronic alcohol intake, 588
*N*-methylnitrosourea (MNU), ACF induced by, 79–80, 81
Methylselenenic acid, and inhibition of cell proliferation, 201
Micronutrients, and cancer risk, 28. *See also specific micronutrients*
Migrant studies, cancer incidence in, 12
Milk products
    and colon cancer, 529
    sphingolipids in, 524
Minerals, effects on cancer of, 194. *See also specific minerals*
Min mice, 531. *See also* Rodent models
Mitogen-activated kinase kinase 1 (MEKK1), and cell signaling pathways, 301

Mitogen-activated kinase phosphatase-1 (MKP-1), 587
4-monomethylsterol, 225, 226
Mortality
    of colorectal cancer, 15
    metastasis and, 43
    and vitamin D synthesis, 90
Multicarotenoids, 82–83
Multiple myeloma, and obesity, 550
Mutations
    ABCG8, 252
    and carcinogenesis, 32
    and folate deficiency, 158
    *Ras,* 39
    with *ras*-p21, 494–495
    and VE analogs, 123–124
Mycotoxins, 46
Myricetin, and colon cancer, 317

**N**

NAC, and chemoprevention, 36
Naphthyl ITC (NITC), 437
Naringin, and lung cancer risk, 412
National Cancer Institute (NCI), 29, 32
National Cholesterol Education Program (NCEP III) guidelines, 240
National Health and Nutritional Survey, Third (NHANES III), 92
Neoplasia. *See also* Tumors
    chemopreventive effect of retinoids on, 67
    nature of, 112
    progression of, 33, 34 (*see also* Progression)
Netherlands, breast cancer study in, 388–389, 389, 392, 393
Netherlands Cohort Study on Diet and Cancer, 254–255, 511
Neural tube defects, and folate supplementation, 166
Neuroblastoma
    effect of α-TOS on, 123
    and isotretinoin, 71
NF-B DNA binding activity, and isoflavone supplementation, 304
Niemann-Pick C1 like 1 (NPC1L1) protein, 236, 251
*N*-nitrosoamines, 46
Nonsteroidal anti-inflammatory drugs (NSAIDs)
    and cancer risk, 45
    and colorectal cancer, 16
N-3 PUFAs
    beneficial effects of, 495

and cancer risk, 489
colon carcinogenesis inhibited by, 492, 493
consumption of, 496
dietary, 491
in fish oils, 488
N-6 PUFAs
    and colon cancer, 492
    tumor-promoting effects of, 490
    in vegetable oils, 488
Nuclear factor KB (NFKB), 352, 356
    blocked by EGCG, 359
    resveratrol suppression of, 374
    and role of genistein, 301
Nude mice, ginseng saponins in, 471
Nutrients
    and cancer prevention, 52
    epigenetic events in, 47–48
    micronutrients, 28
    nuclear acting, 41
    pleiotropic actions of, 48–50
Nuts
    antioxidant capacities of, 45
    phytosterols in, 229, 252

## O

Obesity, 6
    and cancer, 543–550
    and cancer risk, 28, 568
    and carcinogenesis, 38
    causes of, 541
    childhood, 542–543
    defined, 565, 567
    economic impact of, 543
    prevalence of, 542–543, 565
    and prognosis, 546
Olive oil, and colon cancer, 490
Omega fatty acids, chemical structure of, 488.
        *See also* N-3 PUFAs; N-6 PUFAs
Oncogenes
    defined, 32
    *Ras,* 489, 494–495
Oral carcinoma cells, and polyphenols, 333
Oral contraceptive agents (OCAs), 10, 162
Oral leukoplakia, 71
Oral squamous cell carcinoma, and soy
        isoflavones, 335
Organ transplant patients, and chemopreventive
        effect of acitretin, 69
Ornithine decarboxylase (ODC), 372
Ovarian cancer
    and fenretinide, 70
    obesity and, 549

and phytochemical intake, 255
and vitamin E, 120
Ovarian tumors, sphingosines in, 522
Overweight, prevalence of, 542–543
Oxidation
    and carcinogenesis, 424
    and vitamin C, 147
Oxidative stress
    carcinogenic effects of, 142
    and role of isoflavones, 304
    vitamin C protection of, 140

## P

*Panax,* 460
Pancreatic cancer
    effect of genistein on, 335
    incidence of, 320, 321
    and obesity, 549–550
    and polyphenols, 333
Parity, and breast cancer risk, 7
PCR-RFLP analysis, 98
Peanuts, 369, 370
PEB-cancer risk hypothesis, 567, 568
PEITC
    and chemoprevention, 36
    clinical trial for, 448
    effects on cancer of, 443
    lung carcinogens blocked by, 445–446
    pharmacokinetics of, 437
    phase II enzyme induction by, 446
    time profile of, 438
    *in vitro* cytotoxic effects of, 439
Pelargonidin, estrogenic activity of, 421
Perillyl alcohol, and chemoprevention, 36
Peroxisome proliferator-activated receptors
        (PPARs), in lipid metabolism, 510
Pesticides, 46
Petunidin, antitumor promoting effects of,
        420–421
P53 gene
    in colorectal cancer, 33
    mRNA, 48
P53 pathway, loss of function of, 40
pH, and antioxidant activity, 418
Phenethyl isothiocyanate (PEITC), 437
Phenolic acids, 283
Phospholipase C, effects of beta-sitosterol on,
        260
Phospholipids, CLA incorporation in, 509, 511
Physical activity
    and cancer risk, 28
    and carcinogenesis, 38

Phytochemicals
  anticancer activity of, 68
  beneficial effects of, 412
  chemopreventive, 29
  in vegetables, 31
Phytoene, 76, 82
  antioxidative activity of, 84
  in mammalian cells, 84–85
  synthesis, 85
Phytoestrogens
  action of, 387
  cancer and, 315–318
  chemical structure of, 313
  effects of, 403
  lignans as, 387
  and tumor inhibition, 319
Phytopolyphenolics, in food, 354
Phytostanols, 224
Phytosterols, 30. *See also* Sterols
  absorption of, 235–237
  anti-atherogenic effects of, 231–232
  anti-inflammatory effects of, 232
  antioxidant activity of, 232
  apoptosis-promoting activity of, 259–260
  atherogenic studies with, 234
  and cancer, 265
      animal experimentation studies,
          255–258
      epidemiological studies, 253–255
      mechanism of action in, 258–265
  chemical structure of, 224–225
  cholesterol-lowering effect of, 224, 230–231
  classification of, 225, 239–241
  commercial sources of, 228–230
  4-desmethylsterol class, 225
  dietary, 230, 251–253
  effect on cholesterol absorption of, 237–238
  effects on cholesterol biosynthesis of, 261
  effects on membrane-bound enzymes of,
      262
  excretion of, 239
  food sources of, 228, 229
  in human studies, 254
  metabolism of, 235–239
  in NCEP guidelines, 240
  optimal daily dose of, 231
  in plants, 226–228
  positive health effects of, 240
  post-absorptive fate of, 238–239
  properties of, 223
  protective role of, 265
  safety studies on, 233
  and tumor metastasis, 262–263
Piceid, 370, 379

Pickling, and cancer risk, 28
Pinoresinol, 386
Plant stanols, metabolic fate of, 239
Plant sterols. *See also* Phytosterols
  beneficial effects of, 224
  forms of, 226–228
  pharmacology of, 230
Platelet derived growth factor (PDGF), and cell
      proliferation, 39
Platelet derived growth factor (PDGF)-receptor,
      EGCG inhibition of, 359
Pleiotropic actions
  of bioactive compounds, 35
  of nutrients, 48–50
Polycyclic aromatic hydrocarbons, 46
Polyphenolic compounds, antioxidant capacity
      of, 416
Polyphenols. *See also specific polyphenols*
  absorption of, 281, 283
  dietary sources for, 30
Polyprenoic acid, 71
Polyps, and colorectal cancer, 16
Positive energy balance (PEB), 565, 566
  chronic, 574
  effects on carcinogenic response of, 573
  high, 569
  low, 569
  and mammary carcinoma development, 573
Postmenopausal women, and breast cancer
      incidence, 11
Pregnancy
  and breast cancer risk, 7
  vitamin deficiency in, 161
Prevalence, defined, 4
Prevention studies, for colon cancer, 496. *See
      also* Cancer prevention
Proapoptotic effect, of VE analogs, 116, 117.
      *See also* Apoptosis
Procyanidins
  affinity for proteins of, 281
  flavanols and, 278
Progression, 370, 590
  effects of CLA on, 509
  histopathology of, 33
  inhibition through suppressing EGFR
      signaling, 358
  and isoflavones, 304–305
  role of NO in, 492–493
  and sphingolipid administration, 523
Prolactin, and breast cancer risk, 10
Proliferation
  and chronic alcohol intake, 586
  CLA inhibition of, 507–508
  effect of catechins on, 354

effect of ginseng on, 462–463
effect of lignans on, 405
and flaxseed treatment, 400
inhibition through suppressing EGFR
    signaling, 358
and PEB, 570–571, 574
phytosterol inhibition of, 259
protective effect of phytosterols against,
    257–258
unlimited, 520
Promotion, 370, 590
CLA inhibition of, 506, 507–509
flaxseed and lignans and, 396
role of NO in, 492–493
Prostaglandins (PGs)
and carcinogenesis, 45
as mediators of inflammation, 423
and tumor growth, 493, 494
Prostate cancer
CLA in, 506
demographic factors in, 12–13
effect on soy isoflavones on, 334–335
effects of tea polyphenols on, 332–333
endocrine factors in, 13
familial types of, 14
and fenretinide, 67
incidence of, 12, 320, 321
isoflavones and, 298–299
and obesity, 548
and phytosterol diet, 257–258
and selenium supplementation, 195, 196
and soy consumption, 317
and vitamin A, 68
and vitamin B levels, 99–100
and vitamin $D_3$ status, 103
Prostatic hyperplasia, effects of phytosterols on,
    232–233
Prostatic specific antigen (PSA) scores, 99
Protease inhibitors, and chemoprevention, 37
Proteasome, 20S (700-kDa), 361
Protein kinase C (PKC)
CLA modulation of, 508–509
and colon cancer, 492
effects of beta-sitosterol on, 260
and n-6 PUFAs, 494
regulated by selenium, 202
resveratrol inhibition of, 376–377
Proteins, proteasomal degradation of, 362
Protein tyrosine kinase (PTK) inhibitor,
    genistein as, 40
Proteolytic enzymes, and tumor metastasis, 339
Proteomics, 344
Proto-oncogenes, 32
in growth regulation, 39

K-*ras*, 33
and Vitamin D, 49
Provitamin, folic acid, 153
Provitamin A, 76
Purines, in folate deficiency, 163

## Q

Quercetin, 278
antimetastatic activity of, 326, 328, 336–337
and carcinogenesis, 45
jejunal transfer of, 280
and lung cancer risk, 412
metabolism of, 284
and tumor metastasis, 331
tumor metastasis prevented by, 343
Quercetin glucosides, absorption of, 279–280
*Quillaja saponaria,* 458
Quinone reductase, 46

## R

*Raphanus,* 435
*Ras* mutations, 39
*Ras* oncogene, in human colon tumors, 489
*Ras*-p21, 494–495
Rat models. *See also* Rodent models
alcohol consumption in, 586
AOM-Fischer, 489
effect of genistein-containing soy in,
    318–319
flaxseed and lignans in, 397
isoflavone studies with, 297–298
lutein studies in, 80
obesity studies in, 569
SHRSP, 235
Sprague-Dawley, 526
Reactive nitrogen species (RNS), genotoxicity
    of, 140
Reactive oxygen species (ROS), 44
in carcinogenesis, 142
and chronic alcohol consumption, 584
effects of vitamin C on, 146
genotoxicity of, 140
and inflammatory processes, 144–145
and vitamin E, 112
Recommended Dietary Allowance (RDA), 92,
    93
Rectal cancer. *See* Colorectal cancer
Redox-silent analogs, of VE, 116–120
Reduced folate carrier (RFC), 154
Red wine, 369, 370

Resveratrol, 41
    antioxidant activity of, 371
    apoptosis induced by, 373–374
    and cancer prevention, 370–371, 377–379
    and carcinogenesis, 45
    cell cycle and, 372
    and chemoprevention, 36
    and differentiation promotion, 41
    effects of cyclooxygenase on, 375
    estrogen agonist/antagonist activity of, 376,
        378
    and estrogen-dependent gene regulation,
        376
    glucosides of, 370
    NFκB survival pathway suppression by, 374
    nutritional sources of, 370
    pro-oxidant activity, 371
    protein kinase C (PKC) inhibited by,
        376–377
    sources of, 369
Retinoblastoma (Rb) protein, 37
Retinoic acid (RA)
    and chemoprevention, 36
    in chronic alcohol intake, 586–587
    and cutaneous T-cell lymphomas, 69
    and DNA methylation, 47
    genes regulated by, 65
    and hepatic apoptosis, 588
    supplementation, 590
    vitamin A activation into, 65
Retinoic acid receptors (RARs), 63–64, 77, 589
Retinoic acid responsive elements (RARE), 589
Retinoic X receptors (RXR), 63–64
Retinoid deficiency, 62
Retinoids
    anticarcinogenic activity of, 77
    and basal skin cells, 63
    and carcinogenesis, 589
    and chemoprevention, 36, 37, 68
    clinical trials with, 69–70
    and nonsmall cell lung cancer, 70
    signaling by, 64–65
    and skin carcinoma, 67
    and telomerase activity, 42
Retinoid X receptors (RXRs), 77, 493, 589
Retinol
    and cancer, 68
    and squamous cell carcinomas, 69
Retinyl acetate, chemopreventive effect of, 67
Rexinoids, anticarcinogenic activity of, 77
Riboflavin
    in folate deficiency, 165
    and precancerous lesions, 195

Rodent models. *See also* Rat models
    athymic mice, 470–471
    CF1 mice, 525, 530
    for colon cancer study, 525–526
    fatty acid studies in, 491
    Min mice, 531
    nude mice, 471
    for resveratrol study, 378
    vitamin A studies in, 66

**S**

*S*-adenosylmethionine (SAM), 47
Safflower oil, and colon cancer, 490
Saliva, high levels of acetaldehyde in, 580
Salting, and cancer risk, 28
Saponins, 31
    and cancer risk, 476
    cultured cell experiments with, 474–476
    hemolytic activity of, 467–468
    and membrane function, 467
    in plants, 459
    properties of, 458
SCCVII/SF tumors, 102
Screening, for colorectal cancer, 15
SECO, 392–393
Secoisolarciresinol diglycoside (SDG),
            chemical structure of, 386
Seeds
    lignans and isoflavones in, 320
    phytosterols in, 252
Selective estrogen receptor modulators
            (SERMs), 314
Selenium, 30, 31
    as antiangiogenic agent, 204
    anticarcinogenicity of, 208
    and apoptosis, 201–203
    beneficial effects of, 412
    and cancer, 190, 192–193
    and carcinogen metabolism, 199
    and chemoprevention, 36
    in chronic alcohol consumption, 589
    and DNA methylation, 47
    and DNA repair, 203
    in foods, 204–207
    human trials with, 193–196
    and immunity, 200
    mechanisms of cancer reduction by,
            197–204
    nutritive benefit from, 207
    in plasma, 207
    and precancerous lesions, 195
    properties of, 190

RDA for, 208
regulation of protein kinase C (PKC) by, 202
in supplements, 204–207, 208
in tissue culture models, 197
and tumors in small animals, 196–197
Selenium metabolites, antitumorigenic,
          200–201
Selenobetaine, anticarcinogenic efficacy of,
          204–205
Selenocompounds, 189
in animals, 191–192
as anticarcinogenic agents, 206
metabolism of, 190
in plants, 191–192
Selenoenzymes, in cancer reduction, 198–199
Selenomethionine (Semet), 189
Selenoproteins, 191–192
Selenosis, symptoms of, 207
SeMCYS, 196
anticarcinogenic efficacy of, 204–205
effect on tumors of, 190
and inhibition of cell proliferation, 201
in plants, 191
Semet
disadvantage of, 204, 205
in prostate tissue, 196
topical application of, 196
Se-methylselenocysteine (SeMCYS), 189
Sex hormone-binding globulin (SHBG), 400
Sex hormones, in cancer development, 421–422
Shanghai, breast cancer study in, 388–389, 393
Shanghai breast cancer study, 316
Sigmasterol
in human studies, 254
structure of, 251, 252
Single nucleotide polymorphisms (SNPs), 83
Sirtuins, properties of, 371
Sitostanol, metabolism of, 240
β-sitosterol, 30, 227
chemical structure of, 251, 252
and colon cancer, 256–257, 257
in human studies, 252, 254
and membrane structure, 264–265
and metastasis, 263
potential therapeutic role for, 253–254
Sitosterol, in dietary intake, 234
Sitosterolemia, 233, 251
Skin, vitamin D synthesized by, 90
Skin cancer models, and phytoene, 84
Skin carcinogenesis, and lung cancer, 81
Skin tumorigenesis, and α-Carotene, 78
SMAD2, in colorectal cancer, 33
SMAD4, in colorectal cancer, 33

Smoking
and cancer risk, 28
and carcinogenesis, 38
and chemopreventive effects of RAR, 70
colon cancer and, 160
and ITC intake, 442
and vitamin E, 114
Socioeconomic status (SES), and health
          differences, 13
Somatotropic axis, and prostate cancer, 14
Soy
health-promoting functions of, 458–459
isoflavones of, 313–314
phytosterols in, 252
and prostate cancer, 317
and tumor growth, 399
Soyasaponins, 458, 459
and animal colon cancer model, 476
antioxidant activity of, 472
bioavailability of, 472
cancer preventative properties of, 471–476
cultured cell experiments with, 474–476
effect on immune system of, 474
hepatoprotective effects of, 476
main aglycones of, 473
Soybeans
isoflavones in, 296
sphingolipids in, 524
Soy diet, and prostate cancer, 298
Soy isoflavones, 313–314, 327, 336
antimetastatic activity of, 326, 328, 334
and breast cancer, 315–316, 334
and cancer cell adhesion, 341–342
and chemoprevention, 36, 37
effects on angiogenesis of, 338–339
and MMPs, 340–341
and prostate cancer, 334–335
tumor metastasis prevented by, 343
Soy products, lifelong intake of, 320
Sphingolipid metabolites, 526
generation of, 520
site-directed administration of, 523
Sphingolipids
in cancer cells, 521–523
in cancer prevention, 530–531
and cell regulation, 521
chemical structure of, 521
as chemopreventive agents, 520
in colon cancer, 529
and enzyme activity, 522
intraperitoneal injection of, 523–524
intravenous injection of, 524
metabolism of, 260, 520–521
natural, 524–527

oral administration of, 524–528
regulation of β-catenin by, 532
side effects associated with, 531
synthetic, 527–528
topical administration of, 523
Sphingomyelin
colon tumors suppressed by, 528
phytosterol stimulation of, 265
Sphingomyelinase, effects of beta-sitosterol on, 260
Spices, antioxidant capacities of, 45
Sprague-Dawley rats, and preneoplastic lesions, 526. *See also* Rodent models
Squamous carcinoma, and 1α,25-(OH)$_2$D$_3$, 101
Stanol esters, cholesterol-lowering efficacy of, 231
Stanols, plant, 228
Steroids, and energy balance, 572–573
Sterols, 224–226, 228. *See also* Phytosterols
absorption of, 235–236
4-desmethyl class of, 225
esterified, 227
food-grade, 227–228
free, 227
intracellular handling of, 237
nomenclature, 224–226
plant, 228
Stigmasterol, 227
and colon cancer, 257
metabolism of, 240
Stilbenes, 30
Stomach cancer, incidence of, 320, 321. *See also* Gastric cancer
Stroke-prone spontaneously hypertensive (SHRSP) rats, phytosterol studies in, 235
Suckling, lignan exposure during, 395
Sulforaphane (SF), 437
and caspase activity, 448
effects on cancer of, 443
phase II enzyme induction by, 446
*in vitro* cytotoxic effects of, 439
Sun exposure, and cancer, 95
Sweden, breast cancer study in, 390

**T**

Tabar patterns, 315
TAM
beneficial effects of, 405
in breast cancer, 398–399
Targretin, 77
Taxol toxicity, 522

T-cell lymphomas, and RAR ligands, 69
Tea, and chemoprevention, 36, 355–356
Tea catechins, 353
antimetastatic activity of, 326
antioxidative effects of, 356
chemopreventive agents as, 362
Tea polyphenols, 327. *See also* Catechins
antimetastatic activity of, 328, 332
biological activity of, 354
and cancer cell adhesion, 341
in cancer chemoprevention, 352
effects on angiogenesis of, 338
effects on lung cancer of, 333
FAS expression suppressed by, 360
invasion inhibited by, 333
and melanoma and prostate cancer, 332
and MMPs, 340
and tumor metastasis, 329
tumor metastasis prevented by, 343
Telomerase, human, 42
Terminal transferase end-labeling (TUNEL), 102
Theaflavins, 352
anticancer-promoting effects of, 359
apoptotic inducing effects of, 358
biological activity of, 354–355
and carcinogenesis, 353
FAS expression suppressed by, 360
suppression of fatty acid synthase expression by, 360
TPA-induced transformation inhibited by, 358
Theasinensin A in oolong tea, apoptotic inducing effects of, 358
Thymidylate
in folate deficiency, 163
synthesis, 165
Thymidylate synthase reaction, 156
Tissue inhibitors of metalloproteinases (TIMPs), 339
Tissue invasion, inhibition of, 43–44
TNF-related apoptosis-inducing ligand (TRAIL), 124–125
Tobacco smoke, carcinogens in, 445. *See also* Smoking
Tocopherols, 113, 412
α–tocopherol (α-TOH)
and cancer risk, 114–115
chemical structure of, 112, 113
α-tocopheryl succinate (α-TOS), 111
and angiogenesis, 127
anticancer index of, 112
antimesothelioma effects of, 120–122
apoptogenic activity of, 119, 126

chemical structure of, 112, 113
double-edge activity of, 127, 128
hydrolysis of, 122
intraperitoneal administration of, 127
Tocotrienols, 113
Tofu consumption, and cancer risk, 316–317
Tolerable Upper Level Intake (UL), 92, 93
Tomato intake, and cancer, 81
Tomato paste, 31
TPA, and resveratrol, 377–378
Transgenic adenocarcinoma of the mouse
       prostate (TRAMP), 333
*Trans*-3,5,4′-Trihydroxystilbene. *See*
       Resveratrol
Triterpenoid glycosides, 458, 459
Trolox, in human colon cancer cells, 123
Tumor cell growth, and beta-sitosterol
       supplementation, 262
Tumor growth factor-α (TGF-α), and cell
       proliferation, 39
Tumorigenesis. *See also* Carcinogenesis
    changes leading to, 33–35
    in chronic alcohol consumption, 587–589
    colon, 525
    mammary, 573
    process of, 140
    and Western-style diet, 490
Tumor necrosis factor (TNF), and apoptosis,
       259
Tumor necrosis factor-alpha (TNF-α)
    in alcohol-induced liver damage, 584
    in chronic alcoholism, 585
    and ginseng, 461
Tumor necrosis-related apoptosis-inducing
       ligand receptor (TRAILR), 259
Tumors. *See also* Neoplasia
    epithelial, 51
    human, 35
    and selenium status, 196–197
Tumor suppressor genes, 40
    Apc, 50
    loss of, 33
    and Vitamin D, 49
Tumor suppressor proteins, and antigrowth
       signals, 40

**U**

Ubiquitin-proteasome pathways
    catechin inhibition of, 361
    inhibitors in, 362
UDP-glucuronosyl transferases, 46

Urinary flow parameters, in BPH studies, 254
Urine, selenium in, 207
Urosdiol, and chemoprevention, 36
USA, breast cancer study in, 388–389, 390, 393
UV exposure, and cancer mortality, 90

**V**

*Vaccinum* species, anthocyanins from, 425
Vascular cell adhesion molecule 1 (VCAM),
       231–232
Vascular endothelial growth factor (VEGF),
       319, 572
    and breast cancer risk, 404
    inhibited by genistein, 339
Vascularization, and PEB, 571–572, 574
Vascular smooth muscle cells (VSMC), plant
       sterol studies in, 231
VDR gene, 97
Vegetable oils, 488
    phytosterols in, 229
    plant sterols in, 226, 229, 230
Vegetables
    antioxidant capacities of, 45
    *Brassica,* 435, 442
    and cancer incidence, 412, 435
    and cancer risk, 28
    and colorectal cancer, 496
    cruciferous, 46
    DOA recommendations for, 139
    evaluation of, 344
    flavonoids in, 274
    phytochemicals in, 31
    phytosterols in, 229
Vinblastine (VBL), 439
Vincristine, 522
Vitamin A, 30
    anticarcinogenic activity of, 77
    and cancer, 68
    and cancer in experimental animals, 65–68
    and carcinogenesis, 45
    in chronic alcohol consumption, 589–590
    common dietary sources of, 62
    complexity in signaling by, 64–65
    and differentiation promotion, 41
    excessive intake of, 63
    homeostasis of, 61
    limited intake of, 61–62
    mechanism of action of, 63–64
    and precancerous lesions, 195
    and skin carcinoma, 67
    systematic functions of, 62–63

Vitamin A deficiency
  as cancer risk factor, 76
  symptoms of, 63
Vitamin B$_2$ and DNA methylation, 47
Vitamin B$_6$
  in chronic alcohol intake, 588
  and DNA methylation, 47
  and folate deficiency, 165
Vitamin B$_{12}$ and DNA methylation, 47
Vitamin C, 30, 31
  anti-inflammatory activity of, 144–145
  antimetastatic effects of, 146
  antioxidant effects of, 134–144, 146–147
  chemopreventive effects of, 139–140, 147
  and inhibition of GJIC, 146
  pro-oxidant potential of, 144
Vitamin D, 30
  age and intake for, 94
  and cancer connection, 95–97
  and chemoprevention, 36, 37
  in colon cancer, 48–50
  dietary sources of, 92, 93
  and differentiation promotion, 41
  discovery of, 89
  forms of, 91
  human requirement for, 89
  metabolism of, 90–92
  nutritional assessment in, 91
  nutritional forms of, 90
  recommended intake for, 92–94
  and telomerase activity, 42
Vitamin D insufficiency, 103
Vitamin D receptors (VDRs), 94–95
  and breast cancer, 97–99
  and carcinogenesis, 48–49
  and prostate cancer, 99–100
  tissue distribution, 96
Vitamin D-responsive elements (VDREs),
    48–49
Vitamin E analogs
  as anticancer agents, 120–122
  as antitumor agents, 126–127
  apoptogenic pathway induced by, 124
  clinical application of, 122–123
  and immunological apoptogens, 123–125
  molecular mechanism underlying, 129
  pharmacokinetics of, 127–128
  proapoptotic signaling of, 124
  structure-function relationship for, 116–120
  structures of, 118–119
  unique features of, 128
Vitamin E (VE), 30, 111
  as anticancer agent, 113–116

  and cancer risk, 115, 116
  and carcinogenesis, 45
  and chemoprevention, 36
  and chronic alcohol consumption, 585
Vitamins
  effects on cancer of, 194
  and plant sterols, 234
VLDL particles, plant sterols as lipid
    constituents of, 238

**W**

WAF1/p21, resveratrol induction of, 372
Waist circumference, as obesity measure,
    541–542
Waist-to-hip ratio (WHR), 543
  and cancer risk, 545
  and ovarian cancer, 549
Watercress consumption, and tobacco specific
    carcinogens, 445
Westernization, and cancer, 320. *See also* Diets
Whole blood, selenium in, 207
Whole grains, and cancer risk, 28
Wogonin, and chemoprevention, 36
Women's CARE study, 10, 11

**X**

Xanthine oxidase, 419
Xenobiotic detoxification, in carcinogenesis,
    424–425
Xeroderma pigmentosum, and isotretinoin, 71

**Y**

Yeast, selenium-enriched, 190, 195, 206

**Z**

Zeaxanthin, anticarcinogenic activity of, 80
Zetia (ezetimibe), 251
Zidovudine (ZDV), 462
Zinc
  in chronic alcohol consumption, 589
  and DNA methylation, 47
  and precancerous lesions, 195
Z-VAD-FMK, 373